W9-BMI-779

BRUNNER & SUDDARTH'S
Handbook of Laboratory and Diagnostic Tests

Edition

2

Wolters Kluwer | Lippincott Williams & Wilkins
Health

Philadelphia • Baltimore • New York • London
Buenos Aires • Hong Kong • Sydney • Tokyo

Publisher: Lisa McAllister
Executive Editor: Sherry Dickinson
Product Development Editor: Roxanne Halpine Ward
Editorial Assistant: Dan Reilly
Design Coordinator: Joan Wendt
Art Director, Illustration: Jennifer Clements
Production Project Manager: Cynthia Rudy
Manufacturing Coordinator: Karin Duffield
Prepress Vendor: Aptara, Inc.

2nd Edition

9 8 7 6 5 4 3 2

Printed in China

Library of Congress Cataloging-in-Publication Data

Brunner & Suddarth's handbook of laboratory and diagnostic tests. – Edition 2.
    p. ; cm.
  Brunner and Suddarth's handbook of laboratory and diagnostic tests
  Handbook of laboratory and diagnostic tests
  Complemented by: Brunner & Suddarth's textbook of medical-surgical nursing / Janice L. Hinkle, Kerry H. Cheever. Thirteenth edition. ©2014.
  Includes bibliographical references and index.
  ISBN 978-1-4511-9097-7 (alk. paper)
  I. Brunner & Suddarth's textbook of medical-surgical nursing. Complemented by (work): II. Title: Brunner and Suddarth's handbook of laboratory and diagnostic tests. III. Title: Handbook of laboratory and diagnostic tests.
  [DNLM: 1. Clinical Laboratory Techniques—Handbooks. QY 39]
  RT41
  610.73—dc23
                                                                                    2013030503

Care has been taken to confirm the accuracy of the information presented and to describe generally accepted practices. However, the author(s), editors, and publisher are not responsible for errors or omissions or for any consequences from application of the information in this book and make no warranty, expressed or implied, with respect to the currency, completeness, or accuracy of the contents of the publication. Application of this information in a particular situation remains the professional responsibility of the practitioner; the clinical treatments described and recommended may not be considered absolute and universal recommendations.

The author(s), editors, and publisher have exerted every effort to ensure that drug selection and dosage set forth in this text are in accordance with the current recommendations and practice at the time of publication. However, in view of ongoing research, changes in government regulations, and the constant flow of information relating to drug therapy and drug reactions, the reader is urged to check the package insert for each drug for any change in indications and dosage and for added warnings and precautions. This is particularly important when the recommended agent is a new or infrequently employed drug.

Some drugs and medical devices presented in this publication have Food and Drug Administration (FDA) clearance for limited use in restricted research settings. It is the responsibility of the health care provider to ascertain the FDA status of each drug or device planned for use in his or her clinical practice.

Reviewers

Melody Antoon, BS, BSN, MSN, RN
Instructor of Nursing
Lamar State College – Orange
Orange, Texas

Dana Botz, MSN
Nursing Faculty
North Hennepin Community College
Brooklyn Park, Minnesota

Kristine Carey, MSN
Nursing Faculty
Normandale Community College
Bloomington, Minnesota

Conrad Gordon, MS
Assistant Professor
University of Maryland School of
    Nursing
Baltimore, Maryland

Jacqueline Guhde, MSN
Assistant Professor
University of Akron, School of Nursing
Akron, Ohio

Janice Hausauer, MS-FNP
Assistant Clinical Professor
Montana State University, Department
    of Nursing
Bozeman, Montana

Barbara Hoglund, EdD, MSN
Associate Professor
Bethel University, Department of
    Nursing
St. Paul, Minnesota

Susan Jones, MSN
Assistant Professor of Nursing
Jefferson College of Health Science
Roanoke, Virginia

Tonia Mailow, MSN/ED
Faculty/Lecturer
Murray State University School of
    Nursing
Murray, Kentucky

Kristina McKinney, BSN
Faculty
Galen College of Nursing
Louisville, Kentucky

Nancy Noble, MSN
Associate Professor
Marian University, Department of
    Nursing
Fond du Lac, Wisconsin

Maureen O'Shea, DNP, ANP-BC,
    GNP-BC
Associate Professor
Curry College, Department of Nursing
Milton, Massachusetts

Anthony Pennington, MBA, MSN,
    RN-BC
Assistant Dean and Assistant Professor
Remington College of Nursing
Lake Mary, Florida

Linda Phelps, MSN
Clinical Instructor, Nursing Faculty
Ivy Tech Community College
Indianapolis, Indiana

Maria Rosen, PhD
Associate Professor
Massachusetts College of Pharmacy and
    Health Sciences
Department of Nursing
Worcester, Massachusetts

Carolyn Santiago, MSN, RN, NP-C
Director of Nursing
Santa Barbara Business College
Bakersfield, California

Deborah Trotta, MSN, MEd, RN-BC
Assistant Professor
University of Cincinnati Blue Ash
    College
Department of Nursing
Cincinnati, Ohio

Preface

The second edition of *Brunner & Suddarth's Handbook of Laboratory and Diagnostic Tests* is a concise, portable, full-color handbook of hundreds of test results and their implications for nursing. Designed to accompany *Brunner & Suddarth's Textbook for Medical-Surgical Nursing*, 13th edition, this handbook provides readers with a quick-reference tool for use throughout the nursing curriculum, in clinicals, and in practice.

The two-part organization includes a review of specimen collection procedures in Part I, followed by a concise, alphabetical list of close to 300 tests and their implications in Part II.

Organization

The consistent and easy-to-use outline format enables readers to gain quick access to vital information on

- Reference values or normal findings
- Abnormal findings with associated nursing implications
- Critical values
- Purpose
- Description
- Interfering factors
- Nursing considerations for patient care before, during, and after the test, as appropriate

Special Features

In addition to the consistent outline format, the handbook includes features to highlight important information:

- ▶ **Quality and Safety Nursing Alerts**—Tips for best clinical practice and red-flag safety warnings about priority care issues and hazardous or potentially life-threatening situations.
- **Tables**, **Boxes**, and **Figures**— At-a-glance presentations of diseases, disorders, measurements, testing equipment, and examples of results.

For readers requiring more in-depth information, the *Handbook of Laboratory and Diagnostic Tests* includes a list of selected references, in print and online, where readers can find out more.

Mobile Format Available

The *Handbook of Laboratory and Diagnostic Tests* is available in print or as an enhanced ebook, offering full access to the handbook's quick-reference content, along with instant search capability to quickly locate information needed on the go. For more information, please visit thePoint.

We hope you will find this *Handbook of Laboratory and Diagnostic Tests* to be helpful, and we wish you every success in your studies and future profession.

The Publisher

Contents

Specimen
Collection

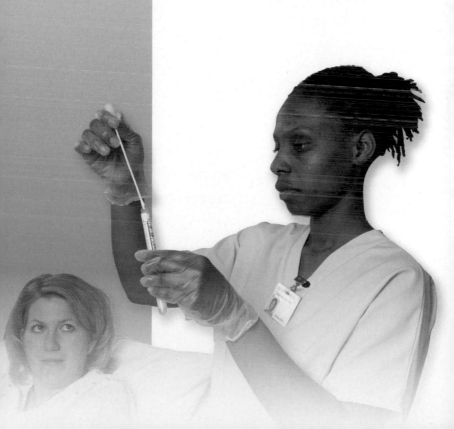

INTRODUCTION

The nurse's prompt and accurate collection of specimens is vital to the correct diagnosis, treatment, and recovery of the patient. Often, the nurse alone is responsible for specimen collections; at other times, the nurse's responsibility focuses on scheduling the patient's tests, assisting the health care provider in performing them, and caring for the patient afterward. Your clinical setting and your facility's policies, along with your state's nurse practice act, will determine your responsibilities.

Patient Preparation

By thoroughly understanding the diagnostic tests you'll perform or assist with, you'll be better prepared to explain them to the patient with clarity and compassion, put the patient at ease, gain the patient's trust and cooperation, and thus ensure more accurate results. Helping the patient understand a procedure also paves the way for consent that's truly informed.

When preparing the patient, your explanations should be clear, straightforward, and complete. For example, before a difficult or painful procedure, such as a bone marrow biopsy, explain that the patient will probably feel discomfort, explain how long the procedure takes, and when the results can be expected. By letting the patient know exactly what to expect, you can help the patient better tolerate such a procedure.

If you're assisting the health care provider with a test, speak to the patient throughout the procedure to comfort and encourage and to prepare for sensations that may be experienced, if necessary. Afterward, watch for adverse reactions or complications, and be prepared to implement appropriate care.

Some tests require detailed instructions to promote cooperation and to ensure accurate specimen collection, especially when the patient must modify behavior beforehand or when the patient will collect the specimen personally. For example, you may need to instruct the patient to observe a special diet, suspend taking certain medications, or learn a special collection technique.

Whenever possible, reinforce verbal explanations with appropriate written instructions and give the patient enough time to read the information before beginning to prepare for the test or procedure. Many facilities also have videocassettes, recorded lectures, and films available to augment the patient-teaching process.

Informed Consent

Informed consent is a fundamental patient right. It provides that the patient (or a responsible family member, if the patient is legally incompetent or a minor) must fully understand what will be done during a test, surgery, or medical procedure and must understand its risks and implications *before* the patient can legally consent to it.

Explaining a procedure, its purpose, how it will be performed, and its potential risks are primarily the health care provider's responsibility. The nurse typically reinforces the health care provider's explanation, confirms that the patient understands it, and verifies that written consent was obtained, when necessary. Written consent isn't always needed for a test—informed consent may be enough—and the patient always retains the legal right to withdraw oral or written consent at any time and for any reason, and to refuse care or treatment.

Ensuring Patient Safety

The Joint Commission requires that before any procedure, test, or surgery is performed, the patient's identity must be verified by two identifiers, neither of which may be the patient's room number. Facilities' policies differ on which patient identifiers are considered acceptable, so always check beforehand.

Using personal protective equipment, as necessary, helps ensure proper specimen collection and test results, and is mandated by the Occupational Safety and Health Administration. Before you're exposed to the patient's body fluids, make sure you take appropriate standard precautions.

PROCEDURES FOR OBTAINING SPECIMENS

Arterial Puncture for Blood Gas Analysis

Obtaining an arterial blood sample requires percutaneous puncture of the brachial, radial, or femoral artery or withdrawal of a sample from an arterial line. The radial artery is usually the preferred site, but the brachial and femoral arteries may be used as well. Once collected, the sample can be analyzed to determine arterial blood gas (ABG) values.

ABG analysis measures blood pH and arterial oxygen (PaO_2) and carbon dioxide ($PaCO_2$) partial pressures. Blood pH measures the blood's acid–base balance, PaO_2 indicates oxygen levels delivered to the lungs, and $PaCO_2$ shows the lungs' capacity to eliminate carbon dioxide. ABG samples can also be analyzed for oxygen content and saturation and for bicarbonate values.

Typically, ABG analysis is ordered to assess for adequate oxygenation and ventilation, assess acid–base balance by measuring the respiratory and metabolic components, and to monitor effectiveness of treatment for patients with chronic obstructive pulmonary disease, pulmonary edema, acute respiratory distress syndrome, myocardial infarction, or pneumonia. It's also performed when a patient is in shock and after coronary artery bypass surgery, resuscitation from cardiac arrest, changes in respiratory therapy or status, and prolonged anesthesia.

Arterial puncture is contraindicated when the patient:
- has a failed Allen's test result,
- has hemophilia or another clotting disorder,
- had arterial spasms following previous punctures,
- has severe peripheral vascular disease,
- exhibits abnormal or infectious skin conditions at or near the puncture site.

In addition, if the patient has a surgical graft, arterial puncture should not be performed distal to the site. Arterial puncture may also be a relative contraindication if the patient is taking anticoagulation therapy.

Most ABG samples can be drawn by a respiratory technician or specially trained nurse. Collection from the femoral artery, however, usually is performed by the health care provider. Before attempting a radial puncture, Allen's test should be performed. (See the *Performing Allen's Test* box.)

Equipment
- 10-mL glass syringe or plastic Luer-Lok syringe specially made for drawing blood for ABG analysis • 1-mL ampule of aqueous heparin (1:1,000) • 20G 1-inch needle • 22G 1-inch needle • gloves • antiseptic pad • two 2 × 2-inch gauze pads • rubber cap for syringe hub or rubber stopper for needle • a clean emesis basin • ice-filled plastic bag • label • laboratory request form • adhesive bandage • 1% lidocaine solution without epinephrine (optional)

Many health care facilities use a commercial ABG kit that contains all the equipment listed above, except the adhesive bandage and ice. If your facility doesn't use such a kit, obtain a sterile syringe specially made for drawing blood for ABG values and use a clean emesis basin filled with ice instead of the plastic bag to immediately transport the sample to the laboratory.

Performing Allen's Test

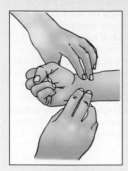 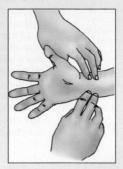 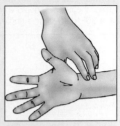

Rest the patient's arm on the mattress or bedside stand and support the wrist with a rolled towel. Have the patient clench a fist. Then, using your index and middle fingers, press on the radial and ulnar arteries. Hold this position for a few seconds.

Without removing your fingers from the patient's arteries, ask the patient to unclench the fist and hold the hand in a relaxed position. The palm will be blanched because pressure from your fingers has impaired the normal blood flow.

Release pressure on the patient's ulnar artery. If the hand becomes flushed, which indicates blood filling the vessels, you can safely proceed with the radial artery puncture. If the hand doesn't flush, perform the test on the other arm.

Equipment Preparation

- Prepare the collection equipment before entering the patient's room.
- Wash your hands thoroughly.
- Open the ABG kit and remove the sample label and the plastic bag.
- Record the patient's name and room number on the label, as well as the date and collection time and the health care provider's name.
- Fill the plastic bag with ice and set it aside.
- Heparinize the syringe, if needed. To do so, attach the 20G needle to the syringe and open the heparin ampule. Draw all the heparin into the syringe to prevent the sample from clotting. Hold the syringe upright, and pull the plunger back slowly to about the 7-mL mark. Rotate the barrel while pulling the plunger back to allow the heparin to coat the inside surface of the syringe. Then, slowly force the heparin toward the hub of the

syringe and expel all but about 0.1 mL of it.
- Heparinize the needle, if needed. To do so, replace the 20G needle with the 22G needle. Then, hold the syringe upright, tilt it slightly, and eject the remaining heparin. Excess heparin in the syringe alters blood pH and PaO_2 values.

Essential Steps

- Confirm the patient's identity using two patient identifiers and confirmation of the patient's identification bracelet according to facility policy.
- Tell the patient that you need to collect an arterial blood sample and explain the procedure to help ease anxiety and promote cooperation.
- Explain that the patient may feel discomfort from the needle stick but must remain still during the procedure.
- Wash your hands and put on gloves.

Arterial Puncture Technique

The needle penetration angle in arterial blood gas sampling varies depending on the artery being used for the sample. For the radial artery, the most commonly used, the needle should enter bevel-up at a 30- to 45-degree angle.

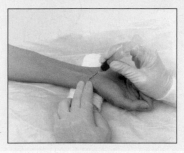

- Place a rolled towel under the patient's wrist for support.
- Locate the artery and palpate it for a strong pulse.
- Clean the puncture site with antiseptic solution, working outward in a side-to-side motion.
- Allow the skin to dry.
- Palpate the artery with the index and middle fingers of one hand while holding the syringe over the puncture site with the other hand.
- Hold the needle bevel up at a 30- to 45-degree angle. When puncturing the brachial artery, hold the needle at a 60-degree angle. (See the *Arterial Puncture Technique* box.)
- Puncture the skin and the arterial wall in one motion, following the artery path.
- Watch for blood backflow in the syringe. Don't pull back on the plunger because arterial blood should enter the syringe automatically.
- Fill the syringe to the 3-mL mark.
- After collecting the sample, press a gauze pad firmly over the puncture site for 5 to 10 minutes, until the bleeding stops.

Quality and Safety Nursing Alert

If the patient is receiving anticoagulant therapy or has a blood dyscrasia, apply pressure for 10 to 15 minutes. If necessary, ask a coworker to hold the gauze pad in place while you prepare the sample for transport to the laboratory. Don't ask the patient to hold the pad: if the patient fails to apply sufficient pressure, a large, painful hematoma may form, hindering future arterial punctures at that site.

- Check the syringe for air bubbles. If any appear, remove them by holding the syringe upright and slowly ejecting some of the blood onto a 2 × 2 gauze pad.
- Insert the needle into a rubber stopper or remove the needle and place a rubber cap directly on the syringe tip. This prevents the sample from leaking and keeps air out of the syringe.
- Put the labeled sample in the ice-filled plastic bag or emesis basin.
- Attach a properly completed laboratory request form and send the sample to the laboratory immediately.
- When bleeding stops, apply a small adhesive bandage to the site.
- Discard syringes, needles, and gloves in the appropriate containers.
- Monitor the patient's vital signs and observe for signs of circulatory impairment, such as swelling, discoloration, pain, numbness, or tingling in the arm or leg.
- Watch for bleeding at the puncture site.

Special Considerations

- If the patient is receiving oxygen, make sure that therapy has been under way for at least 15 minutes before collecting an arterial blood sample.
- Unless ordered, don't turn off existing oxygen therapy before collecting arterial blood samples.

- Indicate on the laboratory request slip the amount and type of oxygen therapy the patient is receiving.
- If the patient isn't receiving oxygen, indicate that he's breathing room air.
- If the patient has been recently suctioned or placed on a ventilator, wait at least 15 minutes before drawing the sample.

▶ *Quality and Safety Nursing Alert*

If the patient has received a nebulizer treatment, wait about 20 minutes before collecting the sample.

- If necessary, you can anesthetize the puncture site with 1% lidocaine solution without epinephrine. Consider lidocaine use carefully because it delays the procedure, the patient may be allergic to the drug, or the resulting vasoconstriction may prevent successful puncture.
- When filling out a laboratory request form for ABG analysis, include the following information to help the laboratory staff calibrate the equipment and evaluate results correctly:
  - the patient's current temperature
  - most recent hemoglobin level
  - current respiratory rate
  - fraction of inspired oxygen, tidal volume, and ventilatory frequency (if the patient is on a ventilator).
- Instruct the patient to notify the nurse if bleeding occurs at the puncture site.
- Tell the patient to report tingling or numbness that occurs in the extremity where the procedure was done.

Complications

If too much force is used when attempting an arterial puncture, the needle may touch the periosteum of the bone, causing the patient considerable pain, or the needle may pass through the artery's opposite wall. If this happens, slowly pull the needle back a short distance and check to see if you obtain a blood return.

If blood still fails to enter the syringe, withdraw the needle completely and start with a fresh heparinized needle.

▶ *Quality and Safety Nursing Alert*

Don't make more than two attempts to withdraw blood from the same site. Probing the artery may injure it and the radial nerve. Also, hemolysis will alter test results.

- If arterial spasm occurs, blood won't flow into the syringe, and you won't be able to collect the sample. If this happens, replace the needle with a smaller one and try the puncture again. A smaller bore needle is less likely to cause arterial spasm.

Documentation

Record:
- Allen's test results
- time the sample was drawn
- patient's temperature
- arterial puncture site
- length of time that pressure was applied to the site to control bleeding
- type and amount of oxygen therapy the patient was receiving.

Blood Culture

Normally bacteria-free blood can be infected through infusion lines, as well as from thrombophlebitis, infected shunts, or bacterial endocarditis from prosthetic heart valve replacements. Bacteria may also invade the vascular system from local tissue infections through the lymphatic system and the thoracic duct.

Blood cultures are done to detect bacterial invasion (bacteremia) and the systemic spread of an infection (septicemia) through the bloodstream. Samples may be taken by the laboratory technician, health care provider, or nurse through venipuncture at the patient's bedside; they're transferred into two bottles: one containing an anaerobic

Isolator Blood-Culturing System

A single-tube blood-culturing system, the Isolator uses lysis and centrifugation to help detect septicemia and monitor the effectiveness of antibacterial drug therapy.

The Isolator is an evacuated tube that contains a substance that lyses red blood cells. Then, centrifugation concentrates bacteria and other organisms in the sample onto an inert cushioning pad; the concentrate can then be applied onto four agar plates.

The Isolator has several advantages over conventional blood-culturing methods. This system:

• eliminates the bottle method's lengthy incubation period, providing faster results
• improves bacterial survival
• results in more valid positive results through direct application onto agar plates, which greatly dilutes any antibiotic present in the sample
• detects more yeast and polymicrobial infections
• improves the laboratory's ability to detect organisms that are difficult to grow
• is easier to use at the patient's bedside and to transport because blood is drawn directly into the Isolator tube.

medium and the other an aerobic medium. The bottles are incubated to encourage any organisms in the sample to grow in the media. Blood cultures identify about 67% of pathogens within 24 hours and up to 90% within 72 hours. (See the *Isolator Blood-Culturing System* box.)

Although some authorities consider the timing of culture collections debatable and possibly irrelevant, others advocate drawing three blood samples at least 1 hour apart. The first sample should be collected as soon as bacteremia or septicemia is suspected. To check for suspected bacterial endocarditis, three or four samples may be collected at 5- to 30-minute intervals before starting antibiotic therapy.

Equipment

• Tourniquet • gloves • antiseptic pad • 10-mL syringe for an adult, 6-mL syringe for a child • three or four 20G 1½-inch needles • two or three blood culture bottles (50-mL bottles for adults, 20-mL bottles for infants and children) with sodium polyethanol sulfonate added (one aerobic bottle containing a suitable medium, such as Trypticase soy broth with 10% carbon dioxide atmosphere; one anaerobic bottle with prereduced medium; and, possibly, one hyperosmotic bottle with 10% sucrose medium) • laboratory request form • 2 × 2-inch gauze pads • small adhesive bandages • labels

Essential Steps

• Check the expiration dates on the culture bottles and replace outdated bottles.
• Confirm the patient's identity using two patient identifiers and confirmation of the patient's identification bracelet according to facility policy.
• Tell the patient that you need to collect a series of blood samples to check for infection.
• Explain the procedure to ease anxiety and promote cooperation. Explain that the procedure usually requires three blood samples collected at different times and different sites.
• Wash your hands and put on gloves.
• Tie a tourniquet 2 inches (5 cm) proximal to the area chosen. (See Venipuncture, page 22).
• Clean the venipuncture site with an antiseptic pad, starting at the site and working outward in a side-to-side motion. Wait 30 to 60 seconds for the skin to dry.
• Perform a venipuncture, drawing 10 mL of blood from an adult.

 Quality and Safety Nursing Alert

Draw 1 to 5 mL of blood from a child.

• Remove the tourniquet.
• Apply pressure to the venipuncture site using a 2 × 2-inch dressing.
• Cover the site with a small adhesive bandage.

- Wipe the diaphragm tops of the culture bottles with a povidone–iodine pad and change the needle on the syringe used to draw the blood.
- Inject 5 mL of blood into each 50-mL bottle or 2 mL into a 20-mL pediatric culture bottle. (Bottle sizes may vary with the facility's protocol, but the sample dilution should always be 1:10.)
- Label the culture bottles with the patient's name, room number, age, and isolation category; the health care provider's name; date and time of collection; and number of the culture.
- Indicate the suspected diagnosis and the patient's temperature, and note on the laboratory request form any recent antibiotic therapy.
- Send the samples immediately to the laboratory.
- Discard syringes, needles, and gloves in the appropriate containers.

Special Considerations
- Obtain each set of cultures from a different site. Infants will rarely have three separate blood cultures run, they will usually have one.
- Avoid using existing blood lines for cultures unless the sample is drawn when the line is inserted or catheter sepsis is suspected.

Complications
Hematomas are the most common venipuncture complication. If a hematoma develops, apply direct pressure to the site.

Documentation
Record:
- blood sample collection date and time
- test name
- amount of blood collected
- number of bottles used
- patient's temperature
- adverse reactions to the procedure.

Sputum Collection

Secreted by mucous membranes lining the bronchioles, bronchi, and trachea, sputum helps protect the respiratory tract from infection. When expelled, sputum carries saliva, nasal and sinus secretions, dead cells, and normal oral bacteria from the respiratory tract.

Sputum may be cultured to identify respiratory pathogens. Expectoration, the usual sputum collection method, may require ultrasonic nebulization, hydration, or chest percussion and postural drainage. Less common methods include tracheal suctioning and, rarely, bronchoscopy. Tracheal suctioning provides a more reliable diagnostic specimen, but generally isn't used, unless expectoration fails to provide a sample.

Tracheal suctioning is contraindicated within 1 hour of eating and in patients with esophageal varices, nausea, facial or basilar skull fractures, laryngospasm, or bronchospasm. It should be performed cautiously in patients with heart disease because it may precipitate arrhythmias.

Equipment
For Expectoration
- Sterile specimen container with tight-fitting cap • gloves • label laboratory request form • aerosol (10% sodium chloride, propylene glycol, acetylcysteine, or sterile or distilled water)

For Tracheal Suctioning
#12 to #14 French sterile suction catheter • water-soluble lubricant • laboratory request form • sterile gloves • mask • goggles • sterile in-line specimen trap (Lukens trap) • normal saline solution • portable suction machine, if wall suction is unavailable • oxygen therapy equipment

Commercial suction kits have all equipment except the suction machine and an in-line specimen container.

Essential Steps
Collecting by Expectoration
- Confirm the patient's identity using two patient identifiers and confirmation of the patient's identification bracelet according to facility policy.

- Inform the patient that you need to collect a sputum specimen by expectoration.
- Explain the procedure.
- Plan to collect the specimen early in the morning, before breakfast.
- Instruct the patient to sit on a chair or at the edge of the bed. If unable sit up, place the patient in high Fowler's position.
- Ask the patient to rinse mouth with water to reduce specimen contamination. Avoid mouthwash or toothpaste because they may affect the mobility of organisms in the sputum sample.
- Then tell the patient to cough deeply and expectorate directly into the specimen container.
- Ask the patient to produce at least 15 mL of sputum. Check the specimen carefully to make sure it includes thick mucus.
- If the patient is unable to hold the specimen container, put on gloves and place it near the patient's mouth.
- Cap the container and, if necessary, clean its exterior.
- Remove and discard your gloves, then wash your hands thoroughly.
- Label the container with the patient's name and room number, the health care provider's name, date and time of collection, and initial diagnosis.
- Include on the laboratory request form whether the patient was febrile or taking antibiotics and whether sputum was induced.
- Send the specimen to the laboratory immediately.

Collecting by Tracheal Suctioning

- Collect a specimen by suctioning if the patient can't produce an adequate specimen by coughing.
- Explain the suctioning procedure to the patient. Explain that the patient may cough, gag, or feel short of breath during the procedure.
- Check the suction equipment to be sure it's functioning properly.
- Place the patient in high Fowler's or semi-Fowler's position.
- Administer oxygen to the patient before beginning the procedure.
- Wash your hands thoroughly.
- Position a mask and goggles over your face.
- Put on sterile gloves. Consider one hand sterile and the other hand clean to prevent cross-contamination.
- Connect the suction tubing to the male adapter of the in-line specimen trap.
- Attach the sterile suction catheter to the rubber tubing of the trap. (See the *Attaching a Specimen Trap to a Suction Catheter* box.)
- Tell the patient to tilt the head back slightly.
- Lubricate the catheter with normal saline solution.
- Gently pass the catheter through the patient's nostril without suction. When the catheter reaches the larynx, the patient will cough. As the patient coughs, quickly advance the catheter into the trachea.
- Tell the patient to take several deep breaths through the mouth.
- Apply suction for 5 to 10 seconds, but never longer than 15 seconds. (Prolonged suction can cause hypoxia.)
- If the procedure must be repeated, let the patient rest for four to six breaths.
- When collection is completed, discontinue the suction.
- Gently remove the catheter.
- Administer oxygen.
- Detach the catheter from the in-line trap and gather it up in your dominant hand.
- Pull the glove cuff inside-out and down around the used catheter to enclose it for disposal. Remove and discard the other glove, your mask, and goggles.
- Detach the trap from the tubing connected to the suction machine.

Attaching a Specimen Trap to a Suction Catheter

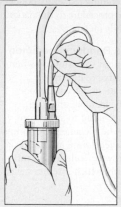 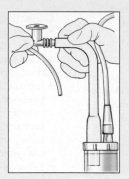 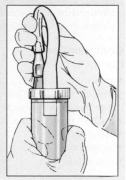

Wearing gloves, push the suction tubing onto the male adapter of the in-line trap.

Insert the suction catheter into the rubber tubing of the trap.

After suctioning, discon-nect the in-line trap from the suction tubing and catheter. To seal the con-tainer, connect the rubber tubing to the male adapter of the trap.

• Seal the trap tightly by connecting the rubber tubing to the male adapter of the trap.
• Examine the specimen to make sure it's really sputum.
• Label the trap's container as an expectorated specimen. Send it to the laboratory immediately with a completed laboratory request form.
• Offer the patient a glass of water or mouthwash.

Special Considerations
• If tracheal suctioning doesn't produce a sputum specimen, perform chest percussion to loosen and mobilize secretions.
• Position the patient for optimal drainage.
• If unsuccessful during the first attempts, wait 20 to 30 minutes and repeat the tracheal suctioning procedure.
• Before sending the specimen to the laboratory, examine it to make sure it's actually sputum, not saliva.

(Saliva will produce inaccurate test results.) Look for thick mucus.
• Remove the catheter immediately if the patient becomes hypoxic or cyanotic, and administer oxygen.
• Watch for aggravated bronchospasms if using an aerosol with more than a 10% concentration of sodium chlo-ride or acetylcysteine in patients with asthma or chronic bronchitis.
• Don't use more than 20% propylene glycol with water when inducing a sputum specimen in someone suspected of having tuberculosis. A higher concentration of propylene glycol inhibits growth of the patho-gen and causes erroneous test results.
• Use 10% to 20% acetylcysteine with water or sodium chloride if propylene glycol isn't available.
• When obtaining a sputum specimen from a patient that is being mechani-cally ventilated, a closed or in-line suction system may be used. Closed suctioning technique involves the

attachment of a sterile, closed, in-line suction catheter to the ventilator circuit, which allows the passage of a suction catheter through the artificial airway without disconnecting the patient from the ventilator.

Complications
Patients may develop:
- arrhythmias, especially in a patient with cardiac disease when the specimen is obtained by suctioning
- tracheal trauma or bleeding
- vomiting
- aspiration
- hypoxemia

Documentation
Record:
- collection method
- collection time and date
- patient's tolerance of the procedure
- color and consistency of the specimen.

Stool Collection

Stool is collected to determine the presence of blood, parasites and their ova, bile, fat, pathogens, or substances such as ingested drugs. Gross examination of stool characteristics, including color, consistency, and odor, can reveal such conditions as gastrointestinal (GI) bleeding and steatorrhea.

Stool specimens are collected randomly or for specific periods. Because stool specimens can't be obtained on demand, proper collection requires careful patient instructions.

Equipment
- Specimen container with lid • gloves • two tongue blades • paper towel • bedpan or portable commode • two patient-care reminders (for timed specimens) • laboratory request form • enema (optional)

Essential Steps
- Confirm the patient's identity using two patient identifiers and confirma-

tion of the patient's identification bracelet according to facility policy.
- Explain the procedure to the patient and his family members.

Collecting a Random Specimen
- Tell the patient to notify you when feeling the urge to defecate.
- Have the patient defecate into a clean, dry bedpan or commode.
- Instruct the patient to avoid contaminating the specimen with urine or toilet tissue. (Urine inhibits fecal bacterial growth. Toilet tissue contains bismuth, which interferes with test results.)
- Put on gloves.
- Using a tongue blade, transfer the most representative stool specimen from the bedpan to the container. Then cap the container.
- Include any blood, mucus, or pus that is produced with the stool.
- Wrap the tongue blade in a paper towel and discard it.
- Remove and discard your gloves.
- Wash your hands thoroughly to prevent cross-contamination.

Collecting a Timed Specimen
- Place a patient-care reminder stating "Save all stool" over the patient's bed, in the patient's bathroom, and in the utility room.
- Put on gloves.
- Collect the first specimen and include this in the total specimen.
- Obtain the timed specimen as you would a random specimen, transferring all stool to the specimen container.
- If stool must be obtained with an enema, use only tap water or normal saline solution.
- Send each specimen to the laboratory immediately with a laboratory request form or, if permitted, refrigerate the specimens collected during the test period and send them when collection is complete.
- Remove and discard gloves.

- Make sure the patient is comfortable after the procedure.
- Provide the patient the opportunity to thoroughly clean the hands and perianal area.
- Perform perineal care, if necessary.

Special Considerations
- Never place a stool specimen in a refrigerator that contains food or medication.
- Notify the health care provider if the stool specimen looks unusual.
- For at-home collections, instruct the patient to collect the specimen in a clean container with a tight-fitting lid, to wrap the container in a brown paper bag, and to keep it in the refrigerator (separate from any food items) until it can be transported.

Documentation
Record:
- specimen collection and laboratory transport times
- stool color, odor, and consistency
- any unusual characteristics
- if the patient had difficulty passing the stool.

Swab Specimens

Proper collection and handling of swab specimens helps minimize contamination from normal bacterial flora, which increases the laboratory staff's accuracy in identifying pathogens.

Normally, sterile cotton swabs or other absorbent materials are used to collect inflamed tissue samples and exudates from the throat, nasopharynx, eyes, ears, rectum, or wounds. The swab type depends on the body part affected. For example, a cotton-tipped swab is used to collect a nasopharyngeal specimen.

After the specimen is collected, the swab is placed immediately into a sterile tube containing a transport medi-

um, such as an inert gas when sampling for anaerobes. Swab specimens usually are collected to identify pathogens or asymptomatic carriers of certain easily transmitted disease organisms. When collecting swab specimens, be aware that:
- *Corynebacterium diphtheriae* requires two swabs and special growth medium.
- *Bordetella pertussis* requires a nasopharyngeal culture and special growth medium.
- *Neisseria meningitides* requires enriched selective medium.

Equipment
For a Throat Specimen
- Gloves • tongue blade • penlight • sterile cotton-tipped swab • sterile culture tube with transport medium (or commercial collection kit) • label • laboratory request form

For a Nasopharyngeal Specimen
- Gloves • penlight • sterile, flexible cotton-tipped swab • tongue blade • sterile culture tube with transport medium • label • laboratory request form • small open-ended Pyrex tube or nasal speculum (optional)

For a Wound Specimen
- Sterile gloves • sterile forceps • alcohol or povidone–iodine pads • sterile swabs • sterile 10-mL syringe • sterile 21G needle • sterile culture tube with transport medium (or commercial collection kit for aerobic culture) • labels • special anaerobic culture tube containing carbon dioxide or nitrogen • fresh dressings for the wound • laboratory request form • rubber stopper for needle (optional)

For an Ear Specimen
- Gloves • normal saline solution • two 2 × 2-inch gauze pads • sterile swabs • sterile culture tube with transport medium • label • 10-mL syringe and 22G 1-inch needle (for tympanocentesis) • label • laboratory request form

For an Eye Specimen
• Sterile gloves • sterile normal saline solution • two 2 × 2-inch gauze pads • sterile swabs • sterile wire culture loop (for corneal scraping) • sterile culture tube with transport medium • label laboratory request form

For a Rectal Specimen
• Gloves • soap and water • washcloth • sterile swab • normal saline solution • sterile culture tube with transport medium • label • laboratory request form

Essential Steps
• Confirm the patient's identity using two patient identifiers and confirmation of the patient's identification bracelet according to facility policy.
• Explain the procedure to the patient.

Collecting a Throat Specimen
• Explain that the patient may gag during the swabbing, but the procedure will probably take less than 1 minute. The swabbing will take 10 to 15 seconds maximum, whereas the entire procedure will take approximately 1 minute.
• Instruct the patient to sit erect at the edge of the bed or in a chair, facing you.
• Wash your hands and put on gloves.
• Ask the patient to tilt the head back.
• Depress tongue with the tongue blade.
• Illuminate throat with the penlight to check for inflamed areas.
• If the patient starts to gag, withdraw the tongue blade and ask the patient to breathe deeply. Once relaxed, reinsert the tongue blade but not as deeply as before.
• Using the cotton-tipped wire swab, wipe the tonsillar areas from side to side.
• Include any inflamed or purulent sites. Don't touch the tongue, cheeks, or teeth with the swab.

• Withdraw the swab and immediately place it in the culture tube.
• When using a commercial kit, crush the culture medium ampule at the bottom of the tube. Push the swab into the medium to keep it moist.
• Remove and discard gloves, then wash your hands.
• Label the specimen with the patient's name and room number; the health care provider's name; and the date, time, and site of collection.
• Indicate on the laboratory request form whether any organism is strongly suspected.
• Immediately send the specimen to the laboratory.

Collecting a Nasopharyngeal Specimen
• Explain that the patient may gag or feel the urge to sneeze during the swabbing but that the procedure takes less than 1 minute. The swabbing will take 10 to 15 seconds maximum, whereas the entire procedure will take approximately 1 minute.
• Have the patient sit erect at the edge of the bed or on a chair, facing you.
• Wash your hands and put on gloves.
• Ask the patient to blow the nose to clear nasal passages.
• When obtaining a sputum specimen from a patient who is being mechanically ventilated, a closed or in-line suction system may be used.
• Use a sterile in-line suction catheter for culture collection.
• Check nostrils for patency with a penlight.
• Tell the patient to occlude one nostril and then the other while exhaling. Listen for the more patent nostril.
• Ask the patient to cough to bring organisms to the nasopharynx.
• While it's still in the package, bend the sterile swab in a curve. Open the package without contaminating the swab.
• Ask the patient to tilt the head back.

Obtaining a Nasopharyngeal Specimen

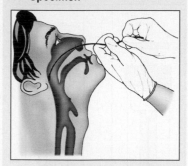

After you've passed the swab into the nasopharynx, quickly and gently rotate the swab to collect the specimen. When removing the swab, be careful not to injure the nasal mucous membrane.

- Gently pass the swab into the patent nostril about 3 to 4 inches (about 8–10 cm) into the nasopharynx. Keep the swab near the septum and floor of the nose. Rotate the swab quickly and remove it. (See the *Obtaining a Nasopharyngeal Specimen* box.)
- If the nostril is narrow, use a nasal speculum for better access. Alternatively, depress the patient's tongue with a tongue blade, pass the bent swab up behind the uvula, then rotate the swab and withdraw it.
- Remove the cap from the culture tube. Insert the swab and break off the contaminated end. Then close the tube tightly.
- Remove and discard your gloves and wash your hands.
- Label the specimen with the patient's name and room number; the health care provider's name; and the date, time, and site of collection.
- Complete a laboratory request form.
- Immediately send the specimen to the laboratory.
- If the specimen is obtained to isolate a possible virus, check with the laboratory for the recommended collection technique.

Collecting a Wound Specimen
- Wash your hands.
- Prepare a sterile field, then put on sterile gloves.
- Remove the dressing with sterile forceps to expose the wound.
- Properly dispose of the soiled dressings.
- Clean the area around the wound with an alcohol or povidone–iodine pad. Allow the area to dry.
- For an aerobic culture, use a sterile cotton-tipped swab to collect as much exudate as possible or insert the swab deeply into the wound and gently rotate it. Remove the swab from the wound and immediately place it in the aerobic culture tube. Label the tube with the patient's name and room number; the health care provider's name; and the date, time, and site of collection. Immediately send it to the laboratory with a completed laboratory request form.

▶ *Quality and Safety Nursing Alert*

Never collect exudate from the skin and then insert the same swab into the wound.

- For an anaerobic culture, insert the sterile cotton-tipped swab deeply into the wound, rotate it gently, then remove it and immediately place it in the anaerobic culture tube. (See the *Anaerobic Specimen Collection* box.)
- Alternatively, insert a sterile 10-mL syringe, without a needle, into the wound, and aspirate 1 to 5 mL of exudate into the syringe. Attach the 21G needle to the syringe and immediately inject the aspirate into the anaerobic culture tube. If an anaerobic culture tube is unavailable, obtain a rubber stopper, attach the needle to the syringe, and gently push all the air out of the syringe.

Anaerobic Specimen Collection

Most anaerobes die when exposed to oxygen, so they must be transported in tubes filled with carbon dioxide or nitrogen. The anaerobic specimen collector (shown here) includes a rubber-stoppered tube filled with carbon dioxide, a small inner tube, and a swab attached to a plastic plunger.

Before specimen collection, the small inner tube containing the swab is held in place with the rubber stopper (shown near right). After collecting the specimen, quickly replace the swab in the inner tube and depress the plunger to separate the inner tube from the stopper (shown far right), forcing it into the larger tube and exposing the specimen to a carbon dioxide-rich environment.

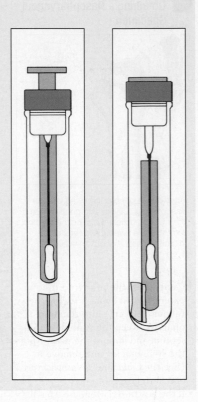

Stick the needle tip into the rubber stopper.
- Remove and discard your gloves.
- Label the syringe with the patient's name and room number; the health care provider's name; and the date, time, and site of collection.
- Immediately send the syringe of aspirate to the laboratory with a completed laboratory request form.
- Put on sterile gloves and apply a new dressing to the wound.

Collecting an Ear Specimen
- Wash your hands and put on gloves.
- Gently clean excess debris from the patient's ear with normal saline solution and gauze pads.

- Insert the sterile swab into the ear canal. Rotate it gently along the walls of the canal to avoid damaging the eardrum.
- Withdraw the swab, being careful to avoid touching other surfaces to prevent contamination.
- Place the swab in the culture tube with transport medium.
- Remove and discard your gloves, then wash your hands.
- Label the specimen with the patient's name and room number; the health care provider's name; and the date, time, and site of collection.
- Complete a laboratory request form.
- Immediately send the specimen to the laboratory.

Collecting a Middle Ear Specimen

- Put on gloves.
- Clean the outer ear with normal saline solution and gauze pads.
- Remove and discard your gloves.
- After the health care provider punctures the patient's eardrum with a needle and aspirates fluid into the syringe and places it in the container with the transport medium, label the container with the patient's name and room number; the health care provider's name; and the date, time, and site of collection.
- Complete a laboratory request form.
- Immediately send the specimen to the laboratory.

Collecting an Eye Specimen

- Wash your hands and put on sterile gloves.
- Gently clean excess debris from the outside of the eye with normal saline solution and gauze pads. Wipe from the inner to the outer canthus.
- Retract the lower eyelid to expose the conjunctival sac. Gently rub a sterile swab over the conjunctiva, taking care not to touch other surfaces. Hold the swab parallel to the eye to prevent corneal irritation or trauma due to sudden movement.
- If a corneal scraping is required, the health care provider will collect the specimen using a wire culture loop. Immediately place the swab or wire loop in the culture tube with transport medium.
- Remove and discard your gloves, then wash your hands.
- Label the specimen with the patient's name and room number; the health care provider's name; and the date, time, and site of collection.
- Complete a laboratory request form.
- Immediately send the specimen to the laboratory.

Collecting a Rectal Specimen

- Wash your hands and put on gloves.

- Clean the area around the patient's anus using a washcloth and soap and water.
- Moisten the swab with normal saline solution or sterile broth medium.
- Insert the swab through the anus and advance it about ⅜-inch (1 cm) for infants or 1½ inches (4 cm) for adults.
- While withdrawing the swab, gently rotate it against the walls of the lower rectum to sample a large area of the rectal mucosa.
- Place the swab in a culture tube with transport medium.
- Remove and discard your gloves, and wash your hands.
- Label the specimen with the patient's name and room number; the health care provider's name; and the date, time, and site of collection.
- Complete a laboratory request form.
- Immediately send the specimen to the laboratory.

Special Considerations

- Note whether the patient has had recent antibiotic therapy on the laboratory request form.
- Avoid cleaning a perineal wound with alcohol, because this could irritate sensitive tissues. Make sure that antiseptic doesn't enter the wound.
- Don't use an antiseptic before taking an eye specimen for culturing to avoid irritating the eye and inhibiting growth of organisms in the culture.
- When collecting an eye specimen from a child or an uncooperative adult, restrain the patient's head to prevent eye trauma from sudden movement.

Documentation

Record:

- time, date, and site of specimen collection
- recent or current antibiotic therapy
- if the specimen has an unusual appearance or odor.

Urine Collection

A random urine specimen, usually collected as part of the physical examination or during hospitalization, permits screening for urinary and systemic disorders, as well as for drugs. A clean-catch midstream specimen is replacing random collection because it provides a virtually uncontaminated specimen without the need for catheterization.

An indwelling catheter specimen—obtained by clamping the drainage tube and emptying the accumulated urine into a container or by aspirating a specimen with a syringe—requires sterile collection technique to prevent catheter contamination and urinary tract infection.

Equipment

For a Random Specimen

Clean bedpan or urinal with cover, if necessary • gloves • graduated container • specimen container with lid • label • laboratory request form

For a Clean-Catch Midstream Specimen

Soap and water • gloves • graduated container • three sterile 2 × 2-inch gauze pads • povidone–iodine solution • sterile specimen container with lid • label • bedpan or urinal • laboratory request form (if necessary)

Commercial clean-catch kits containing antiseptic towelettes, sterile specimen container with lid and label, and instructions for use in several languages are widely used.

For an Indwelling Catheter Specimen

Gloves • alcohol pad • 10-mL syringe • 21G or 22G 1½-inch needle • tube clamp • sterile specimen container with lid • label • laboratory request form

Essential Steps

• Confirm the patient's identity using two patient identifiers and confirmation of the patient's identification bracelet according to facility policy.

• Inform the patient that you need a urine specimen for laboratory analysis.
• Explain the procedure to promote cooperation and prevent accidental disposal of specimens.

Collecting a Random Specimen

• Provide privacy. Instruct the patient on bed rest to void into a clean bedpan or urinal or ask the ambulatory patient to void into either one in the bathroom.
• Put on gloves.
• Pour at least 120 mL of urine into the specimen container and cap the container securely.
• If the patient's urine output must be measured and recorded, pour the remaining urine into the graduated container. Otherwise, discard the remaining urine.
• If you inadvertently spill urine on the outside of the container, clean and dry it to prevent cross-contamination.
• After you label the sample container with the patient's name and room number, and the date and time of collection, attach the request form and send it to the laboratory immediately.

> **Quality and Safety Nursing Alert**
> Delayed transport of the specimen may alter test results.

• Clean the graduated container and urinal or bedpan and return them to their proper storage.
• Discard disposable items.
• Wash your hands thoroughly to prevent cross-contamination.
• Offer the patient a washcloth and soap and water to wash hands.

Collecting a Clean-Catch Midstream Specimen

• Because the goal is a virtually uncontaminated specimen, explain the procedure to the patient carefully.

- Provide illustrations, if possible, to emphasize the correct collection technique.
- Instruct the patient to remove all clothing from the waist down and to stand in front of the toilet as for urination or, if female, to sit far back on the toilet seat and spread her legs.
- Instruct the patient to clean the peri-urethral area (tip of the penis or labial folds, vulva, and urethral meatus) with soap and water and then wipe the area three times, each time with a fresh 2 × 2-inch gauze pad soaked in povidone–iodine solution or with the wipes provided in a commercial kit.
  - Instruct the female patient to sepa-rate her labial folds with the thumb and forefinger. Advise her to strad-dle the bedpan or toilet to allow labial spreading and to continue to keep her labia separated while void-ing. Tell her to wipe down one side with the first pad and discard it, to wipe the other side with the second pad and discard it, and, finally, to wipe down the center over the uri-nary meatus with the third pad and discard it. Stress the importance of cleaning from front to back to avoid contaminating the genital area with fecal matter.
  - For the uncircumcised male patient, emphasize the need to retract his foreskin to effectively clean the meatus and to keep it retracted during voiding.
- Instruct the patient to begin voiding into the bedpan, urinal, or toilet. Then, without stopping the urine stream, the patient should move the collection container into the stream, collecting about 30 to 50 mL at the midstream portion of the voiding. Tell the patient to finish voiding into the bedpan, urinal, or toilet.
- Put on gloves before discarding the first and last portions of the voiding, and measure the remaining urine in a graduated container for intake and

output records, if necessary. Be sure to include the amount in the specimen container when recording the total amount voided.
- Take the sterile container from the patient and cap it securely. Avoid touching the inside of the container or the lid.
- If the outside of the container is soiled, clean it and wipe it dry. Remove gloves and discard them properly.
- Wash your hands thoroughly. Tell the patient to wash his or her hands also.
- Label the container with the patient's name and room number, name of the test, type of specimen, collec-tion time, and suspected diagnosis, if known.
- If a urine culture has been ordered, note any current antibiotic therapy on the laboratory request form.
- Send the container to the laboratory immediately, or place it on ice to prevent specimen deterioration and altered test results.

Collecting an Indwelling Catheter Specimen

- About 30 minutes before collecting the specimen, clamp the drainage tube to allow urine to accumulate.
- Put on gloves.
- If the drainage tube has a built-in sampling port, wipe the port with an alcohol pad. Uncap the needle on the syringe and insert the needle into the sampling port at a 90-degree angle to the tubing. Then aspirate the specimen into the syringe. (See the *Aspirating a Urine Specimen* box.)
- If the drainage tube doesn't have a sampling port and the catheter is made of rubber, obtain the specimen from the catheter. (Other types of catheters will leak after you withdraw the needle.) To withdraw the speci-men from a rubber catheter, wipe it with an alcohol pad just above where it connects to the drainage tube.

Aspirating a Urine Specimen

- If the patient has an indwelling urinary catheter in place, clamp the tube distal to the aspiration port for about 30 minutes. Wipe the port with an alcohol pad and insert a needle with a 20- or 30-mL syringe into the port perpendicular to the tube. Aspirate the required amount of urine and expel it into the specimen container. Remove the clamp on the drainage tube.
- Many indwelling catheters now use a port that does not require needle aspiration of the urine. Using a Luer-Lok syringe, attach it to the port after cleansing with an antiseptic pad and aspirate urine from the tubing after clamping.

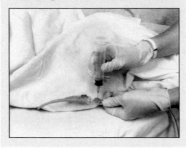

Insert the needle into the rubber catheter at a 45-degree angle and withdraw the specimen. Transfer the specimen to a sterile container, label it, and send it to the laboratory immediately or place it on ice. If a urine culture is to be performed, be sure to list any current antibiotic therapy on the laboratory request form.

 Quality and Safety Nursing Alert

Never insert the needle into the shaft of the catheter because this may puncture the lumen leading to the catheter balloon.

- If the catheter isn't made of rubber or has no sampling port, wipe the area where the catheter joins the drainage tube with an alcohol pad. Disconnect the catheter and allow urine to drain

into the sterile specimen container. (Avoid touching the inside of the sterile container with the catheter and, to avoid contamination, don't touch anything with the catheter drainage tube.) When you've collected the specimen, wipe both connection sites with an alcohol pad and join them, then cap the specimen container and label it. Label the container with the patient's name and room number, name of test, type of specimen, collection time, and suspected diagnosis, if known. Send it to the laboratory immediately or place it on ice.

 Quality and Safety Nursing Alert

Make sure you unclamp the drainage tube after collecting the specimen to prevent urine backflow, which may cause bladder distention and infection.

Special Considerations
- If the patient will be collecting the specimen at home, instruct the patient to collect the specimen in a clean container with a tight-fitting lid.
- Instruct the patient to keep the sample on ice or in the refrigerator (separate from food items) for up to 24 hours.

Documentation
- Record the times of specimen collection and transport to the laboratory.
- Specify the test, as well as the appearance, odor, color, and any unusual characteristics of the specimen.
- If necessary, record the urine volume on the intake and output record.

Urine Collection, Timed

Because hormones, proteins, and electrolytes are excreted in small, variable amounts in urine, specimens for measuring these substances must typically be collected over an extended period to yield quantities of diagnostic value.

A 24-hour specimen is used most commonly because it provides an average excretion rate for substances eliminated during this period. Timed specimens may also be collected for shorter periods, such as 2 or 12 hours, depending on the specific information needed.

A timed urine specimen may also be collected after administering a challenge dose of a chemical—insulin, for example—to detect various renal disorders.

Equipment

Large collection container with a cap or stopper, or a commercial plastic container • preservative (if necessary) • gloves • bedpan or urinal (if patient doesn't have an indwelling catheter) • graduated container (if patient requires intake and output measurement) • gloves • ice-filled container (if a refrigerator isn't available) • label • laboratory request form • four patient-care reminders

Check with the laboratory to see what preservatives may be needed in the urine specimen or if a dark collection container is required.

Essential Steps

- Confirm the patient's identity using two patient identifiers and confirmation of the patient's identification bracelet according to facility policy.
- Explain the procedure to the patient and family, as necessary, to enlist their cooperation and to prevent accidental disposal of urine during the collection period. Emphasize that failure to collect even one specimen during the collection period invalidates the test and requires that it begin again.
- Place patient-care reminders over the patient's bed, in the bathroom, on the bedpan hopper in the utility room, and on the urinal or indwelling catheter collection bag. Include the patient's name and room number, the date, and the collection interval.

- Instruct the patient to save all urine during the collection period, to notify you after each voiding, and to avoid contaminating the urine with stool or toilet tissue.
- Explain any dietary or drug restrictions and make sure they are understood and that the patient is willing to comply with them.

For 2-Hour Collection

- If possible, instruct the patient to drink two to four 8-oz glasses (473–946 mL) of water about 30 minutes before collection begins. After 30 minutes, instruct the patient to void.
- Put on gloves and discard this first specimen so the patient starts the collection period with an empty bladder.
- If ordered, administer a challenge dose of medication (such as glucose solution or corticotropin) and record the time.
- If possible, offer the patient a glass of water at least every hour during the collection period to stimulate urine production.
- After each voiding, put on gloves and add the specimen to the collection container.
- Instruct the patient to void about 15 minutes before the end of the collection period, if possible, and add this specimen to the collection container.
- At the end of the collection period, remove and discard gloves and send the appropriately labeled collection container to the laboratory immediately, along with a properly completed laboratory request form.

For 12- and 24-Hour Collection

- Put on gloves and ask the patient to void. Then discard this urine so the patient starts the collection period with an empty bladder.
- Record the time.
- After putting on gloves and pouring the first urine specimen into the collection container, add the required preservative. Then refrigerate the

bottle or keep it on ice until the next voiding, as appropriate.

• Collect all urine voided during the prescribed period.

• Just before the collection period ends, ask the patient to void again, if possible.

• Add this last specimen to the collection container, pack it in ice to inhibit deterioration of the specimen, and remove and discard gloves.

• Label the collection container and send it to the laboratory with a properly completed laboratory request form.

Special Considerations

• Keep the patient well hydrated before and during the test to ensure adequate urine flow.

• Before collection of a timed specimen, make sure the laboratory will be open when the collection period ends to help ensure prompt, accurate results.

▶ *Quality and Safety Nursing Alert*

Never store a specimen in a refrigerator containing food or medication to avoid contamination.

• If the patient has an indwelling catheter in place, put the collection bag in an ice-filled container at the bedside.

• Instruct the patient to avoid exercise and ingestion of coffee, tea, or any drugs (unless directed otherwise by the health care provider) before the test to avoid altering test results.

• If you accidentally discard a specimen during the collection period, you'll need to restart the collection. This may result in an additional day of hospitalization, which may cause the patient personal and financial hardship. Therefore, emphasize the need to save all the patient's urine during the collection period to everyone

involved in the patient's care, as well as to family and other visitors.

• If the patient must continue collecting urine at home, provide written instructions for the appropriate method.

• Tell the patient to keep the collection container in a brown bag in the refrigerator at home, separate from other refrigerator contents.

Documentation
Record:

• the date and intervals of specimen collection

• when the collection container was sent to the laboratory.

Venipuncture

Performed to obtain a venous blood sample, venipuncture involves piercing a vein with a needle and collecting blood in a syringe or evacuated tube. Typically, venipuncture is performed using the antecubital fossa. If necessary, however, it can be performed on a vein in the dorsal forearm, the dorsum of the hand or foot, or another accessible location. The inner wrist isn't advised because of the high risk of damage to the underlying structures. Although laboratory personnel usually perform this procedure in the hospital setting, you may perform it occasionally.

Equipment
Tourniquet • gloves • syringe or evacuated tubes and needle holder • antiseptic pads • 20G or 21G needle (for the forearm) or 25G needle (for the wrist, hand, and ankle, and for children) • color-coded collection tubes containing appropriate additives • labels • 2 × 2-inch gauze pads • laboratory request form • adhesive bandage

Essential Steps
• Confirm the patient's identity using two patient identifiers and confirmation of the patient's identification bracelet according to facility policy.

- Wash your hands thoroughly and put on gloves.
- Inform the patient that you're about to take a blood sample and explain the procedure to ease anxiety and ensure cooperation. Inquire if the patient has ever felt faint, sweaty, or nauseated when having blood drawn.
- Ask the patient who is on bed rest to lie supine, with head slightly elevated and arms at sides. Ask the ambulatory patient to sit in a chair and support the arm securely on an armrest or table.
- Assess the patient's veins to determine the best puncture site. (See the *Common Venipuncture Sites* box.)
- Observe the skin for the vein's blue color or palpate the vein for a firm rebound sensation.
- Tie a tourniquet 2 inches (5 cm) proximal to the area chosen. By impeding venous return to the heart while still allowing arterial flow, a tourniquet produces venous dilation. If arterial perfusion remains adequate,

you'll be able to feel the radial pulse. (If the tourniquet fails to dilate the vein, have the patient open and close a fist a few times. Then ask the patient to close the fist as you insert the needle and to open it again when the needle is in place.)

> ### ▶ *Quality and Safety Nursing Alert*
>
> A tourniquet is not always recommended for the elderly patient due to the possibility of capillary rupture.

- Clean the venipuncture site with an antiseptic pad. Wipe in a side-to-side motion, working outward from the site to avoid introducing potentially infectious skin flora into the vessel during the procedure.
- Allow the skin to dry before performing venipuncture.
- If you're using evacuated tubes, open the needle packet, attach the needle to its holder, and select the appropriate tubes.

■ Common Venipuncture Sites

The illustrations show the anatomic locations of veins commonly used for venipuncture. The most commonly used sites are on the forearm, followed by those on the hand. (From Lynn P. Taylor's Clinical Nursing Skills, 3rd ed. Philadelphia: Wolters Kluwer Health | Lippincott Williams & Wilkins, 2011, page 929.)

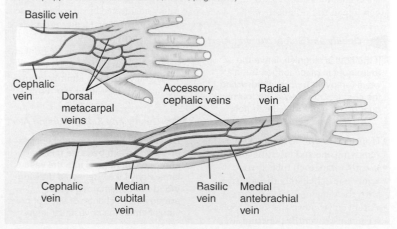

Quality and Safety Nursing Alert

Be sure to check the expiration date on the tubes and discard if expired.

• If you're using a syringe, attach the appropriate needle to it.
• Choose a syringe large enough to hold all the blood required for the test.
• Immobilize the vein by pressing just below the venipuncture site with your thumb and drawing the skin taut.
• Position the needle holder or syringe with the needle bevel-up and the shaft parallel to the path of the vein and at a 30-degree angle to the arm.
• Insert the needle into the vein.
• If you're using a syringe, venous blood will appear in the hub; withdraw the blood slowly, pulling the plunger of the syringe gently to create steady suction until you obtain the required sample. Pulling the plunger too forcibly may collapse the vein.
• If you're using a needle holder and an evacuated tube, grasp the holder securely to stabilize it in the vein and push down on the collection tube until the needle punctures the rubber stopper. Blood will flow into the tube automatically.
• Remove the tourniquet as soon as blood flows adequately to prevent stasis and hemoconcentration, which can impair test results.

Quality and Safety Nursing Alert

If the flow is sluggish, leave the tourniquet in place longer, but always remove it before withdrawing the needle. Don't leave the tourniquet on for more than 3 minutes.

• Continue to fill the required tubes, removing one and inserting another.
• Gently rotate each tube as you remove it to help mix the additive with the sample.
• After you've drawn the sample, place a gauze pad over the puncture site,

and slowly and gently remove the needle from the vein.
• When using an evacuated tube, remove it from the needle holder to release the vacuum before withdrawing the needle from the vein.
• Apply gentle pressure to the puncture site for 2 or 3 minutes or until bleeding stops, keeping the arm straight. Doing so prevents extravasation into the surrounding tissue, which can cause a hematoma.
• After bleeding stops, apply an adhesive bandage.
• If you've used a syringe, transfer the sample to a collection tube.
• Detach the needle from the syringe, open the collection tube, and gently empty the sample into the tube, being careful to avoid foaming, which can cause hemolysis.
• Check the venipuncture site to see if a hematoma has developed. If one has, apply pressure until you're sure the bleeding has stopped.
• Discard syringes, needles, and used gloves in the appropriate containers.
• Label all collection tubes clearly with the patient's name and room number, the health care provider's name, and the date and time of collection.

Special Considerations

• Today, many manufacturers make safety-engineered blood collection sets. If available in your facility, use a safety set to prevent needle sticks.
• Never draw a venous sample from an arm or leg that's already being used for IV therapy or blood administration, because this may affect test results.

Quality and Safety Nursing Alert

Don't collect a venous sample from an infection site because this may introduce pathogens into the vascular system. Likewise, avoid drawing blood from edematous areas, arteriovenous shunts, or sites of previous hematoma or vascular injury.

- If the patient has large, distended, highly visible veins, perform venipuncture without a tourniquet to minimize the risk of hematoma formation.
- If the patient has a clotting disorder or is receiving anticoagulant therapy, maintain firm pressure on the venipuncture site for at least 5 minutes after withdrawing the needle to prevent hematoma formation.
- Avoid using veins in the patient's legs for venipuncture, if possible, because this increases the risk of thrombophlebitis. Some facilities require a health care provider's order to collect blood from a leg or foot vein. Check the policy and procedure at your facility.

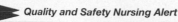 Quality and Safety Nursing Alert

Remember to use pediatric tubes for collecting specimens on infants and children; the volumes are much less than volumes collected on adults. Pediatric tubes may also be used in select patient populations, such as with elderly patients or those with low blood volumes, as indicated. Check your facility's policy.

Complications
- A hematoma at the needle insertion site is the most common complication of venipuncture.
- Infection may result from poor technique.

Documentation
Record:
- date, time, and site of venipuncture
- name of the test
- time the sample was sent to the laboratory
- amount of blood collected
- patient's temperature
- adverse reactions to the procedure.

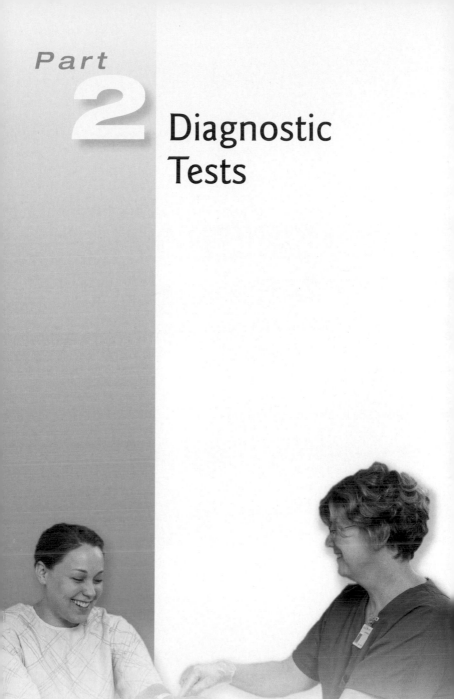

Part

2

Diagnostic
Tests

Acetaminophen Level

Reference Values
Therapeutic dose: 10 to 20 mcg/mL, based on relief of symptoms (SI, 66.2 132.4 mcmol/L)

Critical Values
Greater than 300 mcg/mL (SI, 1.986 mcmol/L)

Abnormal Findings
Elevated Levels
• Results greater than 200 mcg/mL (SI, greater than 1.324 mcmol/L) 4 hours after ingestion or greater than 50 mcg/mL (SI, greater than 331 mcmol/L) 12 hours after ingestion; signifying toxicity and potential for liver damage

Nursing Implications
• Prepare to administer acetylcysteine (Mucomyst, Mucosil, Parvolex) as an antidote to acetaminophen. This agent is effective only within a restricted timeframe. Please check with health care provider for this determination.
• Prepare the patient for hemodialysis to remove acetaminophen from the body.
• Monitor the patient's vital signs closely.
• Monitor serum acetaminophen levels and liver function studies.
• Monitor intake and output to assess renal function.

Purpose
• To monitor for acetaminophen overdose

Description
Acetaminophen is an analgesic used for fever and pain relief, but high levels can be toxic and cause liver toxicity. It's rapidly absorbed in the GI tract; peak concentration occurs 30 to 60 minutes after ingestion. Intoxication doesn't become apparent until 24 to 48 hours after ingestion.

Precautions
• Maintain standard precautions during sample collection.
• Transport the specimen to the laboratory immediately after collection.

Nursing Considerations
Before the Test
• Confirm the patient's identity using two patient identifiers and confirmation of the patient's identification bracelet according to facility policy.
• Explain to the patient that this test shows the amount of acetaminophen in the blood.
• Inform the patient that there is no need to restrict food or fluid intake.
• Tell the patient that the test requires a blood sample.
• Advise the patient that there may be slight discomfort from the tourniquet and the needle puncture.

During the Test
• Perform a venipuncture and collect the sample in a 5-mL tube.

After the Test
• Observe the venipuncture site for bleeding or hematoma formation.
• Apply direct pressure to avoid development of a hematoma.

Activated Clotting Time

Reference Values

Nonanticoagulated patient: 107 seconds, plus or minus 13 seconds (SI, 107 plus or minus 13 seconds)

During cardiopulmonary bypass: 400 to 600 seconds (SI, 400–600 seconds)

During extracorporal membrane oxygenation (ECMO): 220 to 260 seconds (SI, 220–260 seconds)

Abnormal Findings

- Clotting times out of the normal range during cardiopulmonary bypass or ECMO
- Clotting factor deficiencies

Nursing Implications

- Report abnormal findings to the health care provider.
- During cardiopulmonary bypass, heparin should be titrated to maintain an activated clotting time of 400 to 600 seconds (SI, 400–600 seconds).

Purpose

- To monitor heparin's effect
- To monitor protamine sulfate's effect in heparin neutralization
- To detect severe deficiencies in clotting factors (except factor VII)

Description

Activated clotting time, or *automated coagulation time*, measures whole blood clotting time. It's commonly performed when a procedure requires extracorporeal circulation, such as during cardiopulmonary bypass or during ultrafiltration, hemodialysis, and ECMO. It may also be used during invasive procedures, such as cardiac catheterization and percutaneous transluminal coronary angioplasty.

Interfering Factors

- Failure to fill the collection tube completely, to use proper anticoagulant, or to adequately mix the sample and the anticoagulant
- Failure to send the sample to the laboratory immediately or to place it on ice
- Hemolysis from rough handling of the sample or excessive probing at the venipuncture site
- Failure to draw at least 5 mL waste to avoid sample contamination when drawing the sample from a venous access device that's used for heparin infusion

Nursing Considerations

Before the Test

- Confirm the patient's identity using two patient identifiers and confirmation of the patient's identification bracelet according to facility policy.
- Explain to the patient that the activated clotting time test monitors the effect of heparin on the blood's ability to coagulate.
- Explain who will perform the test, when, and where it will occur (usually at the bedside).
- Inform the patient that the test requires two blood samples but, because they'll be drawn from an existing vascular access site, no venipuncture will be necessary.
- Explain that the first blood sample will be discarded so that any heparin in the tubing won't interfere with the results.

During the Test

- Before drawing a sample from a line with a continuous infusion, stop the infusion.
- Withdraw 5 to 10 mL of blood and discard it.
- Take a second blood sample and add it into the special tube containing celite from the activated clotting time unit.
- Start the activated clotting time unit, wait for the signal, and insert the tube.
- Flush the vascular access site according to your facility's policy.

After the Test
- Instruct the patient to report discomfort at the site.
- Monitor the venipuncture site for bleeding.

Alanine Aminotransferase (ALT) (formerly SGPT)

Reference Values
Males: 10–40 U/mL (SI, 0.17–0.68 mckat/L); Females: 8–35 U/mL (SI, 0.14–0.60 mckat/L)

Abnormal Findings
Elevated Levels
- Extensive liver damage from toxins or drugs, viral hepatitis, skeletal–muscle disease, lack of oxygen, usually resulting from very low blood pressure or myocardial infarction (MI) (levels above 1,000 international units/L)
- Acute or chronic hepatitis (300–1,000 international units/L)

Decreased Levels
- Any kind of liver disease (levels below 300 international units/L)

Nursing Implications
- Report abnormal findings to the health care provider.
- Educate the patient about the diagnosis and treatment options.
- In patients with elevated levels, observe standard precautions to prevent disease transmission.

Purpose
- To detect and evaluate treatment of acute hepatic disease, especially hepatitis and cirrhosis without jaundice
- To distinguish between myocardial and hepatic tissue damage (used with aspartate aminotransferase)
- To assess the hepatotoxicity of some drugs

Description
The alanine aminotransferase (ALT) test uses the spectrophotometric method to screen for liver damage by measuring how much of the ALT enzyme is in the liver. ALT, which is necessary for tissue energy production, is found primarily in the liver, with lesser amounts in the kidneys, heart, and skeletal muscles.

ALT is a sensitive indicator of acute hepatocellular disease and is released from the cytoplasm into the bloodstream, typically before jaundice appears, resulting in abnormally high serum levels that may not return to normal for days or weeks.

Interfering Factors
- Barbiturates, chlorpromazine (Thorazine), griseofulvin, isoniazid, methyldopa (Aldomet), nitrofurantoin (Furadantin), para-aminosalicylic acid, phenothiazine, phenytoin (Dilantin), salicylates, tetracycline, and other drugs that cause hepatic injury by competitively interfering with cellular metabolism (false high)
- Opioid analgesics, such as codeine, meperidine (Demerol), and morphine (Duramorph) (possible false high due to increased intrabiliary pressure)
- Lead ingestion or exposure to carbon tetrachloride (sharp increase due to direct injury to hepatic cells)
- Acetaminophen and aspirin therapy

Nursing Considerations
Before the Test
- Confirm the patient's identity using two patient identifiers and confirmation of the patient's identification bracelet according to facility policy.
- Explain to the patient that the ALT test is used to assess liver function and that it requires a blood sample.
- Advise the patient that there may be slight discomfort from the tourniquet and needle puncture.
- Inform the patient that there is no food or fluid restriction.

- Notify the laboratory and health care provider about any medications being taken by the patient that may affect test results; restrict the use of these drugs, if necessary.

During the Test
- Perform a venipuncture and collect the sample in a 4-mL tube without additives.
- Apply direct pressure to the venipuncture site until bleeding stops.

After the Test
- Apply direct pressure to avoid the formation of a hematoma.
- Instruct the patient that he or she may resume medications discontinued before the test, as ordered.

Albumin

Reference Values
Adults: 3.5 to 4.8 g/dL (SI, 35–48 g/L)
Children: 2.9 to 5.5 g/dL (SI, 29–55 g/L)

Abnormal Findings
Elevated Levels (Hyperalbuminemia)
- Dehydration
- Severe vomiting
- Severe diarrhea

Decreased Levels (Hypoalbuminemia)
- Cirrhosis, liver disease, alcoholism
- Severe burns, severe skin disease (Stevens-Johnson)
- Severe malnutrition, malabsorption, anorexia
- Inflammatory bowel disease (Crohn's disease and ulcerative colitis)
- Thyroid disease, Cushing disease

Nursing Implications
- Report abnormal elevated findings to the health care provider.
- Prepare to administer IV fluids to restore volume and electrolytes in patients with elevated levels.

- Prepare to administer IV albumin to restore decreased levels.
- Educate the patient about the disease and treatment options.
- Explain the need for possible further testing of diminished albumin levels.

Purpose
- To help determine whether a patient has liver or kidney disease
- To determine whether enough protein is being absorbed by the body

Description
The test measures the amount of albumin in serum. Albumin is the most abundant protein in human blood, comprising almost 54% of plasma proteins.

Interfering Factors
- Penicillin, sulfonamides, aspirin, and ascorbic acid (decrease)
- Heparin (increase)
- Last-trimester pregnancy (due to increase in plasma volume)
- Estrogens (oral birth control)
- Prolonged bed rest
- IV fluids, rapid hydration, overhydration

Nursing Considerations
Before the Test
- Confirm the patient's identity using two patient identifiers and confirmation of the patient's identification bracelet according to facility policy.
- Inform the patient that there are no food or fluid restrictions.
- Describe the venipuncture procedure to the patient.
- Explain to the patient that he or she may experience slight discomfort from the tourniquet and the needle puncture.
- Explain that certain medications can increase albumin measurements, including anabolic steroids, androgens, growth hormones, and insulin. The patient may need to stop taking these drugs before the test.

During the Test
- Perform a venipuncture and collect 5 to 10 mL in a red-top tube.
- Follow standard precautions when collecting the sample.

After the Test
- Apply direct pressure to the venipuncture site until bleeding stops.
- Encourage the patient to eat a high-protein diet, if not contraindicated.

Aldosterone (Serum, Urine)

Reference Values

Serum Levels
Taken in upright position after 2 hours: 7 to 30 ng/dL (SI, 190–832 pmol/L)
Taken supine: 3 to 16 ng/dL (SI, 80–440 pmol/L)

Urine Levels
3 to 19 mcg/24 hours (SI, 8–51 nmol/day)

Abnormal Findings

Elevated Levels
- Primary aldosteronism (Conn's syndrome), possibly resulting from adrenocortical adenoma or bilateral adrenal hyperplasia
- Secondary aldosteronism resulting from renovascular hypertension, congestive heart failure, cirrhosis of the liver, nephrotic syndrome, idiopathic cyclic edema, third-trimester of pregnancy, salt depletion, potassium loading, laxative abuse, diuretic abuse

Decreased Levels
- Primary hypoaldosteronism
- Salt-losing syndrome
- Eclampsia
- Addison's disease

Nursing Implications
- Report abnormal findings to the health care provider.
- Prepare the patient for further testing to confirm the diagnosis.

- Educate the patient about the disease and possible treatment options.
- Because aldosterone levels affect sodium levels, educate the patient about salt and water intake.

Purpose
- To help diagnose primary and secondary aldosteronism, adrenal hyperplasia, hypoaldosteronism, and salt-losing syndrome (plasma)
- To help diagnose primary and secondary aldosteronism (urine)

Description
The serum aldosterone test measures aldosterone blood levels by quantitative analysis and radioimmunoassay. It identifies aldosteronism and, when supported by serum renin levels, distinguishes between the primary and secondary forms of this disorder. The urine aldosterone test measures urine levels of aldosterone through radioimmunoassay. Levels are usually evaluated after measurement of serum electrolyte and renin levels.

Aldosterone, the principal mineralocorticoid secreted by the zona glomerulosa of the adrenal cortex, regulates ion transport across cell membranes in the renal tubules to promote reabsorption of sodium and chloride in exchange for potassium and hydrogen ions. Consequently, aldosterone helps to maintain blood pressure and volume and to regulate fluid and electrolyte balance.

Aldosterone secretion is controlled primarily by the renin–angiotensin concentration of potassium. As a result, high serum potassium levels cause aldosterone secretion through a potent feedback system, as well as causing hyponatremia, hypovolemia, and other disorders that trigger renin and stimulate aldosterone secretion.

Interfering Factors
- Failure to maintain normal dietary sodium intake, as well as excess intake of licorice or glucose

- Failure to avoid strenuous physical exercise and emotional stress before the test (possible increase due to stimulation of adrenocortical secretions)
- Radioactive scan performed within 1 week before the test
- Antihypertensive drugs (possible decrease due to sodium and water retention)
- Diuretics and most steroids (possible increase due to sodium excretion)
- Some corticosteroids, such as fludrocortisone, which mimic mineralocorticoid activity (possible decrease)

Precautions
- Handle blood samples gently to prevent hemolysis.

Nursing Considerations
Before the Test
- Confirm the patient's identity using two patient identifiers and confirmation of the patient's identification bracelet according to facility policy.
- Explain to the patient that the aldosterone test evaluates hormonal balance.
- Instruct the patient to maintain a normal-sodium diet (3 g/day) before the test and to avoid sodium-rich foods found in processed foods such as corned beef, bouillon cubes or powder, pickles, snack foods (such as potato chips), canned or frozen foods, and olives.
- Notify the laboratory and health care provider about any medications the patient is taking that may affect test results; restrict the use of these drugs, if necessary.

Serum Aldosterone
- Inform the patient that the serum aldosterone test requires a blood sample.
- Advise the patient that there may be slight discomfort from the needle puncture and the tourniquet.

- Advise the patient to maintain a low-carbohydrate, normal-sodium diet for at least 2 weeks or, preferably, for 30 days before this test.
- Provide these additional instructions:
  - Withhold drugs that alter fluid, sodium, and potassium balance (especially diuretics, antihypertensives, steroids, hormonal contraceptives, and estrogens) for at least 2 weeks or, preferably, for 30 days before the test, as ordered.
  - Withhold all renin inhibitors for 1 week before the test, as ordered.
  - Avoid licorice for at least 2 weeks before the test because it produces an aldosteronelike effect.
- If renin inhibitors must be continued, note this information on the laboratory request.

Urine Aldosterone
- Explain to the patient that the test requires collection of urine during a 24-hour period, and teach the patient the proper collection technique.
- Advise the patient to avoid strenuous physical exercise and stressful situations during the urine collection period.

During the Test
Serum Aldosterone
- Perform a venipuncture after a night's rest while the patient is still supine. Collect this sample in a 7-mL clot activator tube and send it to the laboratory immediately.
- Draw another sample 4 hours later, while the patient is standing and after he or she has been up and about, to evaluate the effect of postural change. Collect this second sample in a 7-mL clot activator tube. Send the specimen to the laboratory immediately.
- Make sure to record on the laboratory request slip whether the patient was supine or standing during the venipuncture.

- If the female patient is premenopausal, specify the phase of her menstrual cycle on the laboratory slip because serum aldosterone levels may fluctuate.

Urine Aldosterone
- Collect the patient's urine over a 24-hour period, discarding the first specimen and retaining the last. Use a bottle containing a preservative, such as boric acid, to keep the specimen at a pH of 4.0 to 4.5.
- Refrigerate the specimen or place it on ice during the collection period.
- Send the specimen to the laboratory as soon as collection is complete.

After the Test
- Apply direct pressure to the venipuncture site until bleeding stops. Apply direct pressure to avoid development of a hematoma.
- Instruct the patient to resume usual activities, diet, and medications, as ordered.

Alkaline Phosphatase

Reference Values
30 to 85 international units/mL (SI, 42–128 units/L)

Abnormal Findings
Elevated Levels
- Skeletal disease
- Extrahepatic or intrahepatic biliary obstruction
- Active cirrhosis
- Mononucleosis
- Viral hepatitis
- Complete biliary obstruction by malignant or infectious infiltrations or fibrosis (sharp elevation); most common in Paget's disease
- Osteomalacia and deficiency-induced rickets (moderate increases)

Decreased Levels
- Hypophosphatasia (rarely)
- Protein or magnesium deficiency (rarely)
- Hypothyroidism

Nursing Implications
- Report abnormal findings to the health care provider.
- Prepare the patient with elevated levels for additional liver function studies to identify hepatobiliary disorders.
- Educate the patient about the disease and possible treatment options.

Purpose
- To detect and identify skeletal diseases primarily characterized by marked osteoblastic activity
- To detect focal hepatic lesions causing biliary obstruction, such as a tumor or an abscess
- To assess the patient's response to vitamin D in the treatment of rickets
- To supplement information from other liver function studies and GI enzyme tests

Description
The alkaline phosphatase (ALP) test is used to measure serum levels of ALP, an enzyme that influences bone calcification, as well as to measure lipid and metabolite transport. The measurement reflects the combined activity of several ALP isoenzymes found in the liver, bones, kidneys, intestinal lining, and placenta. Bone and liver ALP always are present in adult serum, with liver ALP most prominent except during the third trimester of pregnancy (when the placenta accounts for one-half). Intestinal ALP can be a normal component (in less than 10% of normal patients; almost exclusively in the sera of blood groups B and O), or it can be an abnormal finding associated with hepatic disease.

The ALP test is particularly sensitive to mild biliary obstruction, and its results can provide a primary indication of space-occupying hepatic lesions. Although skeletal and hepatic diseases can raise ALP levels, diagnosing metabolic bone disease is the primary use of this test. Additional liver function studies are usually required to identify hepato-biliary disorders.

> ▶ **Quality and Safety Nursing Alert**
>
> Alkaline phosphatase levels may increase by 8 to 10 international units/mL in elderly patients, possibly due to declining liver function or vitamin D malabsorption and bone demineralization.

Interfering Factors

- Failure to analyze the sample within 4 hours
- Recent ingestion of vitamin D (possible increase due to the effect on osteoblastic activity)
- Recent infusion of albumin prepared from placental venous blood (marked increase)
- Drugs that influence liver function or cause cholestasis, such as barbiturates, chlorpropamide (Diabinese), hormonal contraceptives, isoniazid (Nydrazid), methyldopa (Aldomet), phenothiazines, phenytoin (Dilantin), and rifampin (Rifadin) (possible mild increase)
- Halothane sensitivity (possible drastic increase)
- Clofibrate (Abitrate) (decrease)
- Healing long-bone fractures and the third trimester of pregnancy (possible increase)
- Age and gender (increase in infants, children, adolescents, and individuals older than age 45)
- Delay in sending the sample immediately to the laboratory (ALP activity increases at room temperature due to a rise in pH)
- Ingestion of fatty meals (increase)

Precautions

- Handle the sample gently to prevent hemolysis.

Nursing Considerations

Before the Test

- Confirm the patient's identity using two patient identifiers and confirmation of the patient's identification bracelet according to facility policy.
- Explain to the patient that the ALP test is used to assess liver and bone function.
- Instruct the patient to fast for at least 8 hours before the test because fat intake stimulates intestinal ALP secretion.
- Tell the patient that this test requires a blood sample.
- Advise the patient that there may be slight discomfort from the tourniquet and needle puncture.

During the Test

- Perform a venipuncture and collect the sample in a 4-mL clot activator tube.

After the Test

- Apply direct pressure to the venipuncture site until bleeding stops and to prevent hematoma formation.
- Instruct the patient to resume a usual diet.

Alpha₁-Antitrypsin (AAT)

Reference Values

110 to 200 mg/dL (SI, 1.1–2 g/L)

Abnormal Findings

Elevated Levels

- Chronic inflammatory disorders
- Necrosis
- Pregnancy
- Acute pulmonary infections
- Respiratory distress syndrome in infants
- Hepatitis
- Systemic lupus erythematosus
- Rheumatoid arthritis

Decreased Levels

- Early-onset emphysema (in adults)
- Cirrhosis (in children)
- Nephrotic syndrome

- Malnutrition
- Congenital alpha₁-globulin deficiency

Nursing Implications
- Report abnormal findings to the health care provider.

Purpose
- To screen the patient at high risk for emphysema
- To use as a nonspecific method of detecting inflammation, severe infection, and necrosis
- To test for congenital alpha₁-antitrypsin (AAT) deficiency

Description
A protein produced by the liver, AAT (also known as alpha₁-AT) is believed to inhibit the release of protease into body fluids by dying cells and is a major component of alpha₁-globulin. AAT is measured using radioimmunoassay or isoelectric focusing. Congenital absence or deficiency of AAT has been linked to high susceptibility to emphysema in adults and cirrhosis in children.

Interfering Factors
- Corticosteroids and hormonal contraceptives (possible false high)
- Smoking or failure to fast for 8 hours before the test (possible false high)

Precautions
- Handle the sample gently to prevent hemolysis.

Nursing Considerations
Before the Test
- Confirm the patient's identity using two patient identifiers and confirmation of the patient's identification bracelet according to facility policy.

> **Quality and Safety Nursing Alert**
>
> If the patient is a child, explain to the parents that the AAT test is used to diagnose respiratory or liver disease, as well as to diagnose inflammation, infection, or necrosis.

- Inform the patient that the AAT test requires a blood sample. Advise the patient that there may be slight discomfort from the tourniquet and needle puncture.
- Instruct the patient to avoid smoking because irritants in tobacco stimulate leukocytes in the lungs to release protease.
- Advise the patient to avoid hormonal contraceptives and steroids for 24 hours before the test.
- Remind the patient to fast for at least 8 hours before the test.
- Be aware that the patient with an AAT level lower than 125 mg/dL (SI, 1.25 g/L) should be phenotyped to confirm homozygous and heterozygous deficiencies. (The heterozygous patient doesn't appear to be at increased risk for early emphysema.)

During the Test
- Perform a venipuncture and collect the sample in a 4-mL tube without additives.

> **Quality and Safety Nursing Alert**
>
> In a child, puncture the clean area with a sharp needle or lancet, then collect the blood sample in a pipette or a small container, or onto a slide.

After the Test
- Apply direct pressure to the venipuncture site until bleeding stops.
- Instruct the patient to resume usual diet and medications that were discontinued before the test, as ordered.
- Send the sample to the laboratory promptly.

Alpha₁-Globulin

Reference Values
0.1 to 0.3 g/dL (SI, 1–3 g/L)

Abnormal Findings

Elevated Levels

- Chronic inflammatory disease (e.g., rheumatoid arthritis, systemic lupus erythematosus)
- Acute inflammatory disease
- Malignancy

Decreased Levels

- Alpha$_1$-antitrypsin deficiency

Nursing Implications

- Report abnormal findings to the health care provider.

Purpose

- To help rule out inflammatory disease

Description

Alpha$_1$-globulin, a serum protein, approximately measures the various protein fractions in a blood sample.

Interfering Factors

- Drugs that can affect the measurement of total proteins, including chlorpromazine (Thorazine), corticosteroids, isoniazid (Nydrazid), neomycin (Mycifradin), salicylates, sulfonamides, and tolbutamide (Orinase)

Nursing Considerations

Before the Test

- Confirm the patient's identity using two patient identifiers and confirmation of the patient's identification bracelet according to facility policy.
- Inform the patient that the test requires a venipuncture.
- Advise the patient that there may be slight discomfort from the tourniquet and needle puncture.

During the Test

- Perform the venipuncture according to protocol.

After the Test

- Apply direct pressure to the venipuncture site until bleeding stops.

Alpha$_2$-Globulin

Reference Values

0.6 to 1 g/dL (SI, 6–10 g/L)

Abnormal Findings

Elevated Levels

- Acute or chronic inflammation

Decreased Levels

- Hemolysis

Nursing Implications

- Report abnormal findings to the health care provider.
- Educate the patient about the disease and possible treatment options for elevated levels.
- Prepare to administer antibiotics in patients with elevated levels, as ordered by the health care provider.
- Repeat the test, if instructed to do so by the health care provider, to confirm decreased levels.
- Be aware that hemolysis may occur as a result of leaving the tourniquet on for an extended period of time, slow blood flow, using large-bore needles for venipuncture, or forcing a syringe blood draw into a tube at too fast a rate.

Purpose

- To quantitate the alpha$_2$-globulin protein factor in the blood
- To help detect the presence of inflammation

Description

Alpha$_2$-globulin, a serum protein, approximately measures the various protein fractions in a blood sample.

Interfering Factors

- Chlorpromazine (Thorazine), corticosteroids, isoniazid (Nydrazid), neomycin (Mycifradin), phenacemide, salicylates, sulfonamides, and tolbutamide (Orinase)

Nursing Considerations

Before the Test
- Confirm the patient's identity using two patient identifiers and confirmation of the patient's identification bracelet according to facility policy.
- Inform the patient that the test requires a venipuncture.
- Advise the patient that there may be slight discomfort from the tourniquet and the needle puncture.

During the Test
- Perform the venipuncture according to protocol.

After the Test
- Apply direct pressure to the venipuncture site until bleeding stops.

Alveolar-to-Arterial Oxygen Gradient (A-aDO$_2$)

Reference Values
At rest: Less than 10 mm Hg (SI, less than 1.33 kPa)
At maximum exercise: 20 to 30 mm Hg (SI, 2.7–4 kPa)

Abnormal Findings

Elevated Levels
- Mucus plugs
- Bronchospasm
- Airway collapse (asthma, bronchitis, emphysema)

Decreased Levels
- Pneumothorax
- Atelectasis
- Emboli
- Edema

Nursing Implications
- Report abnormal findings to the health care provider.

Purpose
- To evaluate the efficiency of gas exchange
- To assess the integrity of the ventilatory control system
- To monitor respiratory therapy

Description
The alveolar-to-arterial oxygen gradient (A-aDO$_2$) test uses calculations based on the patient's laboratory values to approximate the partial pressure of alveolar and arterial oxygenation pressure to help identify the cause of hypoxemia and intrapulmonary shunting. It may help differentiate the cause as ventilated alveoli but no perfusion, unventilated alveoli with perfusion, or collapse of the alveoli and capillaries.

Interfering Factors
- Exposing the sample to air (increase or decrease)
- Age and increasing oxygen concentration (increase)

Nursing Considerations

Before the Test
- Confirm the patient's identity using two patient identifiers and confirmation of the patient's identification bracelet according to facility policy.
- Explain to the patient that the A-aDO$_2$ test is used to evaluate how well the lungs are delivering oxygen to the blood and eliminating carbon dioxide.
- Inform the patient that the test requires a blood sample.
- Inform the patient that there is no need to restrict food and fluids.
- Instruct the patient to breathe normally during the test, and warn the patient of possible cramping or throbbing pain at the puncture site.
- Record the patient's rectal temperature (See arterial blood gas, p. 57).

During the Test
- Perform an arterial puncture or draw blood from an existing arterial line using a heparinized blood gas syringe.
- Eliminate all air from the sample and place the sample on ice immediately.
- Note on the laboratory slip whether the patient was breathing room air

or receiving oxygen therapy when the sample was collected. If the patient was receiving oxygen therapy, indicate the flow rate and delivery method. If the patient was on a ventilator, note the fraction of inspired oxygen, tidal volume, mode, respiratory rate, and positive end-expiratory pressure.

After the Test
- Apply pressure to the arterial puncture site for 3 to 5 minutes.
- Place a gauze pad over the site and tape it in place, but don't tape the entire circumference.
- Monitor the patient's vital signs and observe for signs of circulatory impairment, such as swelling, discoloration, pain, numbness, and tingling in the bandaged arm or leg.
- Watch for bleeding at the puncture site.

Ammonia, Plasma

Reference Values
15 to 56 mcg/dL (SI, 9–33 mcmol/L)

Critical Values
Greater than 68.1 mcg/dL (SI, greater than 40 mcmol/L)

Abnormal Findings
Elevated Levels
- Severe hepatic disease (cirrhosis and acute hepatic necrosis)
- Reye's syndrome
- Severe heart failure
- GI hemorrhage
- Erythroblastosis fetalis
- Renal disease
- Total parenteral nutrition

Nursing Implications
- Report abnormal findings to the health care provider.
- Educate the patient about the disease and possible treatment options.
- Employ safety measures for the patient with elevated ammonia levels related to altered mental status.

Purpose
- To help monitor the progression of severe hepatic disease and the effectiveness of therapy
- To recognize impending or established hepatic coma

Description
The plasma ammonia test measures plasma levels of ammonia, a nonprotein nitrogen compound that helps maintain acid–base balance. In diseases such as cirrhosis of the liver, ammonia can bypass the liver and accumulate in the blood. Plasma ammonia levels may help indicate the severity of hepatocellular damage.

Interfering Factors
- Acetazolamide (Dazamide), ammonium salts, furosemide (Lasix), and thiazides (increase)
- Kanamycin (Kantrex), lactulose (Chronulac), and neomycin (Mycifradin) (decrease)
- Parenteral nutrition or a portacaval shunt (possible increase)
- Smoking, poor venipuncture technique, and exposure to ammonia-containing cleaning agents in the laboratory (possible increase)
- Tight tourniquet or by tightly clenching the fist while samples are drawn (increase)

Precautions
- Handle the sample gently to prevent hemolysis, pack it in ice, and send it to the laboratory immediately.

Nursing Considerations
Before the Test
- Confirm the patient's identity using two patient identifiers and confirmation of the patient's identification bracelet according to facility policy.
- Explain to the patient (or family member, if the patient is comatose) that the plasma ammonia test is used to evaluate liver function.
- Tell the patient that the test requires a blood sample.

- Advise the patient that there may be slight discomfort from the tourniquet and needle puncture.
- Notify the laboratory and health care provider about any medications the patient is taking that may affect test results; these may need to be restricted.
- Notify the laboratory before performing the venipuncture so that preliminary preparations can begin.

During the Test
- Perform a venipuncture and collect the sample in a 10-mL heparinized tube.

After the Test
- Apply direct pressure to the venipuncture site until bleeding stops and to prevent formation of a hematoma.
- Monitor for signs of impending or established hepatic coma if plasma ammonia levels are high.

Amylase, Serum

Reference Values
Adults age 18 and older: 25 to 125 units/L (SI, 0.4–2.1 mckat/L)
Adults older than age 60: 24 to 151 units/L (SI, 0.4–2.5 mckat/L)

Critical Values
Greater than 200 units/L

Abnormal Findings
Elevated Levels
- Acute pancreatitis (levels begin to rise within 2 hours, peak within 12 to 48 hours, and return to normal within 3 to 4 days)

Moderately Elevated Levels
- Obstruction of the common bile duct, pancreatic duct, or ampulla of Vater; pancreatic injury from a perforated peptic ulcer; pancreatic cancer; and acute salivary gland disease
- Impaired kidney function

Decreased Levels
- Chronic pancreatitis
- Pancreatic cancer

- Cirrhosis
- Hepatitis
- Toxemia of pregnancy

Nursing Implications
- Report abnormal findings to the health care provider.
- Determination of urine levels should follow normal serum alpha-amylase (AML) test results to rule out pancreatitis.

Purpose
- To diagnose acute pancreatitis
- To distinguish between acute pancreatitis and other causes of abdominal pain that require immediate surgery
- To evaluate possible pancreatic injury caused by abdominal trauma or surgery

Description
An enzyme that is synthesized primarily in the pancreas and salivary glands and is secreted in the GI tract, amylase (or AML) helps to digest starch and glycogen in the mouth, stomach, and intestine. In cases of suspected acute pancreatic disease, serum or urine AML measurement is the most important laboratory test.

Interfering Factors
- Ingestion of ethyl alcohol in large amounts (possible false high)
- Aminosalicylic acid, asparaginase (Elspar), azathioprine (Imuran), corticosteroids, cyproheptadine (Periactin), hormonal contraceptives, opioid analgesics, rifampin (Rifadin), sulfasalazine (Azulfidine), and thiazide or loop diuretics (possible false high)
- Recent peripancreatic surgery, perforated ulcer or intestine, abscess, spasm of the sphincter of Oddi or, rarely, macroamylasemia (possible false high) (See the *Understanding Macroamylasemia* box.)

Precautions
- If the patient has severe abdominal pain, draw the sample before diagnostic

Understanding Macroamylasemia

An uncommon, benign condition, macroamylasemia doesn't cause any symptoms, but it occasionally causes elevated serum amylase (AML) levels. This condition occurs when macroamylase—a complex of AML and an immunoglobulin or other protein—is present in a patient's serum.

A patient with macroamylasemia typically has an elevated serum AML level and a normal or slightly decreased urine AML level. This characteristic pattern helps differentiate macroamylasemia from conditions in which serum and urine AML levels rise, such as pancreatitis. However, it doesn't differentiate macroamylasemia from hyperamylasemia due to impaired renal function, which may raise serum AML levels and lower urine AML levels. Chromatographic, ultracentrifugation, or precipitation tests are necessary to detect macroamylase in serum and definitively confirm macroamylasemia.

or therapeutic intervention. For accurate results, it's important to obtain an early sample.
• Handle the sample gently to prevent hemolysis.

Nursing Considerations

Before the Test
• Confirm the patient's identity using two patient identifiers and confirmation of the patient's identification bracelet according to facility policy.
• Explain to the patient that the serum AML test is used to assess pancreatic function.
• Inform the patient that this test requires a blood sample, which will involve venipuncture.
• Advise the patient that there may be slight discomfort from the tourniquet and needle puncture.
• Inform the patient that there is no need to fast before the test but that the patient must abstain from alcohol.
• Notify the laboratory and the health care provider about any medications that the patient is taking that may

affect test results; these may need to be restricted.

During the Test
• Perform a venipuncture and collect the sample in a 4-mL clot activator tube.

After the Test
• Apply direct pressure to the venipuncture site until bleeding stops and to prevent hematoma formation.
• Instruct the patient to resume medications that were discontinued before the test, as ordered.

Amylase, Urine

Reference Values
Various units of measure are used, and these differ among laboratories.
The Mayo Clinic's normal urinary excretion: 1 to 17 units/hour (SI, 0.017–0.29 mckat/hour)

Abnormal Findings

Elevated Levels
• Acute pancreatitis (obstruction of the pancreatic duct, intestines, or salivary duct; carcinoma of the head of the pancreas)
• Mumps
• Acute spleen injury
• Renal disease
• Perforated peptic or duodenal ulcer
• Gallbladder disease

Decreased Levels
• Pancreatitis
• Cachexia
• Alcoholism
• Liver cancer
• Cirrhosis
• Hepatitis
• Hepatic abscess

Nursing Implications
• Report abnormal findings to the health care provider.
• Prepare the patient for possible surgery.
• Educate the patient about the diagnosis and possible treatment options.

• If the patient with decreased levels has cachexia, provide nutritional supplementation, as appropriate.

Purpose

• To diagnose acute pancreatitis when serum amylase levels are normal or borderline
• To aid in the diagnosis of chronic pancreatitis and salivary gland disorders

Description

Amylase is a starch-splitting enzyme produced primarily in the pancreas and salivary glands and usually secreted into the alimentary tract and absorbed into the blood. Small amounts are also absorbed into the blood directly from these organs. Following glomerular filtration, amylase is excreted in the urine.

When renal function is adequate, serum and urine levels usually rise together. However, within 2 to 3 days of the onset of acute pancreatitis, serum amylase levels fall to normal, whereas elevated urine amylase persists for 7 to 10 days. One method for determining urine amylase levels is the dye-coupled starch method.

Interfering Factors

• Salivary amylase in the urine due to coughing or talking over the sample (possible increase)
• High levels of bacterial contamination of the specimen or blood in the urine
• Bethanechol (Myotonachol), codeine, indomethacin (Indocin), meperidine (Demerol), morphine, pentazocine (Talwin), thiazide diuretics, or alcohol within 24 hours of the test (possible increase)
• Fluorides and glucose (possible decrease)

Nursing Considerations

Before the Test

• Confirm the patient's identity using two patient identifiers and confirmation of the patient's identification bracelet according to facility policy.

• Explain to the patient that the urine amylase test evaluates the function of the pancreas and salivary glands.
• Inform the patient that no food or fluid restriction is necessary.
• Tell the patient that the test requires urine collection for 2, 6, 8, or 24 hours, and teach the patient how to collect a timed specimen.
• Instruct the patient to empty the bladder and then begin timing the collection.
• Instruct the patient not to contaminate the specimen with toilet tissue or stool.
• Instruct the patient to inform caregivers if a voided sample is inadvertently discarded because test will need to start over.
• Notify the laboratory and health care provider about any medications the patient is taking that may affect test results; these medications may need to be restricted.

During the Test

• Collect the patient's urine over a 2-, 6-, 8-, or 24-hour period. (A 2-hour test is usually performed because collecting urine for a 2-hour period produces fewer errors than a more diagnostic 24-hour collection.)
• Cover and refrigerate the specimen during the collection period.
• If the patient is catheterized, keep the collection bag on ice.

After the Test

• Send the specimen on ice to the laboratory as soon as collection is complete.

Amyloid Beta Protein Precursor

Reference Values
Greater than 450 units/L

Abnormal Findings

Decreased Levels
• Alzheimer's disease

Nursing Implications

- Report abnormal findings to the health care provider.
- Educate the patient about the diagnosis and possible treatment options.

Purpose

- To assist in the diagnosis of Alzheimer's disease

Description

Amyloid beta proteins have neurotrophic and neuroprotective properties and have been found in the plaque covering the brain in Alzheimer's patients. In familial Alzheimer's, a genetic defect is seen on chromosome 21, which is the gene responsible for encoding the synthesis of the amyloid beta protein precursor.

Specimen collection for amyloid beta protein precursor is performed by the health care provider as follows:

- The patient is positioned on the side at the edge of the bed with knees drawn up to the abdomen and the chin tucked against the chest (the fetal position). Alternatively, the patient may be positioned leaning over a bedside table while seated. If the patient is supine, pillows will be placed to support the spine on a horizontal plane.
- The skin site is prepared and draped, and a local anesthetic is injected.
- The health care provider then inserts a spinal needle in the midline between the spinous processes of the vertebrae (usually between the third and fourth lumbar vertebrae or between the fourth and fifth). After the stylet is removed from the needle, cerebrospinal fluid will drip out of the needle if it's properly positioned.
- Specimens are collected and placed in the appropriate containers.
- After the needle is removed, a small sterile dressing is applied.

Precautions

- Maintain sterile technique during the procedure.
- Carefully observe the patient during the procedure for adverse reactions, such as elevated pulse rate, pallor, or clammy skin. Report any significant changes immediately.

Nursing Considerations

Before the Test

- Explain to the patient that this test may help determine the presence of Alzheimer's disease.
- Inform the patient that the test requires a sample of cerebrospinal fluid and that this will be obtained by a lumbar puncture. Explain who will perform the test, where, and when.
- Tell the patient that there are no dietary restrictions with this test.
- Advise the patient that a headache may occur after the test, but that cooperation during the test will help minimize it.
- Make sure the patient or a responsible family member has signed an informed consent form.

After the Test

- Record the collection time on the test request form. Send the form and labeled specimen to the laboratory immediately.
- Keep the patient lying flat for 4 to 6 hours. The patient may turn from side to side.
- Encourage the patient to drink fluids, and assist as needed.
- Administer prescribed analgesics.
- Monitor the patient's vital signs, neurologic status, and fluid intake and output.

▶ **Quality and Safety Nursing Alert**

Watch the patient for complications of lumbar puncture, including reaction to the anesthetic, signs and symptoms of meningitis, bleeding into the spinal canal, cerebellar tonsillar herniation, and medullary compression.

- Monitor the puncture site for redness, swelling, and drainage.

Anion Gap

Reference Values
8 to 14 mEq/L (SI, 8–14 mmol/L)

Abnormal Findings
When bicarbonate loss in the urine or other body fluids causes acidosis, the anion gap remains unchanged. This condition is known as *normal anion gap acidosis*. (See the *Anion Gap and Metabolic Acidosis* box.) It may occur in hyperchloremic acidosis, renal tubular acidosis, and severe bicarbonate-wasting conditions, such as biliary or pancreatic fistulas and poorly functioning ileal loops.

Elevated Levels
- Alcoholic ketoacidosis
- Fasting and starvation
- Lactic acidosis
- Poisoning by salicylates, ethylene glycol (antifreeze), methanol, or propyl alcohol

Anion Gap and Metabolic Acidosis

Metabolic acidosis with a normal anion gap (8 to 14 mEq/L) occurs in conditions characterized by loss of bicarbonate, such as:
- hypokalemic acidosis due to renal tubular acidosis, diarrhea, or ureteral diversions
- hyperkalemic acidosis due to acidifying agents (for example, ammonium chloride, hydrochloric acid), hydronephrosis, or sickle cell nephropathy

Metabolic acidosis with an increased anion gap (greater than 14 mEq/L) occurs in conditions characterized by accumulation of organic acids, sulfates, or phosphates, such as:
- renal failure
- ketoacidosis due to starvation, diabetes, or alcohol abuse
- lactic acidosis
- ingestion of toxins, such as salicylates, methanol, ethylene glycol (antifreeze), and paraldehyde
- diabetic ketoacidosis
- starvation

Decreased Levels
- Multiple myeloma
- Bromide ingestion (hyperchloremia)
- Hyponatremia
- Chronic vomiting or gastric suctioning

Nursing Implications
- Report abnormal findings to the health care provider.

Purpose
- To distinguish types of metabolic acidosis
- To monitor renal function and total parenteral nutrition

Description
Total cation and anion concentrations usually are equal, making serum electrically neutral. Measuring the gap between the concentrations provides information about the level of anions (including sulfate; phosphate; organic acids, such as ketone bodies and lactic acid; and proteins) that aren't routinely measured in laboratory tests. In metabolic acidosis, the anion gap measurement helps to identify the acidosis type and possible causes. Further tests are usually needed to determine the specific cause of metabolic acidosis.

Interfering Factors
- Chlorpropamide (Diabinese), diuretics, lithium (Eskalith), and vasopressin (Pitressin) (possible decrease due to decreased serum sodium levels)
- Antihypertensives and corticosteroids (possible increase due to increased serum sodium levels)
- Ammonium chloride, acetazolamide (Diamox), dimercaprol, ethylene glycol, methicillin, methyl alcohol, paraldehyde, and salicylates (possible increase due to decreased serum bicarbonate levels)
- Adrenocorticotropic hormone, cortisone, mercurial or chlorothiazide diuretics, and excessive ingestion of alkali or licorice (possible decrease due to increased serum bicarbonate levels)

- Ammonium chloride, boric acid, cholestyramine (Prevalite), oxyphen-butazone, phenylbutazone, and excessive IV infusion of sodium chloride (possible decrease due to increased serum chloride levels)
- Bicarbonates, ethacrynic acid, furosemide (Lasix), thiazide diuretics, and prolonged IV infusion of dextrose 5% in water (possible increase due to decreased serum chloride levels)
- Iodine absorption from wounds packed with povidone–iodine or excessive use of magnesium-containing antacids, especially in patients with renal failure (possible false low)

Nursing Considerations

Before the Test

- Confirm the patient's identity using two patient identifiers and confirmation of the patient's identification bracelet according to facility policy.
- Explain to the patient that the anion gap test is used to determine the cause of acidosis.
- Tell the patient that the test requires a blood sample.
- Advise the patient that there may be slight discomfort from the tourniquet and needle puncture.
- Inform the patient that there is no need to restrict food and fluids for the test.
- Notify the laboratory and health care provider about any medications the patient is taking that may affect test results; these drugs may need to be restricted.

During the Test

- Perform a venipuncture and collect the sample in a 3- or 4-mL clot activator tube.

After the Test

- Apply direct pressure to the venipuncture site until bleeding stops and to prevent hematoma formation.
- Instruct the patient to resume medications discontinued before the test, as ordered.

Antegrade Pyelography

Normal Findings

- Uniformly filled upper collecting system that's normal in size and course
- Clearly outlined normal structures

Abnormal Findings

- Obstruction (intrarenal pressure greater than 20 cm H_2O)
- Degree of dilation
- Intrarenal reflux
- Hydronephrosis
- Antegrade pyelonephrosis or malignancy (positive cultures)

Nursing Implications

- Report abnormal findings to the health care provider.
- Prepare the patient for further testing or surgery, as appropriate.
- Administer antibiotics and analgesics, as ordered, for several days after the procedure.
- If hydronephrosis is present, monitor the patient's fluid intake and output, edema, hypertension, flank pain, acid–base status, and glucose level.
- Determine preprocedure if the patient is allergic to iodine or shellfish. If the patient is allergic, report this immediately to the health care provider.

Purpose

- To evaluate obstruction of the upper collecting system by stricture, calculus, clot, or tumor
- To evaluate hydronephrosis revealed during excretory urography or ultrasonography and to enable placement of a percutaneous nephrostomy tube
- To evaluate the function of the upper collecting system after ureteral surgery or urinary diversion
- To assess renal functional reserve before surgery

Description

Antegrade pyelography allows upper collecting system examination when ureteral obstruction rules out retrograde ureteropyelography or when cystoscopy is contraindicated. It requires a percutaneous needle puncture to inject contrast medium into the renal pelvis or calyces.

During the procedure, renal pressure can be measured and urine can be collected for cultures and cytologic studies and for evaluation of renal functional reserve before surgery. After radiographic studies are completed, a nephrostomy tube can be inserted to provide temporary drainage or access for other therapeutic or diagnostic procedures.

The procedure, which is performed by the health care provider in the radiology unit, is as follows:

- The patient is placed in a prone position on the X-ray table, and the skin over the kidney is cleaned with antiseptic solution.
- The health care provider injects a local anesthetic.
- Under fluoroscopic guidance or ultrasonography, the health care provider inserts the percutaneous needle below the 12th rib at the level of the transverse process of the second lumbar vertebra. Urine aspiration confirms that the needle has reached the dilated collecting system, which is usually 2¾ to 3¼ inches (7–8 cm) below the skin surface in adults. (Previous urographic films or ultrasound recordings must be studied for anatomic landmarks and to determine if the kidney being examined is in the normal position. If it isn't, the angle of the needle entry must be adjusted during percutaneous puncture.)
- Flexible tubing is connected to the needle to prevent displacement during the procedure. If intrarenal pressure is being measured, the manometer is connected to the tubing as soon as it's in place. Urine specimens are taken, if needed.
- The health care provider withdraws urine equal to the amount of contrast medium being injected to prevent overdistention of the collecting system.

- The health care provider injects the contrast medium under fluoroscopic or ultrasonic guidance. Posteroanterior, oblique, and anteroposterior radiographs are taken. Ureteral peristalsis is observed to evaluate obstruction.
- A percutaneous nephrostomy tube is inserted if drainage is needed because of increased renal pressure, dilation, or intrarenal reflux. If drainage isn't needed, the catheter is withdrawn and a sterile dressing is applied.

Interfering Factors
- Recent barium procedures or stool or gas in the bowel (possible poor imaging)
- Obesity (may make needle placement difficult)

Precautions
- Antegrade pyelography is contraindicated in patients with bleeding disorders and in pregnant patients, unless the benefits outweigh the risks to the fetus.
- Watch for signs of hypersensitivity to the contrast medium.

Nursing Considerations
Before the Test
- Confirm the patient's identity using two patient identifiers and confirmation of the patient's identification bracelet according to facility policy.
- Explain to the patient that antegrade pyelography allows radiographic examination of the kidney. Explain who will perform the test and when it will take place.
- Advise the patient of the possible requirement to fast for 6 to 8 hours before the test and that the patient may receive antimicrobial drugs before and after the procedure.
- Explain to the patient that a needle will be inserted into the kidney after a sedative and local anesthetic are given. Urine may be collected from the kidney for testing, and, if necessary, a tube will be left in the kidney for drainage.

- Advise the patient that there may be mild discomfort during injection of the local anesthetic and contrast medium, and that transient burning and flushing from the contrast medium may also occur.
- Warn the patient that the X-ray machine makes loud, clacking sounds as films are taken.
- Check the patient's history for hypersensitivity reactions to contrast media, iodine, or shellfish. Mark sensitivities clearly on the chart. Also check history and recent coagulation studies for indications of bleeding disorders.
- Make sure that the patient or a responsible family member has signed an informed consent form.
- Administer a sedative just before the procedure, if needed, and check that pretest blood work, such as kidney function, has been performed, if ordered.

After the Test

- Check the patient's vital signs every 15 minutes for the first hour, every 30 minutes for the second hour, and then every 2 hours for the next 24 hours.
- At each vital signs check, examine dressings for bleeding, hematoma, or urine leakage at the puncture site. For bleeding, apply pressure. For a hematoma, apply direct pressure. Report urine leakage or the patient's inability to void (patient should be able to void within 8 hours after the test).
- Monitor the patient's intake and output for 24 hours. Observe each specimen for hematuria. Report hematuria if it persists after the third voiding.
- Watch for and report signs of sepsis or extravasation of contrast medium (chills, fever, rapid pulse or respirations, and hypotension).

> ▶ **Quality and Safety Nursing Alert**
>
> Watch for and report signs that adjacent organs have been punctured, such as pain in the abdomen or flank, or pneumothorax (sudden onset of pleuritic chest pain, dyspnea, tachypnea, decreased breath sounds on the affected side, and tachycardia).

- If a nephrostomy tube is inserted, check to make sure it's patent and draining well. Irrigate with 5 to 7 mL of sterile saline solution, as ordered, to maintain patency.

Anticardiolipin Antibodies

Reference Values
Less than 23 GPL for immunoglobulin (Ig) G
Less than 11 MPL for IgM

Abnormal Findings
- Positive for anticardiolipin antibodies, indicating thrombosis, thrombocytopenia, or spontaneous fetal loss (if the patient is pregnant), systemic lupus erythematosus (SLE), syphilis, or acute infections

Nursing Implications
- Report abnormal findings to the health care provider.
- Educate the patient about the diagnosis and possible treatment options.

Purpose
- To detect the presence of anticardiolipin antibodies

Description
Anticardiolipin antibodies include IgG and IgM. About 40% of patients diagnosed with SLE have positive anticardiolipin antibodies. Patients with these antibodies are at a higher risk to develop antiphospholipid antibody syndrome, which produces recurring thrombosis (venous and arterial), psychiatric disorders, and thrombocytopenia.

Precautions

- Maintain standard precautions while collecting the sample.
- Handle the sample gently to prevent hemolysis.

Nursing Considerations

Before the Test

- Confirm the patient's identity using two patient identifiers and confirmation of the patient's identification bracelet according to facility policy.
- Inform the patient that there is no food or fluid restriction for this test.
- Explain to the patient that the test determines if there are anticardiolipin antibodies present.
- Tell the patient that the test requires a blood sample and that there may be discomfort from the tourniquet and the needle puncture.

During the Test

- Perform a venipuncture and collect 2 to 6 mL of blood in a tube with clot activator.

After the Test

- Apply direct pressure to the venipuncture site until bleeding stops and to prevent hematoma formation.
- Send the sample to the laboratory immediately.

Antideoxyribonucleic Acid Antibodies

Reference Values

Less than 25 international units/mL (SI, less than 25 kIU/L); considered negative for systemic lupus erythematosus (SLE)

Critical Values

Greater than 200 international units/mL (SI, greater than 200 kIU/L); strongly positive for SLE

Abnormal Findings

Elevated Levels

- 31 to 200 international units/mL (SI, 31–200 kIU/L); positive for SLE
- 25 to 30 international units/mL (SI, 25–30 kIU/L); borderline positive for SLE

Decreased Levels

- Effective treatment of SLE with immunosuppressive therapy

Nursing Implications

- Report abnormal findings to the health care provider.
- Educate the patient with elevated levels about the diagnosis and possible treatment options.
- Inform the patient that a decreased value may indicate a positive response to immunosuppressive therapy.

Purpose

- To confirm a diagnosis of SLE
- To monitor the patient with SLE for his response to therapy and determine prognosis

Description

About two-thirds of patients with active SLE have measurable autoantibody levels to double-stranded (native) deoxyribonucleic acid (anti-ds-DNA). These antibodies are rarely detected in patients with other connective tissue diseases.

In autoimmune diseases, such as SLE, native DNA is thought to be the antigen that complexes with antibody and complements, causing local tissue damage where these complexes are deposited. The degree of renal or vascular damage caused by the disease is directly related to serum anti-ds-DNA levels.

The anti-ds-DNA antibody test measures and differentiates these antibody levels in a serum sample using radioimmunoassay, agglutination, complement fixation, or immunoelectrophoresis. If anti-ds-DNA antibodies are present, they combine with native DNA and form complexes that are too large to pass through a membrane filter. The test counts these oversized complexes.

Interfering Factors
• A radioactive scan performed within 1 week before sample collection

Nursing Considerations
Before the Test
• Confirm the patient's identity using two patient identifiers and confirmation of the patient's identification bracelet according to facility policy.
• Explain to the patient that the anti-ds-DNA antibodies test helps to diagnose SLE and determine the appropriate therapy.
• Inform the patient that there is no food or fluid restriction for this test.
• Inform the patient that the test requires a blood sample.
• Advise the patient that there may be slight discomfort from the tourniquet and needle puncture.
• Inquire if patient has had a recent radioactive test, and, if so, note this on the laboratory request slip.

During the Test
• Perform a venipuncture and collect the sample in a 7-mL tube without additives. (Some laboratories may specify a tube with either ethylenediamine tetraacetic acid [EDTA] or sodium fluoride and potassium oxalate added.)

After the Test
• Apply direct pressure to the venipuncture site until bleeding stops and to prevent hematoma formation.

Antidiuretic Hormone, Serum
Reference Values
1 to 5 pg/mL (SI, 1–5 mg/L)
If serum osmolality is less than 285 mOsm/ kg: less than 2 pg/mL (SI, less than 2 mg/L)
If serum osmolality is greater than 290 mOsm/kg: 2 to 12 pg/mL (SI, 2–12 mg/L)

Abnormal Findings
Elevated Levels
• Syndrome of inappropriate antidiuretic hormone (SIADH)
• Nephrogenic diabetes insipidus
• Porphyria
• Guillain-Barré syndrome
• Pulmonary disease (tuberculosis)
• Brain tumor, diseases, injury, neurosurgery
• Pulmonary diseases (tuberculosis)

Decreased (or Absent) Levels
• Pituitary diabetes insipidus
• Nephrotic syndrome
• Psychogenic polydipsia

Nursing Implications
• Report abnormal findings to the health care provider.
• Educate the patient about the diagnosis and possible treatment options.
• Educate the patient with elevated levels about possible urine concentration disorders or porphyria, as appropriate.

Purpose
• To aid in the differential diagnosis of pituitary diabetes insipidus, nephrogenic diabetes insipidus (congenital or familial), and SIADH

Description
Antidiuretic hormone (ADH), also called *vasopressin,* promotes water reabsorption in response to increased osmolality (water deficiency with high concentration of sodium and other solutes). In response to decreased osmolality (water excess), reduced ADH secretion allows increased water excretion to maintain fluid balance. Along with aldosterone, ADH helps regulate sodium, potassium, and fluid balance. It also stimulates vascular smooth muscle contraction, causing an increase in arterial blood pressure.

This relatively rare test, a quantitative analysis of serum ADH levels, may identify diabetes insipidus and other causes of severe homeostatic imbalance.

It may be ordered as part of dehydration or hypertonic saline infusion testing, which determines the body's response to hyperosmolality states.

> **▶ Quality and Safety Nursing Alert**
>
> **Normal ADH levels in the presence of signs of diabetes insipidus (such as polydipsia, polyuria, and hypotonic urine) may indicate the nephrogenic form of the disease, marked by renal tubular resistance to ADH; however, levels may rise if the pituitary gland tries to compensate.**

Interfering Factors
- Anesthetics, carbamazepine (Tegretol), chlorothiazide (Diuril), chlorpropamide (Diabinese), cyclophosphamide (Cytoxan), estrogen, hypnotics, lithium carbonate (Eskalith), morphine, oxytocin (Pitocin), tranquilizers, and vincristine (Oncovin) (increase)
- Stress, pain, and positive-pressure ventilation (increase)
- Alcohol and negative-pressure ventilation (decrease)
- Radioactive scan performed within 1 week before the test

Precautions
- Use a plastic syringe and collection tube because fragile ADH degrades on contact with glass.

Nursing Considerations
Before the Test
- Confirm the patient's identity using two patient identifiers and confirmation of the patient's identification bracelet according to facility policy.
- Explain to the patient that the serum ADH test, used to measure hormonal secretion levels, may aid in identifying the cause of symptoms.
- Instruct the patient to fast and to limit physical activity for 10 to 12 hours before the test.

- Tell the patient that the test requires a blood sample.
- Advise the patient that there may be slight discomfort from the tourniquet and needle puncture.
- Withhold medications that may cause SIADH before the test, as ordered. If they must be continued, note this on the laboratory request slip.
- Make sure the patient is relaxed and recumbent for 30 minutes before the test.

During the Test
- Perform a venipuncture and collect the sample in a plastic collection tube (without additives) or in a chilled EDTA tube.
- Immediately send the sample to the laboratory, where serum must be separated from the clot within 10 minutes.
- Perform a serum osmolality test at the same time to help interpret the results.

After the Test
- Apply direct pressure to the venipuncture site until bleeding stops, to prevent hematoma formation.
- Instruct the patient to resume usual diet, activities, and medications that were discontinued before the test, as ordered.

Anti-insulin Antibodies

Reference Values
Less than 3% binding of the patient's serum with labeled beef, human, and pork insulin

Abnormal Findings
Elevated Levels
- Insulin allergy or resistance
- Factitious hypoglycemia

Nursing Implications
- Report abnormal findings to the health care provider.
- Educate the patient about the diagnosis and possible treatment options.

- Review the patient's diet with him or her, as well as his or her glucose monitoring and insulin dosing.

Purpose
- To determine insulin allergy
- To confirm insulin resistance
- To determine if hypoglycemia is caused by insulin overuse

Description
Some patients with diabetes form antibodies to the insulin they take. These antibodies bind with some of the insulin, making less insulin available for glucose metabolism, resulting in increased insulin dosages. This phenomenon is known as *insulin resistance*.

Performed on the blood of a patient with diabetes who takes insulin, the anti-insulin antibody test detects insulin antibodies, which are immunoglobulins called *anti-insulin Ab*. The most common type of anti-insulin Ab is immunoglobulin (Ig) G, but anti-insulin Ab also is found in the other four classes of immunoglobulins: IgA, IgD, IgE, and IgM. IgM may cause insulin resistance, and IgE has been associated with allergic reactions.

Interfering Factors
- Radioactive test performed within 1 week before the test

Nursing Considerations
Before the Test
- Confirm the patient's identity using two patient identifiers and confirmation of the patient's identification bracelet according to facility policy.
- Explain to the patient that the anti-insulin antibody test is used to determine the most appropriate treatment for diabetes and to determine if there is insulin resistance or an allergy to insulin.
- Tell the patient that the test requires a blood sample.
- Advise the patient that there may be slight discomfort from the tourniquet and needle puncture.

- Inform the patient that there is no food or fluid restriction.
- Inquire if the patient has had a radioactive test recently, and, if so, note this on the laboratory request slip.

During the Test
- Perform a venipuncture and collect the sample in a 7-mL tube without additives.

After the Test
- Apply direct pressure to the venipuncture site until bleeding stops and to prevent hematoma formation.

Antimyocardial Antibodies

Normal Findings
- No antimyocardial antibodies seen
- Positive results titered

Abnormal Findings
- Myocardial injury or disease, most likely due to an autoimmune reaction

Nursing Implications
- Report abnormal findings to the health care provider.
- Educate the patient about the diagnosis and possible treatment options.
- Prepare the patient for additional testing, as appropriate.
- Administer medications, as appropriate.

Purpose
- To detect the presence of antimyocardial antibodies in the blood

Description
Antimyocardial antibodies are present in autoimmune causes of myocardial injury, such as rheumatic heart disease, cardiomyopathy, postthoracotomy syndrome, and post-MI syndrome. Antimyocardial antibodies are associated with pericarditis that can damage the heart tissue. They're found in up to 40% of postcardiac surgery patients and in some post-MI patients.

Nursing Considerations

Before the Test

- Confirm the patient's identity using two patient identifiers and confirmation of the patient's identification bracelet according to facility policy.
- Explain to the patient that this test determines if antimyocardial antibodies are present.
- Inform the patient that there are no food or fluid restrictions.
- Inform the patient that the test requires a blood sample.
- Advise the patient that there may be slight discomfort from the tourniquet and needle puncture.

During the Test

- Perform a venipuncture and collect the sample in a 4-mL tube with no additives.

After the Test

- Apply direct pressure to the venipuncture site until bleeding stops.

Antinuclear Antibodies (ANAs)

Normal Findings

- Positive (with pattern and serum titer noted) or negative; positive result doesn't confirm disease

Abnormal Findings

- Titer typically exceeding 1:256, indicating SLE (the higher the titer, the more specific the test)

Nursing Implications

- Report abnormal findings to the health care provider.
- Educate the patient about the diagnosis and possible treatment options.

Purpose

- To screen for SLE
- To monitor the effectiveness of immunosuppressive therapy for SLE

Description

In conditions such as SLE, scleroderma, and certain infections, the body's immune system may perceive portions of its own cell nuclei as foreign and may produce antinuclear antibodies (ANAs). Specific ANAs include antibodies to deoxyribonucleic acid, nucleoprotein, histones, nuclear ribonucleoprotein, and other nuclear constituents.

Because they don't penetrate living cells, ANAs are harmless, but they sometimes form antigen–antibody complexes that cause tissue damage (as in SLE). Because of multiorgan involvement, test results aren't diagnostic and can only partially confirm clinical evidence.

About 99% of patients with SLE exhibit ANAs, and a large percentage of them show high titers. Although this test isn't specific for SLE, it's a useful screening tool. Failure to detect ANAs essentially rules out active SLE.

> ◤ **Quality and Safety Nursing Alert**
>
> Although the ANA test is a sensitive indicator of ANAs, it isn't specific for SLE. Low titers may occur in patients with viral diseases, chronic hepatic disease, collagen vascular disease, and autoimmune diseases and in some healthy adults; the incidence increases with age.

Interfering Factors

- Procainamide (Procanbid) and hydralazine (Apresoline) (positive result)

Nursing Considerations

Before the Test

- Confirm the patient's identity using two patient identifiers and confirmation of the patient's identification bracelet according to facility policy.
- Explain to the patient that the ANA test evaluates the immune system and that further testing usually is required for diagnosis.
- Inform the patient that the test will be repeated to monitor response to therapy, if appropriate.

- Inform the patient that there are no food or fluid restrictions.
- Tell the patient that the test requires a blood sample.
- Advise the patient that there may be slight discomfort from the tourniquet and needle puncture.
- Check the patient's history for drugs that may affect test results, such as isoniazid and procainamide. Note findings on the laboratory request slip.

During the Test
- Perform a venipuncture and collect the sample in a 7-mL tube without additives.

After the Test
- Because a patient with an autoimmune disease has a compromised immune system, observe the venipuncture site for signs of infection and report changes to the health care provider immediately.
- Keep a clean, dry bandage over the site for at least 24 hours.
- Apply direct pressure to the venipuncture site until bleeding stops and to prevent hematoma formation.

Anti-Sjögren's Syndrome (SS) Antibodies

Normal Findings
- Negative anti-SS antibody titers

Abnormal Findings
- Presence of anti-SS antibodies; anti-SS-antibody titer decreases with therapy for Sjögren's syndrome
- Anti-SS-A antibodies (possible presence of Sjögren's syndrome or lupus)
- Anti-SS-B antibodies (primary Sjögren's syndrome)
- Anti-SS-C antibodies (Sjögren's syndrome along with other autoimmune disorders)

Nursing Implications
- Report abnormal findings to the health care provider.

- Educate the patient about the diagnosis and possible treatment options.
- Prepare to instill artificial tears as often as every 30 minutes, as prescribed, to prevent eye damage from insufficient tear secretions.
- Provide the patient with plenty of fluids to promote oral moisture.

Purpose
- To diagnose Sjögren's syndrome
- To differentiate between primary and secondary Sjögren's syndrome

Description
Anti-SS-A, anti-SS-B, and anti-SS-C antibodies are types of antinuclear antibodies that are used to diagnose Sjögren's syndrome. Anti-SS-A antibodies are present in 70% of patients who have Sjögren's syndrome without the occurrence of another autoimmune disorder (primary Sjögren's syndrome). Anti-SS-B antibodies are present in 50% of patients with primary Sjögren's syndrome; they aren't regularly found with any other disorders. Anti-SS-C antibodies are found in 75% of patients who have Sjögren's syndrome and rheumatoid arthritis; they're used to differentiate between primary and secondary Sjögren's syndrome.

Nursing Considerations

Before the Test
- Confirm the patient's identity using two patient identifiers and confirmation of the patient's identification bracelet according to facility policy.
- Explain to the patient that this test helps diagnose Sjögren's syndrome and to determine if it occurs alone or with another autoimmune disorder.
- Inform the patient that there are no food or fluid restrictions.
- Inform the patient that the test requires a blood sample.
- Advise the patient that there may be slight discomfort from the tourniquet and needle puncture.

During the Test

- Perform a venipuncture and collect the sample in a 7-mL tube without additives.

After the Test

- Apply direct pressure to the venipuncture site until bleeding stops.

Antithyroid Antibodies

Reference Values

Less than 1:100 for antithyroglobulin and antimicrosomal antibodies

Abnormal Findings

Elevated Levels

- Subclinical autoimmune thyroid disease
- Graves' disease
- Idiopathic myxedema
- Hashimoto's thyroiditis (titers of 1:400 or greater)
- SLE
- Rheumatoid arthritis
- Autoimmune hemolytic anemia
- Thyroid carcinoma

Nursing Implications

- Report abnormal findings to the health care provider.
- Educate the patient about the diagnosis and possible treatment options.

Purpose

- To detect circulating antithyroglobulin antibodies when clinical evidence indicates Hashimoto's thyroiditis, Graves' disease, or other thyroid diseases

Description

In autoimmune disorders—such as Hashimoto's thyroiditis and Graves' disease (hyperthyroidism)—thyroglobulin, the major colloidal storage compound, is released into the blood. Because thyroxine usually separates from thyroglobulin before it's released into the blood, thyroglobulin doesn't normally enter the circulation. When it does, antithyroglobulin antibodies are formed to attack this foreign substance; the ensuing autoimmune response damages the thyroid gland. The serum of a patient whose autoimmune system produces antithyroglobulin antibodies usually contains antimicrosomal antibodies, which react with the microsomes of the thyroid epithelial cells.

The tagged red cell hemagglutination test detects antithyroglobulin and antimicrosomal antibodies. Another laboratory technique, indirect immunofluorescence, can detect antimicrosomal antibodies.

Nursing Considerations

Before the Test

- Confirm the patient's identity using two patient identifiers and confirmation of the patient's identification bracelet according to facility policy.
- Explain to the patient that the antithyroid antibody test evaluates thyroid function.
- Inform the patient that there are no food or fluid restrictions.
- Tell the patient that the test requires a blood sample.
- Advise the patient that there may be slight discomfort from the tourniquet and needle puncture.

During the Test

- Perform a venipuncture and collect the sample in a 7-mL tube without additives.

After the Test

- Apply direct pressure to the venipuncture site until bleeding stops and to prevent hematoma formation.

Apolipoprotein A₁

Reference Values

Females: 94 to 172 mg/dL (SI, 0.94–1.72 g/L) (slightly higher levels of high-density lipoprotein [HDL] occur in females, so they have a higher level of apolipoprotein A_1)

Males: 90 to 155 mg/dL (SI, 0.90–1.55 g/L)

Abnormal Findings

Elevated Levels

- Possible familial hyperalphalipoproteinemia

Decreased Levels

- Increased risk for coronary artery disease, ischemic coronary disease, MI, and hypertriglyceridemia
- Apo C-II deficiency
- Apo A-I melanos disease
- Apo A-I-C-III deficiency
- Poorly controlled diabetes
- Nephrotic syndrome
- Renal failure
- Diet high in polyunsaturated fats

Nursing Implications

- Report abnormal findings to the health care provider.
- Educate the patient about the diagnosis and possible treatment options.

Purpose

- To measure the amount of apolipoprotein A_1 in the blood (A_1 is thought to be a better index of arthrogenic risk than is an HDL assay.)

Description

Apolipoproteins are the surface particles of lipoproteins. Apolipoprotein A_1 is the main component of HDL; the less apolipoprotein that's in the blood, the more that's bound to HDL.

Apolipoprotein A_1 deficiency is associated with premature cardiovascular disease.

Interfering Factors

- Pregnancy (may result in an inconclusive test because pregnancy may increase the apolipoprotein A_1 level)

Nursing Considerations

Before the Test

- Confirm the patient's identity using two patient identifiers and confirmation of the patient's identification bracelet according to facility policy.
- Tell the patient that test will help determine the risk for cardiovascular disease.
- Inform the patient to restrict food for 12 hours before the test, but that water is allowed.
- Advise the patient that smoking is not permitted before the test.

- Tell the patient that the test requires a blood sample.
- Advise the patient that there may be slight discomfort from the tourniquet and needle puncture.

During the Test

- Perform a venipuncture and collect the sample in a 7-mL tube without additives.

After the Test

- Apply direct pressure to the venipuncture site until bleeding stops.

Apolipoprotein B

Reference Values

Females: 45 to 110 mg/dL (SI, 0.45–1.10 g/L)
Males: 55 to 100 mg/dL (SI, 0.55–1 g/L)

Abnormal Findings

Elevated Levels

- Diabetes
- Hypothyroidism
- Biliary obstruction
- Coronary artery disease
- Increased risk for coronary artery disease
- Diet high in saturated fat and cholesterol (may increase apolipoprotein B levels)

Decreased Levels

- Hyperthyroidism
- Malnutrition
- Inflammatory joint disease
- Chronic anemia
- Type I hyperlipidemia
- Apo C-II deficiency

Nursing Implications

- Report abnormal findings to the health care provider.
- Educate the patient about the diagnosis and possible treatment options.

Purpose

- To measure the amount of apolipoprotein B in the blood

Description

Apolipoproteins are the surface particles of lipoproteins. Apolipoprotein B is the main component of low-density lipoprotein (LDL) and very-low-density lipoprotein (VLDL). Apolipoprotein B helps regulate cholesterol and metabolism, and it plays a role in the catabolism of LDLs. Apolipoprotein B deficiency is associated with premature cardiovascular disease.

Interfering Factors

- Pregnancy (increase)
- Many drugs
- Critically ill patients with conditions such as burns, acute stress reactions, inflammatory disease

Nursing Considerations

Before the Test

- Confirm the patient's identity using two patient identifiers and confirmation of the patient's identification bracelet according to facility policy.
- Tell the patient that the test will help determine the risk for cardiovascular disease.
- Inform the patient to restrict food for 12 hours before the test, but that water is allowed.
- Advise the patient that smoking is not permitted before the test.
- Tell the patient that the test requires a blood sample.
- Advise the patient that there may be slight discomfort from the tourniquet and needle puncture.

During the Test

- Perform a venipuncture and collect the sample in a 7-mL tube without additives.

After the Test

- Apply direct pressure to the venipuncture site until bleeding stops.

Arterial Blood Gas (ABG) Analysis

Reference Values

PaO_2: 80 to 100 mm Hg (SI, 10.6–13.3 kPa)

$PaCO_2$: 35 to 45 mm Hg (SI, 4.7–5.3 kPa)
pH: 7.35 to 7.45 (SI, 7.35–7.45)
O_2CT: 15% to 23% (SI, 0.15–0.23)
SaO_2: 94% to 100% (SI, 0.94–1)
HCO_3^-: 22 to 25 mEq/L (SI, 22–25 mmol/L)

Abnormal Findings

Decreased PaO₂, O₂CT, and SaO₂ Levels, and Increased PaCO₂ Level

- Respiratory muscle weakness or paralysis
- Respiratory center inhibition (from head injury, brain tumor, or drug abuse)
- Airway obstruction (possibly from mucus plugs or a tumor)
- Bronchiole obstruction caused by asthma or emphysema
- Partially blocked alveoli or pulmonary capillaries
- Damaged alveoli
- Alveoli that are filled with fluid because of disease, hemorrhage, or near-drowning

Decreased PaO₂, O₂CT, and SaO₂ Levels and Possible Normal PaCO₂ Level

- Pneumothorax
- Impaired diffusion between alveoli and blood (due to interstitial fibrosis, for example)
- Arteriovenous shunt that permits blood to bypass the lungs

Decreased O₂CT Level and Normal PaO₂, SaO₂, and, Possibly, PaCO₂ Levels

- Severe anemia
- Decreased blood volume
- Reduced hemoglobin oxygen-carrying capacity

Nursing Implications

- Report abnormal findings to the health care provider.
- Educate the patient about the diagnosis and possible treatment options.
- Prepare for nursing interventions regarding abnormal levels.

Purpose

• To evaluate the efficiency of pulmonary gas exchange
• To assess the integrity of the ventilatory control system
• To determine the acid–base level of the blood
• To monitor respiratory therapy

Description

Arterial blood gas (ABG) analysis is used to measure the partial pressure of arterial oxygen (PaO_2), the partial pressure of arterial carbon dioxide ($PaCO_2$), and the pH of an arterial sample. Oxygen content (O_2CT), arterial oxygen saturation (SaO_2), and bicarbonate (HCO_3^-) values also are measured.

A blood sample for ABG analysis may be drawn by percutaneous arterial puncture or from an arterial line.

The PaO_2 indicates how much oxygen the lungs are delivering to the blood. The $PaCO_2$ indicates how efficiently the lungs eliminate carbon dioxide. The pH indicates the acid–base level of the blood or the hydrogen ion (H^+) concentration. Acidity indicates H^+ excess; alkalinity, H^+ deficit. (See the *Balancing pH* box.) O_2CT, SaO_2, and HCO_3^- values also aid diagnosis. (See the *Acid–Base Disorders* table.)

Balancing pH

To measure the acidity or alkalinity of a solution, chemists use a pH scale of 1 to 15 that measures hydrogen ion concentrations. As hydrogen ions and acidity increase, pH falls below 7.0, which is neutral. Conversely, when hydrogen ions decrease, pH and alkalinity increase. Acid–base balance, or homeostasis of hydrogen ions, is necessary if the body's enzyme systems are to work properly.

The slightest change in ionic hydrogen concentration alters the rate of cellular chemical reactions; a sufficiently severe change can be fatal. To maintain a normal blood pH—generally between 7.35 and 7.45—the body relies on three mechanisms.

Buffers

Chemically composed of two substances, buffers prevent radical pH changes by replacing strong acids added to a solution (such as blood) with weaker ones. For example, strong acids capable of yielding many hydrogen ions are replaced by weaker ones that yield fewer hydrogen ions. Because of the principal buffer coupling of bicarbonate and carbonic acid—normally in a ratio of 20:1—the plasma acid–base level rarely fluctuates. Increased bicarbonate, however, indicates alkalosis, whereas decreased bicarbonate points to acidosis. Increased carbonic acid indicates acidosis, and decreased carbonic acid indicates alkalosis.

Respiration

Respiration is important in maintaining blood pH. The lungs convert carbonic acid to carbon dioxide and water. With every expiration, carbon dioxide and water leave the body, decreasing the carbonic acid content of the blood. Consequently, fewer hydrogen ions are formed, and blood pH increases. When the blood's hydrogen ion or carbonic acid content increases, neurons in the respiratory center stimulate respiration.

Hyperventilation eliminates carbon dioxide and hence carbonic acid from the body, reduces hydrogen ion formation, and increases pH. Conversely, increased blood pH from alkalosis—decreased hydrogen ion concentration—causes hypoventilation, which restores blood pH to its normal level by retaining carbon dioxide and thus increasing hydrogen ion formation.

Urinary Excretion

The third factor in acid–base balance is urine excretion. Because the kidneys excrete varying amounts of acids and bases, they control urine pH, which in turn affects blood pH. For example, when blood pH is decreased, the distal and collecting tubules remove excessive hydrogen ions (carbonic acid forms in the tubular cells and dissociates into hydrogen and bicarbonate) and displaces them in urine, thereby eliminating hydrogen from the body. In exchange, basic ions in the urine—usually sodium—diffuse into the tubular cells, where they combine with bicarbonate. This sodium bicarbonate is then reabsorbed in the blood, resulting in decreased urine pH and, more important, increased blood pH.

Acid–Base Disorders

Disorders and ABG Finding	Possible Causes	Signs and Symptoms
Respiratory Acidosis (excess CO_2 retention)		
• pH <7.35 (SI, <7.35) • HCO_3^- >26 mEq/L (SI, >26 mmol/L) (if compensating) • $PaCO_2$ >45 mm Hg (SI, >5.3 kPa)	• Central nervous system depression from drugs, injury, or disease • Asphyxia • Hypoventilation due to pulmonary, cardiac, musculoskeletal, or neuromuscular disease • Obesity • Postoperative pain • Abdominal distention	• Diaphoresis, headache, tachycardia, confusion, restlessness, apprehension
Respiratory Alkalosis (excess CO_2 excretion)		
• pH >7.45 (SI, >7.45) • HCO_3^- <22 mEq/L (SI, <22 mmol/L) (if compensating) • $PaCO_2$ <35 mm Hg (SI, <4.7 kPa)	• Hyperventilation due to anxiety, pain, or improper ventilator settings • Respiratory stimulation caused by drugs, disease, hypoxia, fever, or high room temperature • Gram-negative bacteremia • Compensation for metabolic acidosis (chronic kidney disease)	• Rapid, deep breathing; paresthesia; lightheadedness; twitching; anxiety; fear
Metabolic Acidosis (HCO_3^- loss, acid retention)		
• pH <7.35 (SI, <7.35) • HCO_3^- <22 mEq/L (SI, <22 mmol/L) • $PaCO_2$ <35 mm Hg (SI, <4.7 kPa) (if compensating)	• HCO_3^- depletion due to renal disease, diarrhea, or small-bowel fistulas • Excessive production of organic acids due to hepatic disease; endocrine disorders, including diabetes, hypoxia, shock, and drug intoxication • Inadequate excretion of acids due to renal disease	• Rapid, deep breathing; fruity breath; fatigue; headache; lethargy; drowsiness, nausea; vomiting; coma (if severe)
Metabolic Alkalosis (HCO_3^- retention, acid loss)		
• pH >7.45 (SI, >7.45) • HCO_3^- >26 mEq/L (SI, >26 mmol/L) • $PaCO_2$ >45 mm Hg (SI, >5.3 kPa)	• Loss of hydrochloric acid from prolonged vomiting or gastric suctioning • Loss of potassium due to increased renal excretion (as in diuretic therapy) or steroid overdose • Excessive alkali ingestion • Compensation for chronic respiratory acidosis	• Slow, shallow breathing; hypertonic muscles; restlessness; twitching; confusion; irritability; apathy; tetany; seizures; coma (if severe)

Interfering Factors

- Exposing the sample to air (increase or decrease in PaO_2 and $PaCO_2$)
- Venous blood in the sample (possible decrease in PaO_2 and increase in $PaCO_2$)
- HCO_3^-, ethacrynic acid, hydrocortisone, metolazone, prednisone, and thiazides (possible increase in $PaCO_2$)
- Acetazolamide, methicillin, nitrofurantoin, and tetracycline (possible decrease in $PaCO_2$)
- Fever (possible false-high PaO_2 and $PaCO_2$)

Precautions

- Wait at least 20 minutes before drawing arterial blood after starting, changing, or discontinuing oxygen therapy; after initiating or changing settings of mechanical ventilation; or after extubation.

Nursing Considerations

Before the Test

- Confirm the patient's identity using two patient identifiers and confirmation of the patient's identification bracelet according to facility policy.
- Explain to the patient that ABG analysis is used to evaluate how well the lungs are delivering oxygen to the blood and eliminating carbon dioxide.
- Tell the patient that the test requires a blood sample. Explain who will perform the arterial puncture, where, and when, and which site (radial, brachial, or femoral artery) has been selected for the puncture.
- Inform the patient that there is no need to restrict food and fluids.
- Instruct the patient to breathe normally during the test, and warn the patient that there may be a brief cramping or throbbing pain at the puncture site.
- Record the patient's rectal temperature.
- Perform Allen's test to ensure vascular adequacy (see p. 5).

During the Test

- Perform an arterial puncture or draw blood from an arterial line.
- Use a heparinized blood gas syringe to draw the sample. Eliminate air from the sample.
- Place the sample on ice immediately after collection.

After the Test

- After applying pressure to the puncture site for 3 to 5 minutes or until bleeding has stopped, apply a pressure dressing firmly over it. (If the puncture site is on the arm, don't tape the entire circumference; this may restrict circulation.)
- If the patient is receiving anticoagulants or has coagulopathy, apply pressure to the puncture site longer than 5 minutes, if necessary.
- Monitor the patient's vital signs and observe for signs of circulatory impairment, such as swelling, discoloration, pain, numbness, and tingling in the bandaged arm or leg.
- Observe frequently for bleeding from the puncture site.
- Note on the laboratory request slip whether the patient was breathing room air or receiving oxygen therapy when the sample was collected.
- If the patient was receiving oxygen therapy, note the flow rate and method of delivery. If the patient is on a ventilator, note the fraction of inspired oxygen, tidal volume mode, respiratory rate, and positive end-expiratory pressure.
- Transport the sample to the laboratory.

Arterial-to-Alveolar (a/A) Oxygen Ratio

Reference Values
75%

Abnormal Findings

Elevated Levels
- Mucus plugs
- Bronchospasm

- Airway collapse (asthma, bronchitis, emphysema)
- Hypoxemia caused by arterial septal defects, pneumothorax, atelectasis, emboli, or edema

Nursing Implications
- Report abnormal findings to the health care provider.
- Educate the patient about the diagnosis and possible treatment options.
- Initiate appropriate interventions to correct patient problems, based on ratios.

Purpose
- To evaluate the efficiency of gas exchange
- To assess the integrity of the ventilatory control system
- To monitor respiratory therapy

Description
Using calculations based on the patient's laboratory values, the arterial-to-alveolar oxygen ratio (a/A ratio) test can help identify the cause of hypoxemia and intrapulmonary shunting by approximating the partial oxygenation pressure of the alveoli and arteries. It may help differentiate the cause as ventilated alveoli but no perfusion, unventilated alveoli with perfusion, or collapse of the alveoli and capillaries.

The arterial sample is analyzed for partial pressure of arterial oxygen (PaO_2) and partial pressure of arterial carbon dioxide ($PaCO_2$). It also examines barometric pressure (Pb), water vapor pressure (PH_2O), and fractional concentration of inspired oxygen (FiO_2) (21% for room air). From these values, the alveolar oxygen tension (PAO_2), the a/A ratio, and the alveolar-to-arterial oxygen gradient ($A\text{-}aDO_2$) are derived by solving these mathematical formulas:

$$PaO_2 = FiO_2 (Pb - PH_2O) - 1.25 (PaCO_2)$$
$$a/A \text{ ratio} = PaO_2 \div PAO_2$$
$$A\text{-}aDO_2 = PAO_2 - PaO_2.$$

Interfering Factors
- Exposing the sample to air (increase or decrease)
- Age and increasing oxygen concentration (increase)

Nursing Considerations
Before the Test
- Confirm the patient's identity using two patient identifiers and confirmation of the patient's identification bracelet according to facility policy.
- Explain to the patient that the a/A ratio test is used to evaluate how well the lungs are delivering oxygen to the blood and eliminating carbon dioxide.
- Tell the patient that the test requires a blood sample. Explain who will perform the arterial puncture and when.
- Inform the patient that there are no food or fluid restrictions.
- Instruct the patient to breathe normally during the test, and warn that there may be cramping or throbbing pain at the puncture site.
- Note the patient's rectal temperature.

During the Test
- Perform an arterial puncture or draw blood from an arterial line using a heparinized blood gas syringe.
- Eliminate all air from the sample and place it on ice immediately.

After the Test
- Apply pressure to the puncture site for 3 to 5 minutes or until bleeding stops.
- Apply a pressure dressing over the site and tape it in place, but don't tape the entire circumference of the limb.
- Monitor the patient's vital signs and observe for signs of circulatory impairment, such as swelling, discoloration, pain, numbness, and tingling in the bandaged arm or leg.
- Observe frequently for bleeding from the puncture site.
- Note on the laboratory request slip whether the patient was breathing

room air or receiving oxygen therapy when the sample was collected.

- If the patient was receiving oxygen therapy, note the flow rate and method of delivery. If the patient was on a ventilator, note the FiO_2, tidal volume, mode, respiratory rate, and positive end-expiratory pressure.

Arthrography

Normal Findings
- Visible, characteristic, wedge-shaped shadow pointed toward the interior of the joint (normal medial meniscus)
- Visible bicipital tendon sheath, redundant inferior joint capsule, and intact subscapular bursa
- Normal filling of joint space, bursae, ligaments, articular cartilage, menisci, and tendons

Abnormal Findings
- Medial meniscal tears and lacerations (in 90%–95% of cases)
- Extrameniscal lesions, such as osteochondritis dissecans, chondromalacia patellae, osteochondral fractures, cartilaginous abnormalities, synovial abnormalities
- Tears of the cruciate ligaments
- Disruption of the joint capsule and collateral ligaments
- Shoulder abnormalities, such as adhesive capsulitis, bicipital tenosynovitis or rupture, and rotator cuff tears

Nursing Implications
- Report abnormal findings to the health care provider.
- Educate the patient about the diagnosis and possible treatment options.
- Prepare the patient for possible surgical repair.

Purpose
- To identify acute or chronic tears or other abnormalities of the joint capsule or supporting ligaments of the knee, shoulder, ankle, hips, or wrist
- To detect internal joint derangements
- To locate synovial cysts

Description
Arthrography is typically indicated when a patient has persistent unexplained joint discomfort or pain. Testing involves radiographic examination of a joint after injection of a radiopaque dye, air, or both (double-contrast arthrogram) to outline soft-tissue structures and the contour of the joint. The joint is put through its range of motion while a series of radiographs are taken. (See the *Comparing Normal and Abnormal Arthrograms* box.)

The procedures for knee and shoulder arthrography are as follows:

Knee Arthrography
- The knee is cleaned with an antiseptic solution, and the area around the puncture site is anesthetized. (It isn't usually necessary to anesthetize the joint space itself.)
- The health care provider inserts a #29 needle into the joint space between the patella and femoral condyle, and fluid is aspirated. The aspirated fluid usually is sent to the laboratory for analysis.
- While the needle is still in place, the aspirating syringe is removed and replaced with a syringe containing dye.
- If fluoroscopic examination demonstrates correct placement of the needle, the dye is injected into the joint space.
- After the needle is removed, the site is rubbed with a sterile sponge, and the wound may be sealed with collodion.
- The patient is asked to walk a few steps or to move the knee through a range of motion to distribute the dye in the joint space. A film series is quickly taken with the knee held in various positions.
- If the films are clean and demonstrate proper dye placement, the knee is bandaged, typically with an elastic bandage.

Comparing Normal and Abnormal Arthrograms

The arthrogram on the left shows a normal medial meniscus. The view on the right shows a torn medial meniscus (indicated by the arrow).

Normal Arthrogram of Knee	Abnormal Arthrogram of Knee

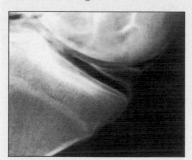 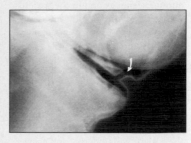

The arthrogram on the left shows a normal shoulder. The arthrogram on the right shows a shoulder with a ruptured rotator cuff. Contrast medium has collected in the subacromial bursa (indicated by the arrows).

Normal Arthrogram of Shoulder	Abnormal Arthrogram of Shoulder

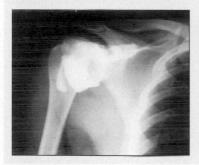 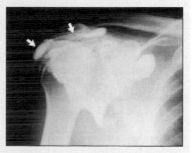

Shoulder Arthrography

- The skin is prepared, and a local anesthetic is injected subcutaneously just in front of the acromioclavicular joint. Additional anesthetic is injected directly onto the head of the humerus.
- A short lumbar puncture needle is inserted until the point is embedded in the joint cartilage.
- The stylet is removed, a syringe of contrast medium is attached, and, using fluoroscopic guidance, about 1 mL of dye is injected into the joint space as the needle is withdrawn slightly.
- If fluoroscopic examination demonstrates correct needle placement, the rest of the dye is injected while the needle is slowly withdrawn, and the site is wiped with a sterile sponge.
- A film series is taken quickly to achieve maximum contrast.

Interfering Factors

- Dilution of the contrast medium due to incomplete aspiration of joint effusion (possible poor imaging)

- Improper injection technique (possible displacement of contrast medium)

Precautions

- Arthrography is contraindicated during pregnancy and in the patient with active arthritis, joint infection, or previous sensitivity to radiopaque media.

Nursing Considerations

Before the Test

- Explain to the patient that this test permits examination of a joint. Describe the specific procedure that the patient will undergo, and answer any questions Tell the patient who will perform the procedure, where, and when.
- Inform the patient that there are no food or fluid restrictions.
- Explain that the fluoroscope allows the health care provider to track the contrast medium as it fills the joint space.
- Inform the patient that standard X-ray films will also be taken after diffusion of the contrast medium.
- Advise the patient that, although the joint area will be anesthetized, there may be a tingling sensation or pressure in the joint when the contrast medium is injected.
- Advise the patient to remain as still as possible during the procedure, except when following instructions to change position. Stress the importance of cooperation in assuming various positions because films must be taken as quickly as possible to ensure optimum quality.
- Check the patient's history to determine hypersensitivity to local anesthetics, iodine, seafood, or dyes used for other diagnostic tests.

After the Test

- Tell the patient to keep the bandage in place for several days, and teach the patient how to rewrap the bandage.

- Tell the patient to rest the joint for at least 12 hours.
- Inform the patient that there may be some swelling, discomfort, or crepitant noises in the joint after the test, but that these symptoms usually disappear after 1 or 2 days; tell the patient to report persistent symptoms.
- Advise the patient to apply ice to the joint if swelling occurs and to take a mild analgesic for pain.
- Instruct the patient to report signs of infection at the needle insertion site, such as warmth, redness, swelling, or foul-smelling drainage.

Arthroscopy

Normal Findings

- Normal knee consisting of a diarthrodial joint surrounded by muscles, ligaments, cartilage, and tendons, and lined with a synovial membrane
- In children, smooth and opaque menisci, with thick outer edges attached to the joint capsule and unattached inner edges lying snugly against the condylar surfaces
- Articular cartilage that's smooth and white
- Ligaments and tendons that are cablelike and silvery
- Synovium that's smooth and marked by a fine vascular network

Abnormal Findings

- Meniscal disease, such as a torn medial or lateral meniscus or other meniscal injuries
- Patellar disease (chondromalacia, dislocation, subluxation, parapatellar synovitis, or fracture)
- Condylar disease (degenerative articular cartilage, osteochondritis dissecans, and loose bodies)
- Extrasynovial disease (torn anterior cruciate or tibial collateral ligaments, Baker's cyst, and ganglionic cyst)
- Synovial disease (synovitis, rheumatoid and degenerative arthritis, and

foreign bodies associated with gout, pseudogout, and osteochondromatosis)

Nursing Implications

- Report abnormal findings to the health care provider.
- Educate the patient about the diagnosis and possible treatment options.
- Depending on test findings, appropriate treatment or surgery can follow arthroscopy. If arthroscopic surgery can't be performed, arthrotomy is the procedure of choice.

Purpose

- To detect and diagnose meniscal, patellar, condylar, extrasynovial, and synovial diseases
- To monitor disease progression
- To perform joint surgery
- To monitor the effectiveness of therapy

Description

Arthroscopy is the visual examination of the interior of a joint (most commonly a major joint, such as a shoulder, hip, or knee) with a specially designed fiberoptic endoscope that's inserted through a cannula in the joint cavity. It usually follows and confirms a diagnosis made through physical examination, radiography, and arthrography.

Arthroscopy may be performed under local anesthesia, but it's usually performed under a spinal or general anesthesia, particularly when surgery is anticipated. A camera may be attached to the arthroscope to photograph areas for later study. (See the *Arthroscopy of the Knee* box.)

Arthroscopic techniques vary depending on the surgeon and the type of arthroscope used. The procedure typically proceeds as follows:

- The patient's leg is elevated and wrapped with an elastic bandage to drain as much blood from the leg as possible, or a mixture of lidocaine with epinephrine and normal saline

solution is instilled into the patient's knee to distend the knee and reduce bleeding.

- The local anesthetic is administered, a small incision is made, and a cannula is passed through the incision and positioned in the joint cavity.
- The arthroscope is inserted, and the knee structures are visually examined and photographed for further study.
- After visual examination, a synovial biopsy or appropriate surgery is performed, as indicated.
- When the examination is completed, the arthroscope is removed, the joint is irrigated, the cannula is removed, and an adhesive strip and compression dressing are applied over the incision site.

Precautions

- Arthroscopy is contraindicated in the patient with fibrous ankylosis with flexion of less than 50 degrees.
- Arthroscopy is contraindicated when the patient has local skin or wound infections with a risk of subsequent joint involvement.

Nursing Considerations

Before the Test

- Explain to the patient that arthroscopy is used to examine the interior of the joint, to evaluate joint disease, or to monitor response to therapy, as appropriate.
- Describe the procedure to the patient and answer any questions.
- If surgery or another treatment is anticipated, explain that this may be accomplished during arthroscopy.
- Obtain procedural consent.
- Instruct the patient to fast after midnight before the procedure.
- Inform the patient who will perform the procedure, and when and where it will be done.
- If local anesthesia is to be used, advise the patient there may be slight discomfort from the local anesthetic

Arthroscopy of the Knee

With the patient's knee flexed to about 40 degrees, the arthroscope is introduced into the joint. The examiner flexes, extends, and rotates the knee to view the joint space. Counterclockwise from the top right, these illustrations show a normal patellofemoral joint with smooth joint surfaces, the articular surface of the patella showing chondromalacia, and a tear in the anterior cruciate ligament.

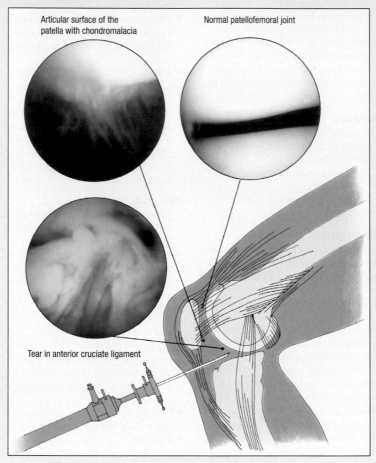

Articular surface of the patella with chondromalacia

Normal patellofemoral joint

Tear in anterior cruciate ligament

injection and the tourniquet pressure on his leg. Also prepare the patient to expect to feel a thumping sensation as the cannula is inserted in the joint capsule.

• Check the patient's history for hypersensitivity to the anesthetic.

• Prepare the surgical site by clipping the area 5 inches (12.7 cm) above and below the joint with electric clippers and administering a sedative, as ordered.

• Prepare the skin with an approved skin preparation from mid-thigh to ankle. Be sure that there is no pooling of the prep solution.

• Position the patient and drape him according to facility policy.

After the Test

• Observe the patient for fever, swelling, increased pain, and localized inflammation at the incision site. If the patient reports discomfort, provide an analgesic, as ordered.

• Monitor the patient's circulation and sensation in his leg.

• Advise the patient to elevate the leg and apply ice for the first 24 hours.

• Instruct the patient to report fever, bleeding, drainage, or increased swelling or pain in the joint.

• Advise the patient to bear only partial weight, using crutches, a walker, or a cane for 48 hours.

• If an immobilizer is ordered, teach the patient how to apply it.

• Tell the patient that showering is permitted after 48 hours, but a tub bath should be avoided until after the postoperative visit.

• Tell the patient to resume his usual diet, as ordered.

Arylsulfatase A

Reference Values

Normal, random: 1.6 to 42 units/g creatinine
24-hour urine: 0.37 to 3.60 units/day creatinine
1-hour test: 2 to 19 units/hour (SI, 2–19 units/hour)
2-hour test: 4 to 37 units/2 hours (SI, 4–37 units/2 hour)
24-hour test: 170 to 2,000 units/24 hours (SI, 2.89–34 mckat/L)

Abnormal Findings

Elevated Levels

• Cancer of the bladder, colon, or rectum
• Myeloid leukemia

Decreased Levels

• Possible metachromatic leukodystrophy (urine studies show metachromatic granules in the urinary sediment)

Nursing Implications

• Report abnormal findings to the health care provider.
• Educate the patient about the diagnosis and possible treatment options.

Purpose

• To help diagnose bladder, colon, or rectal cancer; myeloid (granulocytic) leukemia; and metachromatic leukodystrophy (an inherited lipid storage disease)

Description

This test measures the urine arylsulfatase (ARSA) level by colorimetric or kinetic techniques. The level rises in transitional bladder cancer, colorectal cancer, and leukemia. It's unknown whether elevated levels provoke malignancies or are an enzymatic response to these growths.

Interfering Factors

• Failure to collect all urine during the test period, to properly store the specimen, or to send the specimen to the laboratory immediately after the collection is complete
• Contamination of the specimen with toilet tissue, stool, or menstrual blood
• Surgery within 1 week before the test (possible increase)

Nursing Considerations

Before the Test

• Confirm the patient's identity using two patient identifiers and confirmation of the patient's identification bracelet according to facility policy.
• Inform the patient that this test measures an enzyme that's present throughout the body.
• Explain that the test requires urine collection over a 24-hour period, and teach the patient how to collect a timed specimen.

• Advise the patient that there are no food or fluid restrictions before the test.

During the Test
• Collect the patient's urine over a 24-hour period, discarding the first sample and retaining the last sample in the appropriate container.
• If a female patient is menstruating, anticipate possible test rescheduling.
• Keep the collection container refrigerated or on ice during the collection period.
• If the patient has an indwelling urinary catheter in place, keep the collection bag on ice for the duration of the test.
• Begin the test period with a new, unused continuous urinary drainage apparatus.
• Instruct the patient to avoid contaminating the urine specimen with toilet tissue or stool.

After the Test
• Send the specimen to the laboratory as soon as the collection period is completed.

Aspartate Aminotransferase

Reference Values
Adult females: 7 to 34 units/L (SI, 0.12–0.5 mckat/L)
Adult males: 8 to 46 units/L (SI, 0.14–0.78 mckat/L)
Children: 9 to 80 units/L (SI, 0.15–1.3 mckat/L)
Neonates: 47 to 150 units/L (SI, 0.78–2.5 mckat/L)

Abnormal Findings

Maximum Elevated Levels (More Than 20 Times Normal)
• Acute viral hepatitis
• Severe skeletal muscle trauma
• Extensive surgery
• Drug-induced hepatic injury
• Severe passive liver congestion

High Levels (10–20 Times Normal)
• Severe MI
• Severe infectious mononucleosis
• Alcoholic cirrhosis

Moderate to High Levels (5–10 Times Normal)
• Dermatomyositis
• Duchenne's muscular dystrophy
• Chronic hepatitis

Low to Moderate Levels (2–5 Times Normal)
• Hemolytic anemia
• Metastatic hepatic tumors
• Acute pancreatitis
• Pulmonary emboli
• Delirium tremens
• Fatty liver

Nursing Implications
• Report abnormal findings to the health care provider.
• Educate the patient about the diagnosis and possible treatment options.

Purpose
• To aid detection and differential diagnosis of acute hepatic disease
• To monitor patient progress and prognosis in cardiac and hepatic diseases

Description
Aspartate aminotransferase (AST) is one of two enzymes that catalyze the conversion of the nitrogenous portion of an amino acid to an amino acid residue. It's essential to energy production in the Krebs' cycle. AST is found in the cytoplasm and mitochondria of many cells, primarily in the liver, heart, skeletal muscles, kidneys, pancreas, and red blood cells. It's released into serum in proportion to cellular damage.

Although a high correlation exists between MI and elevated AST levels, this test is sometimes considered superfluous for diagnosing an MI because of its relatively low organ specificity; it doesn't allow differentiation between acute MI and the effects of hepatic congestion due to heart failure.

AST levels fluctuate in response to the extent of cellular necrosis: They're transiently and minimally increased early in the disease process and extremely increased during the most acute phase. AST levels may increase, indicating increasing disease severity and tissue damage, or decrease, indicating disease resolution and tissue repair, depending on the timing of the initial sampling.

Interfering Factors
- Antitubercular agents, chlorpropamide (Diabinese), dicumarol, erythromycin (E-mycin), methyldopa (Aldomet), opioids, pyridoxine (Bendectin), and sulfonamides; large doses of acetaminophen (Tylenol), salicylates, or vitamin A; and many other drugs known to affect the liver (increase)
- Strenuous exercise and muscle trauma due to intramuscular injections (increase)

Precautions
- To avoid missing peak AST levels, draw serum samples at the same time each day.
- Handle the sample gently to prevent hemolysis, and send it to the laboratory immediately.

Nursing Considerations
Before the Test
- Confirm the patient's identity using two patient identifiers and confirmation of the patient's identification bracelet according to facility policy.
- Explain to the patient that the AST test is used to assess heart and liver function.
- Inform the patient that the test usually requires three venipunctures (one on admission and one each day for the next 2 days).
- Inform the patient that there is no food or fluid restrictions.
- Advise the patient there may be slight discomfort from the tourniquet and needle puncture.

- Notify the laboratory and health care provider about any medications the patient is taking that may affect test results; restrict these drugs, if necessary.

During the Test
- Perform a venipuncture and collect the sample in a 4-mL clot activator tube.

After the Test
- Apply direct pressure to the venipuncture site until bleeding stops and to prevent hematoma formation.
- Instruct the patient to resume medications that were discontinued before the test, as ordered.

Atrial Natriuretic Peptides, Plasma

Reference Values
20 to 77 pg/mL (SI, 20–77 ng/L)

Abnormal Findings
Elevated Levels
- Frank heart failure and significantly elevated cardiac filling pressure

Nursing Implications
- Report abnormal findings to the health care provider.
- Educate the patient about the diagnosis and possible treatment options.

Purpose
- To confirm heart failure
- To identify cardiac volume overload that isn't producing symptoms

Description
The test for atrial natriuretic peptides (ANP), also known as plasma atrial natriuretic factor (ANF) or atriopeptins, is a radioimmunoassay that measures the plasma level of ANP. An extremely potent natriuretic agent and vasodilator, ANP rapidly produces diuresis and increases the glomerular filtration rate. ANP's role in regulating extracellular fluid volume, blood pressure, and sodium metabolism appears critical. It promotes sodium excretion, inhibits

the renin–angiotensin system's effect on aldosterone secretion, and decreases atrial pressure by decreasing venous return, thereby reducing blood pressure and volume.

The patient with overt heart failure has highly elevated plasma levels of ANP. The patient with cardiovascular disease and elevated cardiac filling pressure but no heart failure also has markedly elevated ANP levels. ANP may provide a marker for early asymptomatic left ventricular dysfunction and increased cardiac volume.

Interfering Factors
• Cardiovascular drugs, including beta-adrenergic blockers, calcium antagonists, cardiac glycosides, diuretics, and vasodilators

Nursing Considerations
Before the Test
• Confirm the patient's identity using two patient identifiers and confirmation of the patient's identification bracelet according to facility policy.
• Explain the purpose of the plasma ANP test to the patient.
• Tell the patient to fast for 12 hours before the test.
• Tell the patient that the test requires a blood sample and that there may be discomfort from the tourniquet and needle puncture.
• Explain that the test results will be available within 4 days.
• Check the patient's history for medications that can influence test results.
• Withhold beta-adrenergic blockers, calcium antagonists, diuretics, vasodilators, and cardiac glycosides for 24 hours before collection, as ordered.

During the Test
• Perform a venipuncture and collect the sample in a prechilled potassium-EDTA tube.
• After chilled centrifugation, the EDTA plasma should be promptly frozen and sent to the laboratory.

After the Test
• Apply direct pressure to the venipuncture site until bleeding stops and to prevent hematoma formation.
• Instruct the patient to resume a usual diet and medications that were discontinued before the test, as ordered.

Auditory Evoked Potentials
Normal Findings
• Auditory brainstem response (ABR) wave latencies (time of the waveform occurrence after stimulus presentation) occurring at predictable times
• Approximately 4 ms latency between waves I and V (no longer than about 4.4 ms); interaural latency difference of wave V and the I through V interaural latency generally less than 0.3 or 0.4 ms (See the *Auditory Brainstem Response* box).
• ABR threshold typically about 10 to 20 dB nHL for click or high-frequency stimuli; 20 or 30 dB nHL for lower frequency stimuli
• Amplitude ratio of the summating potential and action potential within normal limits for the type of electrocochleography (EcoG or ECohG) electrode used

Abnormal Findings
• With cochlear loss, increased threshold of the ABR response but unaltered wave V latency for stimuli that are well above the threshold, unaffected or shortened time between waves I and V, and possible difficulty establishing wave I
• Prolongation of the I through V interpeak latency, indicating cranial nerve (CN) VIII or lower brainstem pathology (requires confirmation with imaging studies)
• Asymmetry of the I through V interpeak interval between ears, signaling a retrocochlear disorder
• Abnormally large summating potential amplitude compared with action

Auditory Brainstem Response

These graphs illustrate an auditory brainstem response elicited by 100-ms click stimuli. The patient's auditory neural activity is recorded using surface electrodes. The peaks on the graphs represent activity from cranial nerve VIII and brainstem structures. Traces are repeated for accuracy at each intensity. The morphology and time between labeled peaks are evaluated when assessing the patient's neural integrity. Additionally, the symmetry of left and right ear responses are evaluated (not illustrated). When used to estimate the hearing threshold, the stimuli's intensity is decreased. A prolonged wave V occurs. The lowest intensity eliciting an evoked potential is assumed to be slightly supra-threshold.

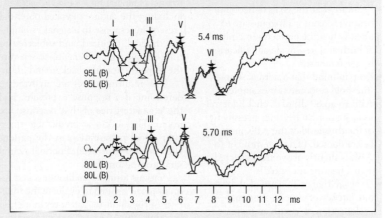

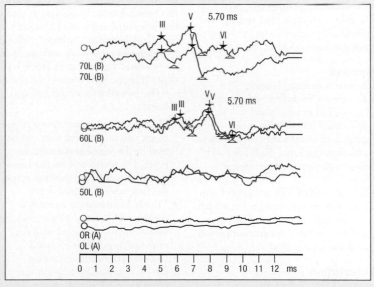

potential amplitude with ECoG testing, indicating Ménière's disease

Nursing Implications

- Report abnormal findings to the health care provider.
- Educate the patient about the diagnosis and possible treatment options.
- Prepare the patient for careful audiologic follow-up.
- Be aware that the goals of neonatal hearing screening programs are to identify hearing problems in children at birth and to provide amplification by age 6 months.
- Keep in mind that a normal suprathreshold response (for example, an ABR to an 80-dB nHL click) doesn't indicate normal hearing; assessment of the threshold of the ABR must be conducted. (The threshold of the ABR is slightly above the expected actual hearing threshold.)
- Be aware that asymmetry of absolute latency of wave V, abnormal prolongation of V with an increase in the stimulus repetition rate, poor replicability or morphology, and atypical amplitude ratios of waves I to V fail to rule out a retrocochlear abnormality.

Purpose

- To screen neonatal hearing
- To estimate or confirm the extent of hearing loss in infants and toddlers
- To estimate threshold in other difficult-to-test patients, such as those with developmental disabilities and those with suspected nonorganic hearing loss
- To evaluate CN VIII and lower brainstem auditory synchronization, which is abnormal with lesions of this area and with auditory dyssynchronization (auditory neuropathy)

Description

Event-related potentials are brain responses that are time-locked to a particular "event." This event may be a sensory stimulus (such as a visual flash or an auditory sound), a mental event (such as recognition of a specified target stimulus), or the omission of a stimulus (such as an increased time gap between stimuli). ABR testing is the most common form of auditory evoked potential testing. It's typically performed by an audiologist and involves attaching electrodes to the surface of the patient's scalp. Electroencephalographic (EEG) activity, including the auditory evoked potential present in response to a signal, is amplified, filtered, digitized, and subjected to time domain signal averaging to separate the response from the background EEG.

The resulting traces are analyzed to determine if a response is present, and the characteristics of that response are noted. They occur at predictable times after signal presentation in the patient with normal hearing and normal neural synchronization.

Various forms of auditory evoked responses can be used to evaluate the function of the auditory pathways in a child or adult suspected of having auditory processing deficits. ECoG can be used in the differential diagnosis of Ménière's disease (endolymphatic hydrops), although its diagnostic sensitivity and specificity is considered by some to be lacking, particularly in the early stages of the disease.

The procedure for ABR testing is as follows:

- Electrodes are connected to a physiologic amplifier so that they can be read by the signal-averaging computer. The waveforms are displayed as the amplitude of the response across the time after the signal begins.
- Threshold estimation typically is conducted by an audiologist, and the signal intensity is varied until the response threshold is obtained.
- In neurodiagnostic testing for CN VIII and auditory brainstem response, click signals are presented at clearly audible intensities to elicit good synchronization of CN VIII. More rapid presentations may reveal

auditory pathology more readily. Assessment of central auditory processing ability typically involves assessing brainstem potentials and one or more of the potentials generated by the neural structures superior to the brainstem.

- In ECoG testing, the recording electrodes are placed in the ear canal of the patient or on the tympanic membrane. In rare instances, a health care provider places the electrode through the tympanic membrane and rests it on the promontory of the middle ear. The cochlear potentials and CN VIII response are recorded.

Interfering Factors

- Hearing loss developed after birth, for instance from such congenital diseases as maternal cytomegalovirus infection and some genetic hearing losses or progressive hearing loss
- Patient movement leading to inaccurate results; for example, if the young child isn't asleep or if the older child or adult is restless
- Threshold testing with click stimuli, possibly creating false-negative results with normal hearing occurring due to a region of residual hearing
- Uncertainty of ABR threshold estimation
- Auditory dyssynchronization, possibly eliminating an ABR even though cochlear function may be normal (The use of otoacoustic emissions testing in conjunction with ABR testing is recommended.)
- Lack of use of age-specific norms (Neonates and infants have longer latency responses than adults.)
- Ménière's disease that isn't producing symptoms, leading to high false-negative results via ECoG. (Normal ECoG findings don't rule out Ménière's disease.)

Precautions

- Accurate test results require passive patient cooperation.

- Skin abrasions from electrode placement may, although rarely, cause irritation and minor allergic reactions.
- A skilled audiologist is needed for ECoG to place the electrode in contact with the tympanic membrane without creating patient discomfort.

Nursing Considerations

Before the Test

- Remove cerumen from the patient's ear before testing begins.

 Quality and Safety Nursing Alert

Depending on the age of the child, sedation may be required. Sedated ABR testing can only be conducted at health care facilities. In other facilities, sleep deprivation of the child may be required to ensure that the patient sleeps during testing.

- Advise the patient to dress comfortably.
- Inform the patient that electrodes will be applied to the skin but that the test is painless.
- Advise the patient that the test takes 1 to 1.5 hours to complete.

After the Test

- If the patient required sedation, observe until recovery is complete.

Avian Flu Virus Ribonucleic Acid

Normal Findings

- 5N1 ribonucleic acid (RNA) not detected

Abnormal Findings

- H5N1 RNA detected (patient has been exposed to the avian flu virus)

Nursing Implications

- Immediately contact the Centers for Disease Control and Prevention (CDC) and the World Health Organization (WHO) and be prepared to

ship specimens to a designated WHO laboratory.
- Report abnormal findings to the health care provider.
- Educate the patient about the diagnosis and possible treatment options.
- After a positive result, further testing will need to be done.

Purpose
- To detect the presence of H5N1 RNA

Description
Avian influenza is a bird infection. Wild birds are carriers of the disease and can transmit it to domesticated birds. The H5N1 virus can be transmitted from a sick bird to humans. More than 100 human cases of H5N1 have been diagnosed, with one-half of those people dying. Genetic studies have shown that H5N1 is able to rapidly mutate, causing concern of a pandemic outbreak of the flu.

Nursing Considerations
Before the Test
- Determine if the patient has been exposed recently to infected poultry.

- Confirm the patient's identity using two patient identifiers and confirmation of the patient's identification bracelet according to facility policy.
- Explain to the patient that this test will help determine exposure to the avian flu.
- Inform the patient that the test is performed with a nasal swab.
- Advise the patient that there is no food or fluid restriction before the test.
- Explain to the patient that, if the test is positive, the results will be reported to the CDC and WHO, and further testing may be done.

During the Test
- Obtain a nasal culture from both nostrils.
- Place each swab into a container containing 3 mL of normal sterile saline solution.
- Place the specimens on ice.

After the Test
- Send the samples to the laboratory immediately.
- Answer the patient's questions about the test.

Bacterial Meningitis Antigen

Normal Findings
- Negative for bacterial antigens

Abnormal Findings
- Positive for specific bacterial antigens, including *Streptococcus pneumoniae*, *Neisseria meningitidis*, *Haemophilus influenzae* type B, or group B streptococci

Nursing Implications
- Report abnormal findings to the health care provider immediately.
- Expect to institute antimicrobial therapy and infection control precautions specific to the identified antigen.

Purpose
- To identify the etiologic agent in meningitis
- To help diagnose bacterial meningitis when the Gram stain smear and culture are negative

Description
The bacterial meningitis antigen test can detect specific antigens of *S. pneumoniae*, *N. meningitidis*, and *H. influenzae* type B, the principal etiologic agents in meningitis. Testing on cerebrospinal fluid (CSF) and urine is preferred, but it can also be done on serum, pleural fluid, and joint fluid samples. CSF specimen collection requires a lumbar puncture.

Interfering Factors
- Previous antimicrobial therapy
- Specimen contamination during collection

Nursing Considerations

Before the Test
- Confirm the patient's identity using two patient identifiers and confirmation of the patient's identification bracelet according to facility policy.
- Explain the purpose of the bacterial meningitis antigen test to the patient, as appropriate.
- Inform the patient that this test requires a specimen of urine or CSF. If a CSF specimen is required, explain the lumbar puncture procedure to the patient.
- Advise the patient requiring a lumbar puncture there may be discomfort from the needle puncture during the test. A headache is a common complication of this procedure but may be alleviated with fluids or an epidural blood patch.
- Make sure the patient or a family member has signed an informed consent form.
- Obtain vital signs prior to lumbar puncture procedure.

During the Test
For Urine Sample
- Wear gloves when obtaining or handling the specimen.
- Maintain specimen sterility during collection.
- Collect a 10-mL urine specimen or a 1-mL CSF specimen in a sterile container.

For CSF Sample
- Assist the patient in maintaining the correct position for lumbar puncture (fetal position with the back bowed,

the head flexed on the chest, and the knees drawn up to the abdomen).
• Encourage the patient to breathe slowly and deeply during the lumbar puncture to help relax.
• Use aseptic technique when handling specimen.

After the Test
• If a lumbar puncture was performed, have the patient lie flat for approximately 4 to 8 hours, as ordered by the health care provider.
• Check vital signs after procedure and at prescribed times (e.g., 30 minutes, 1 hour, 2 hours, 4 hours)
• Encourage the patient to drink plenty of fluids to reduce possible spinal headache after lumbar puncture.
• Assess the lumbar puncture site frequently for leakage; monitor the patient's neurologic status frequently.
• Administer an analgesic as prescribed to relieve headache.
• Make sure the cap is tightly fastened on the specimen containers. There are usually three specimen containers, labeled in the order of collection.
• Place the labeled specimens on a refrigerated coolant and send them to the laboratory immediately.

Barium Enema
Normal Findings
Single Contrast
• Intestine uniformly filled with barium; colonic haustral markings clearly apparent
• Mucosa with a regular, feathery appearance on postevacuation film

Double Contrast
• Intestines uniformly distended with air; thin layer of barium providing excellent detail of the mucosal pattern
• Barium collected on dependent walls of intestine (due to force of gravity) as patient is assisted to various positions

Abnormal Findings
• Localized filling defect, suggesting colon cancer, ulcerative colitis, and granulomatous colitis
• Inflammation characteristic of saccular adenomatous polyps, broad-based villous polyps, structural changes in the intestine (such as intussusception, telescoping of the bowel, sigmoid volvulus, and sigmoid torsion), gastroenteritis, irritable colon, vascular injury caused by arterial occlusion, and, possibly, acute appendicitis, inflammatory bowel disease (Crohn's and ulcerative colitis)

Nursing Implications
• Assist the patient in understanding the results of the barium enema.
• Emphasize the importance of dietary restrictions and bowel preparation.
• Prepare the patient for additional testing such as barium swallow, upper GI and small-bowel series, or biopsy to confirm the results.
• When both a barium enema and barium swallow are prescribed, the barium enema is scheduled prior to the barium swallow procedure.

Purpose
• To help diagnose colorectal cancer and inflammatory disease
• To detect polyps, diverticula, and structural changes in the large intestine

Description
Also called *lower GI examination*, barium enema is the radiographic examination of the large intestine after rectal instillation of barium sulfate (single-contrast technique) or barium sulfate and air (double-contrast technique). It is indicated in patients with histories of altered bowel habits, lower abdominal pain, or the passage of blood, mucus, or pus in the stools. It also may be indicated after colostomy or ileostomy; in these patients, barium (or barium and air) is instilled through the stoma.

Complications include perforation of the colon, water intoxication, barium granulomas, and, rarely, intraperitoneal and extraperitoneal extravasation of barium and barium embolism.

The usual procedure is as follows:

- After the patient is in a supine position on a tilting X-ray table, spot films of the abdomen are taken.
- The patient is assisted to the Sims' position, and a well-lubricated rectal tube is inserted through the anus. If the patient has anal sphincter atony or severe mental or physical debilitation, a rectal tube with a retaining balloon may be inserted.
- The barium is administered slowly, and the filling process is monitored fluoroscopically. To aid filling, the table may be tilted or the patient assisted to supine, prone, and lateral decubitus positions.
- As barium flow is observed, spot films are taken of significant findings. When the intestine is filled with barium, overhead films of the abdomen are taken. The rectal tube is withdrawn, and the patient is escorted to the toilet or provided with a bedpan and is instructed to expel as much barium as possible.
- After evacuation, an additional overhead film is taken to record the mucosal pattern of the intestine and to evaluate the efficiency of colonic emptying.
- A double-contrast barium enema may directly follow this examination or may be performed separately. If it's performed immediately, a thin film of barium remains in the patient's intestine, coating the mucosa, and air is carefully injected to distend the bowel lumen.
- When the double-contrast technique is performed separately, a colloidal barium suspension is instilled, filling the patient's intestine to either the splenic flexure or the middle of the transverse colon. The suspension

is then aspirated and air is forcefully injected into the intestine. If the intestine is filled to the lower descending colon, air is forcefully injected without previous aspiration of the suspension.

- The patient is then assisted to erect, prone, supine, and lateral decubitus positions in sequence. Barium filling is monitored fluoroscopically, and spot films are taken of significant findings.
- After the required films are taken, the patient is escorted to the toilet or provided with a bedpan.

Interfering Factors

- Inadequate bowel preparation (possible poor imaging)
- Retention of barium from previous studies (possible poor imaging)
- The patient's inability to retain barium

Precautions

- Barium enema is contraindicated in patients with tachycardia, fulminant ulcerative colitis associated with systemic toxicity and megacolon, toxic megacolon, or suspected perforation, as well as in pregnant patients because of radiation's possible teratogenic effects.
- This test should be performed cautiously in patients with obstruction, acute inflammatory conditions (such as ulcerative colitis and diverticulitis), acute vascular insufficiency of the bowel, acute fulminant bloody diarrhea, and suspected pneumatosis cystoides intestinalis.

Nursing Considerations

Before the Test

- Explain to the patient that the barium enema test permits examination of the large intestine through x-rays taken after a barium enema.
- Describe the test, including who will perform it, and where and when it will take place.

B

- Because residual fecal material in the colon obscures normal anatomy on X-rays, instruct the patient to carefully follow the prescribed bowel preparation, which may include dietary restrictions, laxatives, or an enema. (Note that for certain conditions, such as ulcerative colitis and active GI bleeding, the use of laxatives and enemas may be prohibited.) Stress that accurate test results depend on full patient cooperation. A typical bowel preparation includes:
  - restricting dairy product intake and following a liquid diet for 24 hours before the test
  - drinking five 8-oz glasses of water or clear liquids 12 to 24 hours before the test
  - administering a bowel preparation supplied by the radiography department (GoLYTELY preparation isn't recommended because it leaves the bowel too wet for the barium to coat the walls of the bowel).
- Advise the patient to administer prescribed enemas until return is clear.
- Instruct the patient not to eat breakfast before the procedure; if the test is scheduled for late afternoon (or delayed), the patient may have clear liquids.
- Inform the patient that he or she will be placed on a tilting X-ray table and adequately draped. Assure that patient that he or she will be secured to the table and will be assisted to various positions.
- Advise the patient that cramping pains or the urge to defecate may occur as the barium or air is introduced into the intestine. Instruct the patient to breathe deeply and slowly through the mouth to ease discomfort.
- Instruct the patient to keep the anal sphincter tightly contracted against the rectal tube; this holds the tube in position and helps prevent leakage of barium. Stress the importance of

retaining the barium enema; if the intestinal walls aren't adequately coated with barium, test results may be inaccurate.
- Assure the patient that the barium enema is fairly easy to retain because of its cool temperature.

During the Test
- Help the patient relax to aid in retaining the barium.
- Tell the patient when he or she will be moving to another position or when the X-ray table will be tilted or moved.

After the Test
- Assist the patient onto the bedpan or to the bathroom as necessary to evacuate the barium.
- Make sure further studies haven't been ordered before allowing the patient food and fluids. Encourage extra fluid intake because bowel preparation and the test itself can cause dehydration.
- Encourage rest because this test and the bowel preparation that precedes it are usually exhausting.
- Because barium retention after this test can cause intestinal obstruction or fecal impaction, administer a mild cathartic or an enema as prescribed.
- Tell the patient that stools will be light colored for 24 to 72 hours.
- Record a description of all stools passed by the patient in the hospital.

Barium Swallow
Normal Findings
- Bolus pouring over the base of the tongue and into the pharynx after the barium sulfate is swallowed
- Peristaltic wave propelling bolus through the entire length of the esophagus in about 2 seconds
- Opening of cardiac sphincter when the peristaltic wave reaches the base of the esophagus

- Bolus entering the stomach, followed by closure of the cardiac sphincter
- Bolus evenly filling and distending the lumen of the pharynx and esophagus; smooth, regular-appearing mucosa

Abnormal Findings

- Hiatal hernia, diverticula, and esophageal varices
- Possible aspiration into the lungs
- Strictures, tumors, polyps, ulcers, and motility disorders (pharyngeal muscular disorders, esophageal spasms, and achalasia)
- Congenital anomalies
- Foreign objects

Nursing Implications

- Reinforce with the patient that definitive diagnosis may require additional testing, such as endoscopic biopsy or manometric studies for motility disorders. (See the GI Motility Study box.)

Purpose

- To diagnose hiatal hernia, diverticula, and esophageal varices
- To detect strictures, ulcers, tumors, polyps, and motility disorders
- To detect congenital anomalies

GI Motility Study

A GI motility study evaluates the intestinal motility and integrity of the mucosal lining by recording the passage of barium through the lower digestive tract. About 6 hours after the patient ingests the barium, the head of the barium column is usually in the hepatic flexure and the tail is in the terminal ileum; 24 hours after ingestion, the barium has completely opacified the large intestine. Spot films taken 24, 48, or 72 hours after ingestion are inferior to barium enema because the amount of barium passing through the large intestine isn't sufficient to fully extend the lumen. However, when spot films suggest intestinal abnormalities, barium enema and colonoscopy can provide more specific results and confirm diagnostic information.

Description

Barium swallow (esophagography) is the cineradiographic, radiographic, or fluoroscopic examination of the pharynx and the fluoroscopic examination of the esophagus after ingestion of thick and thin mixtures of barium sulfate. This test, most commonly performed as part of the upper GI series, is indicated for patients with histories of dysphagia and regurgitation.

The barium swallow procedure is performed in the radiology unit as follows:

- The patient is placed in an upright position behind the fluoroscopic screen, and the heart, lungs, and abdomen are examined.
- The patient is then instructed to take one swallow of the thick barium mixture, and the pharyngeal action is recorded using cineradiography. (This action occurs too rapidly for adequate fluoroscopic evaluation.)
- The patient is then told to take several swallows of the thin barium mixture. The passage of the barium is examined fluoroscopically, and spot films of the esophageal region are taken from lateral angles and from right and left posteroanterior angles. Esophageal strictures and obstruction of the esophageal lumen by the lower esophageal ring are best detected when the patient is upright.
- To accentuate small strictures or demonstrate dysphagia, the patient may be requested to swallow a special "barium marshmallow" (soft white bread that has been soaked in barium) or a barium pill.
- The patient is then secured to the X-ray table and is rotated to the Trendelenburg position to evaluate esophageal peristalsis or demonstrate hiatal hernia and gastric reflux.
- The patient is instructed to take several swallows of barium while the esophagus is examined fluoroscopically, and spot films of significant

findings are taken when indicated. After the table is rotated to a horizontal position, the patient is told to take several swallows of barium so that the esophagogastric junction and peristalsis may be evaluated.

- The passage of the barium is observed fluoroscopically, and spot films of significant findings are taken with the patient in the supine and prone positions.
- During fluoroscopic examination of the esophagus, the cardiac and fundal regions of the stomach are also carefully studied because neoplasms in these areas may invade the esophagus and cause obstruction.

Interfering Factors

- Barium aspiration into the lungs due to poor swallowing reflex
- Retained food or fluids interfere with optimal film clarity

Precautions

- This test is usually contraindicated in patients with intestinal obstruction, as well as in pregnant patients because of radiation's possible teratogenic effects.

Nursing Considerations

Before the Test

- Confirm the patient's identity using two patient identifiers and confirmation of the patient's identification bracelet according to facility policy.
- Explain to the patient that the barium swallow test evaluates the function of the pharynx and esophagus.
- Instruct the patient to fast after midnight the night before the test. Advise that a restricted diet may be necessary for 2 to 3 days before the test.

▶ **Quality and Safety Nursing Alert**

If the patient is an infant, delay feeding to ensure complete digestion of barium.

- Describe the test, including who will perform it, and where and when it will take place.
- Describe the barium preparation's milkshake consistency and chalky taste, and advise the patient that, although the preparation is flavored, it may be unpleasant to swallow. Inform the patient first a thick mixture is given, then a thin one, and that the patient must drink 12 to 14 oz (355–414 mL) during the examination.
- Inform the patient he or she will be placed in various positions on a tilting X-ray table and that X-rays will be taken. Reassure the patient that safety precautions will be maintained.
- Withhold antacids, histamine-2 blockers, and proton pump inhibitors, as ordered, if gastric reflux is suspected.
- Just before the procedure, instruct the patient to put on a gown without snap closures and to remove jewelry, dentures, hair clips, or other radiopaque objects from the X-ray field.

After the Test

- Check that additional spot films and repeat fluoroscopic evaluation haven't been ordered before allowing the patient to resume a usual diet.
- Instruct the patient to drink plenty of fluids, unless contraindicated, to help eliminate the barium.
- Administer a cathartic, if prescribed.
- Inform the patient that stools will be chalky and light colored for 24 to 72 hours.
- Record a description of all stools passed by the patient in the hospital.
- Notify the health care provider if the patient fails to expel barium in 2 or 3 days. Barium retained in the intestine may harden, causing obstruction or fecal impaction. Check the patient for abdominal distention and absent bowel sounds, which are associated with constipation and may suggest barium impaction.

Basal Gastric Secretion Test

Reference Values
Females: 0.2 to 3.3 mEq/hour
Males: 1 to 5 mEq/hour

Abnormal Findings

Elevated Levels
- Duodenal or jejunal ulcer (after partial gastrectomy)
- Zollinger-Ellison's syndrome (markedly elevated)

Decreased Levels
- Gastric carcinoma or benign gastric ulcer
- Pernicious anemia (absence of secretion)

Nursing Implications
- Elevated or decreased levels of basal gastric secretion are nonspecific and must be considered with the results of the gastric acid stimulation test.

Purpose
- To determine gastric output while the patient is fasting

Description
The basal gastric secretion test measures basal secretion during fasting by aspirating stomach contents through a nasogastric (NG) tube. It's indicated in the patient with obscure epigastric pain, anorexia, and weight loss. Because external factors—such as the sight or odor of food—and psychological stress stimulate gastric secretion, accurate testing requires that the patient be relaxed and isolated from all sources of sensory stimulation. Although abnormal basal secretion test results can suggest various gastric and duodenal disorders, a complete evaluation of secretions requires the gastric acid stimulation test.

Interfering Factors
- Failure to observe pretest restrictions (increase)
- Psychological stress (possible increase)
- Adrenergic blockers, adrenocorticosteroids, alcohol, cholinergics, and reserpine (possible increase)
- Antacids, anticholinergics, histamine-2 blockers, and proton pump inhibitors (possible decrease)

Precautions
- The basal gastric secretion test is contraindicated in the patient with a condition that prohibits NG intubation.

> **▶ Quality and Safety Nursing Alert**
>
> During insertion, make sure that the NG tube enters the esophagus and not the trachea. Remove it immediately if the patient develops cyanosis or paroxysmal coughing.

Nursing Considerations

Before the Test
- Confirm the patient's identity using two patient identifiers and confirmation of the patient's identification bracelet according to facility policy.
- Explain to the patient that the basal gastric secretion test measures the stomach's secretion of acid.
- Instruct the patient to restrict food for 12 hours, and fluids and smoking for 8 hours before the test.
- Tell the patient who will perform the test, where and when it will take place, and that the procedure lasts approximately 1¼ hours (or 2¼ hours, if followed by the gastric acid stimulation test).
- Inform the patient that the test requires insertion of a tube through the nose and into the stomach, and that he or she may initially experience discomfort, cough, or gag.
- Notify the laboratory and health care provider about any medications the patient is taking that may affect test results; these may need to be restricted. If these drugs must be continued, note this on the laboratory request slip.

B

- Check the patient's pulse rate and blood pressure just before the test. Then encourage relaxation to minimize gastric secretions.

During the Test
- Position the patient with the head of bed elevated at least 45 degrees.
- Lubricate the NG tube with a water-soluble gel.
- Insert the NG tube.
- Attach a 20-mL syringe to it the tube and aspirate the stomach contents.
- To ensure complete emptying of the stomach, ask the patient to assume three positions in sequence—supine, and right and left lateral decubitus—while stomach contents are aspirated.
- Label the specimen container "Residual contents."
- To prevent contamination of the specimens with saliva, instruct the patient to expectorate excess saliva.
- Connect the NG tube to the suction machine. Aspirate gastric contents by continuous low suction for 1 hour. Aspiration also can be performed manually with a syringe.
- Monitor the patient's vital signs during intubation, and observe the patient carefully for arrhythmias.
- Collect a specimen every 15 minutes, but discard the first two; this eliminates the specimens that could be affected by the stress of the intubation. Label the retained specimens "Basal contents," and number them one through four.
- Record the color and odor of each specimen, and note the presence of food, mucus, bile, or blood.
- Measure secretion volume and acid concentration.
- If the NG tube is to be left in place, clamp it or attach it to low intermittent suction, as ordered.

After the Test
- Send the specimens to the laboratory immediately after the collection is completed.

- Watch for complications, such as nausea, vomiting, and abdominal distention or pain, following removal of the NG tube.
- If the patient complains of a sore throat, provide soothing lozenges.
- Instruct the patient to resume a usual diet and medications, as ordered, unless the gastric acid stimulation test will also be performed.

Basophils

Reference Values
Absolute count: 15 to 50/mm³ (0.02–0.05 × 10⁹/L)
Differential: 0% to 1% of total white blood cell (WBC) count

Abnormal Findings
Elevated Levels
- Leukemia (myelocytic, acute basophilic)
- Hodgkin's disease
- Myeloproliferative disorders

Decreased Levels
- Acute infection
- Hyperthyroidism
- Stress
- Prolonged steroid therapy, chemotherapy, or radiation therapy
- Acute rheumatic fever (children)
- Anaphylactic reaction (rapid decrease)

Nursing Implications
- Elevated basophil counts are correlated with high concentrations of blood histamines.
- Check the patient with elevated findings for history of steroid use, which can mask the basophilia.
- Institute infection control precautions in patients with decreased counts, as indicated.
- Monitor the patient closely for signs and symptoms associated with these disorders.
- Anticipate the need for additional testing to confirm diagnosis.

Purpose

- To determine the number of basophils in a peripheral blood smear
- To aid in determining specific conditions related to basophil counts, such as myeloproliferative disease
- To evaluate chronic inflammation

Description

Basophils are a component of the total WBC count. These cells are phagocytic and accumulate at the site of infection or inflammation, so their numbers increase during infection.

Interfering Factors

- Use of drugs such as desipramine (Norpramin), paroxetine (Paxil), tretinoin (Vesanoid), triazolam (Halcion), and venlafaxine (Effexor) (elevated levels)

Nursing Considerations

Before the Test

- Confirm the patient's identity using two patient identifiers and confirmation of the patient's identification bracelet according to facility policy.
- Explain the purpose of testing, and advise the patient that it requires a venipuncture.
- Advise the patient that there may be discomfort from the tourniquet and the needle puncture.

During the Test

- Perform a venipuncture to collect the sample.

After the Test

- Apply pressure to the venipuncture site until bleeding stops.
- Assess the venipuncture site for hematoma formation; if one develops, apply direct pressure.

Bence Jones Proteins (Urine)

Reference Values

Negative for Bence Jones proteins

Abnormal Findings

Elevated Levels

- Multiple myeloma or Waldenström's macroglobulinemia

Decreased Levels

- Benign monoclonal gammopathy (very low levels in the absence of other symptoms)

Nursing Implications

- Evaluate test results in light of the patient's condition and clinical picture.
- Anticipate the need for additional testing.

Purpose

- To confirm the presence of multiple myeloma in the patient with characteristic clinical signs, such as bone pain (especially in the back and the thorax) and persistent anemia and fatigue

Description

Bence Jones proteins are abnormal light-chain immunoglobulins of low molecular weight that are derived from the clone of a single plasma cell. This globulin appears in the urine of 50% to 80% of patients with multiple myeloma and in most patients with Waldenström's macroglobulinemia.

Screening tests, such as thermal coagulation and Bradshaw's test, can detect Bence Jones proteins, but urine immunoelectrophoresis is usually the method of choice for quantitative studies. Serum immunoelectrophoresis, which is sometimes used, is less sensitive than other tests. Nevertheless, urine and serum studies are usually used when multiple myeloma is suspected.

Interfering Factors

- Connective tissue disease, renal insufficiency, and certain cancers (possible false positive)
- Contamination of the specimen with menstrual blood, prostatic

secretions, or semen (possible false positive)

- Failure to properly store the specimen during the collection period or to send the specimen to the laboratory immediately after the collection is completed (possible false positive from protein deterioration)
- False-positive results from high doses of penicillin or aspirin

Nursing Considerations

Before the Test

- Confirm the patient's identity using two patient identifiers and confirmation of the patient's identification bracelet according to facility policy.
- Inform the patient that the Bence Jones protein test can detect an abnormal protein in the urine.
- Tell the patient that the test requires an early-morning urine specimen; teach how to collect a specimen.
- Instruct the patient not to contaminate the urine specimen with toilet tissue or stools.

During the Test

- Assist with or have the patient collect at least 50 mL of an early-morning, midstream clean-catch urine specimen.

After the Test

- Send the specimen to the laboratory immediately after collection, or refrigerate it if transport is delayed. A refrigerated specimen must be analyzed within 24 hours, or it should be discarded.

Beta-Hydroxybutyrate Assay

Reference Values

Less than 0.4 mmol/L (SI, less than 0.4 mmol/L)

Critical Values

Greater than 2 mmol/L (SI, greater than 2 mmol/L)

Abnormal Findings

Elevated Levels

- Worsening ketosis

Nursing Implications

- Report immediately any levels greater than 2 mmol/L (SI, greater than 2 mmol/L) to the health care provider.

Purpose

- To diagnose carbohydrate deprivation, which may result from starvation, digestive disturbances, dietary imbalances, or frequent vomiting
- To help diagnose diabetes resulting from decreased carbohydrate intake
- To help diagnose glycogen storage diseases, specifically von Gierke's disease
- To diagnose or monitor the treatment of metabolic disorders, such as diabetic ketoacidosis or lactic acidosis

Description

The beta-hydroxybutyrate test is used to measure serum levels of beta-hydroxybutyric acid (beta-hydroxybutyrate), one of the three ketone bodies. The other two ketone bodies are acetoacetate and acetone. An accumulation of all three ketone bodies is referred to as *ketosis;* excessive formation of ketone bodies in the blood is called *ketonemia.*

Interfering Factors

- Presence of lactate dehydrogenase at high concentrations and lactic acid at concentrations greater than 10 mmol/L (SI, greater than 10 mmol/L) (possible increase)
- Increased sodium fluoride concentrations (possible decrease)
- Fasting (increase with extended fasting time)

Nursing Considerations

Before the Test

- Confirm the patient's identity using two patient identifiers and confirmation of the patient's identification bracelet according to facility policy.

- Explain to the patient that this test is used to evaluate ketones in the blood.
- Inform the patient that the test requires a blood sample from a venipuncture.
- Advise the patient that there may be slight discomfort from the needle puncture and the tourniquet.
- Inform the patient that there are no food or fluid restrictions.

During the Test

- Perform a venipuncture and collect the sample in a 5-mL clot activator tube.
- Allow the sample to clot.
- Centrifuge the sample and remove the serum.
- If an acetone level is requested, have this analysis performed first.
- Send the sample to the laboratory immediately.
- Keep in mind that serum beta-hydroxybutyrate remains stable for at least 1 week at 25.6°F to 46.4°F (−3.5°C–8°C). Plasma is also an acceptable sample for beta-hydroxybutyrate analysis.

After the Test

- Apply pressure to the venipuncture site until bleeding stops.
- Assess the venipuncture site for hematoma formation; if one develops, apply direct pressure.

Bilirubin (Serum)

Reference Values

Adults: Indirect serum bilirubin levels, 0.1 to 1.0 mg/dL (SI, 1.7–17.1 mcmol/L); direct serum bilirubin levels, less than 0.5 mg/dL (SI, less than 6.8 mcmol/L)
Neonates: Total serum bilirubin levels, 2 to 12 mg/dL (SI, 34–205 mcmol/L)

Critical Values

Neonates: Greater than 15 mg/dL (SI, greater than 257 mcmol/L)

Abnormal Findings

Elevated Levels

- Hepatic damage or severe hemolytic anemia (elevated indirect serum bilirubin)
- Hemolysis (elevated indirect and direct serum bilirubin levels)
- Congenital enzyme deficiencies such as Gilbert's syndrome
- Biliary obstruction (elevated direct serum bilirubin levels)
- Severe chronic hepatic damage (normal or near-normal direct bilirubin levels and elevated indirect bilirubin levels)

Nursing Implications

- Prepare the patient for additional testing as indicated.

Purpose

- To evaluate liver function
- To aid in the differential diagnosis of jaundice and monitor its progress
- To help diagnose biliary obstruction and hemolytic anemia
- To determine whether a neonate requires an exchange transfusion or phototherapy because of dangerously high unconjugated bilirubin levels

Description

The bilirubin test is used to measure serum levels of bilirubin, the predominant pigment in bile. Bilirubin is the major product of hemoglobin catabolism. Serum bilirubin measurements are especially significant in neonates because elevated unconjugated bilirubin can accumulate in the brain, causing irreparable damage.

Interfering Factors

- Exposure of the sample to direct sunlight or ultraviolet light (possible decrease)
- Hemolytic agents, hepatotoxic drugs, methyldopa, and rifampin (Rifadin) (possible increase)
- Barbiturates and sulfonamides (possible decrease)

B

Precautions
- Protect the sample from strong sunlight and ultraviolet light.
- Handle the sample gently.

Nursing Considerations
Before the Test
- Confirm the patient's identity using two patient identifiers and confirmation of the patient's identification bracelet according to facility policy.
- Explain to the patient that the bilirubin test is used to evaluate liver function and the condition of red blood cells.
- Inform the patient that the test requires a blood sample from a venipuncture.
- Advise the patient there may be slight discomfort from the tourniquet and needle puncture.

▶ *Quality and Safety Nursing Alert*

If the patient is an infant, tell the parents that a small amount of blood will be drawn from the child's heel. Tell them who will be performing the heel stick and when.

- Inform the patient that there is no need to restrict fluids, but the patient should fast for at least 4 hours before the test.

▶ *Quality and Safety Nursing Alert*

Fasting isn't necessary for the neonate.

During the Test
- If the patient is an adult, perform a venipuncture and collect the sample in a 3- or 4-mL clot activator tube.

▶ *Quality and Safety Nursing Alert*

If the patient is an infant, perform a heel stick and fill the microcapillary tube to the designated level with blood.

After the Test
- Apply direct pressure to the venipuncture site until bleeding stops and to prevent hematoma formation.

▶ *Quality and Safety Nursing Alert*

Prepare the neonate for an exchange transfusion if total bilirubin levels are 15 mg/dL (SI, 257 mcmol/L) or more.

Bilirubin (Urine)
Reference Values
Negative for bilirubin

Abnormal Findings
- Positive for bilirubin

Nursing Implications
- The specimen's appearance (dark, with yellow foam) may indicate high direct bilirubin concentrations.
- The presence or absence of direct bilirubin in urine must be correlated with serum test results and with urine and fecal urobilinogen levels. (See the *Comparative Values of Bilirubin and Urobilinogen* table.)

Purpose
- To help identify the cause of jaundice
- To compare urine and serum bilirubin levels and other liver enzyme tests to detect liver disorders

Description
The bilirubin screening test, based on a color reaction with a specific reagent, detects water-soluble direct (conjugated) bilirubin in the urine. Detectable amounts of bilirubin in the urine may indicate liver disease caused by infections, biliary disease, or hepatotoxicity. When combined with urobilinogen measurements, the bilirubin test helps identify disorders that can cause jaundice. The analysis can be performed at the bedside, using a bilirubin reagent strip, or in the laboratory.

Comparative Values of Bilirubin and Urobilinogen

B

	Serum		Urine		Stool
Cause of Jaundice	Indirect Bilirubin	Direct Bilirubin	Bilirubin	Urobilinogen	Urobilinogen
Unconjugated Hyperbilirubinemia					
Hemolytic disorders: hemolytic anemia, erythroblastosis fetalis	↑	N	O	N↑	↑
Gilbert's syndrome: constitutional hepatic dysfunction	↑↑	N	O	N↓	N↓
Crigler-Najjar's syndrome: congenital hyperbilirubinemia	↑↑↑	N	O	N↑	N↓
Conjugated Hyperbilirubinemia					
Extrahepatic obstruction: calculi, tumor, scar tissue in common bile duct or hepatic excretory duct	N	↑	+	↓O	↓O
Hepatocellular disorders: viral, toxic, or alcoholic hepatitis; cirrhosis; parenchymal injury	N	↑	+	↓N↑	N↑
Hepatocanalicular disorders or intrahepatic obstruction: drug-induced cholestasis; some familial defects such as Dubin-Johnson's and Rotor's syndromes; viral hepatitis; and primary biliary cirrhosis	↑	↑	+	↓N↑	N↑

KEY

↑	Increased	O	Absent	
N↑	May be increased	+	Present	
↑↑	Moderately increased	N↓	Normal or reduced	
↑↑↑	Markedly increased	↓O	Decrease or absent	
N	Normal	↓N↑	Variable	

Interfering Factors

- Failure to test the specimen promptly or send it to the laboratory immediately after collection
- Phenazopyridine and phenothiazine derivatives (chlorpromazine and acetophenazine maleate) (false positive)
- Large amounts of ascorbic acid and nitrite (false negative if using dipstick testing, such as Chemstrip or N-Multistix)
- Exposure of specimen to room temperature or light (decrease due to bilirubin degradation)

Precautions

- Use only a freshly voided specimen. Bilirubin disintegrates after 30 minutes of exposure to room temperature or light. If the specimen is to be analyzed in the laboratory, send it there immediately.
- If the specimen is tested at the bedside, make sure 20 seconds elapse before interpreting the color change on the dipstick. Make sure lighting is adequate to make this color determination.

B

Nursing Considerations

Before the Test

- Confirm the patient's identity using two patient identifiers and confirmation of the patient's identification bracelet according to facility policy.
- Explain to the patient that the urine bilirubin test helps determine the cause of jaundice.
- Inform the patient that the test requires a random urine specimen and that there are no food or fluid restrictions before this test.
- Advise the patient that the specimen will be tested at the bedside or in the laboratory.
- Notify the laboratory and health care provider about any medications the patient is taking that may affect test results; these may need to be restricted.

During the Test

- Collect a random urine specimen in the container provided.
- For bedside analysis using a dipstick, follow this procedure:
  - Dip the reagent strip into the specimen and remove it immediately.
  - Compare the strip color with the color standards after 20 seconds.
  - Record the test results on the patient's chart.
- For bedside analysis using the Ictotest method, follow this procedure:
  - Place five drops of urine on the asbestos–cellulose test mat. If bilirubin is present, it will be absorbed into the mat.
  - Put a reagent tablet on the wet area of the mat, and place two drops of water on the tablet. If bilirubin is present, a blue-to-purple coloration will develop on the mat. Pink or red indicates the absence of bilirubin.

After the Test

- Instruct the patient to resume usual medications, as ordered.

Bioterrorism Infectious Agents Testing

Normal Findings

- Cultures negative for the suspected organism
- No increase in response to repetitive nerve stimulation (if an electromyogram is performed for suspected botulism)

Abnormal Findings

- Evidence of causative organism growth
- Guarnieri's bodies present in the lesion scrapings and brick-shaped virions via electron microscopy (for smallpox)

Nursing Implications

- Institute appropriate infection control measures, as indicated.
- Report findings to the appropriate infection control agency, as required.

Purpose

- To isolate and identify the causative organism

Description

Numerous agents can be used to treat the effects of bioterrorism. The most common infections associated with bioterrorism include botulism, anthrax, hemorrhagic fever, Hantaan virus, Ebola virus, yellow fever infections, plague, smallpox, and tularemia. Various specimen collection methods may be used to diagnose a bioterroristic agent infection, depending on the causative agent and site of entry. (See the *Understanding Bioterrorism Infectious Agents* table.) These methods include cultures of blood, sputum, urine, emesis or gastric aspirate, stools, lymph node aspirate, or scrapings from lesions. Regardless of the method used, suspected cases of infection must be reported to local, state, and federal health departments.

Understanding Bioterrorism Infectious Agents

Infectious Agent	Mode of Transmission	Mode of Entry	Specimen for Testing
Clostridium botulinum (spore-forming obligate anaerobe causing botulism)	• Soil • Undercooked food not kept warm	• Mucosal surface (GI tract, lung) • Wound	• Blood, stools, gastric aspirate, emesis • Suspected contaminated food substance
Bacillus anthracis (spore-forming, gram-positive bacillus causing anthrax)	• Undercooked meat from infected animals • Inhalation of animal products such as the animal's wool • Intentional release of spores	• Skin • Inhalation • GI tract	• Blood, sputum, or stools • Fluid from lesion
Viruses for hemorrhagic fever and yellow fever (including Hantaan virus, Ebola virus)	• Bite of infected animal, rodent, or insect	• Skin	• Blood, sputum, tissue, or urine
Yersinia pestis (causing plague)	• Infected flea bite	• Skin	• Blood, sputum, or lymph node aspirate
Variola virus (causing smallpox)	• Airborne via coughing • Direct contact • Contaminated clothing or bedding	• Lungs	• Fluid from lesion
Francisella tularensis (intracellular parasite causing tularemia)	• Infected animals, such as mice, squirrels, or rabbits • Contaminated water, soil, or vegetation	• Skin, mucous membranes • Lungs • GI tract	• Respiratory secretions and blood • Lymph node biopsy • Lesion scrapings

Interfering Factors
• Saline solution in an enema to collect a stool specimen in a patient with botulism
• Anticholinesterase agent use by the patient being tested for botulism

Precautions
• Adhere to standard precautions during collection of all specimens.
• Institute airborne precautions, and use negative-pressure rooms for patients with suspected infection of hemorrhagic fever, Hantaan virus, Ebola virus, and yellow fever.
• Clean contaminated surfaces and spills with appropriate solution, such as a hypochlorite bleach solution.
• Make sure that specimens being examined for smallpox are performed in a biosafety laboratory (level 4); specimens for other infections are studied in a biosafety laboratory (level 2).

B

Nursing Considerations

Before the Test

- Confirm the patient's identity using two patient identifiers and confirmation of the patient's identification bracelet according to facility policy.
- Explain to the patient that the bioterrorism infectious agents test is used to help identify the organism causing the patient's signs and symptoms.
- Wear personal protective equipment prior to collecting any specimen when biologic contaminants are suspected.
- Describe the method and procedure to be used to obtain the sample or specimen, such as blood, stools, or sputum.
- Inform the patient when and where the sample or specimen will be collected, and who will be collecting it. Explain how many samples or specimens will need to be collected.
- Inform the patient that there are no food or fluid restrictions for this test.
- If botulism is suspected, inform the patient that an electromyogram may be done to identify the cause of acute flaccid paralysis.

During the Test

- Obtain the samples or specimens as ordered, based on the suspected infectious agent.
- Place blood samples on ice; refrigerate all samples and specimens for botulinum toxin testing.

> ▶ *Quality and Safety Nursing Alert*
>
> If stools are being cultured for botulism testing and the patient is constipated, administer an enema using sterile water as the solution to ensure that an adequate specimen is obtained.

- Collect vesicular fluid from a previously unopened lesion on at least one culture swab when testing for cutaneous anthrax and smallpox.
- Obtain three blood cultures along with specimens of gastric aspirate, stools, or food if GI anthrax is suspected.
- When obtaining specimens for tularemia, have the patient provide a forced deep cough for a sputum specimen; obtain a lesional specimen from the leading edge of the lesion.

After the Test

- Send the sample or specimen to the laboratory for a "mouse" assay to evaluate for botulinum toxin.
- Send any food that's being tested (for botulism) in its original container.
- Send each sample or specimen to the laboratory immediately.

Bladder Cancer Markers

Reference Values

BTA less than 14 units/mL
NMP22 less than 10 units/mL

Abnormal Findings

Elevated Levels
- Bladder cancer

Nursing Implications
- Prepare the patient for additional testing.
- Provide support to the patient during the diagnosis period.

Purpose

- To monitor and detect bladder cancer recurrence
- To identify individuals at risk for bladder cancer

Description

For bladder cancer, two specific markers in the urine have been identified: BTA and NMP22. BTA is a protein-related substance produced by bladder cancer cells. NMP22 is a nuclear matrix protein that's excreted in the urine when the nucleus of the bladder cancer cells becomes disrupted. In the patient without bladder cancer, these elements are absent or present in only very minimal amounts. However, in the patient with bladder cancer, these elements are elevated.

Bladder cancer markers are helpful in monitoring the patient diagnosed with bladder cancer to evaluate for recurrence after surgical resection. These tests commonly are done in conjunction with a cystoscopy. In addition, NMP22 may also be used to screen individuals who may be at highest risk for recurrence, as well as for those at risk for developing bladder cancer.

Interfering Factors

- Failure to stabilize urine immediately after collection
- Recent urologic surgery, urinary tract infection, or urinary calculi (increase in BTA levels)
- Presence of cancer of the ureters or renal pelvis (increase in both markers)

Nursing Considerations

Before the Test

- Confirm the patient's identity using two patient identifiers and confirmation of the patient's identification bracelet according to facility policy.
- Explain the purpose of the bladder cancer marker test and how it may be helpful in monitoring the patient's disorder, as appropriate.
- Inform the patient that the procedure involves obtaining a urine specimen.
- Tell the patient that there is no need to restrict food or fluids.

During the Test

- Obtain a random voided urine specimen before noon.

After the Test

- Send the urine specimen to the laboratory immediately.
- Refrigerate the specimen if there will be a delay in getting it to the laboratory.
- Provide support to the patient while awaiting results.

Bleeding Time

B

Reference Values

Template method: 3 to 6 minutes (SI, 3–6 minutes)
Ivy method: 3 to 6 minutes
Duke method: 1 to 3 minutes (SI, 1–3 minutes)

Critical Values

Greater than 15 minutes (SI, 15 minutes)

Abnormal Findings

Elevated Levels (Prolonged Bleeding)

- Disorders associated with thrombocytopenia, such as Hodgkin's disease, acute leukemia, disseminated intravascular coagulation, hemolytic disease of the neonate, Schönlein-Henoch purpura, severe hepatic disease (cirrhosis, for example), or severe deficiency of factors I, II, V, VII, VIII, IX, and XI
- Platelet function disorders such as thrombasthenia, thrombocytopathia (prolonged bleeding time with a normal platelet count)
- Severe liver disease
- Advanced renal failure

Nursing Implications

- Anticipate the need for additional testing.
- Prepare the patient with a platelet function disorder for further investigation through clot retraction, prothrombin consumption, and platelet aggregation tests.

Purpose

- To assess overall hemostatic function (platelet response to injury and functional capacity of vasoconstriction)
- To detect congenital and acquired platelet function disorders

Description

Bleeding time is used to measure the duration of bleeding after a measured

B

skin incision. Bleeding time may be measured by one of three methods: template, Ivy, or Duke. The template method is the most commonly used and the most accurate because the incision size is standardized. Bleeding time depends on the elasticity of the blood vessel wall and on the number and functional capacity of platelets.

Although the bleeding time test is usually performed on the patient with a personal or family history of bleeding disorders, it's also useful—along with a platelet count—for preoperative screening.

Interfering Factors
• Anticoagulants, antineoplastics, aspirin and aspirin compounds, nonsteroidal anti-inflammatory drugs, sulfonamides, thiazide diuretics, vitamin E supplementation, and some nonopioid analgesics (can cause prolonged bleeding time)
• Touching the puncture site while performing the test will break off fibrin particles and prolong the bleeding time.
• Edema or cyanosis of the hands
• Extreme hot or cold conditions

Nursing Considerations
Before the Test
• Confirm the patient's identity using two patient identifiers and confirmation of the patient's identification bracelet according to facility policy.
• Confirm that the patient has not been taking anticoagulant, aspirin, or over-the-counter cold medications (may contain salicylates) for 3 days before the test (or as recommended by health care provider).
• Explain to the patient that the bleeding time test involves making tiny incisions or punctures and that it's used to measure the time required to form a clot and stop bleeding. Inform the patient that there are no food or fluid restrictions for the test.

• Advise the patient that there may be some discomfort from the incisions, the antiseptic, and the tightness of the blood pressure cuff. Also, depending on the method used, incisions or punctures may leave tiny scars that should be barely visible when healed.
• Check the patient's baseline platelet count. (The test isn't usually recommended for the patient with a platelet count of less than 75,000/mcL [SI, 75×10^9/L].)
• Notify the laboratory and health care provider about any medications the patient is taking that may affect test results; these may need to be restricted.

During the Test
Template Method
• Wrap the pressure cuff around the upper arm and inflate the cuff to 40 mm Hg, being sure to maintain a cuff pressure of 40 mm Hg throughout the test.
• Select an area on the forearm with no superficial veins and clean it with antiseptic. Allow the skin to dry completely before making the incision.
• Apply the appropriate template lengthwise to the forearm.
• Use the lancet to make two incisions 1 mm deep and 9 mm long.
• Start the stopwatch.
• Without touching the cuts, gently blot the drops of blood with filter paper every 30 seconds until the bleeding stops in both cuts.
• Average the time of the two cuts and record the result.

Ivy Method
• After applying the pressure cuff and preparing the test site, make three small punctures with a disposable lancet.
• Start the stopwatch.
• Taking care not to touch the punctures, blot each site with filter paper every 30 seconds until the bleeding stops.

- Average the bleeding time of the three punctures and record the result.

Duke Method
- Drape the patient's shoulder with a towel.
- Clean the earlobe and let the skin air-dry.
- Make a puncture wound 2 to 4 mm deep on the earlobe with a disposable lancet.
- Start the stopwatch.
- Being careful not to touch the ear, blot the site with filter paper every 30 seconds until bleeding stops.
- Record the bleeding time.

 Quality and Safety Nursing Alert

If the bleeding doesn't diminish after 15 minutes with any test, discontinue the test.

After the Test
- For a patient with a bleeding tendency (such as hemophilia), maintain a pressure bandage over the incision for 24 to 48 hours to prevent further bleeding. Check the test area frequently; keep the edges of the cuts aligned to minimize scarring.
- For other patients, apply a piece of gauze held in place with an adhesive bandage.
- Instruct the patient to resume any medications that were discontinued before the test, as ordered.

Blood Culture

Reference Values
Negative for pathogens

Abnormal Findings

Elevated Levels (Positive Cultures)
- Mild, transient bacteremia infections
- Infections due to *Streptococcus pneumoniae* and other *Streptococcus* species,

Haemophilus influenzae, Staphylococcus aureus, Pseudomonas aeruginosa, Bacteroides spp., *Brucella* spp., Enterobacteriaceae, coliform bacilli, and *Candida albicans*
- *Staphylococcus epidermidis*, diphtheroids, and *Propionibacterium* (in immunocompromised patients)
- *Mycobacterium tuberculosis* and M. *avium* complex (in patients with human immunodeficiency virus infection)

Nursing Implications
- Institute appropriate infection control precautions as indicated by the causative organism.
- Adhere to standard precautions at all times.
- Expect to collect samples over the course of 2 consecutive days.

Purpose
- To confirm bacteremia
- To identify the causative organism in bacteremia and septicemia

Description
A blood culture is performed to isolate and aid in the identification of the pathogens in bacteremia (bacterial invasion of the bloodstream) and septicemia (systemic spread of such infection). It requires inoculating a culture medium with a blood sample and incubating it. Blood cultures can identify about 67% of pathogens within 24 hours and up to 90% within 72 hours.

Bacteremia may be transient, intermittent, or continuous. The timing of sample collection for blood cultures varies; it usually depends on the suspected type of bacteremia (intermittent or continuous) and on whether drug therapy needs to be started regardless of test results.

Interfering Factors
- Previous or current antimicrobial therapy (possible false negative)

- Removal of culture bottle caps at the bedside (possible prevention of anaerobic growth)
- Use of the incorrect bottle and media (possible prevention of aerobic growth)

Precautions
- Avoid drawing blood from an existing IV catheter.
- Use a vein below an IV catheter or in the opposite arm.

Nursing Considerations
Before the Test
- Confirm the patient's identity using two patient identifiers and confirmation of the patient's identification bracelet according to facility policy.
- Explain to the patient that the blood culture procedure is used to help identify the organism causing his or her symptoms.
- Inform the patient that there are no food or fluid restrictions for this test.
- Advise the patient that there may be slight discomfort from the tourniquet and needle punctures.

During the Test
- Put on appropriate personal protective equipment.
- Clean the venipuncture site with an alcohol swab and then with an iodine swab, working in a circular motion from the site outward.
- Wait at least 1 minute for the patient's skin to dry, then remove the residual iodine with an alcohol swab or remove the iodine after venipuncture.
- Apply the tourniquet.
- Perform a venipuncture; draw 10 to 20 mL of blood for an adult.

> ▶ *Quality and Safety Nursing Alert*
>
> If the patient is a child, collect a 2- to 6-mL sample.

- Clean the diaphragm tops of the culture bottles with alcohol or iodine (or other antiseptic agent per facility policy) and change the needle on the syringe.
- If broth is used, add blood to each bottle until a 1:5 or 1:10 dilution is obtained. For example, add 10 mL of blood to a 100-mL bottle. (The size of the bottle varies, depending on facility procedure.)
- If a special resin is used, add blood to the resin in the bottles and invert them gently to mix.
- If the lysis–centrifugation technique (Isolator) is used, draw the blood directly into a special collection and processing tube.
- Indicate the tentative diagnosis on the laboratory request, as well as current or recent antimicrobial therapy.
- Send each sample to the laboratory immediately after collection.

After the Test
- Apply direct pressure to the venipuncture site until bleeding stops and to prevent hematoma formation.
- Prepare to initiate antimicrobial therapy, as ordered.

Blood Smear
Normal Findings
- Red blood cell (RBC), white blood cell (WBC), and platelet numbers within normal parameters
- Normocytic, normochromic RBCs
- WBC differential within normal parameters

Abnormal Findings
- Microcytic, hypochromic RBCs, indicating anemia or thalassemia
- Macrocytic RBCs, indicating vitamin B_{12} or folic acid–deficiency anemia
- Sickle-shaped RBCs, indicating sickle cell anemia
- Small, round RBCs, indicating hereditary spherocytosis

- Heinz bodies, indicating hemoglobin-opathies or hemolytic anemia
- Increased numbers of immature WBCs, indicating leukemia and infection

Nursing Implications
- Anticipate the need for additional testing.
- Institute measures to reduce the patient's risk of infection and bleeding.

Purpose
- To identify the effect of disease on blood cells
- To diagnose congenital and acquired diseases

Description
A blood smear involves obtaining a blood sample and placing it on a slide for microscopic examination of its constituents. Use of a blood smear can aid in the detection of diseases, as well as of a disease's effect on blood components.

Nursing Considerations
Before the Test
- Confirm the patient's identity using two patient identifiers and confirmation of the patient's identification bracelet according to facility policy.
- Explain to the patient that the test is used to identify possible anemia.
- Inform the patient that there are no food or fluid restrictions for this test.
- Advise the patient that the test involves a finger stick or heel stick sample of blood.
- If necessary, a venipuncture may be done to obtain a sample for testing. If this is the case, inform the patient that you'll need to perform a venipuncture and tell him or her what to expect.
- Inform the patient that there may be slight discomfort from the needle puncture.

During the Test
- Perform the finger stick or heel stick.

- Place the sample (drop of blood) in a laboratory-approved device for application to a slide; if necessary, perform a venipuncture to obtain a sample.
- Transport the sample to the laboratory immediately, where it will be studied using an automated calculation device and evaluated by a technologist and pathologist.

After the Test
- Apply direct pressure to the puncture site until bleeding stops and to prevent the formation of a hematoma.

Blood Urea Nitrogen (BUN)
Reference Values
8 to 20 mg/dL (SI, 2.9–7.5 mmol/L)
Elderly patients: Slightly higher, possibly to 69 mg/dL (SI, 25.8 mmol/L)

Critical Values
Less than 2 mg/dL (SI, 0.71 mmol/L)
Greater than 80 mg/dL (SI, 2.85 mmol/L)

Abnormal Findings
Elevated Levels
- Renal disease (greater than 100 mg indicates serious impairment of renal function)
- Reduced renal blood flow (due to dehydration, for example)
- Urinary tract obstruction
- Increased protein catabolism (such as with burns)
- Congestive heart failure
- Diabetes with ketoacidosis

Decreased Levels
- Severe hepatic damage
- Malnutrition
- Overhydration
- Acromegaly
- Nephrotic syndrome

Nursing Implications
- Explain the underlying problem associated with the elevated levels.

B

- Institute measures, as ordered, to correct nutritional and fluid imbalances indicated by decreased levels.
- Prepare the patient for additional testing, as needed.

Purpose
- To evaluate kidney function and aid in the diagnosis of renal disease
- To aid in the assessment of hydration

Description
The blood urea nitrogen (BUN) test is used to measure the nitrogen fraction of urea, the chief end product of protein metabolism. Formed in the liver from ammonia and excreted by the kidneys, urea constitutes 40% to 50% of the blood's nonprotein nitrogen content. BUN level reflects protein intake and renal excretory capacity, but it's a less reliable indicator of uremia than the serum creatinine level.

Interfering Factors
- Chloramphenicol and tetracyclines (possible decrease)
- Anabolic steroids, aminoglycosides, and amphotericin B (possible increase)
- Overhydration and underhydration will affect BUN levels

Nursing Considerations
Before the Test
- Confirm the patient's identity using two patient identifiers and confirmation of the patient's identification bracelet according to facility policy.
- Tell the patient that the BUN test is used to evaluate kidney function.
- Inform the patient to limit meat intake (protein intake affects BUN levels). There are no other food or fluid restrictions.
- Explain to the patient that that the test requires a blood sample from a venipuncture. Advise the patient that there may be slight discomfort from the tourniquet and needle puncture.

- Notify the laboratory and health care provider about any medications the patient is taking that may affect test results; these may need to be restricted.

During the Test
- Perform a venipuncture and collect the sample in a 3- to 4-mL clot activator tube.

After the Test
- Handle the sample gently and send it to the laboratory immediately.
- Apply direct pressure to the venipuncture site until bleeding stops and to prevent the formation of a hematoma.
- Inform the patient to resume medications that were discontinued before the test, as ordered.

Bone Biopsy (Also Called Needle Biopsy)

Normal Findings
- Evidence of normal bone tissue (collagen, osteocytes, and osteoblasts fibers) that may be compact (dense, concentric layers of mineral deposits, or lamellae) or cancellous (widely spaced lamellae, with osteocytes and red and yellow marrow between them)

Abnormal Findings
- Benign tumors, including osteoid osteoma, osteoblastoma, osteochondroma, unicameral bone cyst, benign giant cell tumor, and fibroma
- Malignant tumors, including multiple myeloma, osteosarcoma, and Ewing's sarcoma (most lethal)

Nursing Implications
- Provide support to the patient during the diagnostic phase.
- Anticipate the need for additional testing.

Purpose
- To distinguish between benign and malignant bone tumors

B

Description

Bone biopsy is the removal of a piece or a core of bone for histologic examination. A bone biopsy may be indicated for patients with bone pain and tenderness after bone scan, computed tomography scan, X-ray, or arteriography reveals a mass or deformity. It's performed either by using a special drill needle under local anesthesia or by surgical excision under general anesthesia. Excision provides a larger specimen than does drill biopsy and permits immediate surgical treatment if quick histologic analysis of the specimen reveals cancer.

The usual procedures for bone biopsy are as follows:

Drill Biopsy

- The patient is properly positioned, and the biopsy site is clipped and prepared.
- After local anesthetic is injected, a small incision (usually about 3 mm) is made and the biopsy needle with a pointed trocar is pushed into the bone and then rotated about 180 degrees.
- When the bone core is obtained, the trocar is withdrawn and the specimen is placed in a properly labeled bottle containing 10% formalin solution. Then pressure is applied to the site with a sterile gauze pad.
- After bleeding stops, a topical antiseptic (povidone–iodine ointment) is applied, along with an adhesive bandage or other sterile covering, to close the wound and prevent infection.

Open Biopsy

- The patient is anesthetized and the biopsy site is clipped, cleaned with surgical soap, and disinfected with an iodine wash and alcohol.
- An incision is made and a piece of bone is removed and sent to the histology laboratory immediately for analysis. Further surgery can then be performed, depending on findings.

Interfering Factors

- Failure to obtain a representative bone specimen
- Failure to use the proper fixative

Precautions

- Bone biopsy should be performed cautiously in the patient with coagulopathy to reduce the risk of bleeding.
- Determine whether the patient is on anticoagulant therapy.

Nursing Considerations

Before the Test

- Confirm the patient's identity using two patient identifiers and confirmation of the patient's identification bracelet according to facility policy.
- Explain to the patient that a bone biopsy permits microscopic examination of a bone specimen. Explain the procedure and answer questions.
- Inform the patient who will perform the biopsy, and where and when it will be done.
- Advise the patient undergoing a drill biopsy that there are no food and fluid restrictions; however, if the patient is undergoing open biopsy, an overnight fast is required before the procedure.
- Inform the patient that a local anesthetic will be given, but that discomfort and pressure will be felt when the biopsy needle enters the bone.
- Explain that a special drill forces the needle into the bone; if possible, show a photograph of the bone drill. Stress the importance of cooperation during the biopsy.
- Make sure the patient or a responsible family member has signed an informed consent form.
- Check the patient's history for hypersensitivity to the local anesthetic used.

During the Test

- Assist with specimen collection and patient positioning, if appropriate.

B

After the Test
- Send the specimen to the laboratory immediately.
- Check the patient's vital signs and the dressing at the biopsy site. Determine how much drainage is expected and report excessive amounts.
- If the patient experiences pain, administer an analgesic as ordered.

> ▶ *Quality and Safety Nursing Alert*
>
> **For several days after the biopsy, watch for and report indications of bone infection, including fever, headache, pain on movement, and redness or abscess near the biopsy site. Notify the health care provider if any of these signs or symptoms develop.**

- The patient may resume a usual diet.
- Monitor the patient for possible complications, including bone fracture, damage to surrounding tissue, infection (osteomyelitis) and, possibly, contamination of normal tissue with tumor cells.

Bone Densitometry

Normal Findings
- Negative for osteoporosis or osteopenia
- T-score less than 1 SD below normal (greater than −1)

Abnormal Findings
- 2.5 SD below normal (−1 to −2.5); suggests osteopenia
- Greater than 2.5 SD below normal (less than −2.5) suggests osteoporosis

Nursing Implications
- Prepare the patient for additional testing.

Purpose
- To determine bone mineral density
- To identify the risk of osteoporosis

- To evaluate clinical response to therapy for reducing the rate of bone loss

Description
Bone densitometry assesses bone mass quantitatively. This noninvasive technique, also known as *dual energy X-ray absorptiometry* or *DEXA*, uses an X-ray tube to measure bone mineral density but exposes the patient to only minimal radiation. The images detected are computer analyzed to determine bone mineral status. The computer calculates the size and thickness of the bone, as well as its volumetric density, to determine its potential resistance to mechanical stress. It may be performed in the radiology department of a health care facility, a health care provider's office, or a clinic.

The test involves positioning the patient on a table under the scanning device, with the radiation source below and the detector above. The detector then measures the bone's radiation absorption and produces a digital readout.

Interfering Factors
- Osteoarthritis (possible decrease)
- Fat tissue (poor visualization)
- Fractures
- Size of region to be scanned

Precautions
- Bone densitometry is contraindicated during pregnancy.
- The value and reliability of bone densitometry as a predictor of fractures are still being studied.
- Controversy exists regarding the scanning site and whether bone loss occurs as a general phenomenon or occurs first in the spine; large-scale studies are being conducted to establish an "at-risk" level of bone density to help predict fractures.

Nursing Considerations

Before the Test
- Confirm the patient's identity using two patient identifiers and

B

confirmation of the patient's identification bracelet according to facility
policy.
• Assure the patient that the bone
densitometry test is painless and that
the exposure to radiation is minimal.
• Advise the patient that the test will
take from 10 minutes to 1 hour,
depending on the areas to be scanned.
• Tell the patient who will perform the
test, and where and when it will take
place.
• Instruct the patient to remove all
metallic objects from the area to be
scanned.

Bone Marrow Aspiration and Biopsy

Normal Findings
• Yellow marrow containing fat cells
and connective tissue; red marrow
containing hematopoietic cells, fat
cells, and connective tissue
• +2 level iron stain (used to measure
hemosiderin [storage iron])
• Negative Sudan black B (SBB) fat
stain (which shows granulocytes)
• Negative periodic acid–Schiff
(PAS) stain (used to detect glycogen
reactions)

Abnormal Findings
• See the *Bone Marrow: Normal Values
and Implications of Abnormal Findings*
table.

Nursing Implications
• Anticipate the need for additional
testing.
• Assist the patient in understanding
the implications of the results.

Purpose
• To diagnose thrombocytopenia,
leukemias, and granulomas, as well as
aplastic, hypoplastic, and pernicious
anemias
• To diagnose primary and metastatic
tumors
• To determine the cause of infection
• To aid in the staging of diseases, such
as Hodgkin's disease
• To evaluate the effectiveness of
chemotherapy and monitor myelosup-
pression

Description
Bone marrow is the soft tissue contained
in the medullary canals of the long
bones and in the interstices of cancellous bone. Red marrow, which constitutes about 50% of an adult's marrow,
actively produces stem cells that ultimately evolve into red blood cells, white

Bone Marrow: Normal Values and Implications of Abnormal Findings

| Cell Types | Normal Mean Value | | | Clinical Implications |
	Adults (%)	Children (%)	Infants (%)	
Normoblasts, total	25.6	23.1	8	*Elevated values:* polycythe-mia vera
Pronormoblasts	0.2 to 1.3	0.5	0.1	*Depressed values:* vitamin
Basophilic	0.5 to 2.4	1.7	0.34	B$_{12}$ or folic acid deficien-
Polychromatic	17.9 to 29.2	18.2	6.9	cy; hypoplastic or aplastic
Orthochromatic	0.4 to 4.6	2.7	0.54	anemia
Neutrophils, total	56.5	57.1	32.4	*Elevated values:* acute
Myeloblasts	0.2 to 1.5	1.2	0.62	myeloblastic or chronic
Promyelocytes	2.1 to 4.1	1.4	0.76	myeloid leukemia
Myelocytes	8.2 to 15.7	18.3	2.5	*Depressed values:* lympho-
Metamyelocytes	9.6 to 24.6	23.3	11.3	blastic, lymphatic, or
Bands	9.5 to 15.3	0	14.1	monocytic leukemia;
Segmented	6 to 12	12.9	3.6	aplastic anemia

(continued on page 100)

B

Bone Marrow: Normal Values and Implications of Abnormal Findings (continued)

Cell Types	Normal Mean Value			Clinical Implications
	Adults (%)	Children (%)	Infants (%)	
Eosinophils	3.1	3.6	2.6	*Elevated values:* bone marrow carcinoma, lymphadenoma, myeloid leukemia, eosinophilic leukemia, pernicious anemia (in relapse)
Plasma cells	1.3	0.4	0.02	*Elevated values:* myeloma, collagen disease, infection, antigen sensitivity, malignancy
Basophils	0.01	0.06	0.07	*Elevated values:* no relation between basophil count and symptoms *Depressed values:* no relation between basophil count and symptoms
Lymphocytes	16.2	16.2	49	*Elevated values:* B- and T-cell chronic lymphocytic leukemia, other lymphatic leukemias, lymphoma, mononucleosis, aplastic anemia, macroglobulinemia
Plasma cells	1.3	0.4	0.02	*Elevated values:* myeloma, collagen disease, infection, antigen sensitivity, malignancy
Megakaryocytes	0.1	0.1	0.05	*Elevated values:* advanced age, chronic myeloid leukemia, polycythemia vera, megakaryocytic myelosis, infection, idiopathic thrombocytopenic purpura, thrombocytopenia *Depressed values:* pernicious anemia
Myeloid/erythroid ratio	2:1 to 4:1	2.9:1	4.4:1	*Elevated values:* myeloid leukemia, infection, leukemoid reactions, depressed hematopoiesis *Depressed values:* agranulocytosis, hematopoiesis after hemorrhage or hemolysis, iron deficiency anemia, polycythemia vera

blood cells, and platelets. Yellow marrow contains fat cells and connective tissue and is inactive, but it can become active in response to the body's needs. The histologic and hematologic examination of bone marrow provides reliable diagnostic information about blood disorders. (See the *Common Sites of Bone Marrow Aspiration and Biopsy* box.)

Marrow may be removed by aspiration or needle biopsy under local anesthesia from various sites. In aspiration biopsy, a fluid specimen in which pustulate of marrow is suspended is removed from the bone marrow. In needle biopsy, a core of marrow cells (not fluid) is removed. These methods are typically used concurrently to obtain the best possible marrow specimens.

Bleeding and infection may result from bone marrow biopsy at any site, but the most serious complications occur at the sternum. Such complications are rare but include puncture of the heart and major vessels, causing severe hemorrhage, and puncture of the mediastinum, causing mediastinitis or pneumomediastinum.

The usual procedures for bone marrow removal are as follows:

Aspiration Biopsy
- After the skin over the biopsy site is prepared and the area is draped, a local anesthetic is injected. With a twisting motion, the marrow aspiration needle is inserted through the skin, the subcutaneous tissue, and the cortex of the bone.
- The stylet is removed from the needle and a 10- to 20-mL syringe is attached. The health care provider aspirates 0.2 to 0.5 mL of marrow and then withdraws the needle.
- Pressure is applied to the site for 5 minutes while the marrow slides are being prepared. (If the patient has thrombocytopenia, pressure is applied to the site for 10 to 15 minutes.)
- The biopsy site is cleaned again, and a sterile adhesive bandage is applied.
- If an adequate marrow specimen isn't obtained on the first attempt, the needle may be repositioned within the marrow cavity or removed and reinserted in another site within the anesthetized area. If the second attempt fails, a needle biopsy may be needed.

Needle Biopsy
- After preparing the biopsy site and draping the area, the health care provider marks the skin at the site with an indelible pencil or marking pen.
- A local anesthetic is then injected intradermally, subcutaneously, and at the bone's surface.
- The biopsy needle is inserted into the periosteum, and the needle guard is set as indicated. The needle is advanced with a steady boring motion until the outer needle passes through the bone's cortex.
- The inner needle with a trephine tip is inserted into the outer needle. By alternately rotating the inner needle clockwise and counterclockwise, the health care provider directs the needle into the marrow cavity and then removes a tissue plug.
- The needle assembly is withdrawn, and the marrow is expelled into a labeled bottle containing Zenker's acetic acid solution.
- After the biopsy site is cleaned, a sterile adhesive bandage or a pressure dressing is applied.

Interfering Factors
- Failure to obtain a representative specimen
- Failure to use a fixative for histologic analysis

Precautions
- Bone marrow biopsy is contraindicated in the patient with a severe bleeding disorder.

Nursing Considerations
Before the Test
- Confirm the patient's identity using two patient identifiers and confirmation of the patient's

B

Common Sites of Bone Marrow Aspiration and Biopsy

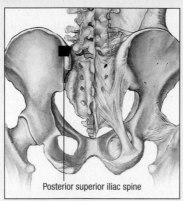

Posterior superior iliac spine

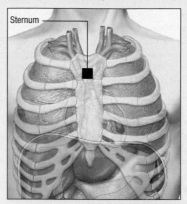

Sternum

The posterior superior iliac spine is usually the preferred site for bone marrow aspiration and biopsy because no vital organs or vessels are located nearby. With the patient in a lateral position with one leg flexed, the health care provider inserts the needle several centimeters lateral to the iliosacral junction, entering the bone plane crest with the needle directed downward and toward the anterior inferior spine or entering a few centimeters below the crest at a right angle to the surface of the bone.

The sternum involves the greatest risk but is commonly used for marrow aspiration because it's near the surface, the cortical bone is thin, and the marrow cavity contains numerous cells and relatively little fat or supporting bone. For this procedure, the patient is in a supine position on a firm bed or examination table with a small pillow beneath the shoulders to elevate the chest and lower the head. The health care provider secures the needle guard 3 to 4 mm from the tip of the needle to avoid accidental puncture of the heart or a major vessel. Then he inserts the needle at the midline of the sternum at the second intercostal space.

identification bracelet according to facility policy.

- Explain to the patient that the bone marrow aspiration and biopsy procedure permit microscopic examination of a bone marrow specimen. Describe the procedure to the patient and answer any questions.
  - Tell the patient which bone—the sternum, anterior or posterior iliac crest, vertebral spinous process, rib, or tibia—will be the biopsy site.
  - Explain that the patient will receive a local anesthetic but will feel pressure on insertion of the biopsy needle and a brief, pulling pain on removal of the marrow.
  - Inform the patient who will perform the biopsy, and where and when it will be done.

- Inform the patient that more than one bone marrow specimen may be required and that a blood sample will be collected before biopsy for laboratory testing.
- Advise the patient that there are no food or fluid restrictions for the test.
- Make sure the patient or a responsible family member has signed an informed consent form.
- Check the patient's history for hypersensitivity to the local anesthetic.
- Administer a mild sedative as prescribed 1 hour before the test.

▶ **Quality and Safety Nursing Alert**

Preparation for children requires additional steps. (See the *Preparing a Child for Bone Marrow Biopsy* box.)

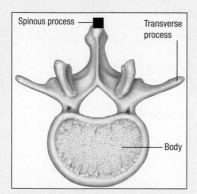

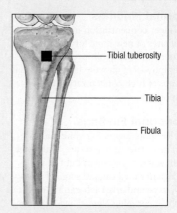

The spinous process is the preferred site if multiple punctures are necessary, marrow is absent at other sites, or the patient objects to sternal puncture. For this procedure, the patient sits on the edge of the bed, leaning over the bedside stand; or, if he's uncooperative, he may be placed in the prone position with restraints. The health care provider selects the spinous process of the third or fourth lumbar vertebra and inserts the needle at the crest or slightly to one side, advancing the needle in the direction of the bone plane.

The tibia is the site of choice for infants younger than age 1 year. The infant is placed in a prone position on a bed or examination table with a sandbag beneath the leg. The foot is taped to the surface of the table, or an assistant holds the leg stationary by placing a hand under it. The health care provider inserts the needle about 3/89 (1 cm) below the tibial tuberosity and slightly toward the medial side, being careful to angle the needle point toward the foot to avoid epiphyseal injury.

Preparing a Child for Bone Marrow Biopsy

To prepare a child for a bone marrow biopsy, give him his own biopsy kit: a syringe without a needle, cotton balls, and adhesive bandages. Act out the procedure by using a doll or a stuffed animal as a model. This will help you gain the child's confidence and answer any questions he or she may have. Be sure to prepare the child by describing the kinds of pressure and discomfort that will be felt during the procedure.

Before the biopsy, explain the equipment on the tray to the child. Encourage the parents to get involved by helping you hold the child still and providing reassurance. Tell the child that there will be some discomfort when the health care provider aspirates the bone marrow and that it's okay to cry or yell if he or she wants to, but that the discomfort will go away quickly.

During the Test
- After positioning the patient, instruct him or her to remain as still as possible.
- Offer emotional support during the biopsy by talking quietly to the patient, describing what's being done, and answering questions.

After the Test
- Send the tissue specimen or slides to the laboratory immediately.
- Check the biopsy site for bleeding and inflammation.
- Observe the patient for signs and symptoms of hemorrhage and infection, such as rapid pulse rate, low blood pressure, and fever, by monitoring vital signs per policy after procedure.
- Bed rest may be prescribed for 30 to 60 minutes after procedure.

Bone Scan

Normal Findings

- Tracer concentration in bone tissue at sites of new bone formation or increased metabolism
- Epiphyses of growing bone as normal sites of high concentration or hot spots

Abnormal Findings

- Hot spots suggesting bone malignancy, infection, fracture, and other disorders if viewed in light of the patient's medical and surgical history, X-rays, and other laboratory tests (See the *Comparing Normal and Abnormal Bone Scans* box.)

Nursing Implications

- Prepare the patient for additional testing, if indicated.
- Assist the patient in understanding the results of the test.
- Provide support in relation to the patient's diagnosis.

Purpose

- To detect or to rule out malignant bone lesions when radiographic findings are normal but cancer is confirmed or suspected
- To detect occult bone trauma due to pathologic fractures
- To monitor degenerative bone disorders
- To detect infection
- To evaluate unexplained bone pain
- To stage cancer

Description

A bone scan involves imaging the skeleton by a scanning camera after IV injection of a radioactive tracer compound. The tracer of choice, radioactive technetium diphosphonate, collects in bone tissue in increased concentrations at sites of abnormal metabolism. When scanned, these sites appear as hot spots that are typically detectable months before an X-ray can reveal a lesion. To promote early detection of lesions, this test may be performed with a gallium scan.

For this procedure, the patient is positioned on the scanner table. As the scanner head moves back and forth over the patient's body, the scanner detects low-level radiation emitted by the skeleton and translates this onto a

Comparing Normal and Abnormal Bone Scans

The scans below compare a normal bone scan with an abnormal scan. The scan on the left is normal because the isotope is distributed evenly throughout the skeletal tissue. The scan on the right is abnormal because the isotope has accumulated in multiple metastases in the ribs and spine.

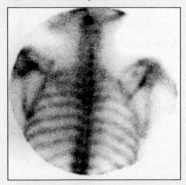
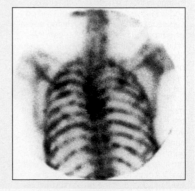

film, paper chart, or both to produce two-dimensional pictures of the area scanned.

Interfering Factors
- Distended bladder (possible obscuring of pelvic detail)
- Improper injection technique (possible seepage of tracer into muscle tissue, creating false hot spots)
- Antihypertensives (invalidate test results)

Precautions
- A bone scan is contraindicated during pregnancy or lactation.
- Allergic reactions to radionuclides may occur.

Nursing Considerations
Before the Test
- Confirm the patient's identity using two patient identifiers and confirmation of the patient's identification bracelet according to facility policy.
- Describe the bone scan procedure to the patient. Explain that this test may detect skeletal abnormalities sooner than is possible with ordinary X-rays.
- Tell the patient who will perform the test, where and when it will take place, and that it may require him or her to assume various positions on a scanner table. Emphasize that he or she must keep still for the scan.
- Assure the patient that the scan itself is painless and that the isotope, although radioactive, emits less radiation than a standard X-ray machine.
- Make sure that the patient or a responsible family member has signed an informed consent form, if required.
- Evaluate the patient's emotional state and offer support if a bone scan is ordered to diagnose cancer.
- Administer prescribed analgesics, as ordered.

- After the patient receives an IV injection of the tracer and imaging agent, encourage increased fluid intake for the next 1 to 3 hours to facilitate renal clearance of the circulating free tracer.
- Instruct the patient to void immediately before the procedure (otherwise, a urinary catheter may be inserted to empty the bladder).

> ### Quality and Safety Nursing Alert
> Anticipate the need to administer sedation to children who can't hold still for the scan.

During the Test
- If appropriate, assist with repositioning the patient several times during the test to obtain adequate views. (The scanner takes as many views as needed to cover the specified area.)

After the Test
- Check the injection site for redness or swelling. If a hematoma develops, apply direct pressure.
- Don't schedule other radionuclide tests for 24 to 48 hours.
- Instruct the patient to drink plenty of fluids and to empty the bladder frequently for the next 24 to 48 hours.
- Provide analgesics for pain resulting from positioning on the scanning table, as needed.

Bone Turnover Biochemical Markers

Reference Values

N-Telopeptide (NTx) Urine
Females: 26 to 124 nm bone collagen equivalents (BCE)/mm creatinine
Males: 21 to 83 nm BCE/mm creatinine

NTx Serum
Females: 6.2 to 19 nm BCE
Males: 5.4 to 24.2 nm BCE

B

Osteocalcin (or Bone G1a Protein [BGP]) Serum
Females: 0.7 to 6.4 ng/mL
Males: 6.4 ng/mL

Pyridinium (PYD)
Females: 15.3 to 33.6 nm/mm
Males: 10.2 to 33.6 nm/mm

Abnormal Findings

Elevated Levels
- Osteoporosis
- Paget's disease
- Primary or metastatic bone tumors
- Acromegaly
- Hyperparathyroidism
- Hyperthyroidism

Decreased Levels
- Hypoparathyroidism
- Hypothyroidism
- Cortisol therapy

Nursing Implications
- Institute measures to prevent injury in patients with elevated levels.
- Anticipate the need for therapy in patients with decreased levels.
- Prepare the patient for possible additional testing.

Purpose
- To identify changes in bone metabolism
- To evaluate effects of therapy for bone conditions

Description
Bone turnover biochemical markers provide information about bone resorption and bone formation. Three specific proteins are evaluated: NTx, a type 1 collagen that's released into the blood when bone is broken down; osteocalcin, a noncollagen protein involved with bone resorption and formation; and PYD crosslinks, which form when type 1 collagen matures. This test is helpful in determining changes in bone density after several months of therapy.

> ►► *Quality and Safety Nursing Alert*
>
> Bone turnover markers are typically elevated in children younger than age 14 because of the increased bone resorption and remodeling that occurs with growth. In addition, marker levels increase after the onset of menopause due to the decrease in estrogen secretion, normally an inhibitor of bone resorption.

Interfering Factors
- Bone volume and time of day testing was done
- Testosterone and other body-building therapies (decreased NTx levels)

Nursing Considerations

Before the Test
- Confirm the patient's identity using two patient identifiers and confirmation of the patient's identification bracelet according to facility policy.
- Explain the test to the patient and why it's being done.
- Ensure that the patient's baseline levels were taken before beginning therapy.
- Tell the patient that a urine specimen or blood sample may be used for the test. Explain that if a blood sample is needed, there may be slight discomfort from the tourniquet and needle puncture.
- Advise the patient that meat intake should be limited, but there are no other food or fluid restrictions for the test.

During the Test
- Obtain the appropriate blood sample or urine specimen.
- If collecting a blood sample, perform a venipuncture and collect the sample, placing it in the appropriate sample container.
- If collecting a urine specimen, obtain a double-voided specimen:

- Collect the first specimen approximately a half hour before the designated time of testing.
- Provide the patient with water to drink to fill the bladder.
- At the designated time, obtain a second urine specimen.

After the Test
- Send the sample or specimen to the laboratory immediately.

<hr>

Breast Biopsy

Normal Findings
- Breast tissue consisting of cellular and noncellular connective tissue, fat lobules, and various lactiferous ducts
- Pink appearance with more fatty than fibrous tissue
- Absence of abnormal cell development or tissue elements

Abnormal Findings
- Benign tumors such as in fibrocystic disease, adenofibroma, intraductal papilloma, mammary fat necrosis, and plasma cell mastitis (mammary duct ectasia)
- Malignant tumors such as in adenocarcinoma, cystosarcoma, intraductal carcinoma, infiltrating carcinoma, inflammatory carcinoma, medullary or circumscribed carcinoma, colloid carcinoma, lobular carcinoma, sarcoma, and Paget's disease

Nursing Implications
- Anticipate the need for additional testing.
- Provide emotional support to the patient during this period.

Purpose
- To differentiate between benign and malignant breast tumors

Description
Breast biopsy is performed to confirm or rule out breast cancer after clinical examination, mammography, or thermography has identified a mass. Common techniques include fine-needle or needle biopsy (performed when a patient has a fluid-filled mass that's been identified by ultrasonography) and open biopsy (performed to allow access to the complete tissue system, which can be sectioned to allow more accurate evaluation). In some cases, stereotactic breast biopsy may be used. This involves immobilizing the breast and allowing a computer to calculate the exact location of the mass based on X-rays from two angles.

A breast biopsy can usually be done on an outpatient basis under local anesthesia; however, an excisional open biopsy may require general anesthesia or monitored anesthesia care with sedation. If sufficient tissue is obtained and the mass is found to be a malignant tumor, specimens are sent for estrogen and progesterone receptor assays to assist in determining future therapy and the prognosis.

The usual procedures for needle and open biopsies are as follows:

Needle Biopsy
- The patient is instructed to undress to the waist and is placed in a sitting or recumbent position with her arms at her sides.
- The biopsy site is prepared, a local anesthetic is administered, and the syringe (Luer-lock syringe for aspiration, Vim-Silverman needle for tissue specimen) is introduced into the lesion.
- Fluid aspirated from the breast is expelled into a properly labeled, heparinized tube; the tissue specimen is placed in a labeled specimen bottle containing normal saline solution or formalin. With fine-needle aspiration, a slide is made for cytology and viewed immediately under a microscope. (Because breast fluid aspiration isn't considered diagnostically accurate, some health care providers aspirate fluid only from cysts. If such fluid is clear yellow and the mass disappears, the aspiration procedure

B

is diagnostic and therapeutic, and the aspirate is discarded. If aspiration yields no fluid or if the lesion recurs two or three times, an open biopsy is then considered appropriate.)

• Pressure is exerted on the biopsy site and, after bleeding stops, an adhesive bandage is applied.

Open Biopsy

• The skin should be prepped with an approved prep solution and allowed to dry.

• After the patient receives a general or local anesthetic, an incision is made in the breast to expose the mass.

• The health care provider may then incise a portion of tissue or excise the entire mass. If the mass is smaller than ¾-inch (2 cm) in diameter and appears benign, it's usually excised; if it's larger or appears malignant, a specimen is usually incised before the mass is excised. Incisional biopsy generally provides an adequate specimen for histologic analysis.

• The specimen is placed in a properly labeled specimen bottle containing 10% formalin solution. Tissue that appears malignant is sent for frozen section and receptor assays. Receptor assay specimens must not be placed in the formalin solution.

• The wound is sutured and an adhesive bandage applied.

Because breast cancer remains the most prevalent cancer in women, genetic researchers are continually working to identify women at risk. (See the *BRCA Testing* box.)

BRCA Testing

Genetic researchers have located two genes, *BRCA1* and *BRCA2*, that are linked to certain forms of breast cancer. BRCA testing can detect the presence of *BRCA* mutations, which may increase an individual's susceptibility to some breast cancers.

The BRCA test, performed on a blood sample, is available for a woman with a family history of breast cancer.

Interfering Factors

• Failure to obtain an adequate tissue specimen

• Failure to place the specimen in the proper solution

Precautions

• Breast biopsy is contraindicated in the patient with a condition that precludes surgery.

Nursing Considerations

Before the Test

• Confirm the patient's identity using two patient identifiers and confirmation of the patient's identification bracelet according to facility policy.

• Describe the procedure to the patient and explain that breast biopsy permits microscopic examination of a breast tissue specimen. Offer emotional support and assure the patient that breast masses don't always indicate cancer.

• Inform the patient scheduled for a needle biopsy of the need to sit still during the procedure.

• If the patient is to receive a local anesthetic, advise that there is no need to restrict food, fluids, and medication. If the patient is to receive a general anesthetic, advise her to fast from midnight before the procedure until after the biopsy.

• Tell the patient who will perform the biopsy, and where and when it will be done. Explain that pretest studies, such as blood tests, urine tests, and chest X-rays, may be required.

• Make sure the patient or a responsible family member has signed an informed consent form.

• Check the patient's history for hypersensitivity to anesthetics.

During the Test

• Remind the patient undergoing a needle biopsy to sit still.

• Assist with the collection of specimens into the appropriate containers, if indicated.

- Send the specimens to the laboratory immediately, if appropriate.

After the Test
- If the patient has received a general or local anesthetic, monitor the patient's vital signs regularly. If she has received a general anesthetic, check her vital signs every 15 minutes for 1 hour, every 30 minutes for 2 hours, every hour for the next 4 hours, and then every 4 hours.
- Administer analgesics for pain, as ordered, and provide ice bags for comfort.
- Instruct the patient to wear a support bra at all times until healing is complete.
- Observe for and report bleeding, tenderness, and redness at the biopsy site.
- Provide emotional support to the patient awaiting diagnosis.

Breast Cancer Tumor Analysis

Normal Findings
- *DNA ploidy:* Two sets of paired chromosomes (diploid)
- *S-phase fraction:* Less than 5.5%
- *Cathepsin D:* Less than 10%
- *HER2 protein:* Partial staining in 10% or less of the cancer cells
- *p53 protein:* Less than 10%
- *Ki67 protein:* Less than 20%

Abnormal Findings
- *DNA ploidy:* Variable number of chromosome sets (aneuploid)
- *S-phase fraction:* Greater than 5.5%
- *Cathepsin D:* Greater than 10%
- *HER2 protein:* Moderate to strong staining of 10% or more of cancer cells
- *p53 protein:* Greater than 10%
- *Ki67 protein:* 10% to 20% (borderline); greater than 20%

Nursing Implications
- Anticipate the need for further testing.

- Provide emotional support to the patient related to the possibility of recurrence.

Purpose
- To identify the risk of recurrence in patients with breast cancer

Description
Breast cancer tumor analysis involves the examination of malignant breast tumor cells to determine their cellular function and growth. The goal is to predict the patient's risk of recurrence even when the entire tumor has been removed and there's no evidence of metastasis to the lymph nodes. During surgery, the surgeon obtains a specimen of the breast tumor tissue. The tissue is then placed on ice or in a preservative solution. The tissue is examined histologically and for levels of markers.

Several markers have been identified as helpful in predicting the risk of recurrence: DNA ploidy, S-phase fraction, cathepsin D, HER2 protein, p53 protein, and Ki67 protein. Each of these markers is associated with aggressive types of breast cancer. (See the *Understanding Breast Tumor Analysis Markers* table.)

Interfering Factors
- Improper or delayed specimen fixing (deterioration of the marker proteins and lower values)
- Chemotherapy use preoperatively (lowers some levels)

Nursing Considerations
Before the Test
- Confirm the patient's identity using two patient identifiers and confirmation of the patient's identification bracelet according to facility policy.
- Describe the procedure to the patient and explain that the test permits microscopic examination of the tumor. Offer emotional support.

Understanding Breast Tumor Analysis Markers

B

Various markers are used to identify the risk of recurrence in patients with breast cancer. This chart describes these markers and each marker's association with breast cancer recurrence.

Marker	Description	Association With Recurrence
DNA ploidy	The number of sets of chromosomes in a cell	• Normally DNA is diploid. • More aggressive cancer results in more rapid cell division, leading to increased or variable numbers of chromosome sets in the cell (aneuploid).
S-phase fraction	The phase of the cell cycle when intracellular protein is being synthesized	• Aggressive cancer cells are most commonly noted in the S-phase.
Cathepsin D	A catabolic protein enzyme	• An increase in the fraction (fraction determined by the number of cells in this phase divided by the total number of cancer cells) suggests a more aggressive cancer and increased likelihood of a recurrence.
HER2 protein	An epidermal growth factor existing on the cell membrane produced by *HER2*	• This enzyme is typically absent in breast cells that are in the resting phase. • With cancer cells, this enzyme is dramatically increased.
p53 protein	A tumor suppressor gene	• Increased levels of HER2 protein reflect overamplification of *HER2* due to aggressive breast cancer.
Ki67 protein	Protein that's encoded by *Ki67*	• This protein has been found to be overexpressed in more aggressive breast cancer. • An increased level of this protein is associated with aggressive breast cancer.

• Tell the patient who will perform the procedure, and where and when it will be done.

• Explain that pretest studies, such as blood tests, urine tests, and chest X-rays, may be required.

• Make sure the patient or a responsible family member has signed an informed consent form.

• Check the patient's history for hypersensitivity to anesthetics.

After the Test

• If the patient has received a general or local anesthetic, monitor vital signs regularly. If the patient has received a general anesthetic, check vital signs every 15 minutes for 1 hour, every 30 minutes for 2 hours, every hour for the next 4 hours, and then every 4 hours.

• Administer analgesics for pain, as ordered, and provide ice bags for comfort.

• Inform the patient that the results usually take approximately 1 week to receive. Reinforce the need for follow-up with the surgeon.

• Provide emotional support to the patient awaiting results.

Bronchography

Normal Findings

- Right mainstem bronchus that's shorter, wider, and more vertical than the left bronchus
- Successive bronchi branches that are smaller in diameter and free from obstruction or lesions

Abnormal Findings

- Bronchiectasis or bronchial obstruction (tumors, cysts, cavities, or foreign objects)

Nursing Implications

- Anticipate the need for additional testing to confirm the diagnosis.
- Keep in mind that findings must be correlated with the physical examination, patient history, and perhaps other pulmonary studies.

Purpose

- To help detect bronchiectasis and map its location for surgical resection
- To detect bronchial obstruction, pulmonary tumors, cysts, and cavities and, indirectly, to pinpoint the cause of hemoptysis
- To provide permanent films of pathologic findings
- To guide procedures such as bronchoscopy

Description

Bronchography is X-ray examination of the tracheobronchial tree after a radiopaque iodine contrast agent is instilled through a catheter into the trachea and bronchi lumens. The contrast agent coats the bronchial tree, permitting visualization of any anatomic deviations. Bronchography of a localized lung area may be accomplished by instilling contrast dye through a fiberoptic bronchoscope placed in the area to be filmed. It may be performed using a local anesthetic instilled through the catheter or bronchoscope, although a general anesthetic may be necessary for children or during a concurrent bronchoscopy.

The usual procedure is as follows:

- After a local anesthetic is sprayed into the patient's mouth and throat, a bronchoscope or catheter is passed into the trachea, and the anesthetic and contrast medium are instilled.
- The patient is placed in various positions during the test to promote movement of the contrast medium into different areas of the bronchial tree.
- After X-rays are taken, the contrast medium is removed through postural drainage and by having the patient cough it up.

Interfering Factors

- Presence of secretions or improper patient positioning (possible poor imaging due to inadequate filling of the bronchial tree)
- Inability to suppress coughing (interferes with bronchial filling and retention of the contrast medium)

Precautions

- Bronchography is contraindicated in pregnant patients and in those who are hypersensitive to iodine or contrast media.
- The test is usually contraindicated in patients with respiratory insufficiency.

Nursing Considerations

Before the Test

- Confirm the patient's identity using two patient identifiers and confirmation of the patient's identification bracelet according to facility policy.
- Explain to the patient that bronchography helps evaluate abnormalities of the bronchial structures. Explain who will perform the test, and where and when it will take place.
- Instruct the patient to fast for 12 hours before the test and to perform good oral hygiene the night before and the morning of the test.

- Check the patient's history for hypersensitivity to anesthetics, iodine, or contrast media.
- Make sure the patient or a responsible family member has signed an informed consent form.
- If the patient has a productive cough, administer a prescribed expectorant and perform postural drainage 1 to 3 days before the test.
- If the procedure is to be performed under a local anesthetic, tell the patient that a sedative will be given to help with relaxation and to suppress the gag reflex. Prepare the patient for the unpleasant taste of the anesthetic spray, as well as for the coughing after instillation of the anesthetic spray.
- Warn the patient that some difficulty in breathing may be experienced during the procedure, Reassure the patient that the airway won't be blocked during the procedure and that oxygen will be administered through the bronchoscope. Tell the patient that the catheter or bronchoscope will pass more easily if he or she relaxes.
- If bronchography is to be performed under a general anesthetic, inform the patient that a sedative will be given before the test to help him or her relax.
- Just before the test, instruct the patient to remove dentures (if present) and to void.

> **Quality and Safety Nursing Alert**

Watch for signs of laryngeal spasms (dyspnea) or edema (hoarseness, dyspnea, laryngeal stridor) secondary to traumatic intubation. Also, immediately report signs of allergic reaction to the contrast medium or anesthetic, such as itching, dyspnea, tachycardia, palpitations, excitation, hypotension, hypertension, or euphoria.

During the Test
- Observe the patient with asthma for laryngeal spasm (such as dyspnea) secondary to the instillation of the contrast medium.
- Observe the patient with chronic obstructive pulmonary disease for airway occlusion secondary to the instillation of the contrast medium.
- Assist with postural drainage and help the patient cough to remove the contrast agent.

After the Test
- Withhold food, fluids, and oral medications until the gag reflex returns (usually in 2 hours).

> **Quality and Safety Nursing Alert**

Fluid intake before the gag reflex returns may cause aspiration.

- Encourage gentle coughing and postural drainage to facilitate clearing of the contrast medium. A postdrainage film usually is acquired in 24 to 48 hours.
- Assess for signs of chemical or secondary bacterial pneumonia—fever, dyspnea, crackles, or rhonchi—the result of incomplete expectoration of the contrast medium.
- If the patient has a sore throat, reassure that it's only temporary and provide throat lozenges or a liquid gargle when the gag reflex returns.
- Advise the outpatient not to resume usual activities until the next day.

Bronchoscopy

Normal Findings
- Trachea consisting of smooth muscle containing C-shaped rings of cartilage at regular intervals and lined with ciliated mucosa
- Bronchi appearing structurally similar to the trachea; the right bronchus slightly larger and more vertical than the left

- Smaller segmental bronchi branching off the main bronchi

Abnormal Findings

- Bronchial wall abnormalities, such as inflammation, swelling, protruding cartilage, ulceration, tumors, and mucous gland orifice or submucosal lymph node enlargement
- Endotracheal abnormalities, such as stenosis, compression, ectasia (dilation of tubular vessel), irregular bronchial branching, and abnormal bifurcation due to diverticulum
- Abnormal substances in the trachea or bronchi, such as blood, secretions, calculi, and foreign bodies
- Evidence of interstitial pulmonary disease, bronchogenic carcinoma, tuberculosis (TB), or other pulmonary infections

Nursing Implications

- Anticipate the need for additional testing, if indicated.
- Radiographic, bronchoscopic, and cytologic findings must be correlated with clinical signs and symptoms.

Purpose

- To visually examine a tumor, an obstruction, secretions, bleeding, or a foreign body in the tracheobronchial tree
- To help diagnose bronchogenic carcinoma, TB, interstitial pulmonary disease, and fungal or parasitic pulmonary infection by obtaining a specimen for bacteriologic and cytologic examination
- To remove foreign bodies, malignant or benign tumors, mucus plugs, and excessive secretions from the tracheobronchial tree

Description

Bronchoscopy allows direct visualization of the larynx, trachea, and bronchi through a flexible fiberoptic bronchoscope or a rigid metal bronchoscope. A more recent approach is the use of

Virtual Bronchoscopy

B

Using a computer and data from a spiral computed tomography (CT) scan, health care providers can now examine the respiratory tract noninvasively with virtual bronchoscopy. Although this test is still in its early stages, researchers believe that it can enhance screening, diagnosis, preoperative planning, surgical technique, and postoperative follow-up.

Unlike its counterpart—conventional bronchoscopy—virtual bronchoscopy is noninvasive, doesn't require sedation, and provides images for examination beyond the segmental bronchi, thus allowing for possible diagnosis of areas that may be stenosed, obstructed, or compressed from an external source. The images obtained from the CT scan include views of the airways and lung parenchyma. Anatomic structures and abnormalities can be precisely identified and therefore can be helpful in locating potential biopsy sites to be obtained with conventional bronchoscopy and provide simulation for planning the optimal surgical approach.

Virtual bronchoscopy does have disadvantages. This technique doesn't allow for specimen collection or biopsies to be obtained from tissue sources. It also can't demonstrate details of the mucosal surface, such as color or texture. Moreover, if an area contains viscous secretions, such as mucus or blood, visualization becomes difficult.

More research on this technique is needed. However, researchers believe that virtual bronchoscopy may play a major role in the screening and early detection of certain cancers, thus allowing for treatment at an earlier, possibly curable stage.

virtual bronchoscopy. (See the *Virtual Bronchoscopy* box.)

Although a flexible fiberoptic bronchoscope allows a wider view and is used more commonly, the rigid metal bronchoscope is required to remove foreign objects, excise endobronchial lesions, and control massive hemoptysis. A brush, biopsy forceps, or catheter may be passed through the bronchoscope to obtain specimens for cytologic examination.

Bronchoscopy may require fluoro-scopic guidance for distal evaluation of lesions for a transbronchial biopsy in alveolar areas. However, the usual bron-choscopy procedure is as follows:

- With the patient sitting upright or lying supine, a local anesthetic is sprayed into the patient's throat.
- Once the anesthetic takes effect, a bronchoscope is introduced through the patient's mouth or nose.
- When the scope is just above the vocal cords, about 3 to 4 mL of 2% to 4% lidocaine is flushed through the scope's inner channel to the vocal cords to anesthetize deeper areas.
- The health care provider inspects the anatomic structure of the trachea and bronchi, observes the color of the mucosal lining, and notes masses or inflamed areas.
- Tissue specimens may be obtained from a suspect area; a bronchial brush to obtain cells from the surface of a lesion and a suction apparatus to remove foreign bodies or mucus plugs may be used. Bronchoalveolar lavage may be performed to diagnose the infectious causes of infiltrates in an immunocompromised patient or to remove thickened secretions.

Interfering Factors
- Failure to place specimens in the appropriate containers

Precautions
- A patient with respiratory failure who can't breathe adequately on his or her own should be placed on a ventilator before bronchoscopy.

Nursing Considerations
Before the Test
- Confirm the patient's identity using two patient identifiers and confirma-tion of the patient's identification bracelet according to facility policy.
- Explain to the patient that bronchos-copy is used to examine the lower airways.

- Describe the procedure, including that it's done in a darkened room. Inform the patient of who will perform the test, and when and where it will occur.
- Inform the patient of the need to fast for 6 to 12 hours before the test and that an IV sedative may be adminis-tered to help the patient relax.
- If the procedure isn't being performed under general anesthesia, inform the patient that a local anesthetic will be sprayed into the nose and mouth to suppress the gag reflex. Warn that the spray has an unpleasant taste and that there may be discomfort during the procedure.
- Reassure the patient that the airway won't be blocked during the proce-dure and that oxygen will be adminis-tered through the bronchoscope.
- Make sure that the patient or a responsible family member has signed an informed consent form.
- Check the patient's history for hyper-sensitivity to the anesthetic.
- Obtain the patient's baseline vital signs.
- Administer the preoperative sedative.
- Have the patient remove dentures, if appropriate, before receiving a sedative.

During the Test
- Place the patient in the supine posi-tion or have him or her sit upright in a chair.
- Tell the patient to remain relaxed with arms at the sides and to breathe through the nose.
- Provide supplemental oxygen by nasal cannula, if necessary.
- Assist with tissue specimen collec-tion, as indicated.
- After collection, place the specimens in their respective, properly labeled containers in accordance with labora-tory and pathology guidelines, and send them to the laboratory at once. Instillation of normal saline may be required for bronchial washings in order to obtain specimens.

After the Test

• Monitor the patient's vital signs per facility policy, or at least every 15 minutes until the patient is stable and then every 30 minutes for 4 hours, every hour for the next 4 hours, and then every 4 hours for 24 hours. Immediately notify the health care provider of adverse reactions to the anesthetic or sedative.

• Place the conscious patient in semi-Fowler's position; place the unconscious patient on his or her side with the head slightly elevated to prevent aspiration.

• Provide an emesis basin and instruct the patient to spit out saliva rather than swallow it. Observe sputum for blood and report excessive bleeding immediately.

• Tell the patient who has had a biopsy to refrain from clearing the throat and coughing, which may dislodge the clot at the biopsy site and cause hemorrhaging.

• Immediately report subcutaneous crepitus around the patient's face and neck, because this may indicate tracheal or bronchial perforation.

> ▶ *Quality and Safety Nursing Alert*
>
> Watch for, listen for, and immediately report symptoms of respiratory difficulty resulting from laryngeal edema or laryngospasm, such as laryngeal stridor and dyspnea. Observe for signs and symptoms of hypoxemia, pneumothorax, bronchospasm, and bleeding.

• Restrict food and fluids to avoid aspiration until the gag reflex returns (usually in 1 to 2 hours). The patient may then resume a usual diet, beginning with sips of clear liquid or ice chips.

• Reassure the patient that hoarseness, loss of voice, and sore throat are temporary. Provide lozenges or a soothing liquid gargle to ease discomfort when the gag reflex returns.

B-Type Natriuretic Peptide Assay

B

Reference Values
Less than 100 pg/mL (SI, less than 100 ng/L)

Abnormal Findings
Elevated Levels
• Heart failure with concentrations greater than 100 pg/mL (BNP blood level is related to heart failure severity; the higher the level, the worse the heart failure symptoms.)

Nursing Implications
• Anticipate the need for additional testing.
• Assess the patient for signs and symptoms associated with heart failure.

Purpose
• To help diagnose and determine the severity of heart failure

Description
Brain (B-type) natriuretic peptide (BNP) is a neurohormone that helps regulate blood pressure and fluid volume. It is primarily secreted from the ventricles in response to increased preload with resulting elevated ventricular pressure. The level of BNP in the blood increases as the ventricular walls expand from increased pressure, making it a helpful diagnostic, monitoring, and prognostic tool in the setting of heart failure. Because this serum laboratory test can be quickly obtained, BNP levels are useful for prompt diagnosis of heart failure in settings such as the ED. Elevations in BNP can occur from a number of other conditions, such as pulmonary embolus, myocardial infarction, and ventricular hypertrophy. Therefore, the clinician correlates BNP levels with abnormal physical assessment findings and other diagnostic tests before making a definitive diagnosis of heart failure.

Nursing Considerations

Before the Test

- Confirm the patient's identity using two patient identifiers and confirmation of the patient's identification bracelet according to facility policy.
- Explain to the patient that the BNP assay is used to identify the presence and severity of heart failure and that it requires a blood sample from a venipuncture.
- Explain to the patient there may be slight discomfort from the tourniquet and needle puncture.
- Inform the patient that there are no food or fluid restrictions for this test.

During the Test

- Perform a venipuncture and collect the sample in a 3.5-mL EDTA tube.

After the Test

- Send the sample to the laboratory immediately.
- Apply direct pressure to the venipuncture site until bleeding stops and to prevent hematoma formation.

Calcitonin

Reference Values
Females: 20 pg/mL (SI, 20 ng/L); after 4-hour calcium infusion, 130 pg/mL (SI, 130 ng/L); after testing with penta-gastrin infusion, 30 pg/mL (SI, 30 ng/L)
Males: 40 pg/mL (SI, 40 ng/L); after 4-hour calcium infusion, 190 pg/mL (SI, 190 ng/L); after testing with pentagas-trin infusion, 110 pg/mL (SI, 110 ng/L)

Abnormal Findings
Elevated Levels
- Thyroid medullary carcinoma (in absence of hypocalcemia)
- Lung oat cell carcinoma (ectopic calcitonin production) or breast carcinoma (occasionally)
- Chronic kidney disease
- Alcoholic cirrhosis
- Hypercalcemia

Nursing Implications
- Anticipate the need for additional testing, including screening of family members.
- Some patients with thyroid medullary carcinoma don't respond to the stimulation test.
- Thyroid medullary carcinoma is an autosomal dominant trait.

Purpose
- To help diagnose thyroid medullary carcinoma and ectopic calcitonin-producing tumors (rare)

Description
Plasma calcitonin is a radioimmunoassay that measures calcitonin (thyrocalcitonin) plasma levels. The exact role of calcitonin in normal human physiology hasn't been fully defined, but it's known to act as an antagonist to parathyroid hormone and to lower serum calcium levels.

This test usually is indicated for suspected thyroid medullary carcinoma, which causes calcitonin hypersecretion (without associated hypocalcemia). Equivocal results require provocative testing with IV pentagastrin or calcium to rule out disease.

Interfering Factors
- Food or fluid ingestion before the test
- Gross lipemia
- Pregnancy (levels normally elevated at term) and newborns
- Estrogens, octreotide, and phenytoin (decreased levels)

Nursing Considerations
Before the Test
- Confirm the patient's identity using two patient identifiers and confirmation of the patient's identification bracelet according to facility policy.
- Explain to the patient that the plasma calcitonin test helps evaluate thyroid function.
- Instruct the patient to fast overnight because food may interfere with calcium homeostasis and, subsequently, calcitonin levels. The patient may have water.
- Tell the patient that the test requires a blood sample.
- Explain that the patient may experience slight discomfort from the tourniquet and the needle puncture.
- Tell the patient that the laboratory requires several days to complete the analysis.

During the Test
- Perform a venipuncture and collect the sample in a 7-mL heparinized tube.

After the Test
- Apply direct pressure to the venipuncture site until bleeding stops and to prevent hematoma formation.
- Send the sample to the laboratory immediately.
- Instruct the patient to resume a usual diet.

Calcium, Serum; Calcium and Phosphates, Urine

Reference Values
Total serum calcium levels (adults): 8.2 to 10.2 mg/dL (SI, 2.05–2.54 mmol/L)
Total serum calcium levels (children): 8.6 to 11.2 mg/dL (SI, 2.15–2.79 mmol/L)
Ionized calcium levels: 4.65 to 5.28 mg/dL (SI, 1.1–1.25 mmol/L)
Urine calcium levels: 100 to 300 mg/24 hours (SI, 2.5–7.5 mmol/L) for normal diet
Normal phosphate excretion: Less than 1,000 mg/24 hours

Critical Values
Total serum calcium: Less than 4.4 mg/dL (SI, less than 1.1 mmol/L), leading to tetany and convulsions; greater than 13 mg/dL (SI, greater than 3.25 mmol/L), leading to cardiotoxicity, arrhythmias, and coma
Ionized calcium levels: Less than 2 mg/dL (SI, less than 0.5 mmol/L), producing tetany or life-threatening complications; 2 to 3 mg/dL (SI, 0.5–0.75 mmol/L, signaling the need to administer calcium if multiple blood transfusions have occurred); greater than 7 mg/dL (SI, greater than 1.75 mmol/L), possibly leading to coma

Abnormal Findings

Elevated Levels (Hypercalcemia)
Total Serum Calcium
- Hyperparathyroidism and parathyroid tumors, Paget's disease of the bone, multiple myeloma, metastatic carcinoma, multiple fractures, and prolonged immobilization
- Inadequate excretion of calcium, such as adrenal insufficiency and renal disease
- Excessive calcium ingestion
- Overuse of antacids such as calcium carbonate

Ionized Calcium
- Malignant neoplasm of bone, lung, breast, bladder, or kidney

Urine Calcium
- Numerous disorders (See the *Disorders That Affect Urine Calcium and Urine Phosphate Levels* box.)

Nursing Implications
- Monitor the patient for signs and symptoms of hypercalcemia (nausea and vomiting, excessive thirst, frequent urination, constipation, abdominal pain, muscle weakness, muscle and joint aches, confusion, lethargy, and fatigue).
- Calcitonin solution may need to be administered rapidly if the patient's total serum calcium is above 13 mg/dL.
- Calcium may need to be administered if the patient's ionized calcium level is between 2 and 3 mg/dL.

Decreased Levels (Hypocalcemia)
Total Serum Calcium
- Hypoparathyroidism, total parathyroidectomy, and malabsorption
- Cushing syndrome, renal failure, acute pancreatitis, peritonitis, malnutrition with hypoalbuminemia, and multiple blood transfusions (during which citrate binds ionized calcium)

Ionized Calcium
- Diarrhea, malabsorption of calcium, burns, alcoholism, pancreatitis, chronic kidney disease, hypoparathyroidism, vitamin D deficiency, and multiple organ failure

Urine Calcium
- Numerous disorders

Disorders That Affect Urine Calcium and Urine Phosphate Levels

Disorder	Urine Calcium Level	Urine Phosphate Level
Hyperparathyroidism	Elevated	Elevated
Vitamin D intoxication	Elevated	Suppressed
Metastatic carcinoma	Elevated	Normal
Sarcoidosis	Elevated	Suppressed
Renal tubular acidosis	Elevated	Elevated
Multiple myeloma	Elevated or normal	Elevated or normal
Paget's disease	Normal	Normal
Milk-alkali syndrome	Suppressed or normal	Suppressed or normal
Hypoparathyroidism	Suppressed	Suppressed
Acute nephrosis	Suppressed	Suppressed or normal
Chronic nephrosis	Suppressed	Suppressed
Acute nephritis	Suppressed	Suppressed
Renal insufficiency	Suppressed	Suppressed
Osteomalacia	Suppressed	Suppressed
Steatorrhea	Suppressed	Suppressed

Nursing Implications

- Monitor the patient closely for signs and symptoms of hypocalcemia (abnormal heart rhythms, numbness and tingling in the fingers, convulsion, lethargy, poor appetite, and mental confusion).
- Monitor the patient for circumoral and peripheral numbness and tingling, muscle twitching, Chvostek's sign (facial muscle spasm), tetany, muscle cramping, Trousseau's sign (carpopedal spasm), seizures, arrhythmias, laryngeal spasm, decreased cardiac output, prolonged bleeding time, fractures, and a prolonged Q interval.

Purpose

- To evaluate endocrine function, calcium metabolism and excretion, and acid–base balance
- To guide therapy in patients with renal failure, renal transplant, endocrine disorders, malignancies, cardiac disease, and skeletal disorders
- To monitor treatment of calcium or phosphate deficiency (urine testing)

Description

Calcium and phosphates are essential for bone formation and resorption. Normally absorbed in the upper intestine and excreted in stool and urine, calcium and phosphates help maintain tissue and fluid pH, electrolyte balance in cells and extracellular fluids, and permeability of cell membranes. Calcium promotes enzymatic processes, aids blood coagulation, and lowers neuromuscular irritability; phosphates aid carbohydrate metabolism.

The bone and teeth contain about 99% of the body's calcium. Approximately 1% of the body's total calcium circulates in the blood. About 50% of this amount is bound to plasma proteins and 40% is ionized, or free.

Serum calcium level measures the total amount of calcium in the blood. Ionized calcium level measures the fraction of serum calcium that's in the ionized form. Urine calcium and phosphate levels generally parallel serum levels.

Interfering Factors

- Venous stasis caused by prolonged tourniquet application (possible false-high total serum calcium)
- Excessive ingestion of vitamin D or its derivatives (dihydrotachysterol, calcitriol) or use of androgens, asparaginase, calciferol-activated calcium salts, progestins–estrogens, or thiazide diuretics (increased total serum calcium)

- Acetazolamide, corticosteroids, hormonal contraceptives, plicamycin, chronic laxative use, and excessive citrated blood transfusions (possible total serum calcium increase or decrease)
- Antibiotics, magnesium products, laxatives, and heparin (decreased ionized calcium)
- Alkaline antacids (increased ionized calcium)
- Excessive milk ingestion (increased ionized calcium)
- Parathyroid hormones (decreased urine calcium)
- Medications containing estrogen, lithium carbonate, and thiazide diuretics (decreased urine calcium excretion)
- Prolonged inactivity and ingestion of corticosteroids, sodium phosphate, and calcitonin (increased urine calcium)
- Thiazide diuretics (decreased urine calcium)

Precautions

- Handle the serum sample gently to prevent hemolysis.
- Tell the patient not to contaminate the urine specimen with toilet tissue or stool.

Nursing Considerations

Before the Test

- Confirm the patient's identity using two patient identifiers and confirmation of the patient's identification bracelet according to facility policy.
- Explain the test to the patient and the reason for it.
- Tell the patient whether the test involves blood or urine samples.
- For total serum calcium level, explain to the patient that there may be slight discomfort from the tourniquet and the needle puncture.
- Instruct the patient undergoing an ionized serum calcium level test to fast for 6 hours before the test.

- If the urine calcium level is being tested, encourage the patient to be as active as possible before the test.
- Tell the patient that the urine test requires urine collection over a 24-hour period. If the patient is collecting the specimen, teach the proper technique.
- Provide a diet that contains about 130 mg of calcium/24 hours for 3 days before the urine test or provide a copy of the diet for the patient to follow at home. Check the laboratory for parameters related to dietary instructions.
- Notify the laboratory and health care provider of medications the patient is taking that may affect test results; these may need to be restricted.

During the Test

- Perform a venipuncture (without a tourniquet, if possible) and collect the sample in a 3- or 4-mL clot activator tube (for total serum calcium), or collect 5 to 10 mL of venous blood in a red-top tube (for ionized calcium).
- Collect the patient's urine over 24 hours, discarding the first specimen and retaining the last.

After the Test

- Apply direct pressure to the venipuncture site until bleeding stops and to prevent hematoma formation.
- Observe the patient with low urine calcium levels for tetany.
- Inform the patient to resume usual diet, activities, and medications, as ordered.

> **Quality and Safety Nursing Alert**
>
> Observe the patient with hypercalcemia for deep bone pain, flank pain caused by renal calculi, and muscle hypotonicity. Hypercalcemic crisis begins with nausea, vomiting, and dehydration, leading to stupor and coma, and can end in cardiac arrest.

Cancer Tumor Markers (CA 15-3 [27, 29], CA 19-9, CA-125, and CA-50)

Reference Values

CA 15-3 (27, 29): Less than 30 units/mL
CA 19-9: Less than 70 units/mL
CA-125: Less than 34 units/mL
CA-50: Less than 17 units/mL

Abnormal Findings

Elevated Levels

- Metastatic breast cancer, pancreas, lung, colorectal, ovarian, and liver cancers (CA 15-3 [27, 29])
- Pancreas, hepatobiliary, and lung cancers (CA 19-9)
- Gastric and colorectal cancers (mild increase CA 19-9)
- Epithelial ovary, fallopian tube, endometrial, endocervix, pancreatic, and liver cancers (CA-125)
- Colon, breast, lung, and GI cancers (increased, but to a lesser degree, CA-125)
- GI and pancreatic cancers (CA-50)

Decreased Levels

- Progressive disease (decreased CA 15-3 [27, 29] despite therapy)

Nursing Implications

- Assist with explaining possible disease progression.
- Provide emotional support to the patient and family.
- Assist with measures to cope with the disease.
- Prepare the patient for additional testing and treatment as indicated.

Purpose

- To assist tumor staging and identify possible metastasis
- To monitor and detect disease
- To assess the patient's response to therapy recurrence

Description

Tumor markers, which are found in the serum of cancer patients, are substances produced and secreted by tumor cells that help determine tumor activity. The type of cancer the patient has determines which test is ordered. The CA 15-3 antigen (breast–cystic fluid protein, or BCFP) in conjunction with the carcinoembryonic antigen is particularly helpful in diagnosing tumor activity in patients with breast cancer (CA 27, metastatic breast cancer, breast–cystic fluid protein 29, BCFP). The CA 19-9 carbohydrate antigen test may be ordered in the patient with pancreatic, hepatobiliary, or lung cancer. The CA-125 glycoprotein antigen and serum carbohydrate antigen are commonly associated with types of ovarian cancers. The CA-50 may be ordered in the patient with GI or pancreatic cancer.

Interfering Factors

- Benign breast or ovarian disease (increased CA 15-3 [27, 29])
- Cholecystitis, cirrhosis, cystic fibrosis, gallstones, and pancreatitis (minimal elevations in CA 19-9)
- Acute and chronic hepatitis, ascites, endometriosis, GI disease, Meigs' syndrome, menstruation, pancreatitis, pelvic inflammatory disease, peritonitis, pleural effusion, pregnancy, and pulmonary disease (increased CA-125)

Precautions

- Transport the specimen as directed.
- Handle the sample gently to prevent hemolysis.

Nursing Considerations

Before the Test

- Consult the laboratory or cancer center about specific patient preparation procedures, such as whether the patient needs to fast or whether interfering factors need to be identified.
- Confirm the patient's identity using two patient identifiers and confirmation of the patient's identification bracelet according to facility policy.
- Explain the purpose of the particular tumor marker test ordered and that it may be helpful in diagnosing or

C

treating the patient's disorder, as appropriate.

- Follow the specific directions from the laboratory or cancer center for the test ordered. Note interfering factors on the appropriate laboratory requests.
- Tell the patient that the test requires a blood sample.
- Explain to the patient that there may be slight discomfort from the tourniquet and the needle puncture.

During the Test
- Obtain a 10-mL venous sample, as ordered, in the tube specified by the laboratory or cancer center and transport the sample as directed.

After the Test
- Apply direct pressure to the venipuncture site until bleeding stops and to prevent hematoma formation.

Candida Antibodies

Normal Findings
- Negative for *Candida* antibodies

Abnormal Findings
- Positive, indicating disseminated candidiasis

Nursing Implications
- This test yields a significant percentage of false-positive results.
- Prepare the patient for additional testing and follow-up therapy.

Purpose
- To help diagnose candidiasis when culture or histologic study can't confirm the diagnosis

Description
Commonly present in the body, *Candida albicans* is a saprophytic yeast that can become pathogenic when the environment favors proliferation or the host's defenses have been weakened significantly.

Candidiasis is usually limited to the skin and mucous membranes but may cause life-threatening systemic infection.

Susceptibility to candidiasis is associated with antibacterial, antimetabolic, and corticosteroid therapy, as well as with immunologic defects, pregnancy, obesity, diabetes, and debilitating diseases. Oral candidiasis is common and benign in children; in adults, it may be an early indication of acquired immune deficiency syndrome (AIDS).

Candidiasis diagnosis usually is made by culture or histologic study. When such diagnosis can't be made, identifying *Candida* antibodies may be helpful in diagnosing systemic candidiasis. Serologic testing to detect antibodies in candidiasis isn't reliable, and investigators continue to disagree about its usefulness.

Precautions
- Handle the sample gently to prevent hemolysis.
- Note recent antimicrobial therapy on the laboratory request form.
- Because the patient's immune system may be compromised, keep the venipuncture site clean and dry.

Nursing Considerations

Before the Test
- Confirm the patient's identity using two patient identifiers and confirmation of the patient's identification bracelet according to facility policy.
- Explain the purpose of the *Candida* antibodies test to the patient, as appropriate.
- Inform the patient that there are no food or fluid restrictions for this test.
- Tell the patient that the test requires a blood sample.
- Explain to the patient that there may be slight discomfort from the tourniquet and the needle puncture.

During the Test
- Perform a venipuncture and collect the sample in a 5-mL sterile collection tube without additives.

After the Test
- Send the sample to the laboratory immediately.

• Maintain pressure on the venipuncture site until bleeding stops and to prevent hematoma formation.

Capsule Endoscopy
Normal Findings
• Normal stomach and small intestine anatomy

Abnormal Findings
• Bleeding sites
• Erosions
• Crohn's disease
• Celiac disease
• Benign and malignant tumors of the small intestine
• Vascular disorders
• Medication-related small-bowel injuries
• Pediatric small-bowel disorders

Nursing Implications
• Report abnormal results to the health care provider.
• Prepare to educate the patient about the diagnosis.

• Prepare to administer medications, as ordered.
• Teach the patient about diet and nutrition specific to the diagnosis.

Purpose
• To detect polyps or cancer
• To detect causes of bleeding and anemia

Description
Capsule endoscopy uses a capsule containing a tiny video camera with a light source and transmitter, allowing recording of images along its path. The capsule endoscope measures 11 × 30 mm and is propelled along the digestive tract by peristalsis. The clear end records images of the stomach walls and, in particular, the small intestine, where many other diagnostic techniques may not reach or otherwise visualize. (See the *Detecting Disorders in the Stomach and Small Intestine* box.) The images are transmitted to a data recorder on a belt placed around the patient's waist. After swallowing the pill, the patient doesn't need to stay at

---

Detecting Disorders in the Stomach and Small Intestine

In capsule endoscopy, the patient swallows the capsule, which then travels through the body by the natural movement of the digestive tract. A receiver worn outside the body records the images. The signal's strength indicates the capsule's location.

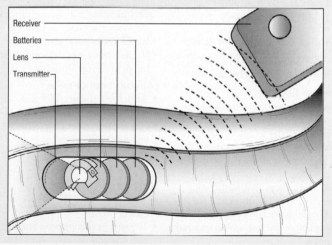

the hospital but can return to work or other activities of daily living.

The typical procedure for capsule endoscopy is as follows:

- The patient ingests the camera pill, as ordered, and a receiver is attached to the patient's belt.
- The pill records images along its path through the stomach, small intestine, and mouth of the large intestine for up to 6 hours, transmitting the information to the receiver.
- The patient returns to the facility, as ordered, so the images can be transmitted into a computer and displayed on the monitor.

Interfering Factors

- Intestinal narrowing or obstruction, causing the pill to become lodged

> **Quality and Safety Nursing Alert**
>
> This procedure is contraindicated in the patient with a suspected obstruction, fistula, or stricture and in the patient who can't swallow (an infant, a young child, or someone with a swallowing impairment).

Precautions

- The battery is short-lived, so images of the large intestine are unobtainable.
- The pill can't be used to stop bleeding, take tissue samples, remove growths, or repair problems it detects. Other invasive studies may be needed.

Nursing Considerations

Before the Test

- Explain to the patient that this test helps visualize the stomach and small intestine, helping to detect disorders.
- Tell the patient who will perform the test, and when and where it will take place.
- Inform the patient that fasting may be required for 12 hours before the test, but fluids are allowed for up to 2 hours before the test, unless ordered otherwise.

- Explain that the patient will need to swallow the camera pill and that the pill will send information to a receiver worn on the belt.
- Tell the patient that the procedure is painless. After swallowing the pill, the patient can go home or go to work.
- Explain to the patient that walking helps facilitate movement of the pill.

After the Test

- Explain that the patient will need to return to the facility in 24 hours (or as directed) so the recorder can be removed from the belt.
- Tell the patient that the pill will be excreted in stool in 8 to 72 hours.
- Tell the patient to resume a usual diet after the images are obtained, as ordered.

Carcinoembryonic Antigen

Reference Values
Less than 5 ng/mL (SI, less than 5 mg/L)

Abnormal Findings

Elevated Levels

- Residual or recurrent tumor (persistently elevated levels)
- Endodermally derived neoplasms of the GI organs and lungs and in certain nonmalignant conditions, such as benign hepatic disease, cirrhosis, alcoholic pancreatitis, inflammatory bowel disease, and renal failure
- Nonendodermal carcinomas, such as breast and ovarian cancers

Nursing Implications

- Anticipate the need for additional testing.
- Prepare the patient for follow-up testing as indicated.
- Provide emotional support to the patient and family.

Purpose

- To monitor the effectiveness of cancer therapy
- To assist in preoperative staging of colorectal cancers, assess the

adequacy of surgical resection, and test for the recurrence of colorectal cancers

Description

Carcinoembryonic antigen (CEA) is a protein normally found in embryonic endodermal epithelium and fetal GI tissue. CEA production stops before birth, but it may begin again if a neoplasm develops. Because CEA levels also are raised by biliary obstruction, alcoholic hepatitis, chronic heavy smoking, and other conditions, this test can't be used as a general indicator of cancer. Measuring enzyme CEA levels by immunoassay is useful for staging and monitoring treatment of certain cancers. (See the *Using CEA to Monitor Cancer Treatment* box.)

Interfering Factors

- Chronic cigarette smoking (possible increase)

Precautions

- Handle the sample gently to prevent hemolysis.

Nursing Considerations

Before the Test

- Confirm the patient's identity using two patient identifiers and confirmation of the patient's identification bracelet according to facility policy.
- Explain to the patient that the CEA test detects and measures a special protein that isn't normally present in adults.
- Inform the patient that the test will be repeated to monitor the effectiveness of therapy, if appropriate.

Using CEA to Monitor Cancer Treatment

Because many patients in the early stages of colorectal cancer have normal or low levels of carcinoembryonic antigen (CEA), the CEA test doesn't screen successfully for early malignancy. It's a good tool, however, for monitoring response to cancer therapy.

After a patient's serum CEA level has dropped following surgery, chemotherapy, or other treatment, an increase suggests recurrence of cancer or diminished effectiveness of treatment.

Both charts below illustrate CEA levels in patients during and after treatment for colorectal cancer. In the left chart, initial results show the usual dramatic drop in response to treatment; the subsequent rise in CEA indicates a diminishing response to chemotherapy. In the right chart, the progressive rise in CEA signals a recurrence of cancer 8 months before clinical symptoms or radiologic evidence.

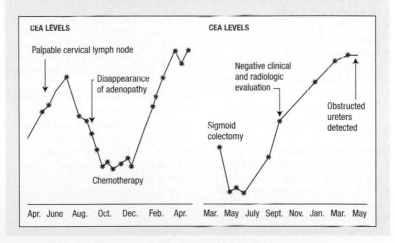

- Inform the patient that there are no food, fluid, or medication restrictions.
- Tell the patient that the test requires a blood sample.
- Explain to the patient that there may be slight discomfort from the tourniquet and the needle puncture.

During the Test
- Perform a venipuncture and collect the sample in a 7-mL tube without additives.

After the Test
- Send the specimen to the laboratory immediately.
- Apply direct pressure to the venipuncture site until bleeding stops and to prevent hematoma formation.

Cardiac Blood Pool Imaging

Normal Findings
- Symmetric left ventricle contractions and an evenly distributed isotope
- Ejection fraction of 55% to 65%

Abnormal Findings
- Asymmetric blood distribution to the myocardium, which produces segmental abnormalities of ventricular wall motion; such abnormalities may also result from preexisting conditions such as myocarditis (in patients with coronary artery disease)
- Globally reduced ejection fractions (patients with cardiomyopathy)
- Prolonged downslope of the scintigraphic data curve caused by the recirculating radioisotope (patients with left-to-right shunt)
- Early arrival of activity in the left ventricle or aorta (patients with right-to-left shunt)

Nursing Implications
- Anticipate the need for additional testing and follow-up.
- Assist with explaining results to the patient and family.
- Prepare the patient for additional testing as indicated.

Purpose
- To evaluate left ventricular function
- To detect aneurysms of the left ventricle and other motion abnormalities of the myocardial wall (areas of akinesia or dyskinesia)
- To detect intracardiac shunting

Description
Cardiac blood pool imaging evaluates regional and global ventricular performance after IV injection of human serum albumin or red blood cells (RBCs) tagged with the isotope technetium 99m (^{99m}Tc) pertechnetate. A scintillation camera records the radioactivity emitted by the isotope in its initial pass through the left ventricle. Higher radioactivity counts occur during diastole because there's more blood in the ventricle; lower counts occur during systole as the blood is ejected. The portion of isotope ejected during each heartbeat can then be calculated to determine the ejection fraction; the presence and size of intracardiac shunts can also be determined.

Cardiac blood pool imaging is more accurate in assessing cardiac function and involves less risk to the patient than left ventriculography.

The procedure for cardiac blood pool imaging is as follows:

- The patient is placed in a supine position beneath the scintillation camera's detector and 15 to 20 millicuries of albumin or RBCs tagged with ^{99m}Tc pertechnetate are injected IV.
- During the next minute, the scintillation camera records the isotope's first pass through the heart, and the aortic and mitral valves are located.
- Then, using an electrocardiogram (ECG), the camera is gated for selected 60-msec intervals, representing end systole and end diastole, and 500 to 1,000 cardiac cycles are recorded on X-ray or Polaroid film.

• To observe septal and posterior wall motion, the patient may be assisted to a modified left anterior oblique position or to a right anterior oblique position and given 0.4 mg of nitroglycerin sublingually. The scintillation camera then records additional gated images to evaluate abnormal contraction in the left ventricle.

• The patient may be asked to exercise as the scintillation camera records gated images.

Precautions

• Cardiac blood pool imaging is contra-indicated during pregnancy.

Nursing Considerations

Before the Test

• Explain to the patient that cardiac blood pooling imaging permits assessment of the heart's left ventricle.

• Describe the test, including who will perform it, when and where it will take place, and its expected duration.

• Tell the patient that there are no food or fluid restrictions before this test.

• Explain that the patient will receive an IV injection of a radioactive tracer and that a detector positioned above the chest will record the circulation of this tracer through the heart.

• Assure the patient that the tracer poses no radiation hazard and rarely produces adverse effects.

• Inform the patient that there may be slight discomfort from the needle puncture but that the imaging itself is painless.

• Instruct the patient to remain silent and motionless during imaging, unless otherwise instructed.

• Make sure that the patient or a responsible family member has signed an informed consent form.

During the Test

• Assist with patient positioning as indicated.

After the Test

• Assess the venipuncture site where the isotope was injected.

> ▶ **Quality and Safety Nursing Alert**

If the patient is elderly or physically compromised, assist to a sitting position and allow legs to dangle until any dizziness passes. Then help the patient get off the examination table.

• Observe for any bruising, redness, irritation, or hematoma formation.

• Dispose of the patient's body fluids and excretions routinely unless directed otherwise.

Cardiac Catheterization

Normal Findings

• No abnormalities of heart chamber size or configuration, wall motion or thickness, blood flow, or valve motion

• Smooth and regular outline of coronary arteries with patent vessels

• Normal pressure curves (See the *Upper Limits of Normal Pressures in Cardiac Chambers and Great Vessels in Recumbent Adults* table, and the *Normal Pressure Curves* box.)

Abnormal Findings

• Constriction of the lumen of the coronary arteries, indicating coronary artery disease (CAD)

• Impaired wall motion, suggesting myocardial incompetence from CAD, aneurysm, cardiomyopathy, or congenital anomalies

• Ejection fraction of less than 35%, suggesting increased risk of complications and decreased probability of successful surgery

• Difference in pressures above and below a heart valve, indicating valvular heart disease

Upper Limits of Normal Pressures in Cardiac Chambers and Great Vessels in Recumbent Adults

This table details the upper limits of normal pressures within the cardiac chambers and great vessels in recumbent adults. Higher-than-normal pressures usually are clinically significant.

Chamber or Vessel	Pressure (mm Hg)
Right atrium	6 (mean)
Right ventricle	30/6*
Pulmonary artery	30/12* (mean, 18)
Left atrium	12 (mean)
Left ventricle	140/12*
Ascending aorta	140/90* (mean, 105)
Pulmonary artery wedge	Almost identical (±1 to 2 mm Hg) to left atrial mean pressure

*Peak systolic and end-diastolic.

- Septal defects (atrial and ventricular) causing altered blood oxygen content on both sides of the heart, elevated blood oxygen levels on the right side (left-to-right atrial or ventricular shunt), or decreased oxygen levels on the left side (right-to-left shunt)

Nursing Implications
- Anticipate the need for additional testing or surgical intervention.
- Prepare the patient for follow-up treatment, including surgery.
- Offer emotional support and patient teaching as indicated.

Normal Pressure Curves

Chambers of the Right Side of the Heart

Two pressure complexes are represented for each chamber. Complexes at the far right in the diagram below represent simultaneous recordings of pressures from the right atrium, right ventricle, and pulmonary artery.

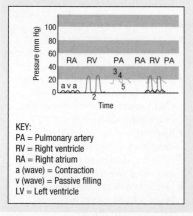

KEY:
PA = Pulmonary artery
RV = Right ventricle
RA = Right atrium
a (wave) = Contraction
v (wave) = Passive filling
LV = Left ventricle

Chambers of the Left Side of the Heart

Overall pressure configurations are similar to those of the right side of the heart, but pressures in the left side of the heart are significantly higher because systemic flow resistance is much greater than pulmonary resistance.

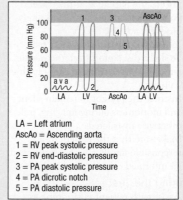

LA = Left atrium
AscAo = Ascending aorta
1 = RV peak systolic pressure
2 = RV end-diastolic pressure
3 = PA peak systolic pressure
4 = PA dicrotic notch
5 = PA diastolic pressure

Purpose

- To evaluate valvular insufficiency or stenosis, septal defects, congenital anomalies, myocardial function and blood supply, and cardiac wall motion
- To help diagnose left ventricular enlargement, aortic root enlargement, ventricular aneurysms, and intracardiac shunts

Description

Cardiac catheterization involves passing a catheter into the right or left side of the heart. Catheterization can determine blood pressure and blood flow in the chambers of the heart, permit blood sample collection, and record films of the heart's ventricles (contrast ventriculography) or arteries (coronary arteriography or angiography). Catheterization of the heart's left side assesses the patency of the coronary arteries, mitral and aortic valve function, and left ventricular function. Catheterization of the heart's right side assesses tricuspid and pulmonic valve function and pulmonary artery pressures.

▶ Quality and Safety Nursing Alert

Coronary artery constriction of greater than 70% is especially significant, particularly in proximal lesions. Narrowing of the left main coronary artery and occlusion or narrowing high in the left anterior descending artery are common indications for revascularization surgery.

The procedure for cardiac catheterization is as follows:

- The patient is placed in the supine position on a tilt-top table and secured by restraints. Electrocardiogram leads are applied for continuous monitoring, and an IV line, if not already in place, is started with dextrose 5% in water or normal saline solution at a keep-vein-open rate.

- After a local anesthetic is injected at the catheterization site, a small incision or percutaneous puncture is made into the artery or vein and the catheter is passed through the needle into the vessel; the catheter is guided to the cardiac chambers or coronary arteries using fluoroscopy.

- In catheterization of the left side of the heart, a catheter is inserted into an artery in the antecubital fossa or into the radial or femoral artery through a puncture or cutdown procedure. Guided by fluoroscopy, the catheter is advanced retrograde through the aorta into the coronary artery orifices and left ventricle.

- In catheterization of the right side of the heart, the catheter is inserted into an antecubital vein or the femoral vein and is advanced through the inferior vena cava or right atrium into the right side of the heart and the pulmonary artery.

- When the catheter is in place, the contrast medium is injected through it to visualize the cardiac vessels and structures.

- The patient may be asked to cough or breathe deeply. Coughing helps counteract nausea or light-headedness caused by the contrast medium and can correct arrhythmias produced by its depressant effect on the myocardium; deep breathing can ease catheter placement into the pulmonary artery or the wedge position and moves the diaphragm downward, making the heart easier to visualize.

- The patient may be given nitroglycerin to eliminate catheter-induced spasm or to measure its effect on the coronary arteries.

- Cardiac output can be measured by analyzing blood oxygen levels in the cardiac chambers. This analysis may be accomplished by drawing blood from cardiac chambers or by injecting contrast medium into the venous circulation and measuring its concentration as it moves past a thermodilution catheter.

• After the procedure is completed, the catheter is removed and pressure should be applied to the incision site for about 30 minutes, either manually or with a mechanical compression device. An adhesive bandage or clear occlusive dressing is applied to protect the site and permit visualization for detection of bleeding or hematoma formation.

Interfering Factors
• Equipment malfunction and poor technique
• Patient anxiety (increased heart rate, blood pressure, and cardiac chamber pressures)

Precautions
• Coagulopathy, impaired renal function, and debilitation usually contraindicate catheterization of both sides of the heart. Unless a temporary pacemaker is inserted to counteract induced ventricular asystole, left bundle-branch block contraindicates catheterization of the right side of the heart.
• If the patient has valvular heart disease, prophylactic antimicrobial therapy may be indicated to guard against subacute bacterial endocarditis.

Nursing Considerations
Before the Test
• Confirm the patient's identity using two patient identifiers and confirmation of the patient's identification bracelet according to facility policy.
• Explain to the patient that cardiac catheterization evaluates the function of the heart and its vessels.
• Instruct the patient to restrict food and fluids for at least 6 hours before the test but to continue prescribed drug regimen unless directed otherwise.
• Describe the test, who will perform it, and when and where it will take place. Tell the patient that the

catheterization team will wear gloves, masks, and gowns to protect the patient from infection.
• Make sure that the patient or a responsible family member has signed an informed consent form.
• Explain that the patient may receive a mild sedative and will remain conscious during the procedure, lying on a padded table as the camera rotates so that the heart can be examined from different angles.
• Inform the patient that an IV needle will be inserted in the arm to administer medication. Assure the patient that the ECG electrodes attached to the chest during the procedure won't cause discomfort.
• Tell the patient that the catheter will be inserted into an artery or a vein in the arm or leg; if the skin above the vessel is hairy, it will be clipped and cleaned with an antiseptic.
• Explain to the patient that there may be a slight stinging sensation when a local anesthetic is injected to numb the incision site for catheter insertion and there may be pressure or a fluttering sensation as the catheter moves along the blood vessel. Assure the patient that these sensations are normal.
• Inform the patient that injection of a contrast medium through the catheter may produce a hot, flushing sensation or nausea that quickly passes; instruct the patient to follow directions to cough or breathe deeply.
• Explain to the patient that medication will be administered if chest pain is experienced during the procedure. The patient may also receive nitroglycerin periodically to dilate coronary vessels and aid visualization. Assure the patient that complications, such as a myocardial infarction (MI) or thromboembolism, are rare.
• Check the patient's history for hypersensitivity to iodine or the contrast

media used in other diagnostic tests; notify the health care provider of any hypersensitivities.

- Discontinue any anticoagulant therapy, as ordered, to reduce the risk of complications from venous bleeding.
- Just before the procedure, tell the patient to void and put on a gown.

After the Test

- Monitor the patient's heart rate and rhythm, respiratory and pulse rates, and blood pressure frequently.
- Monitor the patient's vital signs every 15 minutes for 2 hours after the procedure, every 30 minutes for the next 2 hours, and then every hour for 2 hours. If no hematoma or other problems arise, begin checking every 4 hours. If vital signs are unstable, check every 5 minutes and notify the health care provider.
- Observe the insertion site for a hematoma or blood loss. Additional compression may be necessary to control bleeding.
- Check the patient's color, skin temperature, and peripheral pulse below the puncture site. The brachial approach is associated with a higher incidence of vasospasm (characterized by cool fingers and hands and weak pulses on the affected side); this condition usually resolves within 24 hours.
- Enforce bed rest for 8 hours. If the femoral route was used for catheter insertion, keep the patient's leg extended for 6 to 8 hours; if the antecubital fossa was used, keep the patient's arm extended for at least 3 hours.
- If medications were withheld before the test, check with the health care provider about resuming their administration.
- Administer prescribed analgesics.
- Make sure a posttest ECG is scheduled to check for possible myocardial damage.

Cardiolipin Antibodies

Reference Values
Absent or not detected

Abnormal Findings
- Positive result along with a history of recurrent spontaneous thrombosis, fetal loss, or thrombocytopenia, indicating cardiolipin antibody syndrome
- Positive in connective tissue diseases
- False-positive results can occur from prior history of syphilis.

Nursing Implications
- Anticipate the need for additional testing.
- Be prepared to institute therapy involving anticoagulant or platelet inhibitor agents.

Purpose
- To help diagnose cardiolipin antibody syndrome in the patient with or without lupus erythematosus (LE) who experiences recurrent episodes of spontaneous thrombosis, fetal loss, or thrombocytopenia

Description
The cardiolipin antibodies test measures serum concentrations of immunoglobulin (Ig) G and IgM antibodies in relation to the phospholipid cardiolipin. These antibodies appear in some patients with LE whose serum also contains a coagulation inhibitor (lupus anticoagulant). They also appear in some patients who don't fulfill all the diagnostic criteria for LE but who experience recurrent episodes of spontaneous thrombosis, fetal loss, or thrombocytopenia. Serum concentrations of cardiolipin antibodies are measured by enzyme-linked immunosorbent assay (ELISA).

Precautions
- Handle the sample gently to prevent hemolysis.

Nursing Considerations
Before the Test
- Confirm the patient's identity using two patient identifiers and confirmation of the patient's identification bracelet according to facility policy.
- Tell the patient that the cardiolipin antibodies test helps diagnose cardiolipin antibody syndrome and LE.
- Inform the patient that there are no food or fluid restrictions for this test.
- Tell the patient that the test requires a blood sample.
- Explain to the patient that there may be slight discomfort from the tourniquet and the needle puncture.

During the Test
- Perform a venipuncture and collect the sample in a 5-mL tube without additives.

After the Test
- Send the sample to the laboratory immediately.
- Apply direct pressure to the venipuncture site until bleeding stops and to prevent hematoma formation.

Carotid Artery Duplex Scanning
Normal Findings
- Normal vascular anatomy and blood flow through internal and external carotid arteries and vertebral arteries
- Absence of occlusion or stenosis with normal flow patterns
- Normal vascular wall thickness

Abnormal Findings
- Plaque, stenosis, or occlusion
- Dissection
- Aneurysm
- Tumor of carotid body
- Arteritis

Nursing Implications
- Anticipate the need for additional testing and follow-up.
- Prepare the patient for follow-up treatment.

- Provide emotional support to the patient and family.

Purpose
- To detect occlusive disease of the carotid arterial system
- To evaluate cerebrovascular blood flow

Description
Carotid artery duplex scanning involves two methods of ultrasonic evaluation: Doppler ultrasound and B-mode ultrasound. Doppler ultrasound evaluates the direction and velocity of the blood flow in the arterial system; B-mode ultrasound provides an image of the carotid artery. These ultrasounds are used to evaluate patients with complaints of headache or such neurologic symptoms as dizziness, paresthesias, hemiparesis, and disturbances of speech and vision.

The carotid artery duplex scanning procedure is as follows:
- The patient is placed in a supine position on the examination table with the head slightly extended.
- The patient's head is turned to the opposite side of the examination site.
- Water-soluble gel is applied liberally to the neck area.
- A transducer is moved up and down the area, images are obtained, and the procedure is repeated on the opposite side.

Interfering Factors
- Severe obesity and patient movement (poor quality results)
- Cardiac arrhythmias or cardiac disease (possibly changing hemodynamic patterns)

Nursing Considerations
Before the Test
- Explain to the patient that the test allows examination of the carotid arteries that supply blood to the brain.
- Tell the patient that there are no food or fluid restrictions for this test.

However, advise the patient to refrain from smoking or drinking caffeinated fluids for at least 2 hours before the test.

- Tell the patient who will perform the test, when and where it will take place, that the lights may be dimmed, and there may be only slight pressure felt. Inform the patient that the test takes between 30 and 60 minutes.
- Describe the procedure. Tell the patient that a gel, which may feel cool or wet, will be applied to the neck and that a transducer will pass over the skin, directing safe, painless, and inaudible sound waves into the vessels. Tell the patient that one side will be done at a time.
- Assure the patient that no radiation or contrast medium is used and that there should be no pain felt.
- Advise the patient that any earrings or necklaces will need to be removed before the test.

After the Test
- Remove the conductive gel from the patient's skin.

Catecholamines, Plasma

Reference Values (Fractional Analysis)
Standing: Epinephrine, undetectable to 140 pg/mL (SI, undetectable to 764 pmol/L); norepinephrine, 200 to 1,700 pg/mL (SI, 1,182–10,047 pmol/L)
Supine: Epinephrine, undetectable to 110 pg/mL (SI, undetectable to 600 pmol/L); norepinephrine, 70 to 750 pg/mL (SI, 413–4,432 pmol/L)

Abnormal Findings
Elevated Levels
- Pheochromocytoma, neuroblastoma, ganglioneuroblastoma, or ganglioneuroma
- Thyroid disorders, hypoglycemia, and cardiac disease
- Shock resulting from hemorrhage, endotoxins, and anaphylaxis

Decreased Levels
- Autonomic nervous system dysfunction (normal or low baseline catecholamine levels that don't show an increase in the sample taken after standing)

Nursing Implications
- Anticipate the need for additional testing, as for urine catecholamines.
- Prepare the patient for treatment and follow-up.

Purpose
- To rule out pheochromocytoma (adrenal medullary or extra-adrenal) in the patient with hypertension
- To help identify neuroblastoma, ganglioneuroblastoma, and ganglioneuroma
- To distinguish between adrenal medullary tumors and other catecholamine-producing tumors through fractional analysis (Urinalysis for catecholamine degradation products is recommended to support the diagnosis.)
- To help diagnose autonomic nervous system dysfunction, such as idiopathic orthostatic hypotension

Description
The plasma catecholamines test, a quantitative (total or fractionated) analysis of plasma catecholamines, has clinical importance in the patient with hypertension and signs of adrenal medullary tumor, as well as in the patient with a neural tumor that affects endocrine function. Elevated plasma catecholamine levels necessitate supportive confirmation by urinalysis.

Plasma levels commonly fluctuate in response to temperature, stress, postural change, diet, smoking, anoxia, volume depletion, renal failure, obesity, and many drugs.

Interfering Factors
- Amphetamines, decongestants, epinephrine, levodopa, phenothiazines, sympathomimetics, and tricyclic antidepressants (increase)

- Reserpine (decrease)
- Radioactive scan performed within 1 week before the test

Nursing Considerations

Before the Test

- Confirm the patient's identity using two patient identifiers and confirmation of the patient's identification bracelet according to facility policy.
- Explain to the patient that the plasma catecholamines test helps determine whether hypertension or other symptoms are related to improper hormonal secretion.
- As ordered, instruct the patient to refrain from using self-prescribed medications, especially cold and allergy remedies that may contain sympathomimetics, for 2 weeks before the test.
- Tell the patient to exclude amine-rich foods and beverages, such as bananas, avocados, cheese, coffee, tea, cocoa, beer, and Chianti, from the diet for 48 hours; to maintain vitamin C intake, which is necessary for formation of catecholamines; to abstain from smoking for 24 hours; and to fast for 10 to 12 hours before the test.
- Tell the patient that the test requires one or two blood samples.
- Explain to the patient that there may be slight discomfort from the tourniquet and the needle puncture.
- If the patient is in your facility, withhold medications that affect catecholamine levels, such as amphetamines, phenothiazine (chlorpromazine), sympathomimetics, and tricyclic antidepressants, as ordered.
- Insert an intermittent venous access device (heparin lock or saline lock) 24 hours before the test because the stress of the venipuncture itself may significantly raise catecholamine levels.
- Make sure the patient is relaxed and recumbent for 45 to 60 minutes before the test.

- If necessary, provide blankets to keep the patient warm; low temperatures stimulate catecholamine secretion.

During the Test

- Perform a venipuncture between 6 AM and 8 AM.
- Collect the sample in a 10-mL chilled EDTA tube (sodium metabisulfite solution), which can be obtained from the laboratory on request.
- If a second sample is requested, have the patient stand for 10 minutes, then draw the sample into another tube exactly like the first.
- If a heparin lock is used, it may be necessary to discard the first 1 or 2 mL of blood. Check with the laboratory for the preferred procedure.
- After collecting each sample, roll the tube slowly between your palms to distribute the EDTA without agitating the blood.
- Pack the tube in crushed ice to minimize deactivation of catecholamines and send it to the laboratory immediately.
- Indicate on the laboratory request whether the patient was supine or standing during the venipuncture and the time the sample was drawn.

After the Test

- Apply direct pressure to the venipuncture site until bleeding stops and to prevent hematoma formation.
- Instruct the patient to resume a usual diet and any medications that were discontinued before the test, as ordered.

Catecholamines, Urine

Reference Values (Fractionation)

Dopamine: 65 to 400 mcg/24 hours (SI, 425–2,610 nmol/24 hours)

Epinephrine: 0 to 20 mcg/24 hours (SI, 0–109 nmol/24 hours)

Norepinephrine: 15 to 80 mcg/24 hours (SI, 89–473 nmol/24 hours)

Abnormal Findings

Elevated Levels

- Pheochromocytoma (in the patient with undiagnosed hypertension following a hypertensive episode)
- Neuroblastoma or a ganglioneuroma (elevated levels without marked hypertension)
- Severe systemic situations (burns, peritonitis, shock, and septicemia), cor pulmonale, manic depressive disorders, or depressive neurosis
- Myasthenia gravis and progressive muscular dystrophy (test rarely used to diagnose these disorders)

Decreased Levels

- Dysautonomia (malfunction of the autonomic nervous system) marked by orthostatic hypotension (consistently low-normal catecholamine levels)

Nursing Implications

- Anticipate the need for additional testing.
- Assess the patient's blood pressure when levels are decreased, noting any fluctuations in readings with position changes.
- In patients with increased levels, if tests indicate a pheochromocytoma, the patient may also be tested for multiple endocrine neoplasia.
- In treating patients with increased levels, note that, with the exception of homovanillic acid (HVA)—a dopamine metabolite—catecholamine metabolites may also be elevated. Abnormally high HVA levels rule out a pheochromocytoma because this tumor mainly secretes epinephrine, whose primary metabolite is vanillylmandelic acid (VMA), not HVA.

Purpose

- To help diagnose pheochromocytoma in a patient with unexplained hypertension
- To help diagnose neuroblastoma, ganglioneuroma, and dysautonomia

Description

The test for urine catecholamines uses spectrophotofluorimetry to detect urine levels of the major catecholamines: epinephrine, norepinephrine, and dopamine. For a complete diagnostic workup of catecholamine secretion, urine levels of catecholamine metabolites are also measured. These metabolites—metanephrine, normetanephrine, HVA, and VMA—normally appear in the urine in greater quantities than catecholamines.

Epinephrine is secreted by the adrenal medulla; dopamine, by the central nervous system (CNS); and norepinephrine, by both. Catecholamines help regulate metabolism and prepare the body for the fight-or-flight response to stress. Certain tumors can also secrete catecholamines.

Interfering Factors

- Excessive physical exercise or emotional stress (increase)
- Aminophylline, B-complex vitamins, caffeine, chloral hydrate, insulin, isoproterenol, levodopa, methyldopa, monoamine oxidase inhibitors, nitroglycerin, quinidine, quinine, sympathomimetics, tetracycline, and tricyclic antidepressants (possible increase)
- Clonidine, guanethidine, contrast media containing iodine, and reserpine (possible decrease)
- Erythromycin, methenamine compounds, and phenothiazines (possible increase or decrease)

Precautions

- The preferred specimen is a 24-hour urine specimen because catecholamine secretion fluctuates diurnally and in response to pain, heat, cold, emotional stress, physical exercise, hypoglycemia, injury, hemorrhage, asphyxia, and drugs.
- A random specimen may be useful for evaluating catecholamine levels after a hypertensive episode.

Nursing Considerations

Before the Test

- Confirm the patient's identity using two patient identifiers and confirmation of the patient's identification bracelet according to facility policy.
- Explain to the patient that the urine catecholamine test evaluates adrenal function.
- Inform the patient to avoid amine-rich foods and beverages, such as chocolate, coffee, bananas, avocados, cheese, tea, cocoa, beer, and Chianti for 7 hours before the test and to avoid stressful situations and excessive physical activity during the collection period.
- Tell the patient that the test requires either the collection of urine over 24 hours or a random specimen; explain the collection procedure.
- Notify the laboratory and health care provider of medications the patient is taking that may affect test results; these may need to be restricted.

During the Test

- Collect the patient's urine over a 24-hour period. Use a bottle containing a preservative to keep the specimen acidified to a pH of 3.0 or less. (If a random specimen is ordered, collect it immediately after a hypertensive episode.)
- Refrigerate a 24-hour specimen or place it on ice during the collection period.

After the Test

- Send the specimen to the laboratory as soon as the collection is complete.
- Instruct the patient to resume usual activities, diet, and medications, as ordered.

CD4/CD8 Enumeration

Reference Values

CD4/CD8 ratio: Greater than 1.0

Abnormal Findings

Elevated Levels
- Therapeutic drug effectiveness
- Diurnal variation

Decreased Levels
- Immune dysfunction, including AIDS
- Acute minor viral infections

Nursing Implications

- Anticipate the need for additional testing in patients with elevated levels, including a differential count of lymphocytes. Patients with decreased levels may also require additional testing.
- Determine the specimen collection time in patients with increased levels. (Evening specimen values may be twice as high as specimens obtained in the morning.)

Purpose

- To assist in the identification of immune disorders, primarily AIDS, and possible opportunistic infections
- To help determine when to start antiviral therapy, in combination with viral load testing

Description

The CD4/CD8 enumeration refers to the ratio of CD4 helper T cells to CD8 suppressor T cells. The ratio is based on the CD4 cell count, which is determined by the total number of white blood cells (WBCs) multiplied by the percentage of lymphocytes, and is multiplied by the percentage of lymphocytes that stain positive for CD4. The CD4/CD8 ratio is considered a reliable marker for opportunistic infection in AIDS.

Interfering Factors

- Exercise, emotional stress, and menstruation (increased lymphocytes)
- Recent viral illness (decreased lymphocytes)
- Some antibiotics, such as cefaclor, ceftazidime, and ofloxacin (increased lymphocytes)
- Immunosuppressing agents (decreased lymphocytes)

Precautions

- Institute infection control precautions as indicated.

- Maintain specimen sterility during collection.
- Wear gloves when obtaining or handling the specimen.

Nursing Considerations

Before the Test
- Confirm the patient's identity using two patient identifiers and confirmation of the patient's identification bracelet according to facility policy.
- Explain the purpose of testing to the patient.
- Explain that the testing involves a venipuncture. Explain that there may be discomfort from the tourniquet and the needle puncture.
- Tell the patient that there are no food or fluid restrictions for this test.

During the Test
- Perform a venipuncture; collect a 5-mL sample and place it in an EDTA collection tube.
- Place the specimen in a biohazard bag.

After the Test
- Send the specimen to the laboratory immediately. The specimen must be analyzed within 24 hours.
- Apply pressure to the venipuncture site until bleeding stops and to prevent hematoma formation.
- Assess the venipuncture site for signs and symptoms of infection.
- Teach the patient how to identify infection and when to notify the health care provider.

Celiac and Mesenteric Arteriography

Normal Findings
- Evidence of the three phases of perfusion: arterial, capillary, and venous
- Arteries tapering regularly, becoming gradually smaller with subsequent divisions
- Contrast medium spreading evenly within the sinusoids

- Portal vein emptying 10 to 20 seconds after contrast medium injection as contrast medium empties from the spleen into the splenic vein or from the intestine into the superior mesenteric vein and the portal vein

Abnormal Findings
- Extravasation of contrast medium from the damaged vessels, indicating upper GI hemorrhage from such conditions as Mallory-Weiss syndrome, a gastric or peptic ulcer, hemorrhagic gastritis, or an eroded hiatal hernia, or lower GI hemorrhage resulting from bleeding diverticula, carcinoma, or angiodysplasia
- Neovasculature appearing as abnormal vascular areas or areas of necrosis appearing as puddles of contrast medium, tumor blush, or stain, indicating a neoplasm
- Diminished portal venous flow with dilated tortuous hepatic artery and branches and collateral circulation, indicating progressive cirrhosis
- Displacement of intrasplenic arterial branches, causing the contrast medium to leak from splenic arteries into the splenic pulp, indicating splenic rupture
- Splenic enlargement displacing the splenic artery and vein along with a large, avascular mass that stretches intrasplenic arteries and compresses the splenic pulp away from the capsule, indicating splenic rupture with subcapsular hematoma
- Displacement of the common hepatic artery and extrahepatic branches or displacement of intrahepatic and subcapsular hematomas and stretching of intrahepatic arteries, indicating hepatic injury
- Narrowing of arterial lumen and possible occlusion with formation of collateral circulation, indicating atherosclerotic plaques or atheromas—lipid deposits on the intima
- Aneurysms, thrombi, and emboli

C

Nursing Implications
- Anticipate the need for additional testing.
- Prepare the patient for surgery, if indicated.
- Monitor the patient's vital signs closely for changes.
- Assess the abdomen for increasing girth and pain. Palpate the abdomen for tenderness, rigidity, and rebound tenderness. Note: Don't palpate the abdomen if an abdominal aortic aneurysm is suspected.

Purpose
- To locate the source of GI bleeding
- To help distinguish between benign and malignant neoplasms
- To evaluate cirrhosis and portal hypertension
- To evaluate vascular damage after abdominal trauma
- To detect vascular abnormalities

Description
Celiac and mesenteric arteriography involves the radiographic examination of the abdominal vasculature after intra-arterial injection of a contrast medium through a catheter, which usually is passed through the femoral artery into the aorta and then, using fluoroscopy, positioned in the celiac, superior mesenteric, or inferior mesenteric artery. Injecting contrast medium into one or more of these arteries provides a map of abdominal vasculature; injection into specific arterial branches, called *superselective angiography*, permits detailed visualization of a particular area. As the contrast medium flows through the abdominal vasculature, serial radiographs outline abdominal vessels in the arterial, capillary, and venous phases of perfusion.

Because arteriography can demonstrate the portal vein even when portal venous flow is reversed, it's used more often than splenoportography. Complications associated with this test include hemorrhage, venous and intracardiac thrombosis, cardiac arrhythmia, and emboli caused by dislodging atherosclerotic plaques.

The procedure for celiac and mesenteric arteriography is as follows:
- After the patient is placed in a supine position on the X-ray table, an IV infusion is started to maintain hydration and to permit emergency administration of medication. The patient is attached to a heart monitor and pulse oximeter, and blood pressure is monitored according to the facility's policy.
- Spot films of the patient's abdomen are taken, and the peripheral pulses are palpated and marked.
- The puncture site is cleaned with soap and water; the area is clipped, cleaned with povidone–iodine preparation, and surrounded by sterile drapes.
- A local anesthetic is injected, and the femoral artery is located by palpation. The needle is gently inserted until a pulsing blood flow is obtained.
- A guide wire is passed through the needle into the aorta and then the needle is removed, leaving the guide wire in place.
- The catheter is inserted over the guide wire and then withdrawn to inject the contrast medium to check for catheter placement. The guide wire is again inserted into the selected artery for fluoroscopic guidance.
- When the wire is in position, the catheter is advanced over it into the artery. The wire is then removed and placement verified by hand injection of contrast medium.
- The automatic injector is then attached to the catheter. As the contrast medium is injected, a series of films is taken in rapid sequence.
- After injecting into one or more major arteries, superselective catheterization may be performed. Using fluoroscopy, the catheter is repositioned in a specific branch of a major

artery, contrast medium is injected, and rapid-sequence films are taken. If necessary, several specific branches may be catheterized.

- If an occlusion is detected, balloon angioplasty is performed.
- After filming, the catheter is withdrawn and firm pressure is applied to the puncture site for about 15 minutes.

Interfering Factors

- The patient's inability to remain still during the procedure
- Gas, stool, or barium from a previous procedure (possible poor imaging)
- Presence of an atherosclerotic lesion in the vessel to be cannulated (prevents the entry and passage of the catheter)

Precautions

- Celiac and mesenteric arteriography should be performed cautiously in the patient with coagulopathy.
- This test is contraindicated in the pregnant patient because of radiation's possible teratogenic effects.
- Temporarily discontinue metformin in patients undergoing radiologic studies in which intravascular iodinated contrast media are utilized.

Nursing Considerations

Before the Test

- Explain to the patient that celiac and mesenteric arteriography permits examination of the abdominal blood vessels after injection of a contrast medium.
- Instruct the patient to fast for 8 hours.
- Explain that the patient will receive IV conscious sedation and a local anesthetic and that there may be a brief, stinging sensation as the anesthetic is injected. The patient may also feel pressure when the femoral artery is palpated, but the local anesthetic will minimize pain when the needle is introduced into the artery.

- Tell the patient that there may be a transient burning as the contrast medium is injected.
- Tell the patient that the X-ray equipment makes a loud, clacking sound as the films are taken.
- Instruct the patient to lie still during the test to avoid blurring the films. Restraints may be used to help the patient remain still.
- Warn that the patient may feel some temporary stiffness after the test from lying still on the hard X-ray table.
- Tell the patient who will perform the test, when and where it will take place, and that it takes 30 minutes to 3 hours, depending on the number of vessels studied.
- Make sure that the patient or a responsible family member has signed an informed consent form.
- Check the patient's history for hypersensitivity to iodine or the contrast medium.

> ▶ **Quality and Safety Nursing Alert**
>
> Most reactions to the contrast medium occur within 30 minutes. Watch the patient carefully for cardiovascular shock or arrest, flushing, laryngeal stridor, or urticaria.

- Make sure blood studies (hemoglobin and hematocrit levels; clotting, prothrombin, and partial thromboplastin times; and platelet count) have been completed.
- Just before the procedure, instruct the patient to put on a gown and to remove jewelry and other objects that might obscure anatomic detail on X-ray films.
- Tell the patient to void and then record baseline vital signs.
- Administer a sedative, if prescribed.

After the Test

- Check peripheral pulses.
- Explain that the patient will be on bed rest for 4 to 6 hours and must

C

keep the leg with the puncture site straight. Don't raise the bed more than 30 degrees. The patient will be able to log roll and may use the unaffected leg to reposition to use the bedpan.

• Monitor the patient's vital signs until stable and check peripheral pulses. Note the color and temperature of the leg that was used for the test.

• Check the puncture site for bleeding and hematoma. If bleeding develops, apply pressure to the site. If a hematoma develops, apply warm soaks.

• Confirm whether the patient can resume a usual diet. If the patient isn't receiving IV infusions, encourage intake of fluids to speed excretion of the contrast medium.

► *Quality and Safety Nursing Alert*

The nurse should anticipate the need for administration of acetylcysteine for patients who may have renal compromise to prevent contrast-induced nephropathy.

Cerebral Angiography

Normal Findings

• *During the arterial phase of perfusion:* Contrast medium filling and opacifying superficial and deep arteries and arterioles

• *During venous phase:* Contrast medium opacifying superficial and deep veins

• Symmetric cerebral vasculature

Abnormal Findings

• Changes in the caliber of vessel lumina, suggesting spasms, plaques, fistulas, arteriovenous malformation, or arteriosclerosis

• Diminished blood flow to vessels, possibly related to increased intracranial pressure (ICP) (See the *Comparing Normal and Abnormal Cerebral Angiograms* box.)

• Vessel displacement or changes in circulation, indicating tumor, edema, or obstructed cerebrospinal fluid (CSF) pathway

Nursing Implications

• Anticipate the need for additional testing.

Comparing Normal and Abnormal Cerebral Angiograms

The angiograms below show the differences between normal and abnormal cerebral vasculature. The cerebral angiogram on the left is normal. The cerebral angiogram on the right shows occluded blood vessels caused by a large arteriovenous malformation.

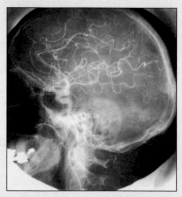 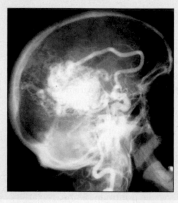

- Prepare the patient for surgery, if indicated.
- Provide emotional support to the patient and family.

Purpose

- To detect cerebrovascular abnormalities, such as aneurysm or arteriovenous malformation, thrombosis, narrowing, or occlusion
- To study vascular displacement caused by tumor, hematoma, edema, herniation, vasospasm, ICP, or hydrocephalus
- To locate clips applied to blood vessels during surgery and to evaluate the postoperative status of affected vessels

Description

Cerebral angiography involves injecting a contrast medium to allow radiographic examination of the cerebral vasculature. Possible injection sites include the femoral and brachial arteries. Because it allows visualization of four vessels (the carotid and vertebral arteries), the femoral artery is used most commonly.

Usually, this test is performed on patients with suspected abnormality of the cerebral vasculature; abnormalities may be suggested by intracranial computed tomography (CT), lumbar puncture, magnetic resonance imaging (MRI), or magnetic resonance angiography.

The procedure for cerebral angiography is as follows:

- The patient is assisted to recline on an X-ray table and instructed to lie still with arms at sides.
- The injection site is prepped and cleaned with alcohol and povidone–iodine.
- A local anesthetic is injected, then the artery is punctured with the appropriate needle and catheterized.
- In the femoral artery approach, a catheter is threaded to the aortic arch.
- In the brachial artery approach (least common), a blood pressure cuff is placed distal to the puncture site and

inflated before injection to prevent the contrast medium from flowing into the forearm and hand.
- After X-rays or fluoroscopy verifies placement of the needle or catheter, the contrast medium is injected. The patient is observed for an adverse reaction, such as hives, flushing, or laryngeal stridor.
- An initial series of lateral and anteroposterior X-rays is taken, developed, and reviewed. Depending on the results, more contrast medium may be injected and another series taken.
- During the test, arterial catheter patency is maintained by continuous or periodic flushing. The patient's vital and neurologic signs are monitored closely.
- When a satisfactory series of X-rays is obtained, the needle (or catheter) is withdrawn and firm pressure is applied to the puncture site for 15 minutes.

Interfering Factors

- Head movement during the test (possible poor imaging)
- Metal objects in X-ray field (possible poor imaging)

Precautions

- Cerebral angiography is contraindicated in patients with hepatic, renal, or thyroid disease and in patients who are hypersensitive to iodine or contrast media.

Nursing Considerations

Before the Test

- Explain to the patient that cerebral angiography shows blood circulation in the brain.
- Describe the test, including who will administer it and when and where it will take place.
- Check the patient's history for hypersensitivity to iodine, iodine-containing substances (such as shellfish), or other contrast media. Note hypersensitivities on the chart, and report them as appropriate.

C

- Tell the patient to fast for 8 to 10 hours before the test.
- Make sure that any pretest blood work results are on the chart to determine bleeding tendency or kidney function.
- Ask the patient about medication use, specifically anticoagulants. These may need to be discontinued for 3 days before testing.
- Explain that the patient will wear a gown and must remove all jewelry, dentures, hairpins, and other metallic objects in the radiographic field.
- If ordered, administer a sedative and an anticholinergic drug 30 to 45 minutes before the test.
- Make sure the patient voids prior to the test.
- Describe the patient's position on the X-ray table with head immobilized and emphasize that the patient should remain still.
- Explain that a local anesthetic will be administered; however, some patients—especially children—receive a general anesthetic.
- Explain that the patient will feel a transient burning sensation as the medium is injected; a warm, flushed feeling; a transient headache; a salty or metallic taste in the mouth; or nausea and vomiting after the dye is injected.
- Make sure that the patient or a responsible family member has signed an informed consent form.

After the Test
- Observe the patient for bleeding, check distal pulses, and apply a pressure bandage.

> **Quality and Safety Nursing Alert**

If the patient has been receiving aspirin or other anticoagulants (such as warfarin) daily, take extra care when compressing the puncture site.

- Maintain bed rest as ordered. Typically, the patient will be on bed rest for 6 to 8 hours.
- Administer prescribed pain medications and monitor the patient's vital signs and neurologic status for 6 hours. The patient is usually discharged the same day.
- Monitor the catheter puncture site frequently and closely for hemorrhage or hematoma formation. If either occurs, notify the health care provider immediately. If bleeding occurs, apply firm pressure to the puncture site and inform the health care provider. Also observe the puncture site for signs of extravasation (redness, swelling) and apply an ice bag to ease the patient's discomfort and minimize swelling.

> **Quality and Safety Nursing Alert**

If the femoral approach was used, keep the patient's affected leg straight for 6 hours or longer and routinely check pulses distal to the site (dorsalis pedis, popliteal). Monitor the leg for temperature, color, and sensation. Thrombosis or hematoma can occlude blood flow; extravasation can also impede blood flow by exerting pressure on the artery.

- If the brachial approach was used, immobilize the affected arm for 6 hours or longer and routinely check the radial pulse.
- Monitor the patient for disorientation and weakness or numbness in the extremities (signs of thrombosis or hematoma) and for arterial spasms, which may produce symptoms of transient ischemic attacks.
- Place a sign near the patient's bed warning personnel not to take blood.
- Observe the patient's arm and hand for changes in color, temperature, or sensation. If they become pale, cool, or numb, report these changes at once.
- Tell the patient to resume a usual diet; encourage the patient to drink fluids to help pass the contrast medium.

Cerebrospinal Fluid Analysis

Normal Findings
- Clear colorless fluid
- No RBCs; 0 to 5 WBCs

- No organisms on Gram stain
- Pressure range of 50 to 180 mm H$_2$O
  (See the *Findings in Cerebrospinal Fluid Analysis* table.)

C

Findings in Cerebrospinal Fluid Analysis

Test	Normal	Abnormality	Implications
Pressure	50 to 180 mm H$_2$O	Increase	Increased intracranial pressure
		Decrease	Spinal subarachnoid obstruction above puncture site
Appearance	Clear, colorless	Cloudy	Infection
		Xanthochromic or blood	Subarachnoid, intracerebral, or intraventricular hemorrhage; spinal cord obstruction; traumatic tap (usually noted only in initial specimen)
		Brown, orange, or yellow	Elevated protein levels, red blood cell (RBC) breakdown (blood present for at least 3 days)
Protein	IS to 50 mg/dL (SI, 0.15–0.5 g/L)	Marked increase	Tumors, trauma, hemorrhage, diabetes, polyneuritis, blood in cerebrospinal fluid (CSF)
		Marked decrease	Rapid CSF production
Gamma globulin	3% to 12% of total protein	Increase	Demyelinating disease, neurosyphilis, Guillain-Barré syndrome
Glucose	50 to 80 mg/dL (SI, 2.8–4.4 mmol/L)	Increase	Systemic hyperglycemia
		Decrease	Systemic hypoglycemia, bacterial or fungal infection, meningitis, mumps, postsubarachnoid hemorrhage
Cell count	0 to 5 white blood cells	Increase	Active disease: meningitis, acute infection, onset of chronic illness, tumor, abscess, infarction, demyelinating disease
	No RBCs	RBCs	Hemorrhage or traumatic lumbar puncture
Venereal Disease Research Laboratories (VDRL), test for syphilis, and other serologic tests	Nonreactive	Positive	Neurosyphilis
Chloride	118 to 130 mEq/L (SI, 118–130 mmol/L)	Decrease	Infected meninges
Gram stain	No organisms	Gram-positive or gram-negative organisms	Bacterial meningitis

C

Abnormal Findings
- Cloudy, bloody, brown, orange, or yellow fluid
- Positive for RBCs; increased WBCs
- Gram-positive or gram-negative organisms
- Increased or decreased pressure

Nursing Implications
- Anticipate the need for additional testing.
- Prepare the patient for follow-up treatment.
- Monitor for signs and symptoms of meningitis or ICP and report them immediately to the health care provider.
- Assess for decreasing level of consciousness, changes in pupil size and reactivity, altered vital signs, and respiratory failure suggesting cerebral herniation.

Purpose
- To measure CSF pressure as an aid in detecting a CSF circulation obstruction
- To help diagnose viral or bacterial meningitis, subarachnoid or intracranial hemorrhage, tumors, and brain abscesses
- To help diagnose neurosyphilis and chronic CNS infections
- To assist in the diagnosis of Alzheimer's disease

Description
CSF, a clear substance that circulates in the subarachnoid space, protects the brain and spinal cord from injury and transports products of neurosecretion, cellular biosynthesis, and cellular metabolism through the CNS.

For qualitative analysis, CSF is obtained most commonly by lumbar puncture (usually between the third and fourth lumbar vertebrae) and, rarely, by cisternal or ventricular puncture. A CSF specimen may also be obtained during other neurologic tests, such as myelography.

The procedure for CSF analysis is as follows:

- The patient is positioned on one side with knees drawn up to the abdomen and the chin on the chest. The patient may also be positioned sitting up with the head and chest bent toward the knees.
- After the skin is prepared for injection, the area is draped.
- The anesthetic is injected, and the spinal needle is inserted in the midline, between the spinous processes of the vertebrae (usually between the third and fourth lumbar vertebra). Next, initial (or opening) CSF pressure is measured and a specimen is obtained and placed in the appropriate containers.
- CSF pressure is recorded, and the appearance of the specimen is checked.
- Three tubes are collected routinely and are sent to the laboratory for protein, sugar, and cell analysis, and for serologic testing (Venereal Disease Research Laboratory [VDRL] test for neurosyphilis). A separate specimen is sent for culture and sensitivity testing.
- Electrolyte analysis and Gram stain may be ordered as supplementary tests. CSF electrolyte levels are of special interest in the patient with abnormal serum electrolyte levels or CSF infection and in the patient receiving hyperosmolar agents.
- A final pressure reading is taken, and the needle is removed.

Interfering Factors
- Patient position and activity (possible increase or decrease in CSF pressure)
- Crying, coughing, or straining (possible increase in CSF pressure)
- Delay between collection time and laboratory testing (possible invalidation of test results, especially cell counts)
- Blood in the spinal fluid from traumatic puncture

Precautions

- Infection at the puncture site contra-indicates CSF removal; in the patient with ICP, CSF should be removed with extreme caution because fluid withdrawal can cause a rapid reduction in pressure and cerebellar tonsillar herniation and medullary compression.

Nursing Considerations

Before the Test

- Confirm the patient's identity using two patient identifiers and confirmation of the patient's identification bracelet according to facility policy.
- Describe the procedure to the patient and explain that CSF analysis analyzes the fluid around the spinal cord.
- Inform the patient that there are no food or fluid restrictions for this test.
- Tell the patient who will perform the procedure, and when and where it will take place.
- Advise the patient that a headache is the most common adverse effect of a lumbar puncture, but assure the patient that cooperation during the test helps minimize this effect.
- Make sure that the patient or a responsible family member has signed an informed consent form.

During the Test

- If the patient is positioned on the side, provide pillows to support the spine on a horizontal plane. This position allows full flexion of the spine and easy access to the lumbar subarachnoid space. Help the patient maintain this position by placing one arm around the knees and the other arm around the neck.
- If the sitting position is used, help the patient maintain this position throughout the procedure.
- Warn the patient that experiencing a transient burning sensation when the local anesthetic is injected is likely.
- Tell the patient that when the spinal needle is inserted, there may be slight local pain as the needle transverses the dura mater.
- Ask the patient to report pain or sensations that differ from or continue after this expected discomfort because such sensations may indicate irritation or puncture of a nerve root, requiring needle repositioning.
- Instruct the patient to remain still and breathe normally; movement and hyperventilation can alter pressure readings or cause injury.
- Observe closely for adverse reactions, such as elevated pulse rate, pallor, or clammy skin. Report any significant changes immediately.
- After the specimen is collected, label the containers in the order in which they were filled and find out whether specific instructions are required for the laboratory.
- Record the collection time on the test request form. Send the form and labeled specimens to the laboratory immediately after collection.
- Clean the puncture site with a local antiseptic, such as povidone–iodine solution, and apply a small adhesive bandage.

After the Test

- Check whether the patient must lie flat or if the head of the bed may be slightly elevated. In most cases, you'll be instructed to keep the patient lying flat for 6 hours after lumbar puncture. Some health care providers, however, allow a 30-degree elevation at the head of the bed.
- Explain that the patient's head must lie back and should not be raised, but it may be turned from side to side.
- Encourage the patient to drink fluids. Provide a flexible straw.
- Check the puncture site for redness, swelling, and drainage every hour for the first 4 hours, and then every 4 hours for the first 24 hours.
- If CSF pressure is elevated, assess the patient's neurologic status every 15 minutes for 4 hours. If the patient

is stable, assess every hour for 2 hours and then every 4 hours or according to the pretest schedule.

▶ Quality and Safety Nursing Alert

Watch the patient for complications of lumbar puncture, such as reaction to the anesthetic, meningitis, bleeding into the spinal canal, cerebellar tonsillar herniation, and medullary compression. Signs of meningitis include fever, neck rigidity, and irritability; signs of herniation include decreased level of consciousness, changes in pupil size and equality, altered vital signs (including widened pulse pressure, decreased pulse rate, and irregular respirations), and respiratory failure.

Ceruloplasmin

Reference Values
- 22.9 to 43.1 g/dL (SI, 0.22–0.43 g/L)

Abnormal Findings

Elevated Levels
- Hepatic diseases and infections

Decreased Levels
- Wilson's disease, Menkes' syndrome, nephrotic syndrome, and hypocupremia caused by total parenteral nutrition

Nursing Implications
- Anticipate the need for additional testing, including, in patients with decreased levels, iron levels.
- Prepare the patient for follow-up treatment.
- Monitor the patient's total parenteral nutrition as indicated.
- Provide emotional support to the patient and family.

Purpose
- To help diagnose Wilson's disease, Menkes' syndrome, and copper deficiency

Description

The ceruloplasmin test is used to measure serum levels of ceruloplasmin, an alpha$_2$-globulin that binds about 95% of serum copper, usually in the liver. Ceruloplasmin is thought to regulate iron uptake by transferrin, making iron available to reticulocytes for heme synthesis.

Interfering Factors
- Estrogen, methadone, phenytoin (possible increase)
- Pregnancy (possible increase)

Nursing Considerations

Before the Test
- Confirm the patient's identity using two patient identifiers and confirmation of the patient's identification bracelet according to facility policy.
- Explain to the patient that this test is used to determine the copper content of blood.
- Tell the patient that the test requires a blood sample.
- Explain to the patient that there may be slight discomfort from the needle puncture and the tourniquet.
- Notify the laboratory and health care provider of medications the patient is taking that may affect test results; these may need to be restricted.

During the Test
- Perform a venipuncture; collect the sample in a 7-mL clot activator tube.

After the Test
- Send the sample to the laboratory immediately.
- Apply direct pressure to the venipuncture site until bleeding stops and to prevent hematoma formation.
- Explain that the patient may resume usual medications that were discontinued before the test, as ordered.

Cervical Punch Biopsy

Normal Findings
- Cervical tissue composed of columnar and squamous and epithelial cells, loose connective tissue, and smooth muscle fibers
- No dysplasia or abnormal cell growth

Abnormal Findings
• Dysplasia or abnormal cells, indicating intraepithelial neoplasia or invasive cancer

Nursing Implications
• Anticipate the need for additional testing.
• Prepare the patient for possible cone biopsy under general anesthesia to obtain a larger tissue specimen and to allow a more accurate evaluation of dysplasia.
• Provide emotional support to the patient and family during and after testing.
• Help the patient cope with a possible cancer diagnosis.

Purpose
• To evaluate suspicious cervical lesions
• To diagnose cervical cancer

Description
Cervical punch biopsy or cervical biopsy is the excision by sharp forceps of a tissue specimen from the cervix for histologic examination. Generally, multiple biopsies are done to obtain specimens from all areas with abnormal tissue or from the squamocolumnar junction and other sites around the cervical circumference. The biopsy site is selected by direct visualization of the cervix with a colposcope or by Schiller's test, which stains normal squamous epithelium a dark mahogany but fails to color abnormal tissue. Other biopsies are done to detect other gynecologic disorders. The biopsy is performed when the cervix is least vascular, usually 1 week after menses.

The procedure for cervical punch biopsy is as follows:

• The patient is placed in the lithotomy position, and an unlubricated speculum is inserted.
• For direct visualization, the colposcope is inserted through the speculum, the biopsy site is located, and the cervix is cleaned with a swab soaked in 3% acetic acid solution.

• The biopsy forceps are inserted through the speculum or the colposcope, and tissue is removed from a lesion or from selected sites, starting from the posterior lip to avoid obscuring other sites with blood.
• Each specimen is immediately put in 10% formalin solution in a labeled bottle.
• To control bleeding after biopsy, the cervix is swabbed with 5% silver nitrate solution (cautery or sutures may be used instead). If bleeding persists, the examiner may insert a tampon.
• For Schiller's test, an applicator stick saturated with iodine solution is inserted through the speculum. This stains the cervix to identify lesions for biopsy.

Interfering Factors
• Nonrepresentative specimens obtained
• Delay in placing specimen in preservative

Nursing Considerations
Before the Test
• Confirm the patient's identity using two patient identifiers and confirmation of the patient's identification bracelet according to facility policy.
• Assess the date of the patient's last menses.
• Describe the procedure to the patient, and explain that it provides a cervical tissue specimen for microscopic study.
• Tell the patient who will perform the biopsy and when and where it will be done.
• Tell the patient that she may experience mild discomfort and cramping during and after the biopsy.
• Advise the outpatient to have someone accompany her home after the biopsy.
• Make sure the patient or a responsible family member has signed an informed consent form.
• Ask the patient to void just before the biopsy.

During the Test

- Assist the patient into the lithotomy position, and tell her to relax as the unlubricated speculum is inserted.
- Ensure that specimens are placed in the preservative immediately.

After the Test

- Record the patient's and health care provider's names and the biopsy sites on the laboratory request.
- Send the specimens to the laboratory immediately.
- Instruct the patient to avoid strenuous exercise for 24 hours after the biopsy.
- Encourage the outpatient to rest briefly before leaving the office.
- If a tampon was inserted after the biopsy, tell the patient to leave it in place for 8 to 24 hours. Inform her that some bleeding may occur, but tell her to report heavy bleeding (heavier than menses). Warn the patient to avoid using additional tampons, which can irritate the cervix and provoke bleeding.
- Tell the patient to avoid douching and intercourse for 2 weeks, or as directed, if she has undergone such treatments as cryotherapy or laser treatment during the procedure.
- Tell the patient that a foul-smelling, gray-green vaginal discharge is normal for several days after the biopsy and may persist for 3 weeks.
- If no tampon was used after the procedure, have the patient use a sanitary pad to avoid soiling clothes with discharge. In rare cases, the patient may experience cramping.

Chest Radiography

Normal Findings

- Translucent and tubelike trachea visible midline in the anterior mediastinal cavity
- Heart in the anterior left mediastinal cavity, appearing solid because of its blood content
- Aortic knob visible as water density
- Mediastinum (mediastinal shadow) visible as the space between the lungs, appearing shadowy and widened at the hilum
- Ribs visible as a thoracic cavity encasement
- Spine with visible midline in the posterior chest, clearest on a lateral view
- Clavicles visible in the upper thorax, appearing intact and equidistant in properly centered films
- Hila (lung roots appearing as small, white, bilateral branching densities) visible above the heart where pulmonary vessels, bronchi, and lymph nodes join the lungs
- Translucent, tubelike mainstem bronchus visible as part of the hila
- Hemidiaphragm rounded and visible with right side to ¾-inch (1–2 cm) higher than the left side

Abnormal Findings

- Deviation of the trachea from midline, indicating possible tension pneumothorax or pleural effusion
- Right-sided hypertrophy of the heart, indicating cor pulmonale or heart failure
- Tortuous aortic knob, indicating atherosclerosis
- Gross widening of the mediastinum, suggesting neoplasm or aortic aneurysm
- Break or misalignment of bones, indicating fracture
- Visible bronchi, indicating bronchial pneumonia
- Flattening of the diaphragm, indicating emphysema or asthma
- Irregular, patchy infiltrates in the lung fields, indicating pneumonia (See the *Selected Clinical Implications of Chest X-ray Films* table.)

Nursing Implications

- Anticipate the need for additional testing to support or confirm the diagnosis.

Selected Clinical Implications of Chest X-Ray Films

C

Normal Anatomic Location and Appearance	Possible Abnormality	Implications
Trachea		
Visible midline in the anterior mediastinal cavity; translucent tubelike appearance	• Deviation from midline	• Tension pneumothorax, atelectasis, pleural effusion, consolidation, mediastinal nodes or, in children, enlarged thymus
	• Narrowing with hourglass appearance and deviation to one side	• Substernal thyroid or stenosis secondary to trauma
Heart		
Visible in the anterior left mediastinal cavity; solid appearance due to blood contents; edges possibly clear in contrast to surrounding air density of the lung	• Shift	• Atelectasis, pneumothorax
	• Hypertrophy	• Cor pulmonale, heart failure
	• Cardiac borders obscured by stringy densities ("shaggy heart")	• Cystic fibrosis
Aortic Knob		
Visible as water density; formed by the arch of the aorta	• Solid densities, possibly indicating calcifications	• Atherosclerosis
	• Tortuous shape	• Atherosclerosis
Mediastinum (mediastinal shadow)		
Visible as the space between the lungs; shadowy appearance that widens at the hilum of the lungs	• Deviation to nondiseased side; deviation to diseased side by traction	• Pleural effusion or tumor, fibrosis or collapsed lung
	• Gross widening	• Neoplasms of esophagus, bronchi, lungs, thyroid, thymus, peripheral nerves, lymphoid tissue; aortic aneurysm; mediastinitis; cor pulmonale
Rib		
Visible as thoracic cage	• Break or misalignment	• Fractured sternum or ribs
	• Widening of intercostal spaces	• Emphysema
Spine		
Visible midline in the posterior chest; straight bony structure	• Spinal curvature	• Scoliosis, kyphosis
	• Break or misalignment	• Fractures
Visible in upper thorax; intact and equidistant in properly centered X-ray film	• Break or misalignment	

(continued on page 150)

Selected Clinical Implications of Chest X-Ray Films (continued)

Normal Anatomic Location and Appearance	Possible Abnormality	Implications
Hila (lung roots)		
Visible above the heart, where pulmonary vessels, bronchi, and lymph nodes join the lungs; appear as small, white, bilateral densities	• Accentuated shadows • Shift to one side	• Atelectasis • Pneumothorax, emphysema, pulmonary abscess, tumor; enlarged lymph nodes
Mainstem bronchus		
Visible; part of the hila with translucent tube-like appearance	• Spherical or oval density	• Bronchogenic cyst
Bronchi		
Usually not visible	• Visible	• Bronchial pneumonia
Lung Fields		
Usually not visible throughout, except for the blood vessels	• Visible • Irregular	• Atelectasis • Resolving pneumonia, infiltrates, silicosis, fibrosis, neoplasm
Hemidiaphragm		
Rounded, visible; right side ⅜ to ¾ inch (1 to 2 cm)	• Elevation of diaphragm (difference in elevation can be measured on inspiration and expiration to detect movement) • Flattening of diaphragm • Unilateral elevation of either side • Unilateral elevation of left side only	• Active tuberculosis, pneumonia, pleurisy, acute bronchitis, active disease of the abdominal viscera, bilateral phrenic nerve involvement • Asthma, emphysema • Possible unilateral phrenic nerve paresis • Perforated ulcer (rare), gas distention of stomach or splenic flexure of colon, free air in abdomen

• Prepare the patient for follow-up treatment as indicated.
• Assess cardiopulmonary status for changes.

Purpose
• To detect cardiopulmonary disorders, such as emphysema, pneumonia, atelectasis, pneumothorax, pulmonary bullae, pleurisy, cardiomegaly, heart failure, and tumors
• To detect mediastinal abnormalities, such as tumors, and cardiac disease, such as heart failure
• To determine the correct placement of pulmonary catheters, endotracheal tubes, and other chest tubes
• To determine the location and size of lesions or foreign bodies
• To help assess pulmonary status
• To evaluate the patient's response to interventions

Description

In chest radiography, X-rays or electromagnetic waves penetrate the chest and cause an image to form on specially sensitized film. Air appears radiolucent, whereas normal tissue, bone, and abnormalities—such as infiltrates, foreign bodies, fluids, and tumors—appear as densities. A chest X-ray is most useful when compared with previous films to detect changes.

The procedure for chest radiography is as follows:

• If a stationary X-ray machine is used, the patient stands or sits in front of the machine so films can be taken of the posteroanterior and left lateral views.

• If a portable X-ray machine is used at the patient's bedside, the patient is moved to the top of the bed, if possible. Nipple markers are placed on the patient's areolae to identify nipples, which may have a distinct density and otherwise appear as nodules. The head of the bed is elevated for maximum upright positioning. The patient must take a deep breath and hold it for several seconds.

Interfering Factors

• Portable chest X-rays (possible lower quality image than stationary X-rays)

• Portable chest X-rays taken in the anteroposterior position (possible larger cardiac shadowing than other X-rays because of shorter distance between the beam and anterior structures)

• Excessive movement

• Patient in a supine position (hides fluid levels that are visible in decubitus views)

• Patient's inability to take a full inspiration

• Under- or overexposure of films

• Incorrect view of the area (For example, lateral film views reveal infiltrates [pneumonia, atelectasis] that may not be seen in anteroposterior views or posteroanterior views because of heart obstruction.)

• Extrathoracic structures, such as breast implants or body piercings (may be radiopaque and obscure anatomic area of interest)

Precautions

• Chest radiography usually is contraindicated during the first trimester of pregnancy; however, when radiography is absolutely necessary, a lead apron placed over the patient's abdomen can shield the fetus.

• To avoid exposure to radiation, leave the room or the immediate area while the films are being taken. If you must stay in the area, wear a lead-lined apron or protective clothing.

Nursing Considerations

Before the Test

• Explain to the patient that chest radiography assesses chest anatomy.

• Tell the patient that there are no food or fluid restrictions for this test.

• Describe the test, including who will perform it, and where and when it will take place.

• Provide a gown without snaps and instruct the patient to remove jewelry and other metallic objects that may be in the X-ray field.

• Explain that the patient will be asked to take a deep breath and to hold it momentarily while the film is being taken to provide a clearer view of pulmonary structures.

• Tell the patient that a lead apron may be placed over the abdomen to protect the reproductive organs.

• If the patient is intubated, check that no tubes have been dislodged during positioning.

During the Test

• If the X-ray is done at the bedside, place cardiac monitoring lead wires, IV tubing from central lines, pulmonary artery catheter lines, and safety pins as far from the X-ray field as possible.

After the Test
- If the test is done at the bedside, reposition the patient comfortably. Otherwise, no special care is required.

Chlamydia trachomatis Culture

Normal Findings
- No *Chlamydia trachomatis* in the culture

Abnormal Findings
- Positive culture, confirming *C. trachomatis* infection

Nursing Implications
- Help explain the test results.
- Administer prescribed antimicrobial treatment as ordered.
- Counsel the patient about encouraging sexual partners to be tested.
- Report findings to the local health authority as required.

Purpose
- To confirm infections caused by *C. trachomatis*

Description
The most common sexually transmitted disease in the United States, chlamydia infection is caused by the *C. trachomatis* organism. Identifying this parasite requires cultivation in the laboratory. After incubation, cells infected with chlamydia can be detected by iodine stain or by fluorescein isothiocyanate-conjugated monoclonal antibodies.

Detection in cell cultures of *C. psittaci* and *C. pneumoniae* requires specific technical manipulations and reagents; deoxyribonucleic acid detection may also be performed in women who may be susceptible to the infections, regardless of whether they have symptoms.

Culture is the detection method of choice, but rapid noncultural (antigen detection) procedures are also available.

Interfering Factors
- Use of an antimicrobial drug within a few days before specimen collection

(possible inability to recover *C. trachomatis*)
- In males, voiding within 1 hour of specimen collection; in females, douching within 24 hours of specimen collection (fewer organisms available for culture)
- Contamination of the specimen because of fecal material in a rectal culture
- Menses

Precautions
- Place the male patient in the supine position to prevent him from falling if vasovagal syncope occurs when the cotton swab or wire loop is introduced into the urethra. Observe for profound hypotension, bradycardia, pallor, and sweating.
- Wear gloves when performing the procedures and handling the specimens.
- Collect a urethral specimen at least 1 hour after the patient has voided to prevent loss of urethral secretions.
- After collecting the specimens, carefully dispose of gloves, swabs, and speculum to prevent staff exposure.

Nursing Considerations

Before the Test
- Confirm the patient's identity using two patient identifiers and confirmation of the patient's identification bracelet according to facility policy.
- Explain the purpose of the *C. trachomatis* culture test to the patient.
- Describe the procedure for collecting a specimen for culture.
- If the specimen will be collected from the male patient's genital tract, instruct him not to urinate for 3 to 4 hours before the specimen is taken.
- Tell the female patient not to douche for 24 hours before the test.
- Tell the male patient that he may experience some burning and pressure as the culture is taken, but that the discomfort will subside after a few minutes.

During the Test
- Obtain a specimen of the epithelial cells from the infected site. In adults, these sites may include the eye, urethra (rather than from the purulent exudate that may be present), endocervix, and rectum.
- Obtain a urethral specimen by inserting a cotton-tipped applicator ¾ to 2 inches (2–5 cm) into the urethra.
- To collect a specimen from the endocervix, use a microbiologic transport swab or cytobrush.
- Extract the specimen into 2-sucrose–phosphate (2-SP)-based transport medium.

> **Quality and Safety Nursing Alert**
>
> In cases where sexual abuse of the patient is suspected, process the specimen by culture rather than by antigen detection methods.

After the Test
- Send specimens extracted from the throat, eye, or nasopharynx and aspirates from infants to the laboratory at a temperature of 39.2°F (4°C).
- If the anticipated time between specimen collection and inoculation into cell culture is more than 24 hours, freeze the 2-SP transport medium and send it to the laboratory with dry ice.
- Advise the patient to avoid all sexual contact until after test results are available.
- If the culture confirms infection, counsel the patient about treating sexual partners.

Chloride, Serum

Reference Values
100 to 108 mEq/L (SI, 100–108 mmol/L)

Abnormal Findings
Elevated Levels
- Severe dehydration, complete renal shutdown, head injury (producing neurogenic hyperventilation), and primary aldosteronism
- Hyperchloremic metabolic acidosis caused by excessive chloride retention or ingestion

Decreased Levels
- Hypochloremic metabolic acidosis from excessive loss of gastric juices or other secretions
- Prolonged vomiting, gastric suctioning, intestinal fistula, chronic kidney disease, and Addison's disease leading to decreased chloride levels from low sodium and potassium levels
- Dilutional hypochloremia secondary to heart failure or edema resulting in excess extracellular fluid

Nursing Implications
- Anticipate the need for additional testing.
- Prepare the patient for follow-up treatment; institute therapy as ordered.
- Monitor the patient with increased levels for signs and symptoms of metabolic acidosis associated with hyperchloremia, such as tachypnea, lethargy, weakness, diminished cognitive ability, and Kussmaul's respirations.
- Monitor the patient with decreased levels for signs and symptoms of hypochloremia.

Purpose
- To detect acid–base imbalance (acidosis or alkalosis) and to aid evaluation of fluid status and extracellular cation–anion balance

Description
This test is used to measure serum chloride levels, the major extracellular fluid anion. Chloride helps maintain osmotic pressure of blood and, therefore, helps regulate blood volume and arterial pressure. Chloride levels also affect acid–base balance. Chloride is absorbed from the intestines and excreted primarily by the kidneys.

C

Interfering Factors

- Use of acetazolamide, ammonium chloride, androgens, boric acid, cholestyramine, estrogens, excessive IV infusion of sodium chloride, non-steroidal anti-inflammatory agents, oxyphenbutazone, and phenylbutazone (possible increase)
- Use of bicarbonates, ethacrynic acid, furosemide, or laxatives, thiazide diuretics, and prolonged IV infusion of dextrose 5% in water (decrease)

Nursing Considerations

Before the Test

- Confirm the patient's identity using two patient identifiers and confirmation of the patient's identification bracelet according to facility policy.
- Explain to the patient that the serum chloride test is used to evaluate the chloride content of blood.
- Tell the patient that the test requires a blood sample.
- Explain to the patient that there may be slight discomfort from the tourniquet and the needle puncture.
- Inform the patient that there are no food or fluid restrictions for this test.
- Notify the laboratory and health care provider of medications the patient is taking that may affect test results; these may need to be restricted.

During the Test

- Perform a venipuncture and collect the sample in a 3- or 4-mL clot activator tube.

After the Test

- Apply direct pressure to the venipuncture site until bleeding stops and to prevent hematoma formation.
- Handle the sample gently to prevent hemolysis and send it to the laboratory immediately.
- Instruct the patient to resume any medications that were discontinued before the test, as ordered.

> ▶ *Quality and Safety Nursing Alert*
>
> In the patient with hyperchloremia, watch for signs of developing stupor, rapid deep breathing, and weakness, which may lead to coma. Observe the patient with hypochloremia for hypertonicity of muscles, tetany, depressed respirations, and decreased blood pressure with dehydration.

Chloride, Urine

Reference Values

Adults: 110 to 250 mmoL/24 hours (SI, 110–250 mmol/day)
Children: 15 to 40 mmoL/24 hours (SI, 15–40 mmol/day)
Infants: 2 to 10 mmol/24 hours (SI, 2–10 mmol/day)

Abnormal Findings

Elevated Levels

- Water-deficient dehydration, salicylate toxicity, diabetic ketoacidosis, adrenocortical insufficiency (Addison's disease), or salt-losing renal disease

Decreased Levels

- Excessive diaphoresis, heart failure, hypochloremic metabolic alkalosis, or prolonged vomiting or gastric suctioning

Nursing Implications

- Anticipate the need for additional testing.
- Urine chloride levels parallel urine sodium levels; if both levels are abnormal, more specific testing usually is necessary.
- Expect to obtain serum electrolyte levels; assess the patient for signs and symptoms of sodium and chloride imbalances.

Purpose

- To help evaluate fluid and electrolyte imbalance
- To monitor the effects of a low-sodium diet
- To help evaluate renal and adrenal disorders

Description

The urine chloride test, which is commonly done in conjunction with a urine sodium test, determines the urine level of chloride, the major extracellular anion. (Urine sodium levels determine the urine levels of the major extracellular cation, sodium.) The measurement is used to reevaluate renal conservation of the electrolytes and confirm serum values. Normal values vary greatly with dietary salt intake and perspiration.

Interfering Factors

- Failure to collect all urine during the test period
- Ammonium chloride and potassium chloride (increased chloride)

Nursing Considerations

Before the Test

- Confirm the patient's identity using two patient identifiers and confirmation of the patient's identification bracelet according to facility policy.
- Explain to the patient that the urine sodium and chloride test helps determine the balance of salt and water in the body.
- Advise the patient that no special restrictions are necessary.
- Tell the patient that the test requires urine collection over a 24-hour period.
- If the patient will be collecting the specimen at home, instruct about proper collection technique.
- Notify the laboratory and health care provider of drugs the patient is taking that may affect test results; it may be necessary to restrict these.
- Tell the patient not to contaminate urine specimen with stool or toilet tissue.
- Advise the patient not to use a metal bedpan for specimen collection.

During the Test

- Collect the patient's urine over a 24-hour period, discarding the first specimen and retaining the last.

After the Test

- Send the specimen to the laboratory immediately on completing the collection.
- Instruct the patient to resume usual medications.

Clostridial Toxin Assay

Normal Findings

- Negative

Abnormal Findings

- Positive for *Clostridium difficile*, indicating possible clostridial enterocolitis or pseudomembranous colitis

Nursing Implications

- Institute appropriate infection control precautions.
- Anticipate the need for additional testing.
- Prepare to administer treatment as ordered.
- Monitor the patient's fluid and electrolyte balance and administer fluid replacement therapy as ordered.

Purpose

- To identify *C. difficile* as the organism causing diarrhea

Description

C. difficile, an organism that releases a toxin that causes the intestinal epithelium of the colon to necrose, is responsible for pseudomembranous colitis and subsequent profuse watery diarrhea. This disorder commonly is associated with patients who are immunocompromised and those receiving broad-spectrum antibiotics. These conditions cause a reduction in the normal flora of the intestine, allowing the *C. difficile* bacteria to proliferate.

Interfering Factors

- Contamination of specimen with urine or toilet tissue
- Improper specimen collection or collection container

Precautions

- Adhere to specific infection control precautions at all times.
- Wear personal protective equipment when collecting the specimen.

Nursing Considerations

Before the Test

- Explain the purpose of the test to the patient.
- Inform the patient that the test requires a stool sample.
- Teach the patient how to collect the stool specimen, which includes placing the specimen in a clean container that can be closed securely.

During the Test

- Assist the patient with collection of the stool sample, as necessary.
- Send the specimen to the laboratory immediately. Refrigerate the specimen if immediate transport can't be done.

After the Test

- Continue to provide care as before the test.
- Monitor the patient's intake and output and administer medications and fluid replacement as ordered.

Coagulation Factor Assay

Reference Values

Factor II (prothrombin): 80% to 120% of normal

Factor V (labile factor): 50% to 150% of normal

Factor VII (stable factor): 65% to 140% of normal (SI, 65–135 AU)

Factor VIII (antihemophilic factor): 55% to 145% of normal (SI, 55–145 AU)

Factor IX (Christmas factor): 60% to 140% of normal (SI, 60–140 AU)

Factor X: 45% to 155% of normal (SI, 45–155 AU)

Factor XI: 65% to 135% of normal (SI, 65–135 AU)

Factor XII (Hageman's factor): 50% to 150% of normal (SI, 50–150 AU)

Ristocetin (von Willebrand's factor): 45% to 140% of normal (SI, 45–140 AU)

Factor VIII antigen: 100 mcg/L or 50% to 150% of normal (SI, 50–150 AU)

Factor VIII-related antigen: 45% to 185% of normal (SI, 45–185 AU)

Fletcher's factor (prekallikrein): 80% to 120% of normal (SI, 0.80–1.20 AU)

Critical Value

Any factor less than 10% of normal

Abnormal Findings

Elevated Levels

- Postoperative, following rapid discontinuation of coumarin-based drug therapy, hepatic disease, or thromboembolic conditions (increased factor VIII)

Decreased Levels

- Inherited or acquired disorder of the coagulation system
- Disseminated intravascular coagulation (DIC) (factor X deficiency)
- Severe hepatic disease, DIC, or fibrinogenolysis (factor V deficiency)
- Congenital disorders (factors II, V, VII, and X deficiencies)
- Hemophilia A, von Willebrand's disease, a factor VIII inhibitor, DIC, or fibrinolysis (factor VIII deficiency)
- Hemophilia B, hepatic disease, a factor IX inhibitor, a vitamin K deficiency, or coumarin therapy (factor IX deficiency)
- Postoperative stress response (factor XI deficiency)

Nursing Implications

- Anticipate the need for additional testing.
- Prepare the patient with increased levels for follow-up treatment, such as anticoagulant therapy for thromboembolic conditions.
- Closely assess the patient with increased levels for signs and symptoms associated with thrombus formation and embolism.

- Prepare the patient with decreased levels for follow-up treatment, as indicated, such as blood component therapy or factor replacement.
- Assess the patient with decreased levels closely for bleeding signs and symptoms, especially from any injection and venipuncture sites.
- Institute bleeding precautions in the patient with decreased levels.

Purpose
- To identify a specific factor deficiency in a person with prolonged prothrombin time (PT) or partial thromboplastin time (PTT)
- To study the patient with congenital or acquired coagulation defects
- To monitor the effects of blood component therapy in the factor-deficient patient

Description
The coagulation factor assay is a quantitative analysis identifying the specific amount of each coagulation factor in the patient's blood. These factors are part of the body's extrinsic and intrinsic coagulation system.

 Quality and Safety Nursing Alert

Elevated factor VIII levels are normal during the later part of pregnancy and the neonatal period. A deficiency of all coagulation factors, including factor XI, may appear in the neonate for a short period. This deficiency is usually transient.

Interfering Factors
- Failure to mix the sample and the anticoagulant adequately or to send the sample to the laboratory immediately or to place it on ice
- Hemolysis caused by rough handling of the sample
- Oral anticoagulants (possible increase resulting from inhibition of vitamin K-dependent synthesis and activation of clotting factors II, VII, and X, which form in the liver)

Nursing Considerations
Before the Test
- Confirm the patient's identity using two patient identifiers and confirmation of the patient's identification bracelet according to facility policy.
- Explain to the patient that the one-stage assay test is used to assess the function of the blood coagulation mechanism.
- Tell the patient that a blood sample will be taken.
- Explain to the patient that there may be slight discomfort from the needle puncture and the tourniquet.
- When the patient is factor deficient and receiving blood component therapy, inform the patient that a series of follow-up tests may be needed.
- Notify the laboratory and health care provider of medications the patient is taking that may affect test results; these may need to be restricted.
- Inform the patient that there are no food or fluid restrictions.

During the Test
- Perform a venipuncture and collect the sample in a 3- or 4.5-mL siliconized tube.

Quality and Safety Nursing Alert

If the patient has a suspected coagulation defect, avoid excessive probing during venipuncture, don't leave the tourniquet on too long (it will cause bruising), and apply pressure to the puncture site for 5 minutes or until the bleeding stops. A patient with a bleeding disorder may require a pressure bandage to stop bleeding at the venipuncture site.

- Completely fill the collection tube; invert it gently several times to mix the sample and the anticoagulant.

After the Test
- Send the sample to the laboratory immediately or place it on ice.

- Assess the venipuncture site closely for bruising, continued bleeding, oozing from the site, or hematoma development and apply direct pressure.
- Explain that the patient may resume a usual diet and any medications that were discontinued before the test, as ordered.

Cold Agglutinins

Reference Values
Negative
Positive with a titer less than 1:64

Abnormal Findings

Elevated Levels

- Infectious mononucleosis, cytomegalovirus infection, hemolytic anemia, multiple myeloma, scleroderma, malaria, cirrhosis, congenital syphilis, peripheral vascular disease, pulmonary embolism, trypanosomiasis, tonsillitis, staphylococcemia, scarlatina, influenza, and, occasionally, pregnancy, infections, or lymphoreticular cancer
- Pneumonia and lymphoreticular cancer (chronic elevations)
- Viral infections (typically acute, transient elevations)
- Idiopathic cold agglutinin disease preceding lymphoma (titers greater than 1:2,000)

Nursing Implications

- Anticipate the need for additional testing, including sequential titer evaluations.
- One-half to two-thirds of patients with primary atypical pneumonia exhibit cold agglutinins in serum during the first week of acute infection, with titers becoming positive at 7 days, peaking above 1:32 in 4 weeks, and gradually disappearing after 6 weeks.
- Institute therapy as ordered.

Purpose

- To help confirm primary atypical pneumonia
- To provide additional diagnostic evidence for cold agglutinin disease

associated with many viral infections and lymphoreticular cancer
- To detect cold agglutinins in the patient with suspected cold agglutinin disease

Description

Cold agglutinins are antibodies, usually of the IgM type, that cause RBCs to aggregate at low temperatures. They may occur in small amounts in healthy people. Transient elevations of these antibodies develop during certain infectious diseases, notably primary atypical pneumonia. This test reliably detects such pneumonia within 1 to 2 weeks of its onset.

Patients with high cold agglutinin titers, such as those with primary atypical pneumonia, may develop acute transient hemolytic anemia after repeated exposure to cold; patients with persistently high titers may develop chronic hemolytic anemia.

Interfering Factors

- Refrigeration of the sample before serum is separated from RBCs (possible false-low titer)
- Antimicrobial drugs

Nursing Considerations

Before the Test

- Confirm the patient's identity using two patient identifiers and confirmation of the patient's identification bracelet according to facility policy.
- Explain to the patient that the cold agglutinins test detects antibodies in the blood that attack RBCs after exposure to low temperatures.
- Tell the patient that the test will be repeated to monitor response to therapy, if appropriate.
- Tell the patient that there are no food or fluid restrictions for this test.
- Tell the patient that the test requires a blood sample.
- Explain to the patient that there may be slight discomfort from the tourniquet and the needle puncture.

• If the patient is receiving antimicrobial drugs, note this information on the laboratory request because the use of such drugs may interfere with the development of cold agglutinins.

During the Test
• Perform a venipuncture and collect the sample in a 7-mL tube without additives that has been prewarmed to 98.6°F (37°C).
• If cold agglutinin disease is suspected, keep the patient warm. If he's exposed to low temperatures, agglutination may occur within peripheral vessels, possibly leading to frostbite, anemia, Raynaud's phenomenon, and, rarely, focal gangrene.

> **Quality and Safety Nursing Alert**
>
> Watch for signs of vascular abnormalities, such as mottled skin, purpura, jaundice, pallor, pain or swelling of extremities, and cramping of fingers and toes. Hemoglobinuria may result from severe intravascular hemolysis on exposure to severe cold.

After the Test
• Send the sample to the laboratory immediately.

> **Quality and Safety Nursing Alert**
>
> Don't refrigerate the sample; cold agglutinins will coat the RBCs, leaving none in the serum for testing.

• Apply direct pressure to the venipuncture site until bleeding stops and to prevent hematoma formation.

Colonoscopy
Normal Findings
• Light-pink–orange mucosa of the large intestine beyond the sigmoid colon that's marked by semilunar folds and deep tubular pits

• Visible blood vessels beneath the intestinal mucosa, which glisten from mucus secretions

Abnormal Findings
• Proctitis, granulomatous or ulcerative colitis, Crohn's disease, and malignant or benign lesions
• Diverticular disease or the site of lower GI bleeding (See the *Abnormal Colonoscopy* box.)

Nursing Implications
• Anticipate the need for further testing.
• Prepare the patient for follow-up treatment, including possible surgery.
• Provide emotional support to the patient and family.

Purpose
• To detect or evaluate inflammatory and ulcerative bowel disease
• To locate the origin of lower GI bleeding
• To help diagnose colonic strictures and benign or malignant lesions
• To evaluate the colon postoperatively for recurrence of polyps and malignant lesions

Description
Colonoscopy uses a flexible fiberoptic video endoscope to permit visual examination of the large intestine's lining. It's indicated for patients with a history of constipation or diarrhea, persistent rectal bleeding, and lower abdominal pain when the results of proctosigmoidoscopy and a barium enema test are negative or inconclusive.

The procedure for colonoscopy is as follows:
• The patient is placed on the left side with knees flexed and draped.
• Baseline vital signs are obtained. Vital signs are monitored throughout the procedure. Continuous ECG monitoring should be instituted. Continuous pulse oximetry is advisable, particularly in the high-risk patient with possible respiratory

Abnormal Colonoscopy

These two views, taken with a fiberoptic colonoscope, show ulcerative colitis (below left) and diverticulosis (below right).

Fiberoptic colonoscope

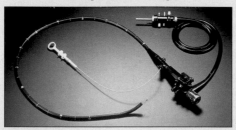

Ulcerative colitis   **Diverticulosis**

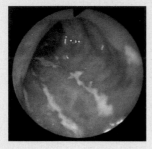   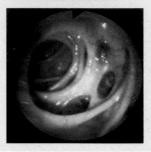

depression secondary to sedation, which may be given.

- The patient is instructed to breathe deeply and slowly through the mouth as the health care provider palpates the mucosa of the anus and rectum and inserts, under direct vision, the lubricated colonoscope through the patient's anus into the sigmoid colon.
- A small amount of air is insufflated to locate the bowel lumen, then the scope is advanced through the rectum.
- When the instrument reaches the descending sigmoid junction, the patient is assisted to a supine position to aid the scope advance, if necessary. After passing the splenic flexure, the scope is advanced through the transverse colon, through the hepatic flexure, and into the ascending colon and cecum.

- Abdominal palpation or fluoroscopy may be used to help guide the colonoscope through the large intestine.
- Suction may be used to remove blood and secretions that obscure vision.
- Biopsy forceps or a cytology brush may be passed through the colonoscope to obtain specimens for histologic or cytologic examination; an electrocautery snare may be used to remove polyps.
- If the physician removes a tissue specimen, it's placed immediately in a specimen bottle containing 10% formalin; cytology smears are immediately placed in a Coplin jar containing 95% ethyl alcohol. Specimens are sent to the laboratory immediately.

Interfering Factors
- Sigmoid colon fixation due to inflammatory bowel disease, surgery, or

C

radiation therapy (may hinder passage of the colonoscope)
- Blood from acute colonic hemorrhage (hinders visualization)
- Insufficient bowel preparation or barium retained in the intestine from previous diagnostic studies (makes accurate visual examination impossible)

Precautions
- Although it's usually a safe procedure, a colonoscopy can cause large intestine perforation, excessive bleeding, and retroperitoneal emphysema.
- The procedure is contraindicated in pregnant women near term, patients who have had recent acute MI or abdominal surgery, and patients with ischemic bowel disease, acute diver-

ticulitis, peritonitis, fulminant granulomatous colitis, perforated viscus, or fulminant ulcerative colitis. For these cases or for screening purposes, a virtual colonoscopy may help visualize polyps before they become concerns. (See the *Virtual Colonoscopy* box.)

Nursing Considerations

Before the Test
- Check the patient's medical history for allergies, medications, and information pertinent to the current complaint.
- Tell the patient that colonoscopy permits examination of the large intestine's lining.
- Describe the procedure and tell the patient who will perform it and when and where it will take place.
- Explain that the large intestine must be thoroughly cleaned to be clearly visible. To do so, tell the patient a clear-liquid diet must be maintained for 24 to 48 hours before the test, to take nothing by mouth after midnight the night before, and to take a laxative, as ordered, or 1 gallon of GoLYTELY solution in the evening (drinking the chilled solutions in 8 oz [236.6 mL] doses every 10 minutes until the entire gallon is consumed).
- Advise the patient that if fecal results aren't clear, a laxative, suppository, or tap water enema is necessary.

Virtual Colonoscopy

Virtual colonoscopy combines computed tomography (CT) scanning and X-ray images with sophisticated image processing computers to generate three-dimensional (3-D) images of the patient's colon. These images are interpreted by a skilled radiologist to recreate and evaluate the colon's inner surface. Although this procedure isn't as accurate as a routine colonoscopy, it's less invasive and is useful in screening the patient with small polyps or in those patients who have strictures.

The colon must be free from residue and fecal material. Bowel preparation consists of following a clear-liquid diet for 24 hours before the procedure. Also, the patient performs GoLYTELY bowel preparation the evening before and takes a rectal suppository on the morning of the test.

Before performing the CT scan, a thin, red rectal tube is placed and air is introduced into the colon to distend the bowel. This insertion may produce mild cramping. The CT scan is done with the patient in the supine position and again while prone. The scans are then shipped over a network to a 3-D image processing computer, and a radiologist evaluates the images obtained. If polyps are identified, a colonoscopy may be scheduled to remove them.

> **Quality and Safety Nursing Alert**
>
> Don't administer a soapsuds enema because doing so irritates the mucosa and stimulates mucus secretions that may hinder the examination.

- Inform the patient that an IV line will be started and a sedative will be administered before the procedure. Because a sedative will be given, advise the patient to arrange for a ride home after the procedure.

C

• Assure the patient that the colono-scope is well lubricated with a water-soluble gel to ease its insertion, that it initially feels cool, and that the patient may feel an urge to defecate when it's inserted and advanced. A rectal exam may be performed prior to the procedure with the application of lidocaine gel to ease the discomfort of scope insertion.

• Explain to the patient that air may be introduced through the colonoscope to distend the intestinal wall and to facilitate viewing the lining and advancing the instrument. Tell the patient that flatus normally escapes around the instrument because of air insufflation and that there's no need to try to control it.

• Tell the patient that suction may be used to remove blood or liquid stool that obscures vision, but that this won't cause discomfort.

• Make sure that the patient or a responsible family member has signed an informed consent form.

• It is more comfortable if the patient voids immediately before the proce-dure.

During the Test

• Assist with patient positioning as necessary.

• Encourage the patient to take slow, deep breaths to aid in relaxation.

> **Quality and Safety Nursing Alert**

Watch the patient closely for ad-verse effects of the sedative. Have available emergency resuscitation equipment and an opioid antago-nist, such as naloxone, for IV use, if necessary. If midazolam is used, have Romazicon available for an antidote if necessary.

After the Test

• Observe the patient closely for signs of bowel perforation. Report such signs immediately.

• Check the patient's vital signs and document them according to your facility's policy.

• After the patient has recovered from sedation, allow him or her to resume a usual diet unless the health care provider orders otherwise.

• Provide privacy while the patient rests after the procedure; explain that the patient may pass large amounts of flatus after insufflation.

• If a polyp is removed but not retrieved during the examination, give enemas and strain stools to retrieve it, if the health care provider requests it.

• If a polyp has been removed, tell the patient that some blood in the stool is normal but that excessive bleeding should be reported immediately.

Colposcopy

Normal Findings

• Smooth and pink surface contour of the cervical vessels
• Grapelike columnar epithelium
• Different tissue types sharply demarcated

Abnormal Findings

• White epithelium (leukoplakia) or punctate and mosaic patterns, indicating cervical intraepithelial neoplasia
• Keratinization in the transformation zone and atypical vessels, indicating possible invasive carcinoma
• Inflammatory changes, indicating infection
• Atrophic changes (from aging or, less commonly, use of hormonal contra-ceptives)
• Erosion (probably from increased pathogenicity of vaginal flora due to changes in vaginal pH)
• Papilloma and condyloma (possibly from viruses)

Nursing Implications

• Anticipate the need for additional testing.

- Because histologic study of the biopsy specimen confirms colposcopic findings, inconsistency between the Papanicolaou (Pap) test and squamocolumnar junction biopsy results may indicate the need for conization of the cervix.
- Prepare the patient for follow-up treatment.
- Provide emotional support to the patient and her family while awaiting confirmation of diagnosis.

Purpose

- To help confirm cervical intraepithelial neoplasia or invasive carcinoma after a positive Pap test
- To evaluate vaginal or cervical lesions
- To monitor conservatively treated cervical intraepithelial neoplasia
- To monitor the patient whose mother received diethylstilbestrol during pregnancy

Description

In colposcopy, the cervix and vagina are examined visually with a colposcope, an instrument containing a magnifying lens and a light. During the examination, a biopsy may be performed and photographs taken of suspicious lesions with the colposcope and its attachments. Risks of biopsy include bleeding (especially during pregnancy) and infection.

The procedure for colposcopy is as follows:

- With the patient in the lithotomy position, the physician inserts the speculum and, if indicated, performs a Pap test.
- The cervix is swabbed with acetic acid solution to remove mucus.
- After the cervix and vagina are examined, biopsy is performed on areas that appear abnormal.
- Bleeding is stopped by applying pressure, by hemostatic solutions, or by cautery.

Interfering Factors

- Presence of menstrual blood or foreign materials in the cervix, such as creams and medications (possible obstruction to visualization)

Nursing Considerations

Before the Test

- Explain to the patient that the colposcopy magnifies the image of the vagina and cervix, providing more information than a routine vaginal examination.
- Inform the patient that she doesn't need to restrict food and fluids.
- Tell the patient who will perform the examination, when and where it will be done, and that it's safe and painless.
- Tell the patient that a biopsy may be performed during colposcopy and that this procedure may cause minimal but easily controlled bleeding and mild cramping.
- Make sure that the patient or a responsible family member has signed an informed consent form.
- It is more comfortable if the patient voids immediately before the procedure.

During the Test

- Provide emotional support to the patient.
- Help the patient relax during insertion by telling her to breathe through her mouth and concentrate on relaxing her abdominal muscles.

After the Test

- After a biopsy, instruct the patient to abstain from intercourse and to avoid inserting anything into her vagina (including a tampon) until healing of the biopsy site is confirmed (in about 10 days).
- Instruct the patient to report danger signs and symptoms, such as elevated temperature and vaginal bleeding, immediately.

Complement Assays

Reference Values

Total complement: 25 to 110 units/mL (SI, 0.25–1.1 g/L)
C3: 70 to 150 mg/dL (SI, 0.7–1.5 g/L)
C4: 15 to 45 mg/dL (SI, 0.15–0.45 g/L)

Abnormal Findings

Elevated Levels

- Obstructive jaundice, thyroiditis, acute rheumatic fever, rheumatoid arthritis, acute MI, ulcerative colitis, and diabetes (elevated total complement levels)
- Autoimmune hemolytic anemia (increased C4)

Decreased Levels

- Hereditary angioedema (C1 esterase inhibitor deficiency), leading to submucosal swelling
- Systemic lupus erythematosus (SLE), acute poststreptococcal glomerulonephritis, and acute serum sickness (decreased total complement levels caused by excessive formation of antigen–antibody complexes, insufficient complement synthesis, inhibitor formation, or increased complement catabolism)
- Recurrent pyogenic infection and disease activation in SLE; immune complex disease; and major necrosis and tissue injury, sepsis, and viremia
- SLE and rheumatoid arthritis (C4 deficiency)
- Advanced cirrhosis of the liver, multiple myeloma, hypogammaglobulinemia, or rapidly rejecting allografts (decreased total complement levels)

Nursing Implications

- Anticipate the need for additional testing.
- Prepare the patient for follow-up treatment.
- Provide emotional support to the patient and family.
- In patients with decreased levels, institute infection control precautions because of the patient's increased susceptibility to infection and monitor vital signs for changes.

Purpose

- To help detect immune-mediated disease and genetic complement deficiency

- To monitor the effectiveness of therapy
- To aid in determining the presence of acute inflammatory processes

Description

Complement is a collective term for a system of at least 20 serum proteins that destroy foreign cells and help remove foreign materials. Complement may be triggered by contact with antigen–antibody complexes or by clotting factor XIIa. A cascade of events follows, which forms a complex that ruptures cell membranes.

Complement components are designated as C1 through C9, with C1 having three subcomponents: C1q, C1r, and C1s. These components constitute 3% to 4% of total serum globulins and play a key role in antibody-mediated immune reactions.

Complement can function as a defense by promoting the removal of infectious agents or as a threat by triggering destructive reactions in host tissues. Therefore, complement deficiency can increase susceptibility to infection and predispose a person to other diseases.

Hemolytic assay, laser nephelometry, and radial immunodiffusion are the most common laboratory methods used to evaluate and measure total complement and its components. Although complement assays provide valuable information about the patient's immune system, the results must be considered in light of serum immunoglobulin and autoantibody tests for a definitive diagnosis of immune-mediated disease or an abnormal response to infection.

Interfering Factors

- Recent heparin therapy

Precautions

- Handle the sample gently to prevent hemolysis. The specimen should be sent to the laboratory for analysis within 1 hour. If the specimen is left at room temperature for more than 1 hour, the C3 level may result in a false low-level finding.

Nursing Considerations

Before the Test

- Confirm the patient's identity using two patient identifiers and confirmation of the patient's identification bracelet according to facility policy.
- Explain to the patient that the complement assay test measures a group of proteins that fight infection.
- Inform the patient that there are no food or fluid restrictions for this test.
- Tell the patient that the test requires a blood sample.
- Explain to the patient that there may be slight discomfort from the tourniquet and the needle puncture.
- If the patient is scheduled for C1q assay, check the history for recent heparin therapy; report such therapy to the laboratory.

During the Test

- Perform a venipuncture and collect the sample in a 7-mL tube without additives.

After the Test

- Send the sample to the laboratory immediately because complement is heat labile and deteriorates rapidly.
- Because many patients with complement defects have a compromised immune system, keep the venipuncture site clean and dry.
- Apply direct pressure to the venipuncture site until bleeding stops and to prevent hematoma; assess for ecchymosis.
- Compare C3 and C4 findings with the results of other lab studies performed for specific disorders.

Computed Tomography of the Abdomen and Pelvis

Normal Findings

- Organs normal in size and position
- No masses or other abnormalities

Abnormal Findings

- Well-circumscribed or poorly defined areas of lower density than normal

parenchyma, suggesting primary and metastatic neoplasms
- Relatively low-density, homogeneous areas, usually with well-defined borders, indicating abscesses
- Sharply defined round or oval structures, with densities less than that of abscesses and neoplasms, indicating cysts
- Dilatation of the biliary ducts, indicating obstructive disease from tumor or calculi

Nursing Implications

- Anticipate the need for additional testing.
- Prepare the patient for follow-up treatment.
- Provide emotional support to the patient and family.
- Promote patient safety (allergic responses).

Purpose

- To evaluate soft tissue and organs of the abdomen, pelvis, and retroperitoneal space
- To evaluate inflammatory disease
- To aid staging of neoplasms
- To evaluate trauma
- To detect tumors, cysts, hemorrhage, or edema
- To evaluate response to chemotherapy

Description

CT of the abdomen and pelvis combines radiologic and computer technology to produce cross-sectional images of various layers of tissue. IV or oral contrast medium can be used to accentuate tissue density differences (dynamic imaging). CT scan of the abdomen may be performed with or without a CT scan of the pelvis.

The procedure for CT is as follows:

- The patient is placed in a supine position with arms above the head on an adjustable table inside a scanning gantry.
- A series of transverse radiographs is taken and recorded. For abdomen CT, the area between the dome of the

diaphragm and iliac crests is scanned. For pelvic CT, the area is between the iliac crests and the perineum. In men, the pelvic scan includes the bladder and prostate; in women, the bladder and adnexa.

- The information is reconstructed by a computer, and selected images are photographed.
- The patient is assisted into the supine position on the X-ray table, and the table is positioned into the imaging machine.
- After the images are reviewed, an IV contrast enhancement may be ordered. Usually, the test requires oral contrast material to outline the intestines.
- Additional images are obtained after the IV contrast injection.
- The patient is observed carefully for adverse reactions to the contrast medium.

Interfering Factors

- Oral or IV contrast media use from previous diagnostic tests (obscures the images)
- Claustrophobia (inability to complete CT scan)
- Excessive patient movement (poor image)
- Metallic objects in the examination field (poor image)

 *Quality and Safety Nursing Alert*

A CT scan isn't recommended during pregnancy because of potential risk to the fetus.

Precautions

- The specific type of CT scan dictates the need for an oral or IV contrast medium.
- The patient may experience strong feelings of claustrophobia or anxiety when inside the CT body scanner. A mild sedative may be ordered to help reduce anxiety.

Nursing Considerations

Before the Test

- Confirm the patient's identity using two patient identifiers and confirmation of the patient's identification bracelet according to facility policy.
- Notify the radiology department if your patient has a peripheral inserted central catheter (PICC) line. Power-PICC is indicated for power injection of contrast media.
- Make sure the patient or a responsible family member has signed an appropriate consent form.
- Check the patient's history for hypersensitivity reactions to iodine, shellfish, or contrast media. If such reactions have occurred, note them in the patient's chart and notify the health care provider, who may order prophylactic medications or choose not to use contrast enhancement.
- For women of childbearing age, assess pregnancy status (i.e., determine last menstrual period [LMP]) for possible pregnancy and notify radiology as needed.
- Patients not receiving a contrast medium don't need to restrict food and fluids. Instruct the patient who will receive a contrast medium to fast for 4 hours before the test.
- Instruct the patient to remove body piercings, jewelry, or other metal objects in the X-ray field to allow for precise imaging.
- Stress to the patient the need to remain still during testing because movement can limit the test's accuracy. The patient may experience minimal discomfort because of lying still.
- Warn about transient discomfort from the needle puncture and a warm or flushed feeling or metallic taste if an IV contrast medium is used.
- Explain that the patient may hear clacking sounds as the table moves into the scanner.
- Explain that the test takes about 35 to 40 minutes.

After the Test

- Monitor the patient for delayed reaction to iodinated contrast medium.
- Allow the patient to resume a normal diet and activities unless otherwise ordered.
- If contrast medium was used, encourage fluids to assist in eliminating the contrast medium.

Computed Tomography of the Bone

Normal Findings

- No pathology in the bones or joints
- Crisp images of the structure with blurred or eliminated details of surrounding structures

Abnormal Findings

- Primary bone tumors, soft-tissue tumors, and skeletal metastasis (differentiation of tissues)
- Bone fracture
- Other bone abnormalities (based on characteristics of tissues and organs)
- Joint abnormalities

Nursing Implications

- Anticipate the need for additional testing.
- Prepare the patient for follow-up treatment, such as repair of fractures or drug therapy.
- Provide emotional support to the patient and family.
- Expect to immobilize any fractured area as ordered.

Purpose

- To determine the existence and extent of primary bone tumors, skeletal metastases, soft-tissue tumors, injuries to ligaments or tendons, and fractures
- To diagnose joint abnormalities that are difficult to detect by other methods

Description

CT of the bone involves a series of tomograms, translated by a computer and displayed on a monitor, that represent cross-sectional images of various layers (or slices) of bone. It can reconstruct cross-sectional, horizontal, sagittal, and coronal plane images. By taking collimated (parallel) radiographs, CT of the bone increases the number of radiation density calculations the computer makes, improving the degree of resolution, specificity, and accuracy. The CT combines hundreds of thousands of readings of radiation levels absorbed by tissues to depict anatomic slices of varying thicknesses.

The procedure for bone CT is as follows:

- The patient is assisted into a supine position on an X-ray table and asked to lie as still as possible.
- The table is slid into the circular opening of the CT scanner. The scanner revolves around the patient, taking radiographs at preselected intervals.
- After the first set of scans is taken, the patient is removed from the scanner and a contrast medium is given, if necessary. The patient is observed for 30 minutes after injection of the contrast medium for signs and symptoms of a hypersensitivity reaction, including pruritus, rash, and respiratory difficulty.
- After the IV injection of contrast medium, the patient is moved back into the scanner and another series of scans is taken. The images obtained from the scan are displayed on a monitor during the procedure and stored on magnetic tape to create a permanent record for subsequent study.

Interfering Factors

- Claustrophobia (inability to complete CT scan)
- Excessive patient movement (poor image)
- Metallic objects in the examination field (poor image)

> ▶ *Quality and Safety Nursing Alert*
>
> A CT scan isn't recommended during pregnancy because of potential risk to the fetus.

Precautions

- The patient may experience strong feelings of claustrophobia or anxiety when inside the CT body scanner. A mild sedative may be ordered to help reduce anxiety.

Nursing Considerations

Before the Test

- Confirm the patient's identity using two patient identifiers and confirmation of the patient's identification bracelet according to facility policy.
- Notify the radiology department if your patient has a PICC line. Power-PICC is indicated for power injection of contrast media.
- Explain to the patient that this type of CT scan allows imaging of bones and joints.
- Make sure that the patient or a responsible family member has signed an informed consent form.
- Check the patient's history for hypersensitivity reactions to iodine or contrast media. Mark such reactions in the chart and notify the health care provider, who may order prophylactic medications or choose not to use a contrast medium.
- For women of childbearing age, assess pregnancy status (i.e., determine LMP) for possible pregnancy and notify radiology as needed.
- Patients not receiving a contrast medium don't need to restrict food and fluids. Instruct the patient who will receive a contrast medium to fast for 4 hours before the test.
- Instruct the patient to remove body piercings, jewelry, hairpins, or other metal objects in the X-ray field to allow for precise imaging.

- Explain that the patient will lie on an X-ray table inside a CT scanner and be asked to lie still; the computer-controlled scanner will revolve around the patient taking multiple scans.
- Stress that the patient should lie as still as possible.
- If the patient is to receive a contrast medium, explain that the patient may feel flushed and warm, and may experience a transient headache, a salty or metallic taste, and nausea or vomiting after its injection.
- If the patient appears restless or apprehensive about the procedure, a mild sedative may be prescribed.

> ▶ *Quality and Safety Nursing Alert*
>
> For the patient with significant bone or joint pain, give analgesics as ordered so that the patient can lie comfortably during the scan.

After the Test

- If contrast medium is used, observe the patient for a delayed allergic reaction and treat as necessary. (Diphenhydramine is the drug of choice.) Encourage fluids to assist in eliminating the contrast medium.
- Tell the patient to resume a usual diet and activities, if appropriate.
- Provide comfort measures and medication to relieve pain caused by prolonged positioning on the table.

Computed Tomography of the Brain

Normal Findings

- Bone that appears white
- Ventricular and subarachnoid CSF that appears black
- Brain matter appearing in shades of gray

Abnormal Findings

- Areas of altered density (appearing lighter or darker), suggesting hydrocephalus, intracranial tumors, subdural and epidural hematomas, acute hemorrhages, arteriovenous malformation, or cerebral atrophy, infarction, or edema

Nursing Implications

• Report abnormal findings to the health care provider.
• Prepare to educate the patient about the diagnosis.
• Prepare the patient for further testing or surgery, as indicated.

Purpose

• To diagnose intracranial lesions and abnormalities
• To monitor the effects of surgery, radiation therapy, or chemotherapy on intracranial tumors
• To serve as a guide for cranial surgery

Description

CT of the brain, or *intracranial CT*, provides a series of tomograms, translated by a computer and displayed on a monitor, representing cross-sectional images of various brain layers. This technique can reconstruct cross-sectional, horizontal, sagittal, and coronal plane images. Hundreds of thousands of readings of radiation levels absorbed by brain tissues may be combined to depict anatomic slices of varying thickness. Specificity and accuracy are enhanced by the degree of resolution, which depends on the number of radiation density calculations made by the computer.

Although MRI has surpassed CT scanning in diagnosing neurologic conditions, the CT scan is more widely available and cost-effective, and it can be performed more easily in acute situations. (See the *Comparing Normal and Abnormal Intracranial CT Scans* box.) Another technology for obtaining brain images is positron emission tomography (PET). (See the *Understanding PET and SPECT* box.)

The procedure for CT of the brain is as follows:

• The patient is placed in a supine position on an X-ray table with the head immobilized by straps, if required, and asked to lie still.

Comparing Normal and Abnormal Intracranial CT Scans

Shown here are two intracranial computed tomography (CT) scans. The scan on the left is normal. The scan on the right shows a large meningioma in the frontal region, represented by the white area.

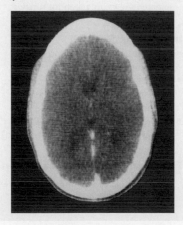 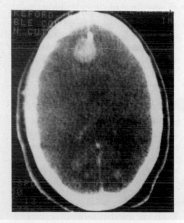

Understanding PET and SPECT

Like computed tomography (CT) scanning and magnetic resonance imaging (MRI), positron emission tomography (PET) and single-photon emission computed tomography (SPECT) provide brain images through sophisticated computer reconstruction algorithms. However, PET and SPECT images detail brain function as well as structure and thus differ significantly from the images provided by these other advanced techniques. PET and SPECT combine elements of CT scanning and conventional radionuclide imaging. For example, they measure the emissions of injected radioisotopes and convert them to a tomographic image of the brain. SPECT scanning uses gamma radiation with radionucleotides within the brain, and PET uses radioisotopes of biologically important elements—oxygen, nitrogen, carbon, and fluorine—that emit particles called positrons.

How It Works

During PET and SPECT, pairs of gamma rays are emitted; the scanner detects them and relays the information to a computer for reconstruction as an image. SPECT scanners use radionucleotides labeled with iodine or hexamethylpropylene aminoxime to detect blood flow. PET scanners emit positrons that can be chemically "tagged"

to biologically active molecules, such as carbon monoxide, neurotransmitters, hormones, and metabolites (especially glucose), enabling study of their uptake and distribution in brain tissue. For example, blood tagged with 11C-carbon monoxide allows study of hemodynamic patterns in brain tissue; tagged neurotransmitters, hormones, and drugs allow mapping of receptor distribution.

Isotope-tagged glucose (which penetrates the blood–brain barrier rapidly) allows dynamic study of brain function because PET scans can pinpoint the sites of glucose metabolism in the brain under various conditions. Researchers expect SPECT and PET scanning to prove useful in the diagnosis of psychiatric disorders, transient ischemic attacks, amyotrophic lateral sclerosis, Parkinson's disease, Wilson's disease, multiple sclerosis, seizure disorders, cerebrovascular disease, and Alzheimer's disease. The reason is that all of these disorders may alter the location and patterns of cerebral glucose metabolism.

Cost Factors

PET scanning is a costly test because the radioisotopes used have very short half-lives and must be produced at an on-site cyclotron and attached quickly to the desired tracer molecules.

- The head of the table is moved into the scanner, which rotates around the patient's head, taking radiographs at 1-degree intervals in a 180-degree arc.
- When this series of radiographs is completed, contrast enhancement is performed. Usually 50 to 100 mL of contrast medium is administered by IV injection or IV drip over 1 to 2 minutes.

 Quality and Safety Nursing Alert

Monitor the patient for hypersensitivity reactions, such as urticaria, respiratory difficulty, or rash. Reactions usually develop within 30 minutes.

- After injection of the contrast medium, another series of scans is

taken. Information from the scans is stored on magnetic tapes, fed into a computer, and converted into images on an oscilloscope. Photographs of selected views are taken for further study.

Interfering Factors
- Patient's head movement (possible poor imaging)
- Failure to remove metal objects from the scanning field (possible poor imaging)
- Hemorrhage (possible false-negative imaging due to change in hematoma)

 Quality and Safety Nursing Alert

A CT scan isn't recommended during pregnancy because of potential risk to the fetus.

Precautions

- Contrast enhancement is contraindicated for the patient who's hypersensitive to iodine or contrast medium.

 Quality and Safety Nursing Alert

Noncontrast scans are conducted in the presence of a head injury.

Nursing Considerations

Before the Test

- Confirm the patient's identity using two patient identifiers and confirmation of the patient's identification bracelet according to facility policy.
- Notify the radiology department if your patient has a PICC line. Power-PICC is indicated for power injection of contrast media.
- Make sure that the patient or a responsible family member has signed an informed consent form.
- Explain to the patient that this type of CT permits assessment of the brain.
- Unless contrast enhancement is scheduled, inform the patient that there are no food or fluid restrictions. If contrast enhancement is scheduled, instruct the patient to fast for 4 hours before the test.
- For women of childbearing age, assess pregnancy status (i.e., determine LMP) for possible pregnancy and notify radiology as needed.
- Tell the patient that a series of X-ray films will be taken of the brain. Describe who will perform the test and when and where it will take place. Explain that the test will cause minimal discomfort.
- Explain that the patient will be positioned on a moving CT bed with the head immobilized and the face uncovered. The head of the table will then be moved into the scanner, which rotates around the head and makes loud clacking sounds.

- If a contrast medium is used, explain that the patient may feel flushed and warm or may experience a transient headache, a salty or metallic taste, or nausea and vomiting after the contrast medium is injected.
- Instruct the patient to wear a gown (outpatients may wear comfortable clothing) and to remove jewelry, hairpins, or other metal objects in the X-ray field to allow for precise imaging.
- Explain that, if the patient is restless or apprehensive, a sedative may be prescribed.
- Check the patient's history for hypersensitivity to iodine or contrast media, and mark your findings in the chart. Inform the health care provider of any sensitivities because prophylactic medications may be ordered or the provider may choose not to use contrast enhancement.

After the Test

- If a contrast medium was used, watch the patient for residual adverse reactions (headache, nausea, and vomiting) and explain that the patient may resume a usual diet.

Computed Tomography of the Kidneys

Normal Findings

- Renal parenchyma of slightly higher density than that of the liver
- Bone that appears white
- Collecting system of low density that appears black, unless a contrast medium is used to enhance it to a higher (whiter) density
- Normal kidney position in relation to surrounding structures
- Normal kidney size and shape, as determined by counting cuts between the superior and inferior poles and following the contour of the kidneys' outline

C

Abnormal Renal CT Scan

This photograph of a renal computed tomography (CT) scan reveals a renal adenocarcinoma that has displaced and distorted the right kidney and now exceeds the kidney in size. The left kidney appears normal, the spine is sharp and white in the center, and the stomach is equally clear at the top.

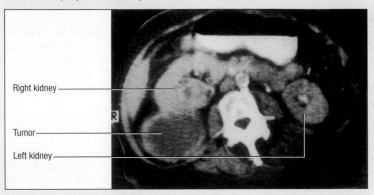

Right kidney ——————

Tumor ——————

Left kidney ——————

Abnormal Findings

- Renal masses (appearing as areas of different density, possibly altering the kidneys' shape or projecting beyond their margins)
- Tumors (appearing as areas of nonuniform density) (See the *Abnormal Renal CT Scan* box.)
- Obstructions
- Calculi
- Polycystic kidney disease
- Congenital anomalies
- Fluid accumulation (hematomas, lymphoceles, abscesses)

Nursing Implications

- Report abnormal findings to the health care provider.
- Prepare to educate the patient about the diagnosis.
- Support the patient and family if surgery is indicated for a neoplasm.
- If calculi are present, strain urine, hydrate the patient, and discuss nutritional adaptations as indicated.

Purpose

- To detect and evaluate renal abnormalities
- To evaluate the retroperitoneum

Description

CT of the kidneys provides images made from a series of cross-sectional slices or tomograms, which are then translated by a computer and displayed on a monitor. The image density reflects the amount of radiation absorbed by renal tissue and permits identification of masses and other lesions. An IV contrast medium may be injected to accentuate the renal parenchyma's density and help differentiate renal masses. This highly accurate test is usually performed to investigate diseases found by other diagnostic procedures such as excretory urography.

The procedure for CT of the kidneys is as follows:

- The patient is placed in a supine position on the X-ray table and secured with straps. The patient is instructed to lie still.
- The table is moved into the scanner. The scanner rotates around the patient, taking multiple images at different angles within each cross-sectional slice.
- When one series of tomograms is complete, IV contrast enhancement

may be performed and another series of tomograms is then taken.

- Information from the scan is stored on a disk or magnetic tape, fed into a computer, and converted into an image for display on a monitor. Radiographs and photographs are taken of selected views.

Interfering Factors

- Patient's inability to remain still (possible poor imaging)
- Presence of contrast media from other recent tests or of foreign bodies, such as catheters or surgical clips (possible poor imaging)

 Quality and Safety Nursing Alert

A CT scan isn't recommended during pregnancy because of potential risk to the fetus.

Precautions

- An IV contrast medium is contraindicated in patients hypersensitive to iodine and in patients with severe renal or hepatic disease.
- A CT scan conducted *without* the use of contrast is indicated in the presence of genitourinary (GU) trauma or other conditions in which acute bleeding might be present.

Nursing Considerations

Before the Test

- Confirm the patient's identity using two patient identifiers and confirmation of the patient's identification bracelet according to facility policy.
- Notify the radiology department if your patient has a PICC line. Power-PICC is indicated for power injection of contrast media.
- Explain to the patient that the CT scan permits examination of the kidneys.
- If contrast enhancement isn't scheduled, inform the patient that there are no food or fluid restrictions. If

contrast enhancement is scheduled, instruct the patient to fast for 4 hours before the test.

- For women of childbearing age, assess pregnancy status (i.e., determine LMP) for possible pregnancy and notify radiology as needed.
- Tell the patient who will perform the test, and when and where it will take place.
- Explain that the patient will be positioned on an X-ray table and that a scanner will take films of the kidneys.
- Warn the patient that the scanner may make loud clacking sounds as it rotates around the body.
- If contrast medium is used, tell the patient that there may be transient adverse effects, such as flushing, a metallic taste, and headache, after contrast medium injection.
- Instruct the patient to remove body piercings, jewelry, or other metal objects in the X-ray field to allow for precise imaging.
- Check the patient's history for hypersensitivity to iodine or contrast media. If such reactions have occurred, note them in the patient's chart and notify the health care provider, who may order prophylactic medications or choose not to use contrast enhancement.
- Make sure that the patient or a responsible family member has signed an informed consent form.
- Instruct the patient to put on a gown and to remove metallic objects that could interfere with the scan.
- Administer sedatives as ordered.

During the Test

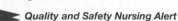 **Quality and Safety Nursing Alert**

Monitor the patient for allergic reactions to contrast medium, such as respiratory difficulty, urticaria, or skin eruptions.

After the Test
- If a sedative was administered, monitor the patient's vital signs.
- If the procedure was performed with contrast enhancement, watch for a delayed hypersensitivity reaction to the contrast medium. Encourage fluids to assist in eliminating the contrast medium. If the patient is at risk for impaired renal function, prepare for the administration of acetylcysteine to assist with renal clearance of contrast medium.
- Inform the patient to resume a usual diet as ordered.

Computed Tomography of the Liver and Biliary Tract

Normal Findings
- Liver of uniform density that's slightly greater than that of the pancreas, kidneys, and spleen; possible linear and circular areas of slightly lower density, representing hepatic vascular structures interrupting this uniform appearance
- Visible portal vein; nonvisible hepatic artery and intrahepatic biliary radicles
- Visible common hepatic and bile ducts (as low-density structures)
- Visible gallbladder as a round or elliptic low-density structure; if contracted, impossible to visualize

Abnormal Findings
- Areas that are less dense than normal parenchyma, indicating focal hepatic lesions
- Well-circumscribed or poorly defined areas of slightly lower density than the normal parenchyma, some with the same density as the liver parenchyma and undetectable, indicating primary and metastatic neoplasms
- Relatively low-density, homogeneous areas, usually with well-defined borders, indicating hepatic abscesses
- Sharply defined round or oval structures with a density lower than abscesses and neoplasms, indicating hepatic cysts

- Crescent-shaped masses that compress the liver away from the capsule, indicating subcapsular hematomas
- Biliary duct dilation, indicating obstructive jaundice, or absence of biliary duct dilation, indicating nonobstructive jaundice

Nursing Implications
- Anticipate the need for additional testing, such as percutaneous transhepatic cholangiography or endoscopic retrograde cholangiopancreatography (less common) to identify the obstruction site.
- Prepare the patient for follow-up treatment as indicated.
- Provide emotional support to the patient and family.

Purpose
- To distinguish between obstructive and nonobstructive jaundice
- To detect intrahepatic tumors and abscesses, subphrenic and subhepatic abscesses, cysts, and hematomas

Description
In CT of the liver and biliary tract, multiple X-rays pass through the upper abdomen and are measured while detectors record differences in tissue attenuation. A computer reconstructs these data as a two-dimensional image on a monitor. CT scanning accurately distinguishes the biliary tract and the liver if the ducts are large. Contrast media use during CT scanning can accentuate different densities.

Although CT scanning and ultrasonography detect biliary tract and liver disease equally well, the latter technique is performed more commonly. CT scanning is more expensive than ultrasonography and requires exposure to moderate amounts of radiation. However, it's the test of choice in patients who are obese and in those with livers positioned high under the rib cage, because bone and excessive fat hinder ultrasound transmission.

The procedure for liver and biliary tract CT is as follows:

- The patient is placed in a supine position on an X-ray table that's positioned within the opening of the scanning gantry.
- A series of transverse X-ray films is taken and recorded on magnetic tape. This information is reconstructed by a computer and appears as images on a monitor.
- The images are studied, and selected ones are photographed. When the first series of films is completed, the images are reviewed.
- Contrast enhancement may be performed. After the contrast medium is injected, a second series of films is taken, and the patient is carefully observed for an allergic reaction.

Interfering Factors

- Presence of oral or IV contrast media, including barium, in the bile duct from earlier tests (possible poor imaging)
- Claustrophobia (inability to complete CT scan)
- Excessive patient movement (poor image)
- Metallic objects in the examination field (poor image)

▶ *Quality and Safety Nursing Alert*

A CT scan isn't recommended during pregnancy because of potential risk to the fetus.

Precautions

- The patient may experience strong feelings of claustrophobia or anxiety when inside the CT body scanner. A mild sedative may be ordered to help reduce anxiety.
- An IV contrast medium is contraindicated in patients hypersensitive to iodine and in patients with severe renal or hepatic disease.

Nursing Considerations

Before the Test

- Confirm the patient's identity using two patient identifiers and confirmation of the patient's identification bracelet according to facility policy.
- Notify the radiology department if your patient has a PICC line. Power-PICC is indicated for power injection of contrast media.
- Explain to the patient that CT scanning helps detect biliary tract and liver disease.
- Check the patient's history for hypersensitivity reactions to iodine or contrast media. If such reactions have occurred, note them in the patient's chart and notify the health care provider, who may order prophylactic medications or choose not to use contrast enhancement.
- Check the patient's history for contrast media used in other diagnostic tests.
- For women of childbearing age, assess pregnancy status (i.e., determine LMP) for possible pregnancy and notify radiology as needed.
- Explain that the patient will be given a contrast medium to drink and then should fast until after the examination. If contrast isn't ordered, fasting isn't necessary.
- Instruct the patient to remove body piercings, jewelry, or other metal objects in the X-ray field to allow for precise imaging.
- Explain to the patient who will perform the test and when and where it will take place.
- Explain that the patient will be placed on an adjustable table positioned inside a scanning gantry. Assure the patient that the test will be painless.
- Tell the patient to remain still during the test and to hold the breath when instructed. Stress the importance of remaining still during the test because movement can cause artifact, thereby

prolonging the test and limiting its accuracy.

- If IV contrast medium is being used, inform the patient that transient discomfort from the needle puncture and a localized feeling of warmth on injection, as well as a salty or metallic taste may be experienced. Tell the patient to immediately report nausea, vomiting, dizziness, headache, or hives.
- If oral contrast medium has been ordered, give the patient the contrast medium supplied by the radiology department.
- Make sure that the patient or a responsible family member has signed an informed consent form.
- If the procedure used contrast enhancement, watch for a delayed hypersensitivity reaction to the contrast medium.

After the Test

- If contrast medium is used, observe the patient for a delayed allergic reaction and treat as necessary. (Diphenhydramine is the drug of choice.) Encourage fluids to assist in eliminating the contrast medium. For the patient who is at risk for renal impairment, prepare to administer acetylcysteine to assist with clearance of the contrast medium.
- Instruct the patient to resume a usual diet as ordered.

Computed Tomography of the Orbit

Normal Findings

- Normal size, shape, and position of orbital structures
- Dense orbital bone in marked contrast to periocular fat
- Clearly defined optic nerve and medial and lateral rectus muscles
- Thin, dense bands of rectus muscles on each side, behind the eye
- Optic canals of equal size
- Absence of foreign body or ocular trauma

Abnormal Findings

- Irregular areas of density, indicating lymphomas or metastatic carcinomas
- Clearly defined masses of consistent density, indicating benign hemangiomas or meningiomas
- Optic nerve thickening, suggesting gliomas
- The presence of trauma or foreign body

Nursing Implications

- Report abnormal findings to the health care provider.
- Prepare to educate the patient about the diagnosis.
- Prepare the patient for further testing or surgery as indicated.
- Provide emotional support to the patient and family.

Purpose

- To evaluate pathologies of the orbit and eye, especially expanding lesions and bone destruction
- To evaluate fractures of the orbit and adjoining structures
- To determine the cause of unilateral exophthalmos
- To determine the presence of ocular trauma or foreign body

Description

CT of the orbit can delineate the size, position, and relationship to adjoining structures of abnormalities not readily seen on standard radiographs. Additionally, orbital CT is most typically used to determine the presence of ocular trauma or foreign body. A series of tomograms reconstructed by a computer and displayed as anatomic slices on a monitor, this type of CT scan identifies space-occupying lesions earlier and more accurately than other radiographic techniques, and it provides three-dimensional images of orbital structures, especially the ocular muscles and the optic nerve.

The procedure for orbital CT is as follows:

- The patient is placed in a supine position on the X-ray table with the head immobilized by straps, if required, and asked to lie still.
- The head of the table is moved into the scanner, which rotates around the patient's head, taking radiographs.
- Information obtained is stored on magnetic tapes. Images are then displayed on a monitor. Photographs may be made if a permanent record is desired.
- When this series of radiographs has been taken, contrast enhancement is performed. The contrast medium is injected IV, and a second series of scans is recorded.

Interfering Factors
- Head movement (possible poor imaging)
- Failure to remove metallic objects from examination field (possible poor imaging)

> ◤ **Quality and Safety Nursing Alert**
>
> A CT scan isn't recommended during pregnancy because of potential risk to the fetus.

Precautions
- Contrast medium is contraindicated in patients with a history of iodine hypersensitivity or in patients with severe renal or hepatic disease.

Nursing Considerations
Before the Test
- Confirm the patient's identity using two patient identifiers and confirmation of the patient's identification bracelet according to facility policy.
- Notify the radiology department if your patient has a PICC line. Power-PICC is indicated for power injection of contrast media.
- Explain that the orbital CT scan visualizes the anatomy of the eye and its surrounding structures.

- Tell the patient that a series of X-ray films will be taken of the eye.
- If contrast enhancement isn't scheduled, the patient need not restrict food and fluids. If contrast enhancement is scheduled, withhold food and fluids from the patient for 4 hours before the test.
- For women of childbearing age, assess pregnancy status (i.e., determine LMP) for possible pregnancy and notify radiology as needed.
- Explain who will perform the test, and when and where it will take place.
- Assure the patient that the procedure is painless, but that having to remain still for a prolonged period of time may be uncomfortable.
- Explain that the patient will be positioned on an X-ray table and that the head of the table will be moved into the scanner, which will rotate around the head and make loud clacking sounds.
- If a contrast medium is being used, tell the patient that a flushed and warm feeling, a transient headache, a salty or metallic taste, and nausea or vomiting after the contrast medium is injected may be experienced. Assure the patient that these reactions are normal.
- Instruct the patient to remove body piercings, jewelry, hairpins, or other metal objects in the X-ray field to allow for precise imaging of the orbital structures.
- Make sure that the patient or a responsible family member has signed an informed consent form if required.
- Check the patient's history for hypersensitivity reactions to iodine or contrast media. If such reactions have occurred, note them in the patient's chart and notify the health care provider, who may order prophylactic medications or choose not to use contrast enhancement.

After the Test

- If a contrast medium was used, watch for its residual adverse effects, including headache, nausea, or vomiting. Encourage fluids to assist in eliminating the contrast medium. If the patient is at risk for impaired renal function, prepare for the administration of acetylcysteine to assist with renal clearance of contrast medium.
- Instruct the patient to resume a usual diet as ordered.

Computed Tomography of the Pancreas

Normal Findings

- Pancreatic parenchyma displaying a uniform density, especially when an IV contrast medium is used
- Normal thickening from tail to head with a smooth surface
- Opacification of adjacent stomach and duodenum with outline of the pancreas (with oral contrast medium) (See the *Normal CT Scan of the Pancreas* box.)

Abnormal Findings

- Change in pancreatic size and shape, initially appearing as a localized swelling of the head, body, or tail of the pancreas that spreads to obliterate the fat plane and dilate the main pancreatic duct and common bile duct and produces low-density focal lesions in the liver from metastasis, indicating pancreatic cancer
- Change in pancreatic size and shape and sharply circumscribed, low-density areas that may contain debris, indicating pseudocysts
- Diffuse pancreatic enlargement with uniform decrease in density, indicating acute edematous (interstitial) pancreatitis
- Diffuse pancreatic enlargement with nonuniform density, indicating acute necrotizing pancreatitis
- Low-density areas most readily detected when they contain gas, indicating abscesses
- Normal, enlarged (localized or generalized), or atrophic pancreas, depending on disease severity; characteristic

Normal CT Scan of the Pancreas

This normal pancreatic computed tomography (CT) scan shows the pancreas opacified by contrast medium.

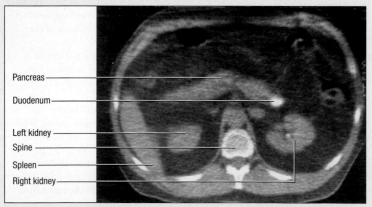

Pancreas
Duodenum
Left kidney
Spine
Spleen
Right kidney

duct calcification and main pancreatic duct dilation, indicating chronic pancreatitis

Nursing Implications
- Anticipate the need for additional testing.
- Prepare the patient for follow-up treatment, including drug therapy or surgery.
- Provide emotional support to the patient and family.

Purpose
- To detect pancreatic carcinoma or pseudocysts
- To detect or evaluate pancreatitis
- To distinguish between pancreatic disorders and disorders of the retroperitoneum

Description
In CT of the pancreas, multiple X-rays penetrate the upper abdomen while a detector records the differences in tissue attenuation, which is then displayed as an image on a monitor. A series of cross-sectional views can provide a detailed look at the pancreas. CT scanning accurately distinguishes the pancreas and surrounding organs and vessels if enough fat is present between the structures. IV or oral contrast medium use can further accentuate differences in tissue density.

CT scanning is replacing ultrasonography as the test of choice for examining the pancreas. Although ultrasonography costs less and involves less risk for the patient, it's less accurate. In retroperitoneal disorders, specifically when pancreatitis is suspected, CT scanning goes beyond ultrasonography by showing the general swelling that accompanies acute inflammation of the gland. In chronic cases, CT scanning easily detects calcium deposits commonly missed by simple radiography, particularly in obese patients.

The procedure is as follows:
- The patient is placed in the supine position on the X-ray table, which is positioned within the opening of the scanning gantry.
- A series of transverse X-rays is taken and recorded on magnetic tape. The varying tissue absorption is calculated by a computer, and the information is reconstructed as images on a monitor. These images are studied, and selected images are photographed.
- After the first series of films is complete, the images are reviewed and a decision may be made to order contrast enhancement.
- After the contrast medium is administered, another series of films is taken and the patient is observed for an allergic reaction, such as itching, hypotension, hypertension, diaphoresis, or dyspnea.

Interfering Factors
- Barium or other contrast media in the GI tract from earlier tests (possible poor imaging)
- Excessive peristalsis or excessive patient movement (poor image)
- Claustrophobia (inability to complete CT scan)
- Metallic objects in the examination field (poor image)

 Quality and Safety Nursing Alert

A CT scan isn't recommended during pregnancy because of potential risk to the fetus.

Precautions
- Contrast medium is contraindicated in patients with a history of iodine hypersensitivity or severe renal or hepatic disease.

Nursing Considerations
Before the Test
- Confirm the patient's identity using two patient identifiers and confirmation of the patient's identification bracelet according to facility policy.

- Notify the radiology department if your patient has a PICC line. Power-PICC is indicated for power injection of contrast media.
- Explain to the patient that CT scanning helps detect disorders of the pancreas.
- Describe the test, including who will perform it and when and where it will take place.
- Explain that the patient will be placed on an adjustable table positioned inside a scanning gantry. Assure the patient that the procedure is painless.
- For women of childbearing age, assess pregnancy status (i.e., determine LMP) for possible pregnancy and notify radiology as needed.
- Instruct the patient to remove body piercings, jewelry, or other metal objects in the X-ray field to allow for precise imaging.
- Explain that the patient will need to remain still during the test and periodically hold the breath.
- Explain that the patient may be given an IV contrast medium, an oral contrast medium, or both to enhance visualization of the pancreas. Describe possible adverse reactions to the medium, such as nausea, flushing, dizziness, and sweating, and tell the patient to report these symptoms.
- Check the patient's history for recent barium studies.
- Check the patient's history for hypersensitivity reactions to iodine or contrast media. If such reactions have occurred, note them in the patient's chart and notify the health care provider, who may order prophylactic medications or choose not to use contrast enhancement.
- Make sure that the patient or a responsible family member has signed an informed consent form.
- Administer the oral contrast medium. Instruct the patient to fast after administration of the oral contrast medium.

After the Test

- Instruct the patient to resume a usual diet as ordered.
- Observe for signs and symptoms of a delayed allergic reaction to the contrast dye, such as urticaria, headache, and vomiting.
- If contrast medium is used, observe the patient for a delayed allergic reaction and treat as necessary. (Diphenhydramine is the drug of choice.) Encourage fluids to assist in eliminating the contrast medium.
- In patients who are at risk for renal impairment, prepare to administer acetylcysteine to assist with renal clearance of contrast medium.

Computed Tomography of the Spine

Normal Findings

- White, black, or gray spinal tissue, depending on its density
- White vertebrae (densest tissues)
- Black CSF
- Gray soft tissues

Abnormal Findings

- Altered density and structural malformation, indicating spinal lesions and tumors
- Degenerative processes and structural changes, such as herniated nucleus pulposus
- Cervical cord compression caused by bony hypertrophy of the cervical spine, indicating cervical spondylosis
- Hypertrophy of the lumbar vertebrae, causing cord compression, indicating lumbar stenosis
- Soft-tissue changes, bony overgrowth, and spurring of the vertebrae, indicating facet disorders
- Dark masses displacing the spinal cord, indicating fluid-filled arachnoidal and other paraspinal cysts
- Masses or clusters, usually on the dorsal aspect of the spinal cord, suggesting vascular malformations

- Abnormally large, dark gaps between the white vertebrae, indicating congenital spinal malformations, such as meningocele, myelocele, and spina bifida

Nursing Implications

- Anticipate the need for additional testing.
- Prepare the patient for follow-up treatment, including medication therapy, surgery, or physical therapy.
- Provide emotional support to the patient and family.
- Assess mobility status and monitor for pain.

Purpose

- To diagnose spinal lesions and abnormalities
- To monitor the effects of spinal surgery or therapy

Description

Much more versatile than conventional radiography, CT of the spine provides detailed high-resolution images in the cross-sectional, longitudinal, sagittal, and lateral planes. Multiple X-ray beams from a computerized body scanner are directed at the spine from different angles; these pass through the body and strike radiation detectors, producing electrical impulses. A computer then converts these impulses into digital information, which is displayed as a three-dimensional image on a monitor. Storage of the digital information allows electronic recreation and manipulation of the image, creating a permanent record of the images to enable reexamination without repeating the procedure.

The procedure for spinal CT is as follows:

- The patient is placed in a supine position on an X-ray table and asked to lie as still as possible.
- The table slides into the CT scanner's circular opening. The scanner revolves around the patient, taking radiographs at preselected intervals.
- After the first set of scans is taken, the patient is removed from the

scanner. Contrast medium may be administered.

- The patient is observed for signs and symptoms of a hypersensitivity reaction, including pruritus, rash, and respiratory difficulty, for 30 minutes after the contrast medium has been injected. Nausea is not uncommon and may last for a few minutes.
- After contrast medium injection, the patient is moved back into the scanner and another series of scans is taken. The images obtained from the scan are displayed on a monitor during the procedure and stored on magnetic tape.

Interfering Factors

- Barium or other contrast media in the GI tract from earlier tests (possible poor imaging)
- Excessive peristalsis or excessive patient movement (poor image)
- Claustrophobia (inability to complete CT scan)
- Metallic objects in the examination field (poor image)

 Quality and Safety Nursing Alert

A CT scan isn't recommended during pregnancy because of potential risk to the fetus.

Precautions

- Use of contrast medium is contraindicated in patients with a history of hypersensitivity to iodine or in patients with severe renal or hepatic disease.

Nursing Considerations

Before the Test

- Confirm the patient's identity using two patient identifiers and confirmation of the patient's identification bracelet according to facility policy.
- Notify the radiology department if your patient has a PICC line. PowerPICC is indicated for power injection of contrast media.

C

- Explain to the patient that spinal CT allows visualization of the spine.
- If contrast medium isn't ordered, tell the patient that there are no food or fluid restrictions for this test. If contrast medium is ordered, instruct the patient to fast for 4 hours before the test.
- For women of childbearing age, assess pregnancy status (i.e., determine LMP) for possible pregnancy and notify radiology as needed.
- Instruct the patient to remove body piercings, jewelry, hairpins, or other metal objects in the X-ray field to allow for precise imaging.
- Tell the patient that a series of scans will be taken of the spine. Explain who will perform the procedure and when and where it will take place.
- Assure the patient that the procedure is painless, but that having to remain still for a prolonged period may be uncomfortable.
- Explain that the patient will be positioned on an X-ray table inside a CT body-scanning unit that will revolve around the patient, taking multiple scans. The patient will be told to lie still because movement during the procedure may cause distorted images.
- If a contrast medium is used, the patient may feel flushed and warm, and may experience a transient headache, a salty taste, and nausea or vomiting after injection of the contrast medium. Assure the patient that these reactions are normal.
- Instruct the patient to wear a radiologic examining gown and to remove all metal objects and jewelry.
- Check the patient's history for hypersensitivity reactions to iodine or contrast media. If such reactions have occurred, note them in the patient's chart and notify the health care provider, who may order prophylactic medications or choose not to use contrast enhancement.

- If the patient appears restless or apprehensive about the procedure, a mild sedative may be prescribed.
- Make sure that the patient or a responsible family member has signed an informed consent form, if required.
- For the patient with significant back pain, administer prescribed analgesics before the scan.

After the Test
- After testing with contrast enhancement, observe the patient for residual effects, such as headache, nausea, and vomiting.
- If contrast medium is used, observe the patient for a delayed allergic reaction and treat as necessary. (Diphenhydramine is the drug of choice.) Encourage fluids to assist in eliminating the contrast medium. In patients who are at risk for renal impairment, prepare to administer acetylcysteine to assist with renal clearance of contrast medium.
- Instruct the patient to resume a usual diet as ordered.

Computed Tomography of the Thorax

Normal Findings
- Air and bone densities as black and white areas, respectively
- Shades of gray corresponding to water, fat, and soft-tissue densities

Abnormal Findings
- Areas of altered density, indicating tumors, nodules, cysts, aortic aneurysms, enlarged lymph nodes, pleural effusion, and accumulations of blood, fluid, or fat

Nursing Implications
- Anticipate the need for additional testing.
- Prepare the patient for follow-up treatment, including drug therapy or surgery.
- Provide emotional support to the patient and family.

Purpose

- To locate suspected neoplasms (such as in Hodgkin's disease), especially with mediastinal involvement
- To differentiate coin-sized calcified lesions (indicating tuberculosis) from tumors
- To differentiate emphysema or bronchopleural fistula from lung abscess
- To distinguish tumors adjacent to the aorta from aortic aneurysms
- To detect the invasion of a neck mass in the thorax
- To evaluate primary malignancy that may metastasize to the lungs, especially in the patient with a primary bone tumor, soft-tissue sarcoma, or melanoma
- To evaluate the mediastinal lymph nodes
- To evaluate the severity of lung disease, such as emphysema
- To detect a dissection or leak of an aortic aneurysm or aortic arch aneurysm
- To plan radiation treatment

Description

CT of the thorax provides cross-sectional views of the chest by passing an X-ray beam from a computerized scanner through the body at different angles. It provides a three-dimensional image and is especially useful in detecting small differences in tissue density. It may replace mediastinoscopy in the diagnosis of mediastinal masses and Hodgkin's disease; its value in the evaluation of pulmonary pathology is proved.

The procedure for CT of the thorax is as follows:

- The patient is assisted into the supine position on the X-ray table and the contrast medium is injected.
- The machine scans the patient at different angles while the computer calculates small differences in densities of various tissues, water, fat, bone, and air.
- Information is displayed as a printout of numerical values and a projection

on a monitor. Images may be recorded for further study.

Interfering Factors

- Barium or other contrast media in the GI tract from earlier tests (possible poor imaging)
- Excessive peristalsis or excessive patient movement (poor image)
- Claustrophobia (inability to complete CT scan)
- Metallic objects in the examination field (poor image)

 Quality and Safety Nursing Alert

A CT scan isn't recommended during pregnancy because of potential risk to the fetus.

Precautions

- Use of contrast medium is contraindicated in the patient with a history of iodine hypersensitivity or severe renal or hepatic disease.

Nursing Considerations

Before the Test

- Confirm the patient's identity using two patient identifiers and confirmation of the patient's identification bracelet according to facility policy.
- Notify the radiology department if your patient has a PICC line. Power-PICC is indicated for power injection of contrast media.
- Explain that the thoracic CT provides cross-sectional views of the chest and distinguishes small differences in tissue density.
- If the patient won't receive a contrast medium, there is no need for food or fluid restriction. If the patient will receive a contrast medium, instruct the patient to fast for 4 hours before the test.
- For women of childbearing age, assess pregnancy status (i.e., determine LMP) for possible pregnancy and notify radiology as needed.
- Instruct the patient to remove body piercings, jewelry, or other metal

C

objects in the X-ray field to allow for precise imaging.

- Explain that the patient will lie on an X-ray table that moves into the center of a large ring-shaped piece of X-ray equipment and that the equipment may be noisy.
- Explain that the patient may be injected with contrast medium and that it may cause nausea, warmth, flushing of the face, and a salty or metallic taste. Assure the patient that these symptoms are normal and that radiation exposure is minimal.
- Tell the patient to remain still during the test, breathing normally until told to follow specific breathing instructions.
- Make sure that the patient or a responsible family member has signed an informed consent form.
- Check the patient's history for hypersensitivity reactions to iodine or contrast media. If such reactions have occurred, note them in the patient's chart and notify the health care provider, who may order prophylactic medications or choose not to use contrast enhancement.

After the Test

- Watch the patient for signs of delayed hypersensitivity to the contrast medium (itching, hypotension or hypertension, or respiratory distress).
- Instruct the patient to resume a usual diet as ordered.
- If contrast medium was used, encourage fluids to assist in eliminating the contrast medium.

Concentration and Dilution Test

Reference Values

Specific gravity: 1.005 to 1.035
Osmolality: 300 to 900 mOsm/kg

Concentration Test

Specific gravity: 1.025 to 1.032; osmolality greater than 800 mOsm/kg of

water (SI, greater than 800 mmol/kg) in the patient with normal renal function Urine-to-serum ratio of 1:1 to 3:1

Dilution Test

Specific gravity less than 1.003; osmolality less than 100 mOsm/kg for at least one specimen; 80% or more of the ingested water eliminated in 4 hours

Abnormal Findings

Decreased Levels

- Tubular epithelial damage, decreased renal blood flow, loss of functional nephrons, or pituitary or cardiac dysfunction (decreased renal capacity to concentrate urine in response to fluid deprivation or to dilute urine in response to fluid overload)

Nursing Implications

- Anticipate the need for additional testing.
- Prepare the patient for follow-up treatment.
- Monitor fluid balance status, including intake and output.

Purpose

- To evaluate renal tubular function
- To detect renal impairment
- To diagnose disorders such as diabetes insipidus

Description

The kidneys normally concentrate or dilute urine according to fluid intake. When such intake is excessive, the kidneys excrete more water in the urine; when intake is limited, they excrete less.

The concentration and dilution test evaluates renal capacity to concentrate urine in response to fluid deprivation or to dilute it in response to fluid overload. This test may also be referred to as the *water loading* or *water deprivation test*.

 Quality and Safety Nursing Alert

In an elderly person, depressed values can be associated with normal renal function.

Interfering Factors

- Use of radiographic contrast agents within 7 days of test (possible increase in osmolality)
- Diuretics and nephrotoxic drugs (possible increase or decrease in specific gravity and osmolality)
- Glycosuria

Precautions

- Testing may be contraindicated in the patient with advanced renal disease or cardiac dysfunction, because fluid overload can precipitate water intoxication, sodium diuresis, or heart failure.

Nursing Considerations

Before the Test

- Confirm the patient's identity using two patient identifiers and confirmation of the patient's identification bracelet according to facility policy.
- Explain to the patient that the concentration and dilution test evaluates kidney function.
- Explain that the test requires multiple urine specimens and how many specimens will be collected and at what intervals.
- Instruct the patient to discard urine voided for a specific time, per laboratory protocol, such as all urine collected during the night.
- Withhold diuretics as needed.
- If the patient is catheterized, empty the drainage bag before the test.

Concentration Test

- Provide a high-protein meal and only 200 mL of fluid the night before the test.
- Instruct the patient to restrict food and fluids for at least 14 hours before the test. (Some concentration tests require that water be withheld for 24 hours, but permit relatively normal food intake.)
- Limit salt intake at the evening meal to prevent excessive thirst.
- Emphasize to the patient that adherence to pretest protocols is necessary to obtain accurate results.

Dilution Test

- Generally, the dilution test directly follows the concentration test and requires no additional patient preparation.
- If this test is performed alone, simply withhold breakfast.

During the Test

- Provide the patient with a clean bedpan, urinal, or toilet specimen pan if the patient is unable to urinate into the specimen containers.
- Rinse the collection device after each use.
- If the patient is catheterized, obtain the specimens from the catheter and clamp the catheter between collections.

Concentration Test

- Collect urine specimens at 6 AM, 8 AM, and 10 AM.

Dilution Test

- Instruct the patient to void and discard the first urine sample.
- Give the patient 1,500 mL of water to drink within a 30-minute period.
- Collect urine specimens every half hour or every hour for 4 hours thereafter.

After the Test

- Send each specimen to the laboratory immediately after collection.
- Provide a balanced meal or a snack after collecting the final specimen.

Coombs' Test, Direct

Normal Findings

- Negative (neither antibodies nor complement appearing on the RBCs)

Abnormal Findings

- Positive result on umbilical cord blood, indicating that maternal antibodies have crossed the placenta and coated fetal RBCs, indicating hemolytic disease of the newborn (HDN)
- Positive (+1 to +4), indicating hemolytic anemia; differentiates between

autoimmune and secondary hemolytic anemia, which can be drug induced or associated with underlying disease
- Positive, indicating sepsis
- Weakly positive, indicating transfusion reaction
- Transfusion reactions

Nursing Implications
- Anticipate the need for additional testing.
- Prepare the patient for follow-up treatment.
- Transfuse compatible blood lacking the antigens to these maternal antibodies, as ordered and indicated, to prevent anemia.

Purpose
- To diagnose HDN
- To investigate hemolytic transfusion reactions
- To aid in the differential diagnosis of hemolytic anemias, which may be congenital or may result from an autoimmune reaction or use of certain drugs

Description
The direct Coombs' test, also called the *direct antiglobulin test,* detects immunoglobulins (antibodies) on the surface of the RBCs. They coat the RBCs when they become sensitized to an antigen such as the Rh factor. Antiglobulin (Coombs') serum added to saline-washed RBCs results in agglutination if immunoglobulins or complement is present. This process is considered direct because it requires only one step—the addition of Coombs' serum to washed cells.

Interfering Factors
- Hemolysis
- Aldomet, cephalosporins, chlorpromazine, diphenylhydantoin, ethosuximide, hydralazine, insulin, isoniazid, levodopa, mefenamic acid, melphalan, methyldopa, penicillin, procainamide, quinidine, rifampin, streptomycin, sulfonamides, and tetracycline (positive test results, possibly from immune hemolysis)

Nursing Considerations
Before the Test
- Confirm the patient's identity using two patient identifiers and confirmation of the patient's identification bracelet according to facility policy.
- If the patient is suspected of having hemolytic anemia, explain that the test determines whether the condition results from an abnormality in the body's immune system, the use of certain drugs, or some unknown cause.
- Inform the adult patient that there are no food or fluid restrictions for this test.
- Tell the patient that the test requires a blood sample.

 Quality and Safety Nursing Alert

If the patient is a neonate, explain the test and its requirements to the neonate's parents.

- Explain to the patient that slight discomfort from the tourniquet and the needle puncture may be experienced.
- Withhold drugs that may interfere with test results, including cephalosporins, chlorpromazine, diphenylhydantoin, ethosuximide, hydralazine, isoniazid, levodopa, mefenamic acid, melphalan, methyldopa, penicillin, procainamide, quinidine, rifampin, streptomycin, sulfonamides, and tetracycline.

During the Test
- Perform a venipuncture and collect the sample in two 5-mL EDTA tubes.

 Quality and Safety Nursing Alert

For a neonate, draw 5 mL of cord blood into a tube with EDTA or additives after the cord is clamped and cut.

- Handle samples gently to prevent hemolysis.
- Label the sample with the patient's full name, the facility or blood bank number, the date, and your initials.

- Send the sample to the laboratory immediately.

After the Test
- Apply direct pressure to the venipuncture site until bleeding stops.
- Explain that the patient may resume medications that were stopped before the test.
- Tell the patient or the parents of the neonate with HDN that further tests will be necessary to monitor anemia.

Coombs' Test, Indirect

Normal Findings
- No agglutination, indicating that the patient's serum contains no circulating antibodies other than anti-A or anti-B

Abnormal Findings
- Positive (+1 to +4), indicating the presence of unexpected circulating antibodies to RBC antigens (donor and recipient incompatibility). Note that drugs, such as antibiotics, including but not limited to the cephalosporins, penicillins, tetracycline, streptomycin, as well as phenytoin (Dilantin), chlorpromazine (Thorazine), the sulfonamides, antiarrhythmics (Pronestyl), and the antituberculins (INH), may result in an increase in the indirect Coombs' test; check all patient medications before the test is completed.

Nursing Implications
- Anticipate the need for additional testing.
- Prepare the patient for follow-up treatment.
- If the patient is pregnant, anticipate the need for repeated testing throughout the pregnancy to evaluate the development of circulating antibody levels. If Rh incompatibility is suspected, anticipate administering Rho (D) immune globulin (RhoGAM) to the mother.
- Be aware of any medications that the patient might be taking that can

interfere with obtaining accurate results.

Purpose
- To detect unexpected circulating antibodies to RBC antigens in the recipient's or donor's serum before transfusion
- To determine the presence of anti-D antibody in maternal blood
- To evaluate the need for Rho (D) immune globulin
- To help diagnose acquired hemolytic anemia

Description
Indirect Coombs' test, also called *antibody screening*, detects unexpected circulating antibodies in the patient's serum. After incubating the serum with group O RBCs, an antiglobulin (Coombs' serum) is added. Agglutination occurs if the patient's serum contains an antibody to one or more antigens on the RBCs. This test detects 95% to 99% of the circulating antibodies. After detection, antibody identification testing can determine the specific identity of the antibodies present.

 Quality and Safety Nursing Alert

A positive result in a pregnant patient with Rh-negative blood may indicate the presence of antibodies to the Rh factor from an earlier transfusion with incompatible blood or from a previous pregnancy with an Rh-positive fetus. A positive result indicates that the fetus may develop HDN.

Interfering Factors
- Previous dextran or IV contrast media administration (causing aggregation resembling agglutination)
- Blood transfusion or pregnancy within the past 3 months (possible presence of antibodies)
- Drugs that may cause false-positive results; these may include cephalosporins, insulin, penicillins, phenytoin, and sulfonamides.

Precautions

- Handle the sample gently to prevent hemolysis.

Nursing Considerations

Before the Test

- Confirm the patient's identity using two patient identifiers and confirmation of the patient's identification bracelet according to facility policy.
- Explain to the patient that the antibody screening test helps to evaluate the possibility of a transfusion reaction or determines whether fetal antibodies are in the patient's blood and whether treatment is necessary.
- If the test is for a patient who's anemic, explain that the test helps identify the type of anemia.
- Inform the patient that there are no food or fluid restrictions for this test.
- Tell the patient that the test requires a blood sample.
- Explain to the patient that there may be slight discomfort from the tourniquet and the needle puncture.
- Check the patient's history for recent blood, dextran, or IV contrast media administration and for any medications that can result in an inaccurate result; note this information.

During the Test

- Perform a venipuncture and collect the sample in two 10-mL tubes. If the antibody screen is positive, antibody identification is performed on the blood.
- Label the sample with the patient's name, the hospital or blood bank number, the date, and your initials.
- Include on the laboratory request the patient's diagnosis and pregnancy status, history of transfusions, and current drug therapy.

After the Test

- Send the sample to the laboratory immediately.
- Apply direct pressure to the venipuncture site until bleeding stops and to prevent hematoma formation.

Corticotropin, Plasma (Adrenocorticotropic Hormone [ACTH], Corticotropin, Corticotropin-Releasing Factor [CRF])

Reference Values

Baseline values: Less than 120 pg/mL (SI, less than 26.4 pmol/L at 6 AM to 8 AM using Mayo Medical Laboratories sets); values may vary with each laboratory

Abnormal Findings

Elevated Levels

- Primary adrenal hypofunction (Addison's disease caused by idiopathic atrophy or partial gland destruction by granuloma, neoplasm, amyloidosis, or inflammatory necrosis)
- Cushing syndrome
- Pituitary-dependent adrenal hyperplasia and nonadrenal tumors such as oat cell carcinoma of the lungs (moderately elevated)

Decreased Levels

- Secondary adrenal hypofunction resulting from pituitary or hypothalamic dysfunction
- Adrenal hyperfunction caused by adrenocortical tumor or hyperplasia

Nursing Implications

- Anticipate the need for additional testing.
- Prepare the patient for follow-up and treatment.
- Provide emotional support to the patient during the diagnostic period.

Purpose

- To facilitate a differential primary and secondary adrenal hypofunction diagnosis of primary and secondary adrenal hypofunction
- To aid a differential diagnosis of Cushing syndrome

Description

The corticotropin test measures corticotropin plasma levels by radioimmunoassay. Corticotropin stimulates the adrenal gland to secrete cortisol and, to a lesser degree, androgens and aldosterone. Corticotropin levels vary diurnally, peaking between 6 AM and 8 AM and ebbing between 6 PM and 11 PM. Emotional and physical stress (pain, surgery, insulin-induced hypoglycemia) stimulate secretion and can override the effects of plasma cortisol levels.

Interfering Factors

- Failure to observe pretest restrictions
- Corticosteroids, including cortisone and its analogues (decrease)
- Drugs that increase endogenous cortisol secretion, such as estrogens, calcium gluconate, amphetamines, spironolactone, and ethanol (decrease)
- Lithium carbonate (decreases cortisol levels and may interfere with corticotropin secretion)
- Menstrual cycle and pregnancy
- Radioactive scan performed within 1 week before the test
- Acute stress (including hospitalization and surgery) and depression (increase)

Precautions

- Proteolytic enzymes in plasma degrade corticotropin. A 39.2°F (4°C) temperature is necessary to retard enzyme activity.

Nursing Considerations

Before the Test

- Confirm the patient's identity using two patient identifiers and confirmation of the patient's identification bracelet according to facility policy.
- Explain to the patient that this test helps determine whether hormonal secretion is normal.
- Advise the patient to fast and limit physical activity for 10 to 12 hours before the test.
- Tell the patient that the test requires a blood sample.
  Explain that the patient may experience slight discomfort from the tourniquet and the needle puncture.

- Check the patient's history for medications that may affect test result accuracy. Withhold these medications for 48 hours or longer before the test. If the patient must continue them, note this on the laboratory request.

During the Test

- For a patient with suspected adrenal hypofunction, perform the venipuncture for a baseline level between 6 AM and 8 AM (peak secretion).
- For a patient with suspected Cushing syndrome, perform the venipuncture between 6 PM and 11 PM (low secretion).
- Collect the sample in a plastic EDTA tube (corticotropin may adhere to glass). The tube must be full because excess anticoagulant will affect results.
- Pack the sample in ice and send it to the laboratory immediately, where plasma must be rapidly separated from blood cells at 39.2°F (4°C). The collection technique may vary, depending on the laboratory.

After the Test

- Apply direct pressure to the venipuncture site until bleeding stops.
- Explain that the patient may resume usual diet, activities, and medications that were stopped before the test.

Cortisol, Plasma and Urine

Reference Values

Morning: 9 to 35 mcg/dL (SI, 250-690 nmol/L)

Afternoon: 3 to 12 mcg/dL (SI, 80–330 nmol/L) (usually half the morning level)

Free cortisol values: Less than 50 mcg/24 hours (SI, less than 138 mmol/24 hours)

Abnormal Findings

Elevated Levels

- Adrenocortical hyperfunction caused by Cushing disease or Cushing syndrome (plasma)

- Cushing syndrome caused by adrenal hyperplasia, adrenal or pituitary tumor, or ectopic corticotropin production (urine)

Nursing Implications

- Anticipate the need for additional testing.
- Provide emotional support to the patient during the diagnostic period.
- Prepare the patient for follow-up and treatment.
- Explain the underlying problem associated with the disorder.
- Keep in mind that hepatic disease and obesity can raise plasma cortisol levels, but generally don't appreciably raise free cortisol urine levels.

Decreased Levels, Plasma

- Primary adrenal hypofunction (Addison's disease), usually caused by idiopathic glandular atrophy (a presumed autoimmune process)
- Secondary adrenal insufficiency, such as hypophysectomy, postpartum pituitary necrosis, craniopharyngioma, and chromophobe adenoma
- Adrenal hyperplasia and hypothyroidism, hypopituitarism (from the anterior pituitary)

Nursing Implications

- Anticipate the need for additional testing.
- Prepare the patient for follow-up and treatment.
- Provide emotional support to the patient during the diagnostic period.
- Explain the underlying problem associated with the disorder.
- Be aware that low urine cortisol levels have little diagnostic significance and don't necessarily indicate adrenocortical hypofunction.

Purpose

- To help diagnose Cushing disease, Cushing syndrome, and Addison's disease
- To evaluate adrenocortical function

Description

Cortisol—the principal glucocorticoid secreted by the zona fasciculata of the adrenal cortex—helps metabolize nutrients, mediate physiologic stress, and regulate the immune system. Cortisol secretion normally follows a diurnal pattern: Levels rise during the early morning hours, peaking around 8 AM, and then decline to very low levels in the evening and during the early phase of sleep. (See the *Diurnal Variations in Cortisol Secretion* box.) Intense heat or cold, infection, trauma, exercise, obesity, and debilitating disease influence cortisol secretion.

Plasma cortisol level measured quantitatively via radioimmunoassay usually is ordered for patients with signs of adrenal dysfunction. Dynamic tests, suppression tests for hyperfunction, and stimulation tests for hypofunction generally are required to confirm the diagnosis. An adrenocorticotropic hormone (ACTH) stimulation blood test may be ordered to determine if the adrenal glands are producing sufficient amounts or cortisol.

Urine-free cortisol is used as a screen for adrenocortical hyperfunction. It measures urine levels of the portion of cortisol not bound to the corticosteroid-binding globulin transcortin. It's one of the best diagnostic tools for detecting Cushing syndrome.

Unlike a single plasma cortisol measurement of plasma cortisol, radioimmunoassay level determinations of free cortisol levels in a 24-hour urine specimen reflect overall secretion levels instead of diurnal variations. Concurrent plasma cortisol and corticotropin measurements, with urine 17-hydroxycorticosteroids and the dexamethasone suppression test, may be used to confirm the diagnosis.

Interfering Factors

Plasma Cortisol

- Pregnancy or hormonal contraceptive use (false high resulting from an

Diurnal Variations in Cortisol Secretion

Cortisol secretion rises in the early morning, peaking after the patient awakens. Levels decline sharply in the evening and during the early phase of sleep. They rise again during the night and peak by the next morning.

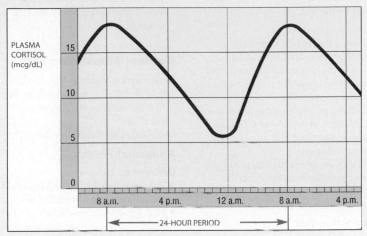

C

increase in cortisol-binding plasma proteins)
• Physical activity, obesity, stress, and severe hepatic or renal disease (possible increase)
• Androgens and phenytoin (possible decrease resulting from a decrease in cortisol-binding plasma proteins)
• Radioactive scan performed within 1 week before the test

Urine Cortisol
• Emotional or physical stress (possible increase)
• Pregnancy (possible increase)
• Aldactone, amphetamines, danazol, hormonal contraceptives, morphine, phenothiazine, prolonged steroid therapy, reserpine, and spironolactone (possible increase)
• Dexamethasone, ethacrynic acid, ketoconazole, and thiazides (decrease)

Nursing Considerations
Before the Test
• Confirm the patient's identity using two patient identifiers and confir-

mation of the patient's identification bracelet according to facility policy.
• Explain to the patient that the plasma and urine cortisol tests help evaluate adrenal gland function.

Plasma Cortisol
• Instruct the patient to maintain a normal sodium diet (2–3 g/day) for 3 days before the test and to fast and limit physical activity for 10 to 12 hours before the test.
• Tell the patient that the test requires a blood sample.
• Explain to the patient that there may be slight discomfort from the tourniquet and the needle puncture.
• Withhold all medications that may interfere with plasma cortisol levels, such as estrogens, androgens, and phenytoin, for 48 hours before the test, as ordered. If the patient is receiving replacement therapy and is dependent on exogenous steroids for survival, note this factor—as

C

well as other medications that must be continued—on the laboratory request.

• Make sure the patient is relaxed and recumbent for at least 30 minutes before the test.

Urine Cortisol

• Inform the patient that there is no need to restrict food and fluids, but to avoid stressful situations and excessive physical exercise during the collection period.

• Tell the patient that the test requires collection of urine over a 24-hour period and teach the proper collection technique.

• Notify the laboratory and the health care provider of medications the patient is taking that may affect test results; these may need to be restricted.

During the Test

Plasma Cortisol

• Perform a venipuncture between 6 AM and 8 AM.

• Collect the sample in a 7-mL heparinized tube, label it appropriately, and send it to the laboratory immediately.

• For diurnal variation testing, draw another sample between 4 PM and 6 PM.

• Collect the second sample in a 7-mL heparinized tube, label it appropriately, and send it to the laboratory immediately.

• Record the blood specimen's collection time on the laboratory request.

• Handle the blood sample gently to prevent hemolysis.

Urine Cortisol

• Collect the patient's urine over a 24-hour period, discarding the first specimen and retaining the last specimen. Use a bottle containing a preservative to keep the specimen at a pH of 4.0 to 4.5.

• Refrigerate the urine specimen or place it on ice during the collection period.

After the Test

• Apply direct pressure to the venipuncture site until bleeding stops.

• Instruct the patient to resume diet, activities, and medications that were discontinued before the test, as ordered.

Cortisol Stimulation Test

Reference Values

18 mg/dL (SI, 500 mmol/L) or greater 30 to 60 minutes after cosyntropin injection

Doubling of the baseline value

Abnormal Findings

Decreased Levels

• Primary adrenal hypofunction (Addison's disease) (levels remain low)

• Hypopituitarism (secondary adrenal insufficiency), adrenal carcinoma, and adenoma

Nursing Implications

• Anticipate the need for additional testing.

• Prepare the patient for follow-up and treatment.

Purpose

• To help identify primary and secondary adrenal hypofunction

Description

The cortisol stimulation test, also known as the *rapid corticotropin test* or the *cosyntropin test,* is gradually replacing the 8-hour corticotropin stimulation test as the most effective diagnostic tool for evaluating adrenal hypofunction. Using cosyntropin, the rapid corticotropin test provides faster results and causes fewer allergic reactions than the 8-hour test, which uses natural corticotropin from animal sources.

This test requires baseline cortisol levels to evaluate the effect of cosyntropin administration on cortisol secretion. A morning cortisol level that's within the reference value range rules out adrenal hypofunction and makes further testing unnecessary.

> **Quality and Safety Nursing Alert**

If test results show subnormal increases in cortisol levels, prolonged stimulation of the adrenal cortex may be required to differentiate between primary and secondary adrenal hypofunction.

Interfering Factors
- Amphetamines and estrogens (increase in plasma cortisol)
- Obesity and smoking (possible increase in plasma cortisol)
- Lithium carbonate (decrease in plasma cortisol)
- Radioactive scan performed within 1 week before the test

Nursing Considerations
Before the Test
- Confirm the patient's identity using two patient identifiers and confirmation of the patient's identification bracelet according to facility policy.
- Explain that the test helps determine whether the patient's condition is caused by a hormonal deficiency.
- Explain that the patient may be required to fast for 10 to 12 hours before the test and must be relaxed and resting quietly for 30 minutes before the test.
- Explain that the test takes at least 1 hour to complete.
- If the patient is an inpatient, withhold corticotropin and all steroid medications, as ordered; if an outpatient, tell the patient to refrain from taking these drugs, if instructed by the health care provider. If the drugs must be continued, note this factor on the laboratory request.
- Tell the patient that the test requires blood samples.
- Explain to the patient that slight discomfort from the tourniquet and the needle puncture may be experienced.

During the Test
- Draw 5 mL of blood for a baseline value. Collect the sample in a 5-mL

heparinized tube. Label this sample "preinjection" and send it to the laboratory.
- Inject 250 mcg (0.25 mg) of cosyntropin IV or IM. (IV administration provides more accurate results because ineffective absorption after IM administration may cause wide variations in response.) Direct IV injection should take about 2 minutes.
- Draw another 5 mL of blood at 30 and 60 minutes after the cosyntropin injection. Collect the samples in 5-mL heparinized tubes. Label the samples "30 minutes postinjection" and "60 minutes postinjection" and send them to the laboratory. Include the collection times on the laboratory request.

After the Test
- Apply direct pressure to the venipuncture site until bleeding stops.
- Observe the patient for signs of a rare allergic reaction to cosyntropin, such as hives, itching, and tachycardia.
- Instruct the patient to resume a usual diet, activities, and medications that were discontinued before the test, as ordered.

C-Peptide

Reference Values
0.78 to 1.89 ng/mL (SI, 0.26–0.63 mmol/L) (fasting values)

Abnormal Findings
Elevated Levels
- Endogenous hyperinsulinism (insulinemia), oral hypoglycemic drug ingestion, pancreas or B-cell transplantation, renal failure, or type 2 diabetes

Decreased Levels
- Factitious hypoglycemia (surreptitious insulin administration), radical pancreatectomy, or type 1 diabetes

Nursing Implications
- Anticipate the need for further testing, including an insulin C-peptide

C

ratio, which differentiates insulinoma from factitious hypoglycemia. A ratio of 1.0 or less indicates increased endogenous insulin secretion; a ratio of 1.0 or more indicates exogenous insulin.
• Prepare the patient for follow-up.
• Provide emotional support to the patient and family.

Purpose
• To determine the cause of hypo-glycemia
• To indirectly measure insulin secretion in the presence of circulating insulin antibodies
• To detect residual tissue after total pancreatectomy for carcinoma
• To determine beta-cell function in the patient with diabetes

Description
Connecting peptide (C-peptide) is a biologically inactive chain formed during the proteolytic conversion of proinsulin to insulin in the pancreatic beta cells. It has no insulin effect either biologically or immunologically. Circulating insulin is measured by immunologic assay. As insulin is released into the bloodstream, the C-peptide chain splits off from the hormone.

Precautions
• Handle the samples gently to prevent hemolysis.

Nursing Considerations
Before the Test
• Confirm the patient's identity using two patient identifiers and confirmation of the patient's identification bracelet according to facility policy.
• Explain to the patient that the C-peptide test helps to evaluate pancreatic function and determine the cause of hypoglycemia.
• Instruct the patient to fast for 8 to 12 hours before the test, restricting all intake except for water.
• Tell the patient that the test requires a blood sample.

• Explain to the patient that slight discomfort from the tourniquet and the needle puncture may be experienced.
• If the patient is scheduled for radioisotope testing, it should take place after blood is drawn for C-peptide levels. Blood glucose levels usually are drawn at the same time as C-peptide levels.
• If the C-peptide stimulation test is done, IV glucagon is administered, as ordered, after a baseline blood sample is drawn.
• Withhold drugs that may interfere with test results, as ordered. If they must be continued, note this factor on the laboratory request.

During the Test
• Perform a venipuncture and collect a 1-mL sample in a chilled clot activator tube. The blood is separated and frozen to be tested later.
• Collect a sample for glucose level in a tube with sodium fluoride and potassium oxalate, if ordered.
• Pack the sample in ice and send it, along with the glucose sample, to the laboratory immediately.

After the Test
• Apply direct pressure to the venipuncture site until bleeding stops and to prevent hematoma formation.
• Instruct the patient to resume usual activities, diet, and medications that were discontinued before the test, as ordered.

C-Reactive Protein

Reference Values
None present; reported as less than 0.8 mg/dL (SI, less than 8 mg/L)
Highly specific (hs-CRP): 0.020 to 0.800 mg/dL (SI, 0.2–8 mg/L)

Abnormal Findings
Elevated Levels
• Rheumatoid arthritis (RA), rheumatic fever, MI, cancer (active, widespread), acute bacterial and

viral infections, inflammatory bowel disease, Hodgkin's disease, SLE
• Increased risk of cardiac events such as MI (elevations of hs-CRP)

Nursing Implications
• Be aware that elevated levels may be present postoperatively, but that levels decline after the fourth day.
• Anticipate the need for further testing.
• Prepare the patient for follow-up.
• Provide emotional support to the patient and family.
• Monitor the patient's cardiac status closely for changes; assess changes in mobility and functional level related to inflammatory conditions.

Purpose
• To evaluate the inflammatory disease course and severity in conditions, including tissue necrosis (MI, malignancy, RA)
• To monitor acute inflammatory phases of RA and rheumatic fever so that early treatment can be initiated
• To monitor the patient's response to treatment or determine whether the acute phase is declining
• To help interpret the erythrocyte sedimentation rate (ESR)
• To monitor the wound-healing process of internal incisions, burns, and organ transplantation

Description
C-reactive protein (CRP) is an abnormal protein that appears in the blood during an inflammatory process. It's absent from the blood of healthy people. This nonspecific protein is mainly synthesized in the liver and is found in many body fluids (pleural, peritoneal, pericardial, and synovial). It appears in the blood 18 to 24 hours after the onset of tissue damage, with levels that increase up to 1,000-fold and then decline rapidly when the inflammatory process regresses. CRP has been found to rise before increases in antibody titers and ESR levels occur. It also decreases sooner than ESR levels.

CRP is also a valuable cardiac marker to evaluate a patient with an MI. Levels correlate with creatine kinase MB (CK-MB) isoenzyme but typically peak 1 to 3 days after CK-MB. However, if CRP doesn't return to normal, it's highly suggestive of ongoing myocardial tissue damage. A more highly specific test for CRP, the hs-CRP, is capable of detecting even low CRP levels, which helps determine the risk of MI in patients with acute coronary syndromes.

Interfering Factors
• Steroids and salicylates (false-normal level)
• Hormonal contraceptives (false increase)
• Intrauterine contraceptive devices (increase) and pregnancy (third trimester)

Nursing Considerations

Before the Test
• Confirm the patient's identity using two patient identifiers and confirmation of the patient's identification bracelet according to facility policy.
• Explain to the patient that the CRP test is used to identify the presence of an inflammatory reaction or to monitor treatment.
• Instruct the patient to restrict all fluids except water for 8 to 12 hours before the test.
• Tell the patient that the test requires a blood sample.
• Explain to the patient that slight discomfort from the tourniquet and the needle puncture may be experienced.
• Notify the laboratory and the health care provider of medications patient is taking that may affect test results; these may need to be restricted.

During the Test
• Perform a venipuncture and collect the sample in a 5-mL clot activator tube.
• Send the specimen to the laboratory immediately; keep the sample away from heat.

After the Test

- Apply direct pressure to the venipuncture site until bleeding stops and to prevent hematoma formation.
- Instruct the patient to resume a usual diet and any medications that were discontinued before the test, as ordered.

Creatine Kinase

Reference Values

Total creatine kinase (CK) (females): 55 to 170 units/L (SI, 0.94–2.89 mkat/L)

Total CK (males): 30 to 135 units/L (SI, 0.51–2.3 mkat/L)

Total CK (infants ages 1 and younger): Levels two to four times higher than adult levels, possibly reflecting birth trauma and striated muscle development

Possibly significantly higher total values in muscular people

CK-BB (females and males): Undetectable

CK-MB (females and males): Less than 5% of total (SI, less than 0.05)

CK-MM (females and males): 96% to 100% of total (SI, 0.9–1.0)

Abnormal Findings

Elevated Levels

- Brain tissue injury, widespread malignant tumors, severe shock, or renal failure (detectable CK-BB isoenzyme)
- MI (CK-MB levels greater than 5% of the total CK level)
- Serious skeletal muscle injury that occurs in certain muscular dystrophies, polymyositis, and severe myoglobinuria (mild CK-MB increase)
- Skeletal muscle damage from trauma, such as surgery and IM injections, from rhabdomyolysis, and from diseases such as dermatomyositis and muscular dystrophy (increasing CK-MM values—50 to 100 times normal)
- Hypothyroidism (moderate increase in CK-MM)
- Severe hypokalemia, carbon monoxide poisoning, malignant hyperthermia, alcoholic cardiomyopathy, seizures, pulmonary or cerebral infarction (total CK levels increased)

Nursing Implications

- Anticipate the need for additional testing.
- Prepare the patient for follow-up and treatment.
- Institute emergency cardiac measures if the patient is experiencing MI.
- Monitor other cardiac enzyme levels as indicated. (See the *Release of Cardiac Enzymes and Proteins* box.)

Purpose

- To detect and assist in the diagnosis of an acute MI and reinfarction (CK-MB primarily used)

> ▶ *Quality and Safety Nursing Alert*
>
> Troponin levels increase within 1 hour of MI and may remain elevated for up to 14 days. Patients with unstable angina and high troponin levels but normal CK, CK-MB, and myoglobin levels are at increased risk for MI or other serious heart problems in the months following diagnosis.

- To evaluate possible causes of chest pain and to monitor the severity of myocardial ischemia after cardiac surgery, cardiac catheterization, and cardioversion (CK-MB primarily used)
- To detect early dermatomyositis and musculoskeletal disorders that aren't neurogenic in origin, such as Duchenne's muscular dystrophy (total CK primarily used)

Description

CK is an enzyme that catalyzes the creatine–creatinine metabolic pathway in muscle cells and brain tissue. Because of its intimate role in energy production, CK reflects normal tissue catabolism; increased serum levels indicate trauma to cells.

Fractionation and measurement of three distinct CK isoenzymes—CK-BB

Release of Cardiac Enzymes and Proteins

Because they're released by damaged tissue, serum proteins and isoenzymes (catalytic proteins that vary in concentration in specific organs) can help identify the compromised organ and assess the extent of damage. After an acute myocardial infarction, cardiac enzymes and proteins rise and fall in a characteristic pattern, as shown in the graph below.

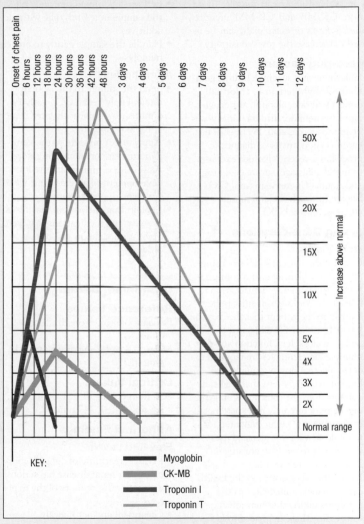

KEY:
- Myoglobin
- CK-MB
- Troponin I
- Troponin T

(CK1), CK-MB (CK2), and CK-MM (CK3)—have replaced the use of total CK levels to accurately localize the site of increased tissue destruction. CK-BB is found most commonly in brain tissue. CK-MM and CK-MB are found primarily in skeletal and heart muscle. In addition, CK-MB and CK-MM subunits, called *isoforms* or *isoenzymes,* can be assayed to increase the test's sensitivity.

Interfering Factors

- Halothane and succinylcholine, gemfibrozil, amphotericin B, chlorthalidone, clofibrate, alcohol, anticoagulants, furosemide, lithium, large doses of aminocaproic acid, IM injections, cardioversion, invasive diagnostic procedures, recent vigorous exercise or muscle massage, severe coughing, and trauma (increase in total CK)
- Surgery through skeletal muscle (increase in total CK)

Nursing Considerations

Before the Test

- Confirm the patient's identity using two patient identifiers and confirmation of the patient's identification bracelet according to facility policy.
- Explain to the patient that the creatine kinase test is used to assess myocardial and musculoskeletal function and that multiple blood samples are required to detect fluctuations in serum levels.
- Explain to the patient that slight discomfort from the tourniquet and the needle puncture may be experienced.
- If the patient is being evaluated for musculoskeletal disorders, advise the patient to avoid exercising for 24 hours before the test.
- Notify the laboratory and the health care provider of medications the patient is taking that may affect test results; these may need to be restricted.
- Draw the sample before giving IM injections or 1 hour after giving them because muscle trauma increases the total CK level.

During the Test

- Obtain the sample on schedule. Note on the laboratory request the time the sample was drawn and the hours elapsed since the onset of chest pain.
- Perform a venipuncture and collect the sample in a 4-mL tube without additives.
- Handle the sample gently to prevent hemolysis.

After the Test

- Send the sample to the laboratory immediately because CK activity diminishes significantly after 2 hours at room temperature.
- Apply direct pressure to the venipuncture site until bleeding stops.
- Assess the venipuncture site for development of a hematoma; if one develops, apply pressure.
- Explain that the patient may resume exercise and medications that were discontinued before the test, as ordered.

Creatinine, Serum

Reference Values

Females: 0.6 to 0.9 mg/dL (SI, 53–97 mmol/L)
Males: 0.8 to 1.2 mg/dL (SI, 62–115 mmol/L)

Critical Values

Less than 0.4 mg/dL (SI, 35 mmol/L) or 2.8 mg/dL (SI, 247 mmol/L)

Abnormal Findings

Elevated Levels

- Plasma creatinine of 2 mg/dL indicates that renal disease has seriously damaged 50% or more of the nephrons
- Gigantism and acromegaly

Decreased Levels

- Liver disease
- Deficient levels of protein in the diet
- Small build
- Loss of muscle mass

Nursing Implications
- Anticipate the need for additional testing.
- Prepare the patient for follow-up and treatment.
- Monitor fluid balance and intake and output.

Purpose
- To assess glomerular filtration
- To screen for renal damage

Description
Serum creatinine levels provide a more sensitive measure of renal damage than do blood urea nitrogen (BUN) levels. Creatinine is a nonprotein end product of creatine metabolism that appears in serum in amounts proportional to the body's muscle mass.

Interfering Factors
- Ascorbic acid, barbiturates, and diuretics (possible increase)
- Exceptionally large muscle mass, such as is found in athletes (possible increase despite normal renal function)
- Phenolsulfonphthalein given within the previous 24 hours (possible increase, if the test is based on Jaffe's reaction)

Nursing Considerations
Before the Test
- Confirm the patient's identity using two patient identifiers and confirmation of the patient's identification bracelet according to facility policy.
- Explain to the patient that the serum creatinine test is used to evaluate kidney function.
- Tell the patient that the test requires a blood sample.
- Explain to the patient that slight discomfort from the tourniquet and the needle puncture may be experienced.
- Instruct the patient that there are no food or fluid restrictions for this test.
- Notify the laboratory and the health care provider of medications the patient is taking that may affect

test results; these may need to be restricted.

During the Test
- Perform a venipuncture and collect the sample in a 3- or 4-mL clot activator tube.
- Handle the sample gently to prevent hemolysis.

After the Test
- Send the sample to the laboratory immediately.
- Apply direct pressure to the venipuncture site until bleeding stops and to prevent hematoma formation.
- Instruct the patient to resume any usual medications that were discontinued before the test, as ordered.

Creatinine, Urine

Reference Values
Females: 11 to 20 mg/kg body weight/ 24 hours (SI, 97–177 mmol/kg body weight/day)
Males: 14 to 26 mg/kg body weight/ 24 hours (SI, 124–230 mmol/kg body weight/day)

Abnormal Findings
Decreased Levels
- Impaired renal perfusion or renal disease resulting from urinary tract obstruction
- Chronic bilateral pyelonephritis, acute or chronic glomerulonephritis, and polycystic kidney disease

Nursing Implications
- Anticipate the need for additional testing.
- Prepare the patient for follow-up and treatment.
- Monitor fluid balance and intake and output.

Purpose
- To help assess glomerular filtration
- To check the accuracy of 24-hour urine collection, based on the relatively constant levels of creatinine excretion

Description

This test measures urine creatinine levels, the chief metabolite of creatine. Produced in amounts proportional to total body muscle mass, creatinine is removed from the plasma primarily by glomerular filtration and is excreted in the urine. Because the body doesn't recycle it, creatinine has a relatively high, constant clearance rate, making it an efficient indicator of renal function. However, the creatinine clearance test, which measures urine and plasma creatinine clearance, is a more precise index than this test. A standard method for determining urine creatinine levels is based on Jaffe's reaction, in which creatinine treated with an alkaline picrate solution yields a bright-orange–red complex.

Interfering Factors

- Amphotericin B, corticosteroids, diuretics, gentamicin, and tetracyclines (possible decrease)

Nursing Considerations

Before the Test

- Confirm the patient's identity using two patient identifiers and confirmation of the patient's identification bracelet according to facility policy.
- Explain to the patient that the urine creatinine test helps evaluate kidney function.
- The patient doesn't need to restrict fluids, but instruct the patient not to eat an excessive amount of meat (protein) before the test.
- Advise the patient to avoid strenuous physical exercise during the collection period.
- Tell the patient that the test usually requires urine collection over a 24-hour period and teach the proper collection technique.
- Notify the laboratory and the health care provider of medications the patient is taking that may affect test results; these may need to be restricted.

During the Test

- Collect the patient's urine over a 24-hour period, discarding the first specimen. Start the timing of the collection at that point, also retaining the last specimen. When possible, use a specimen bottle that contains a preservative to prevent creatinine degradation.
- Refrigerate the specimen or keep it on ice during the collection period.

After the Test

- Send the specimen to the laboratory immediately after the collection is completed.
- Instruct the patient to resume usual activities, diet, and medications, as ordered.

Creatinine Clearance (CrCl)

Reference Values

Adults (<40 years)

Females: 72 to 110 mL/sec/1.73 m^2 (SI, 0.69–1.06 mL/sec/m^2)

Males: 94 to 140 mL/sec/1.73 m^2 (SI, 0.91–1.35 mL/sec/m^2)

Abnormal Findings

Elevated Levels

- Poor hydration
- Exercise
- Pregnancy
- Burns
- Carbon monoxide poisoning
- Hypothyroidism

Decreased Levels

- Reduced renal blood flow (associated with shock or renal artery obstruction), acute tubular necrosis, acute or chronic glomerulonephritis, advanced bilateral chronic pyelonephritis, advanced bilateral renal lesions (which may occur in polycystic kidney disease, renal tuberculosis, and cancer), and nephrosclerosis
- Heart failure
- Severe dehydration

Nursing Implications

- Anticipate the need for additional testing.

- Prepare the patient for follow-up and treatment.
- Monitor intake and output.
- Assess hydration level and encourage fluids as appropriate in patients with elevated levels.
- Assess fluid balance status in patients with decreased levels.

Purpose
- To assess renal function (primarily glomerular filtration rate [GFR])
- To monitor progression of renal insufficiency

Description
A creatine anhydride, creatinine is formed and excreted in constant amounts by an irreversible reaction and functions solely as the main end product of creatine. Creatinine production is proportional to total muscle mass and is relatively unaffected by urine volume or normal physical activity or diet.

An excellent diagnostic indicator of renal function, the creatinine clearance test determines how efficiently the kidneys are clearing creatinine from the blood. The clearance rate is expressed in terms of the volume of blood (in milliliters) that can be cleared of creatinine in 1 minute. Reference values vary with age, but creatinine levels become abnormal when more than 50% of the nephrons have been damaged.

Interfering Factors
- Amphotericin B, aminoglycosides, furosemide, and thiazide diuretics (possible decrease)
- High-protein diet or strenuous exercise (increase)

Nursing Considerations
Before the Test
- Confirm the patient's identity using two patient identifiers and confirmation of the patient's identification bracelet according to facility policy.
- Explain to the patient that the creatinine clearance test assesses kidney function.

- Explain that the patient may need to avoid meat, poultry, fish, tea, or coffee for 6 hours before the test.
- Advise the patient to avoid strenuous physical exercise during the collection period.
- Tell the patient that the test requires a timed or 24-hour urine specimen and at least one blood sample. Tell the patient how the urine specimen will be collected and that some discomfort from the needle puncture may be experienced.
- Notify the laboratory and the health care provider of medications the patient is taking that may affect test results; these may need to be restricted.

During the Test
- Collect a timed urine specimen at 2, 6, 12, or 24 hours in a bottle containing a preservative to prevent creatinine degradation.
- Perform a venipuncture any time during the collection period and collect the sample in a 7-mL tube without additives.
- Refrigerate the urine specimen or keep it on ice during the collection period.

After the Test
- Send the specimen to the laboratory as soon as the collection is completed.
- Apply direct pressure to the venipuncture site until bleeding stops and to prevent hematoma formation.
- Instruct the patient to resume usual activities, diet, and medications, as ordered.

Crossmatching

Normal Findings
- Absence of agglutination (indicating compatibility between the donor's and the recipient's blood)

Abnormal Findings
- Agglutination when the donor's RBCs and the recipient's serum are

C

correctly mixed and incubated (positive crossmatch, indicating incompatibility between the donor's blood and the recipient's blood)

Nursing Implications

• Withhold the donor's blood and continue the crossmatch to determine the cause of the incompatibility and identify the antibody.

Purpose

• To serve as the final check for compatibility between a donor's and a recipient's blood

Description

Crossmatching, also known as *compatibility testing*, establishes compatibility or incompatibility of a donor's and a recipient's blood. It's the best antibody detection test available for avoiding lethal transfusion reactions. After the donor's and the recipient's ABO and Rh factor type are determined, major crossmatching determines compatibility between the donor's RBCs and the recipient's serum. Minor crossmatching determines compatibility between the donor's serum and the recipient's RBCs. (Because all blood donors routinely receive the antibody screening test, minor crossmatching commonly is omitted.) A complete crossmatch may take from 45 minutes to 2 hours, so an incomplete (10-minute) crossmatch may be performed in an emergency, such as severe blood loss due to trauma. In an emergency, transfusion can begin with limited amounts of group O packed RBCs while crossmatching is completed. Incomplete typing and crossmatching increases the risk of complications. After crossmatching, compatible units are labeled and a compatibility record is completed.

> ▶ *Quality and Safety Nursing Alert*
>
> Agglutination (positive crossmatch) indicates an undesirable antigen–antibody reaction. However, the absence of agglutination doesn't guarantee a safe transfusion.

Interfering Factors

• Recent administration of dextran or IV contrast media (causing cellular aggregation resembling antibody-mediated agglutination)
• Previous blood transfusion (possibility of new antibodies to donor blood)
• Hemolysis from rough handling of the sample
• Testing delay of more than 72 hours after sample collection

Precautions

• If more than 72 hours has elapsed since an earlier transfusion, previously crossmatched donor blood must be crossmatched again with a new recipient serum sample to detect newly acquired incompatibilities.
• Handle the sample gently to prevent hemolysis, which can mask hemolysis of the donor's RBCs.

Nursing Considerations

Before the Test

• Confirm the patient's identity using two patient identifiers and confirmation of the patient's identification bracelet according to facility policy.
• In some states, blood transfusions require informed consent.
• Explain to the patient that this test ensures that the blood received matches the patient's own blood, to prevent a transfusion reaction.
• Inform the patient that there are no food or fluid restrictions for this test.
• Tell the patient that the test requires a blood sample.
• Explain to the patient that slight discomfort from the tourniquet and the needle puncture may be experienced.
• Check the patient's history for recent administration of blood, dextran, or IV contrast media.
• If the surgery is rescheduled and the patient has received blood during the past 3 months, the patient's blood will need to be crossmatched again to detect recently acquired incompatibilities.

During the Test

- Perform a venipuncture and collect the sample in a 10-mL tube without additives or EDTA. ABO typing, Rh typing, and crossmatching all occur together.
- Label the sample with the patient's name, the hospital or blood bank number, the date, and your initials.

After the Test

- Indicate on the laboratory request the amount and type of blood component needed.
- Send the sample to the laboratory immediately.
- Apply direct pressure to the venipuncture site until bleeding stops and to prevent hematoma formation.

Cryoglobulins

Reference Values

Negative

Abnormal Findings

- Positive, indicating cryoglobulinemia (reported as a percentage based on the amount of sample cryoprecipitation)

Nursing Implications

- Anticipate the need for additional testing.
- Positive results don't always indicate the presence of disease. (See the *Diseases Associated with Cryoglobulinemia* table.)

Purpose

- To detect cryoglobulinemia in the patient with Raynaud-like vascular symptoms

Diseases Associated with Cryoglobulinemia

Type of Cryoglobulin	Serum Level	
Type I		
Monoclonal cryoglobulin	>5 mg/mL	• Myeloma • Waldenström's macroglobulinemia • Chronic lymphocytic leukemia
Type II		
Mixed cryoglobulin	<1 mg/mL	• Rheumatoid arthritis • Sjögren's syndrome • Mixed essential cryoglobulinemia • Human immunodeficiency virus-1 infection
Type III		
Mixed polyclonal cryoglobulin	>1 mg/mL (50% below 80 mcg/mL)	• Systemic lupus erythematosus • Rheumatoid arthritis • Sjögren's syndrome • Infectious mononucleosis • Cytomegalovirus infection • Acute viral hepatitis • Chronic active hepatitis • Primary biliary cirrhosis • Poststreptococcal glomerulonephritis • Infective endocarditis • Leprosy • Kala-azar • Tropical splenomegaly syndrome

Description

Cryoglobulins are abnormal serum proteins that precipitate at low laboratory temperatures (39.2°F [4°C]) and redissolve after being warmed. Their presence in the blood (cryoglobulinemia) is usually associated with immunologic disease, but can also occur without known immunopathology.

If patients with cryoglobulinemia are subjected to cold, they may experience Raynaud-like symptoms (pain, cyanosis, and cold fingers and toes), which generally result from cryoglobulin precipitation in cooler parts of the body. In some patients, for example, cryoglobulins may precipitate at temperatures as high as 86°F (30°C); such temperatures are possible in some peripheral blood vessels.

The cryoglobulin test involves refrigerating a serum sample at 33.8°F (1°C) for 24 hours and observing for formation of a heat-reversible precipitate. Such a precipitate requires further study by immunoelectrophoresis or double diffusion to identify cryoglobulin components.

Interfering Factors

- Nonadherence to dietary restrictions prior to testing
- Failure to keep the sample at 98.6°F (37°C) before centrifugation (possible loss of cryoglobulins)
- Reading the sample before the 72-hour precipitation period ends (possible incorrect analysis of results because some cryoglobulins take several days to precipitate)

Nursing Considerations

Before the Test

- Confirm the patient's identity using two patient identifiers and confirmation of the patient's identification bracelet according to facility policy.
- Explain to the patient that the cryoglobulins test detects antibodies in blood that may cause sensitivity to low temperatures.
- Instruct the patient that a fast for 4 to 8 hours before the test may be required.
- Tell the patient that the test requires a blood sample.
- Explain to the patient that slight discomfort from the tourniquet and the needle puncture may be experienced.
- Warm the syringe and collection tube to 98.6°F before the venipuncture and keep the tube at that temperature to prevent cryoglobulin loss.

During the Test

- Perform a venipuncture and collect the sample in a prewarmed 10-mL tube without additives.

After the Test

- Send the sample to the laboratory immediately.
- Apply direct pressure to the venipuncture site until bleeding stops and to prevent hematoma formation.
- Instruct the patient to resume a usual diet.
- Tell the patient to avoid cold temperatures or contact with cold objects if the test is positive for cryoglobulins, as ordered.
- Observe for signs of intravascular coagulation, such as decreased color and temperature in distal extremities and increased pain.

Cyclic Adenosine Monophosphate

Reference Values

0.3 to 3.6 mg/day (SI, 100–723 nmol/day) or 0.29 to 2.1 mg/g creatinine (SI, 100–723 nmol/day creatinine)

Abnormal Findings

- Failure to respond to parathyroid hormone (PTH), as evidenced by normal urinary cyclic adenosine monophosphate [cAMP] excretion, indicating type 1 pseudohypoparathyroidism

Nursing Implications

- Anticipate the need for additional testing.
- Prepare the patient for follow-up and treatment.
- Monitor for signs and symptoms of hypoparathyroidism.

Purpose

- To aid in the differential diagnosis of hypoparathyroidism and pseudohypoparathyroidism

Description

The cAMP nucleotide influences the protein synthesis rate within cells. Measuring the urinary excretion of cAMP after infusing a dose of standard PTH IV can show renal tubular resistance in a patient with hypoparathyroid symptoms and high levels of PTH. Such findings suggest type 1 pseudohypoparathyroidism, a rare inherited disorder. Urinary cAMP levels respond normally in type 2 pseudohypoparathyroidism because the defect is beyond the level of cAMP generation.

Interfering Factors

- Contamination or improper storage of the specimen
- Failure to acidify the urine with hydrochloric acid

Precautions

- This test is contraindicated in patients with a positive PTH test result and in patients with high calcium levels.
- Use this test cautiously in patients receiving a cardiac glycoside and in those with sarcoidosis or renal or cardiac disease.

Nursing Considerations

Before the Test

- Confirm the patient's identity using two patient identifiers and confirmation of the patient's identification bracelet according to facility policy.
- Explain to the patient that this test evaluates parathyroid function.
- Tell the patient that the test requires a 15-minute IV infusion of PTH and a 3- to 4-hour urine specimen collection.
- Perform a skin test to detect an allergy to PTH; keep epinephrine or a histamine-1 receptor antagonist, such as diphenhydramine or glucocorticoids (methylprednisolone), readily available in case of an adverse reaction.
- Just before performing the procedure, instruct the patient not to touch the IV line or exert pressure on the arm receiving the infusion.
- Tell the patient that discomfort from the needle puncture may be experienced and to tell you if there is a severe burning sensation or if the site becomes inflamed or swollen.
- Tell the patient to avoid contaminating the urine specimen with toilet tissue or stool.

During the Test

- Instruct the patient to empty the bladder.
- If the patient has an indwelling urinary catheter in place, replace the collection apparatus with an unused one. Send this specimen to the laboratory, if ordered; otherwise, discard the specimen.
- Prepare the PTH for infusion, as directed, using sterile water for dilution.
- Start the infusion with dextrose 5% in water and infuse the PTH over 15 minutes. Record the start of the infusion as time zero.
- Collect a urine specimen 3 to 4 hours after the infusion.
- Stop the IV infusion.
- Keep the collection bag on ice if the patient has a catheter in place.

After the Test

- Send the specimen to the laboratory immediately after the collection is completed; if transport is delayed, refrigerate the specimen.
- Observe the patient for symptoms of hypercalcemia, including lethargy, anorexia, nausea, vomiting, vertigo, and abdominal cramps and report them to the health care provider.

Cystometry (Cystometrogram [CMG])

Normal Findings

- See the *Normal and Abnormal Cystometry Findings* table.

Normal and Abnormal Cystometry Findings

Because cystometry assesses micturition and vesical function, it can aid diagnosis of neurogenic bladder dysfunction. The five main types of neurogenic bladder, as presented in this chart, result from lesions of the central or peripheral nervous system. *Uninhibited neurogenic bladder* results from a lesion to the upper motor neuron and causes frequent, usually uncontrollable micturition in the presence of even a small amount of urine. A complete upper motor neuron lesion characterizes *reflex neurogenic bladder* and causes total loss of conscious sensation and vesical control.

Feature or Response	Normal Bladder Function	Uninhibited Neurogenic Bladder (Mildly Spastic, Incomplete Upper Motor Neuron Lesion)
Micturition		
Start	+	+/0
Stop	+	0
Residual urine	0	0
Vesical sensation	+	+
First urge to void	150 to 200 mL	E (<150 mL)
Bladder capacity	400 to 500 mL	↓
Bladder contractions	0	+
Intravesical pressure	L	↑
Bulbocavernosus reflex	+	+
Saddle sensation	+	+
Bethanechol test (exaggerated response)	0	+
Ice water test	+	+
Anal reflex	+	+
Heat sensation and pain	+	+

KEY:

+ = Present/positive	V = Variable	↑ = Increased
0 = Absent/negative	L = Low 4	↓ = Decreased
D = Delayed	E = Early	

Abnormal Findings

- See the *Normal and Abnormal Cystometry Findings* table.

Nursing Implications

- Anticipate the need for additional testing.
- Prepare the patient for follow-up and treatment.
- Assess urinary function; monitor intake and output.
- Assess neurologic status, including motor and sensory function.
- Obtain informed consent according to facility policy.

Purpose

- To evaluate detrusor muscle function and tonicity
- To help determine the cause of bladder dysfunction

Description

Cystometry assesses the bladder's neuromuscular function by measuring the efficiency of the detrusor muscle reflex, intravesical pressure and capacity, and the bladder's reaction to thermal stimulation. Because cystometry results can be ambiguous, they're typically supported by other test results, such as

In *autonomous neurogenic bladder*, a lower motor neuron lesion produces a flaccid bladder that fills without contracting. The patient can't perceive bladder fullness or initiate and maintain urination without applying external pressure. Lower motor neuron lesions can cause sensory or motor paralysis of the bladder. In sensory *paralysis*, the patient can't perceive bladder fullness and therefore experiences chronic urine retention. In *motor paralysis*, the patient has full sensation but can't initiate or control urination.

Reflex Neurogenic Bladder (Completely Spastic, Complete Upper Motor Neuron Lesion)	Autonomous Neurogenic Bladder (Flaccid, Incomplete Lower Motor Neuron Lesion)	Sensory Paralytic Bladder (Lower Motor Neuron Lesion)	Motor Paralytic Bladder (Lower Motor Neuron Lesion)
0	0	+	0
0	0	+	0
0	0	+	0
0	0	0	++
+	+	D	+
0	0	↑/(<1L)	V
0	0	0	0
↓	↑	↓	L
+	0	+/↓/0	+
↑	↓	V	+
↑	0	+	0
0		0	0
0		V	V
+		0	+

cystourethrography, excretory urography, and voiding cystourethrography.

The procedure for cystometry is as follows:

- The patient is placed in a supine position on the examination table.
- A catheter is passed into the bladder to measure the residual urine level. Any catheter insertion difficulty may reflect meatal or urethral obstruction.
- To test the patient's response to thermal sensation, 30 mL of room-temperature physiologic saline solution or sterile water is instilled into the bladder. Then an equal volume of warm (110°F to 115°F [43.3°C to 6.1°C]) fluid is instilled into the bladder. The patient is asked to report sensations, such as the need to void, nausea, flushing, discomfort, or a feeling of warmth.
- After the fluid is drained from the patient's bladder, the catheter is connected to the cystometer and normal saline solution, sterile water, or gas (usually carbon dioxide) is slowly introduced into the bladder. The gas flow is adjusted automatically to the

C

desired reading (100 mL/minute) by a four-channel cystometer.

- The patient is asked to indicate when he or she first feels an urge to void, and then the need to urinate. The related pressure and volume are plotted automatically on the graph.

- When the bladder reaches its full capacity, the patient is asked to urinate so that the maximal intravesical voiding pressure can be recorded. The patient's bladder is then drained and, if no additional tests are required, the catheter is removed; otherwise, the catheter is left in place to measure the urethral pressure profile or to provide supplemental findings.

- If abnormal bladder function is caused by muscle incompetence or disrupted innervation, an anticholinergic medication (atropine) or cholinergic medication (bethanechol) may be injected and the study repeated in 20 to 30 minutes.

Interfering Factors
- Inability to urinate in the supine position
- Concurrent use of drugs such as antihistamines (possible interference with bladder function)
- Cystometry performed within 6 to 8 weeks after surgery for spinal cord injury (inconclusive results)

Precautions
- Cystometry is contraindicated in the patient with an acute urinary tract infection because uninhibited contractions may cause erroneous readings, and the test may lead to pyelonephritis and septic shock.

Nursing Considerations
Before the Test
- Explain to the patient that cystometry evaluates bladder function.
- Tell the patient that there are no food or fluid restrictions.
- Describe the procedure, including who will perform it, when and where

it will take place, and how long it will last.

- Explain that the patient will feel a strong urge to void during the test and may feel embarrassed or uncomfortable. Provide reassurance.
- Advise the patient not to strain at voiding; it can cause ambiguous cystometric readings.
- Make sure that the patient or a responsible family member has signed an informed consent form.
- Check the patient's medication history for drugs, such as antihistamines, that may affect test results.
- Tell the patient to urinate just before the procedure.
- If the patient has a spinal cord injury that has caused motor impairment, transport on a stretcher so that the test can be performed without transferring to the examination table.

After the Test
- Encourage the patient to drink lots of fluids, unless contraindicated, to relieve burning on urination, a common adverse effect of the procedure.
- Administer short-term antibiotics, as ordered, to prevent infection.
- Administer a sitz bath or warm tub bath if the patient experiences discomfort after the test.
- Measure fluid intake and urine output for 24 hours. Watch for hematuria that persists after the third voiding and for signs of sepsis (such as fever or chills).

Cystourethroscopy (Cystography)
Normal Findings
- Normal size, shape, and position of urethra, bladder, and ureteral orifice
- Smooth and shiny lower urinary tract mucosal lining with no evidence of erythema, cysts, or other abnormalities
- Bladder free of obstructions, tumors, and calculi

Abnormal Findings
- Enlarged prostate gland in older men
- Urethral stricture, calculi, tumors, diverticula, ulcers, and polyps
- Bladder wall trabeculation and various congenital anomalies, such as ureteroceles, duplicate ureteral orifices, or urethral valves in children

Nursing Implications
- Anticipate the need for additional testing.
- Prepare the patient for follow-up and treatment.
- Assess urinary function; monitor intake and output.
- Obtain informed consent according to facility policy.

Purpose
- To diagnose and evaluate urinary tract disorders by direct visualization of urinary structures

Description
Cystourethroscopy, a test that combines two endoscopic techniques, allows visual examination of the bladder and urethra. One of the instruments used in this test is the cystoscope, which has a fiberoptic light source, a magnification system, a right-angled telescopic lens, and an angled beak for smooth passage into the bladder. The other instrument, the urethroscope (or panendoscope), is similar but has a straight-ahead lens and is used to examine the bladder neck and urethra. The cystoscope and urethroscope lenses use a common sheath inserted into the urethra to obtain the desired view.

Other invasive procedures, such as biopsy, lesion resection, calculi removal, constricted urethra dilatation, and ureteral orifice catheterization for retrograde pyelography, may also be performed through this sheath.

Kidney–ureter–bladder radiography and excretory urography usually precede this test. The procedure for cystourethroscopy is as follows:

- After a general or regional anesthetic (as required) is administered, the patient is placed in the lithotomy position on a cystoscopic table. The genitalia are cleaned with an antiseptic solution, and the patient is draped. (Local anesthetic is instilled at this point.)
- The instrument is moved toward the bladder to visually examine the urethra. A urethroscope is inserted into the well-lubricated sheath (instead of an obturator), and both are passed gently through the urethra into the bladder. The urethroscope is then removed, and a cystoscope is inserted through the sheath into the bladder.
- After the bladder is filled with irrigating solution, the scope is rotated to inspect the entire surface of the bladder wall and ureteral orifices with the right-angled telescopic lens.
- The cystoscope is removed, the urethroscope is reinserted, and the urethroscope and sheath are slowly withdrawn, permitting examination of the bladder neck and the various portions of the urethra, including the internal and external sphincters. (See the *Using a Cystourethroscope* box.)
- During cystourethroscopy, a urine specimen is taken routinely from the bladder for culture and sensitivity testing, and residual urine is measured.
- If a tumor is suspected, a urine specimen is sent to the laboratory for cytologic examination; if a tumor is found, biopsy may be performed. If a urethral stricture is present, urethral dilatation may be necessary before cystourethroscopy.
- Patients receiving only a local anesthetic may complain of a burning sensation when the instrument is passed through the urethra. The patient may also feel an urgent need to urinate as the bladder fills with irrigating solution. Assure the patient that these sensations are common and generally transient.

C

Using a Cystourethroscope

This cross-sectional illustration shows how a urologic examination is performed with a cystourethroscope, a device that allows direct visualization of the tissues of the lower urinary tract. The sheath of the cystourethroscope permits passage of a cystoscope and urethroscope for illuminating the urethra, bladder, and ureters. This instrument also provides a channel for minor surgical procedures, such as biopsy, excision of small lesions, and calculi removal.

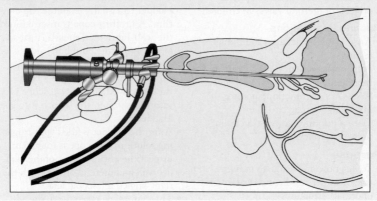

Precautions

- Cystourethroscopy is contraindicated in patients with acute forms of urethritis, prostatitis, or cystitis because instrumentation can lead to sepsis.
- Cystourethroscopy is contraindicated in patients with bleeding disorders because instrumentation can lead to increased bleeding.

Nursing Considerations

Before the Test

- Explain to the patient that cystourethroscopy permits examination of the bladder and urethra.
- Unless a general anesthetic has been ordered, inform the patient that there are no food or fluid restrictions. If a general anesthetic will be administered, instruct the patient to fast for 8 hours before the test.
- Tell the patient who will perform the test, when and where it will take place, and that it takes about 20 to 30 minutes.
- Inform the patient that some discomfort after the procedure, including a

slight burning during urination, may be experienced.

- Make sure that the patient or a responsible family member has signed an informed consent form.
- Before the procedure, administer a sedative, if ordered, and instruct the patient to urinate.

After the Test

- Monitor the patient's vital signs for 15 minutes for the first hour after the test and then every hour until they stabilize.
- If local anesthesia was used, keep the patient supine for several minutes and then help the patient to sit or stand. Watch for orthostatic hypotension.
- Instruct the patient to drink plenty of fluids (or increase IV fluids, if ordered) and to take the prescribed analgesic. Assure that burning and frequency will soon subside.
- Administer antibiotics, as ordered, to prevent bacterial sepsis due to urethral tissue trauma. Inform the patient about signs and symptoms

of urinary sepsis, and instruct the patient to report them immediately.

- Report flank or abdominal pain, chills, fever, an elevated WBC count, or low urine output to the health care provider immediately.
- Record the patient's intake and output for 24 hours and observe for distention. If the patient doesn't void within 8 hours after the test or if bright red blood continues to appear after three voidings, notify the health care provider.
- Instruct the patient to abstain from alcohol for 48 hours.
- Apply heat to the lower abdomen to relieve pain and muscle spasm, if ordered. A warm sitz bath may be ordered.

Cytomegalovirus Antibody Screen

Reference Values
No detectable virus antibodies; immunoglobulin (Ig) G and IgM negative

Abnormal Findings
- Positive for antibodies, indicating cytomegalovirus (CMV) infection

Nursing Implications
- Anticipate the need for additional testing, if indicated.
- Serum samples collected early during the acute phase or late in the convalescent stage may not contain detectable IgG or IgM antibodies to CMV. Therefore, a negative result doesn't preclude recent infection. Multiple samples are needed to ensure accurate results.
- If the patient is immunosuppressed and lacks CMV antibodies, administer blood products from a donor who's a seronegative, and advise patient about organ transplants from such a donor if applicable. The patient with CMV antibodies doesn't require seronegative blood products.
- Institute infection control precautions as indicated.

Purpose
- To detect CMV infection in donors and recipients of organs and blood and in immunocompromised patients
- To screen for CMV infection in infants who require blood transfusions or tissue transplants

Description
After primary infection, CMV remains latent in WBCs. The presence of CMV antibodies indicates past infection with this virus. In an immunocompromised patient, CMV can be reactivated to cause active infection. Blood or tissue administration from a seropositive donor may cause active CMV infection in a CMV-seronegative organ transplant recipient or in a neonate, especially one born prematurely.

CMV antibodies can be detected by several methods, including passive hemagglutination, latex agglutination, enzyme immunoassay, and indirect immunofluorescence. The complement fixation test is only 60% sensitive compared with other assays and shouldn't be used to screen for CMV antibodies. Screening tests for CMV antibodies are qualitative; they detect the presence of antibody at a single low dilution. In quantitative methods, several dilutions of the serum sample are tested to indicate acute CMV infection. Laboratory tests for CMV antibody should be performed by using paired serum samples. One blood sample should be taken upon suspicion of CMV and another one taken within 2 weeks. A virus culture can be performed at any time the patient is symptomatic.

Precautions
- Handle the sample gently to prevent hemolysis.

Nursing Considerations
Before the Test
- Confirm the patient's identity using two patient identifiers and confirmation of the patient's identification bracelet according to facility policy.

C

• Tell the patient that the CMV antibody screen requires a blood sample.
• Explain to the patient that slight discomfort from the tourniquet and the
needle puncture may be experienced.

During the Test
• Perform a venipuncture and collect
the sample in a 5-mL tube designated
by the laboratory.

• Allow the blood to clot for at least
1 hour at room temperature.

After the Test
• Transfer the serum to a sterile tube or
vial and send it to the laboratory.
• If transfer must be delayed, store the
serum at 39.2°F (4°C) for 1 to
2 days or at –4°F (–15.5°C) for longer
periods to avoid contamination.
• Apply direct pressure to the venipuncture site until bleeding stops and
to prevent hematoma formation.
• Because the patient may have a
compromised immune system, keep
the venipuncture site clean and dry.

D

D-Dimer

Reference Values
Negative (no D-dimer fragments present) or less than 250 mcg/L (SI, less than 1.37 nmol/L)

Abnormal Findings
Elevated Levels
- Disseminated intravascular coagulation (DIC), pulmonary embolism, arterial or venous thrombosis, neoplastic disease, surgery occurring up to 2 days before testing, subarachnoid hemorrhage (spinal fluid only), or secondary fibrinolysis
- Pregnancy (late and postpartum)
- Sickle cell anemia

Nursing Implications
- Prepare the patient for further testing.
- Institute safety and bleeding precautions as indicated.
- Apply additional pressure at venipuncture sites to control bleeding.

Purpose
- To diagnose DIC
- To differentiate subarachnoid hemorrhage from a traumatic lumbar puncture in spinal fluid analysis

Description
A D-dimer is an asymmetrical carbon compound fragment formed after thrombin converts fibrinogen to fibrin, factor XIIIa stabilizes it into a clot, and plasma acts on the cross-linked, or clotted, fibrin. The D-dimer test is specific for fibrinolysis because it confirms the presence of fibrin split products.

Interfering Factors
- High rheumatoid factor titers or increased CA-125 levels (possible false positive)
- Spinal fluid analysis in an infant younger than 6 months (possible false negative)

Nursing Considerations
Before the Test
- Confirm the patient's identity using two patient identifiers and confirmation of the patient's identification bracelet according to facility policy.
- Obtain the patient's history of medications being taken, hematologic diseases, recent surgery, and the results of other tests performed.
- Explain to the patient that the D-dimer test is used to determine whether the blood is clotting normally.
- Advise the patient that the test requires a blood sample. Explain that slight discomfort from the tourniquet and the needle puncture may be experienced.
- No fasting required.

During the Test
- Perform a venipuncture and collect the sample in a 4.5-mL tube with sodium citrate added. (For a spinal fluid analysis, the sample is collected during a lumbar puncture and placed in a plastic vial.)
- Completely fill the collection tube, invert it gently several times, and send it to the laboratory immediately.

After the Test
- Apply pressure to the venipuncture site for 5 minutes or until bleeding stops and to prevent hematoma formation.

D

Delayed Hypersensitivity Skin Tests

Normal Findings
- In the recall antigen test, a positive response (5 mm or more of induration at the test site) appearing 48 hours after injection

Abnormal Findings
- Diminished delayed hypersensitivity, as evidenced in the recall antigen test: a positive response to fewer than two of the test antigens, a persistent unresponsiveness to intradermal injection of higher strength antigens, or a generalized diminished reaction (causing less than 10 mm combined induration)
- Diminished delayed hypersensitivity possibly resulting from Hodgkin's disease (common); sarcoidosis; liver disease; congenital immunodeficiency disease, such as ataxia–telangiectasia, DiGeorge's syndrome, and Wiskott-Aldrich's syndrome; uremia; acute leukemia; viral diseases, such as influenza, infectious mononucleosis, measles, mumps, and rubella; fungal diseases, such as coccidioidomycosis and cryptococcosis; bacterial diseases, such as leprosy and tuberculosis (TB); and terminal cancer
- Diminished delayed hypersensitivity possibly from immunosuppressive or steroid therapy or viral vaccination

Nursing Implications
- Anticipate the need for further testing.
- Institute infection control precautions as indicated.
- Assess the patient closely for signs and symptoms of infection or hypersensitivity reactions.

Purpose
- To assess for exposure to or activation of certain diseases, most commonly TB
- To assess the status of a patient's immune system during illness (such as cancer or transplantation)
- To evaluate sensitivity to environmental antigens in the patient with persistent symptoms (for example, asthma, seasonal rhinitis, or recurrent or persistent urticaria)

Description
Skin test for delayed-type hypersensitivity (DTH) that's used to evaluate T-cell-mediated immune response in a patient. (However, positive reactions don't indicate protection against the antigen.) This response requires previous exposure to the antigen and an intact immune system. After initial exposure to the antigen, the body produces antibodies and sensitized T cells. When reexposed to the antigen (recall antigen), the antibodies react immediately, causing a hypersensitivity reaction; however, the T cells respond over the next few days, causing a delayed hypersensitivity reaction. The immediate response is typically erythema, whereas the delayed response is induration (hardening). The lack of response to a recall antigen is called *anergy* and, in the absence of underlying disease or immunosuppressive therapy, may indicate T-cell immunodeficiency disease.

DTH testing can be used to assess the status of an individual's immune system in severe infection, cancer, pretransplantation, and malnutrition. Antigens used for this testing must be those to which the patient has been previously exposed. (For example, *Candida albicans*, tetanus, or mumps may be used.)

> ▶ **Quality and Safety Nursing Alert**
>
> Skin testing has limited value in infants because of their immature immune system and lack of previous sensitization.

DTH testing involves injecting a small amount of antigenic material intradermally or applying it topically and measuring the reaction after 48 to 72 hours. Patch testing may also be used.

This method involves applying antigenic material topically to the skin, helping to confirm allergic contact sensitization and isolate the causative agent.

Interfering Factors

- Use of antigens that have expired or that have been exposed to heat and light or to bacterial contamination
- Poor injection technique (subcutaneous instead of intradermal injection)
- Inaccurate dilution of antigens or an error in reading or timing test results
- A strong immediate reaction to the antigen at the injection site
- Hormonal contraceptives (may cause false-negative results by inhibiting lymphocyte mitosis)

Precautions

- If appropriate, store antigens in lyophilized (freeze-dried) form at 39.2°F (4°C) and protected from light. Reconstitute them shortly before use and check their expiration dates. If the patient has a suspected hypersensitivity to the antigens, apply them first in low concentrations.
- If the forearms aren't free from disease (for example, if the patient has atopic dermatitis), use other sites for testing, such as the back.

Nursing Considerations

Before the Test

- Confirm the patient's identity using two patient identifiers and confirmation of the patient's identification bracelet according to facility policy.
- Explain to the patient that a small amount of antigenic material will be injected superficially or applied to the skin.
- Inform the patient that testing takes only a few minutes for each antigen and that reactions will

be evaluated 48 to 72 hours later. Advise the patient that, occasionally, the test must be repeated in 2 to 3 weeks when a negative result is initially displayed. The first test "reminds" the body that it was previously exposed to the antigen, and a response is noted on retesting. This reminder is commonly done for TB testing and is called the *two-step test*.

- Ask the patient about any known sensitivity to the test antigens, whether the patient has had previous skin testing, and what the outcomes of that testing were. When performing TB testing, ask about previous TB disease or exposure and Bacille Calmette-Guérin vaccination.
- Be aware that the U.S. Food and Drug Administration hasn't approved all vaccines for use in skin testing, although nonapproved substances are commonly used. Currently approved antigens include the purified protein derivative to *Mycobacterium tuberculosis* and mumps.

During the Test

- Perform the test by injecting the antigens intradermally into the patient's forearm, using a separate tuberculin syringe for each antigen to be tested. (See the *Administering Test Antigens* box.)
- Circle each injection site with a pen, and label each according to the antigen given.
- Instruct the patient to avoid washing off the circles until the test is completed.
- Inject the control allergy diluent on the other forearm.
- Inspect the injection sites for reactivity after 48 to 72 hours. Record induration and erythema in millimeters. A negative test at the first concentration of antigen should be confirmed using a higher concentration.

Administering Test Antigens

This illustration shows the arm of a patient undergoing a recall antigen test, which determines whether the patient has previously been exposed to certain antigens. A sample panel of four test antigens has been injected into the patient's forearm, and the test site has been marked and labeled for each antigen.

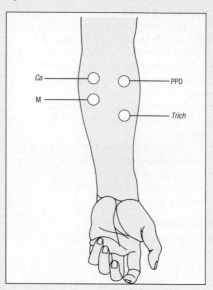

KEY:
Ca = Candida
M = Mumps
PPD = Purified protein derivative
Trich = Trichophyton

> ### Quality and Safety Nursing Alert
>
> Watch the patient closely for severe local reactions that may occur at the test site, such as pain, blistering, swelling, induration, itching, and ulceration. Scarring or hyperpigmentation also may result. Also observe for swelling and tenderness in the lymph nodes at the elbow or axillary region. Check for tachycardia and fever, although these rarely occur. Symptoms typically appear in 15 to 30 minutes.

- Alternatively, perform a patch test. (See the *Performing a Patch Test* box.)

After the Test

- Advise the patient experiencing hypersensitivity that steroids will control the reaction but that skin lesions may persist for 10 to 14 days. Instruct the patient to avoid scratching or otherwise disturbing the affected area.

- Continue to observe the patient carefully for signs of anaphylactic shock—urticaria, respiratory distress, and hypotension. If such signs develop, administer epinephrine, as ordered, and notify the health care provider immediately. Resuscitation equipment should be readily available.

Delta Aminolevulinic Acid

Reference Values

1.5 to 7.5 mg/24 hours (SI, 11–57 mcmol/day)

Abnormal Findings

Elevated Levels

- Lead poisoning, hereditary tyrosinemia, acute porphyria, hepatic carcinoma, or hepatitis
- Diabetic ketoacidosis

Performing a Patch Test

A patch test confirms allergic contact sensitivity and can help identify its cause. In this test, a sample series of common allergens (antigens) is applied to the skin in the hope that one or more will produce a positive reaction. A positive patch test proves that the patient has a contact sensitivity but doesn't necessarily confirm that the test substance caused the clinical eruption.

If the patient has an acute inflammation, the patch test should be postponed until the inflammation subsides to avoid exacerbating the inflammation.

Keep the following points in mind when performing a patch test:

• Use only potentially irritating substances for a patch test. Testing with primary irritants isn't possible.

• To avoid skin irritation, dilute substances that may be irritating to 1% to 2% in petroleum jelly, mineral oil, or water (as a last choice). When there are no clues to a likely allergen in a person with possible contact dermatitis, use a series of common allergens available in standard patch tests.

• Apply the allergens to normal, hairless skin on the back or on the ventral surface of the forearm. First, apply them to a small disk of filter paper attached to aluminum and coated with plastic. Tape the paper to the skin or use a small square of soft cotton and cover it with occlusive tape. Apply liquids and ointments to the disk or cotton. Apply volatile liquids to the skin and allow the areas to dry before covering. Before application, powder solids and moisten powders and fabrics.

• Make sure that patches remain in place for 48 hours. However, remove the patch immediately if pain, pruritus, or irritation develops. Positive reactions may take time to develop, so check findings 20 or 30 minutes after removing the patch and again 96 hours (4 days) after the application.

• Advise the patient to relieve the effects of a positive reaction by applying topical corticosteroids as ordered.

Nursing Implications

• Anticipate the need for additional testing.
• Prepare the patient for follow-up treatment.
• Provide emotional support to the patient and family.

Purpose

• To screen for lead poisoning
• To help diagnose porphyrias and certain hepatic disorders, such as hepatitis and hepatic carcinoma

Description

Using the colorimetric technique, the quantitative analysis of urine delta aminolevulinic acid (ALA) levels helps diagnose porphyrias, hepatic disease, and lead poisoning. In an emergency, a simple qualitative screening test may be performed. ALA, the basic precursor of the porphyrins, normally converts to porphobilinogen during heme synthesis. Impaired conversion, which occurs in porphyrias and lead poisoning, causes urine ALA levels to rise before other chemical or hematologic changes occur.

Interfering Factors

• Failure to collect all urine during the test period, to properly store the specimen and protect it from light, or to send the specimen to the laboratory immediately after the collection is completed

• Barbiturates and griseofulvin (increase because of accumulation of porphyrins in the liver)

• Vitamin E in pharmacologic doses (possible decrease)

• Penicillin may cause increased levels.

Nursing Considerations

Before the Test

• Confirm the patient's identity using two patient identifiers and confirmation of the patient's identification bracelet according to facility policy.

• Explain to the patient or parents that the urine ALA test detects abnormal hemoglobin formation.

- If lead poisoning is suspected, tell the patient (or parents, because the patient is usually a child) that the test helps detect the presence of excessive lead in the body.

Quality and Safety Nursing Alert

Keep in mind that blood levels for lead aren't sensitive indicators of lead poisoning in a child.

- Inform the patient or the patient's parents that there are no food or fluid restrictions for this test.
- Explain to the patient or parents that the test requires urine collection over a 24-hour period and teach the patient or parents the proper collection technique.
- Notify the laboratory and health care provider about any medications the patient is taking that may affect test results; these may need to be restricted.

During the Test
- Collect the patient's urine over a 24-hour period, discarding the first specimen and retaining the last. Use a light-resistant bottle containing a preservative (usually glacial acetic acid) to prevent ALA degradation.
- Refrigerate the specimen or keep it on ice during the collection period.

Quality and Safety Nursing Alert

Protect the specimen from direct sunlight. If the patient has a catheter in place, insert the drainage bag into a dark plastic bag.

- Indicate starting time on container and lab slip.
- Place a sign above the bed or in the bathroom with hours for collection to prevent accidentally discarding specimens.
- Encourage the patient to drink fluids during the 24-hour collection unless contraindicated

- Indicate on lab slip any drug that may affect result.

After the Test
- Send the specimen to the laboratory as soon as the collection is completed.
- Instruct the patient to resume usual medications as ordered.

Dexamethasone Suppression
Reference Values
Less than 5 mcg/dL (less than 138 nmol/L) or less than 50% or 0.50 of baseline

Abnormal Findings
- Failure of dexamethasone suppression, indicating possible major depression, Cushing syndrome, or severe stress
- Helps differentiate causes of elevated cortisol levels

Nursing Implications
- Anticipate the need for additional testing.
- Prepare the patient for treatment, including antidepressant therapy and for Cushing syndrome, if indicated.
- Monitor the patient's status closely, noting any changes in behavior.
- Assess fluid and electrolyte status closely in a patient with Cushing syndrome.

Purpose
- To diagnose Cushing syndrome
- To help diagnose clinical depression

Description
The dexamethasone suppression test requires administration of dexamethasone, an oral steroid. Dexamethasone suppresses levels of circulating adrenal steroid hormones in most people but fails to suppress them in patients with Cushing syndrome and some forms of clinical depression.

Interfering Factors
- Diabetes mellitus, pregnancy, and severe stress, such as trauma, severe weight loss, dehydration, and acute

alcohol withdrawal (possible false positive)
- Certain drugs, particularly barbiturates or phenytoin, within 3 weeks of the test (possible false positive)
- Caffeine consumed after midnight the night before the test (possible false positive)
- Use of corticosteroids, hormonal contraceptives, lithium, methadone, aspirin, diuretics, morphine, or monoamine oxidase inhibitors
- Tetracycline

Nursing Considerations

Before the Test
- Confirm the patient's identity using two patient identifiers and confirmation of the patient's identification bracelet according to facility policy.
- Explain to the patient the purpose of the dexamethasone suppression test.
- Inform the patient that the test requires two blood samples drawn after administration of dexamethasone. Advise that discomfort from the tourniquet and the needle punctures may be experienced.
- Advise the patient to withhold medications for 24 to 48 hours, if possible.
- Restrict food and fluids for 10 to 12 hours before the test.

During the Test
- On the first day, administer 1 mg dexamethasone at 11 PM.
- On the next day, collect blood samples at 4 PM and 11 PM. (More frequent sampling may increase the likelihood of measuring a nonsuppressed cortisol peak.)

After the Test
- Send the sample to the laboratory immediately.
- Apply direct pressure to the venipuncture site to control bleeding and prevent hematoma formation.
- Instruct the patient to resume usual diet and medications, as ordered.

Digital Subtraction Angiography

Normal Findings
- Filling and opacification of all superficial and deep arteries, arterioles, and veins with contrast medium, allowing visualization of normal cerebral vasculature
- Intensification of areas that should receive only contrast medium

Abnormal Findings
- Vascular filling defects (areas of increased vascular opacity), indicating arteriovenous occlusion or stenosis, possibly due to vasospasm, vascular malformation or angiomas, arteriosclerosis, or cerebral embolism or thrombosis
- Outpouchings in vessel lumina, possibly reflecting cerebral aneurysms (Such aneurysms commonly rupture, causing subarachnoid hemorrhage.)
- Vessel displacement or vascular masses, possibly indicating an intracranial tumor

Nursing Implications
- Anticipate the need for additional testing and prepare the patient for follow-up treatment.
- Assess the patient's neurologic status closely for changes.
- Keep in mind that conventional angiography provides a more detailed image of the carotid arteries than does digital subtraction angiography (DSA).
- Provide emotional support to the patient and family.

Purpose
- To visualize extracranial and intracranial cerebral blood flow
- To detect and evaluate cerebrovascular abnormalities
- To aid postoperative evaluation of cerebrovascular surgery, such as arterial grafts and endarterectomies

D

Description

DSA is a sophisticated radiographic technique that uses video equipment and computer-assisted image enhancement to examine the vascular systems. As in conventional angiography, X-ray images are obtained after injecting a contrast medium. However, unlike conventional angiography, in which images of bone and soft tissue commonly obscure vascular detail, DSA provides a high-contrast view of blood vessels without interfering images or shadows.

The usual procedure for DSA is as follows:

• The patient is placed supine on an X-ray table and asked to lie still with arms at sides.

• After an initial series of fluoroscopic pictures (mask images) of the patient's head is taken, the injection site—most commonly the antecubital basilic or cephalic vein—is clipped and cleaned with an antiseptic solution.

• If catheterization is ordered, a local anesthetic is administered, a venipuncture is performed, and a catheter is inserted and advanced to the superior vena cava.

• After placement is verified by X-ray, IV lines from a bag of normal saline solution and from an automatic contrast medium injector are connected. While the saline is administered, the injector delivers the contrast medium at a rate of about 14 mL/sec. If a simple injection of the contrast medium is ordered, a bolus of 40 to 60 mL is administered IV by needle.

• While vital signs and neurologic status are monitored, the patient is observed for signs of a hypersensitivity reaction, such as urticaria, flushing, and respiratory distress.

• After allowing time for the contrast medium to clear the pulmonary circulation and enter the cerebral vasculature, a second series of fluoroscopic

images (contrast images) is taken. The computer digitizes the information received from both series and compares mask and contrast images, subtracting the information (images of bone and soft tissue) common to both. A detailed image of the contrast medium–filled vessels is displayed on a video monitor; the image may be stored on videotape or a disk for future reference.

Interfering Factors

• Patient movement
• Radiopaque objects in the fluoroscopic field
• Vessel overlap of external and internal carotid arteries

Precautions

• DSA may be contraindicated in the patient with hypersensitivity to iodine or contrast media; poor cardiac function; renal, hepatic, or thyroid disease; diabetes; or multiple myeloma.

Nursing Considerations

Before the Test

• Explain to the patient that DSA visualizes cerebral blood vessels.

• Advise the patient to fast for 4 hours before the test but that there are no fluid restrictions.

• Check the patient's history for hypersensitivity to iodine, substances containing iodine such as shellfish, and contrast media. If the patient has had such reactions, note them on the chart and inform the health care provider, who may order prophylactic medications or choose not to perform the test.

• Explain that the patient will receive an injection of a contrast medium, either by needle or through a venous catheter inserted in the arm, and that a series of X-rays will be taken of the head. Explain who will perform the test, where it will take place, and that it will take 30 to 90 minutes.

- Inform the patient that he or she will be positioned on an X-ray table with the head immobilized and that he or she will be asked to lie still.

> ▶ *Quality and Safety Nursing Alert*
>
> Some patients—especially children—may be given a sedative to prevent movement during the procedure.

- Instruct the patient to remove all jewelry, dentures, and other radiopaque objects from the X-ray field.
- Tell the patient that some transient pain from the needle or catheter insertion may be felt and that a feeling of warmth, a headache, a metallic taste, and nausea or vomiting after the contrast agent is injected may be experienced.
- Make sure that the patient or a responsible family member has signed an informed consent form.

After the Test

- Because the contrast medium acts as a diuretic, encourage the patient to increase fluid intake for 24 hours after this test. Advise that extra fluid intake will also speed excretion of the contrast medium. Monitor the patient's intake and output as ordered. Assess vital signs every 15 minutes for 1 hour. Report any deviation from the patient's normal readings to the health care provider.
- Check the venipuncture site for signs of extravasation, such as redness or swelling. If bleeding occurs, apply firm pressure and an ice pack to the puncture site. If a hematoma develops, elevate the arm and apply pressure.
- Observe the patient for a delayed hypersensitivity reaction to the contrast medium. A delayed reaction can occur up to 18 hours after the procedure.
- Tell the patient to resume a usual diet.

Doppler Ultrasonography

Normal Findings

- Triphasic arterial waveforms of the arms and legs, with a prominent systolic component and one or more diastolic sounds
- The ankle–arm pressure index (also known as the *arterial ischemia index, ankle–brachial index,* or *pedal–brachial index*)—the ratio between ankle systolic pressure and brachial systolic pressure—normally equal to or greater than one
- Proximal thigh pressure 20 to 30 mm Hg higher than arm pressure, but with similar pressure measurements at adjacent sites; in the arms, pressure readings unchanged despite postural changes
- Venous blood flow velocity phasic with respiration and of a lower pitch than arterial flow
- Distal compression or release of proximal limb compression increasing blood flow velocity; in the legs, abdominal compression eliminating respiratory variations, but release increasing blood flow; Valsalva's maneuver also interrupting venous flow velocity
- Strong velocity signal in cerebrovascular testing
- Blood flow velocity increasing during diastole in the common carotid artery due to low peripheral vascular resistance of the brain
- Periorbital arterial blood flowing anterograde out of the orbit

Abnormal Findings

- Diminished blood flow velocity signal, with no diastolic sound and a less prominent systolic component distal to the lesion; at the lesion, high-pitched and, occasionally, turbulent signal, indicating arterial stenosis or occlusion
- Absent velocity signal, indicating complete occlusion without collateral circulation

- Pressure gradient exceeding 20 mm Hg at adjacent sites of measurement in the leg, indicating occlusive disease
- Low proximal thigh pressure, indicating common femoral or aortoiliac occlusive disease
- Abnormal gradient between the proximal thigh and the above- or below-knee cuffs, indicating superficial femoral or popliteal artery occlusive disease
- Abnormal gradient between the below-knee and ankle cuffs, indicating tibiofibular occlusive disease
- Abnormal gradient between arm and forearm pressures, indicating brachial artery occlusion
- Inability to identify Doppler signals during cerebrovascular examination, indicating total arterial occlusion
- Reversed periorbital arterial flow, indicating arterial occlusive disease of the extracranial internal carotid artery
- Turbulent signals, indicating internal carotid artery stenosis
- Absent or unchanged venous blood flow velocity in response to respirations, compression, or Valsalva's maneuver, indicating venous thrombosis
- Reversed flow velocity signal, indicating chronic venous insufficiency and varicose veins
- Retrograde blood velocity in the vertebral artery, indicating subclavian steal syndrome
- Weak velocity signal on comparison of contralateral vertebral arteries, indicating diffuse vertebral artery disease

Nursing Implications
- Anticipate the need for additional testing and prepare the patient for follow-up treatment.
- Keep in mind that an abnormal ankle–arm pressure index is directly proportional to the degree of circulatory impairment: mild ischemia, 1.0 to 0.75; claudication, 0.75 to 0.50;

pain at rest, 0.50 to 0.25; and pregangrene, 0.25 to 0.
- Monitor the patient's pulses, skin color, and temperature frequently for changes.
- Assess the patient's neurologic status for changes.

Purpose
- To help diagnose venous insufficiency and superficial and deep vein thrombosis (popliteal, femoral, and iliac)
- To help diagnose peripheral artery disease and arterial occlusion
- To monitor the patient who has had arterial reconstruction and bypass grafts
- To detect abnormalities of carotid artery blood flow associated with such conditions as aortic stenosis
- To evaluate possible arterial trauma

Description
Doppler ultrasonography is a noninvasive test used to evaluate blood flow in the major veins and arteries of the arms and legs and in the extracranial cerebrovascular system. An alternative to arteriography and venography, it's safer, less costly, and faster than invasive tests.

In Doppler ultrasonography, water-soluble conductive gel is applied to the tip of a handheld transducer, which directs high-frequency sound waves to the artery or vein being tested. The sound waves strike moving red blood cells and are reflected back to the transducer, allowing direct listening and graphic recording of blood flow.

Measurement of systolic pressure during this test is used to detect the presence, location, and extent of peripheral arterial occlusive disease. Changes in sound wave frequency during respiration are observed to detect venous occlusive disease. Compression maneuvers detect occlusion of the veins and occlusion or stenosis of carotid arteries. Pulse volume recorder testing may be performed with Doppler ultrasonography to record changes in blood volume or flow in an extremity or organ.

The usual procedures for peripheral arterial and venous evaluation and extracranial cerebrovascular evaluation are outlined here.

Peripheral Arterial Evaluation

- Peripheral arterial evaluation is always performed bilaterally. The usual test sites in each leg are the common femoral, superficial femoral, popliteal, posterior tibial, and dorsalis pedis arteries; in each arm, the test sites are usually the subclavian, brachial, radial, ulnar, and, occasionally, palmar arch and digital arteries.
- The patient is instructed to remove all clothing above or below the waist, depending on the test site, and is placed in a supine position on the examination table or bed, with arms at sides.
- Brachial blood pressure is measured, and the transducer is placed at various points along the test arteries.
- The signals are monitored, and the waveforms are recorded for later analysis.
- Segmental limb blood pressure is obtained to localize arterial occlusive disease.
- During lower extremity tests, a blood pressure cuff is wrapped around the calf, pressure readings are obtained, and waveforms are recorded from the dorsalis pedis and posterior tibial arteries. Then the cuff is wrapped around the thigh, and waveforms are recorded at the popliteal artery.
- In upper extremity tests, examination is performed on one arm, with the patient placed first in a supine position and then sitting; examination is then repeated on the other arm. A blood pressure cuff is wrapped around the forearm, pressure readings are taken, and waveforms are recorded over the radial and ulnar arteries.

Then the cuff is wrapped around the upper arm, pressure readings are taken, and waveforms are recorded with the transducer over the brachial artery.

- Blood pressure readings and waveform recordings are repeated with the arm in extreme hyperextension and hyperabduction to check for possible compression factors that may interfere with arterial blood flow. The upper extremity examination is performed on one arm, with the patient first placed in a supine position and then sitting; it's then repeated on the other arm.

Peripheral Venous Evaluation

- Usual test sites for peripheral venous evaluation include the popliteal, superficial femoral, and common femoral veins in the leg and the posterior tibial vein at the ankle; the brachial, axillary, and subclavian veins in the arm; jugular veins; and, occasionally, the inferior and superior vena cava.
- The patient is instructed to remove all clothing above or below the waist, depending on the test site.
- The patient is placed in a supine position and instructed to breathe normally.
- The transducer is placed over the appropriate vein, waveforms and compressibility are recorded, and respiratory modulations are noted.
- Proximal limb compression maneuvers are performed and augmentation is noted after release of compression, to evaluate venous valve competency.
- Changes in respiration are monitored.
- During lower extremity tests, the patient is asked to perform Valsalva's maneuver and venous blood flow is recorded.
- The procedure is repeated for the other arm or leg. (See the *How to Detect Thrombi with a Doppler Probe* box.)

D

How to Detect Thrombi with a Doppler Probe

The Doppler probe is typically used to detect venous thrombi by first positioning the transducer and then occluding the blood vessel by compression (as shown in the illustration of the normal leg below). Water-soluble conductive gel is applied to the tip of the transducer to provide coupling between the skin and transducer.

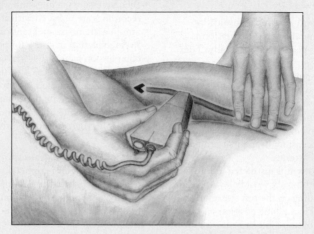

When pressure is released, allowing blood flow to resume, the transducer picks up the sudden augmentation of the flow sound and permits graphic recording of blood flow. If a thrombus is present, a compression maneuver fails to produce the augmented flow sound because the blood flow (as shown below in the femoral vein) is significantly impaired.

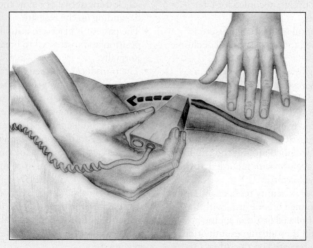

Extracranial Cerebrovascular Evaluation

- Usual test sites for extracranial cerebrovascular evaluation include the supraorbital, common carotid, external carotid, internal carotid, and vertebral arteries.
- The patient is placed in a supine position on the examination table or bed, with a pillow beneath the head for support.
- Brachial blood pressure is then recorded using the Doppler probe.
- The transducer is positioned over the test artery, and blood flow velocity is monitored and recorded.
- The influence of compression maneuvers on blood flow velocity is measured, and the procedure is repeated on the opposite side.

Interfering Factors
- Patient's inability to cooperate

Precautions
- Bradyarrhythmias may occur if the probe is placed near the carotid sinus.
- Make sure that the Doppler probe isn't placed over an open or draining lesion.

Nursing Considerations

Before the Test
- Explain to the patient that Doppler ultrasonography is used to evaluate blood flow in the arms and legs or neck. Explain who will perform the test and where and when.
- Reassure the patient that the test doesn't involve risk or discomfort.
- Explain that the patient will be asked to move the arms to different positions and to perform breathing exercises as measurements are taken. Advise the patient that a small ultrasonic probe resembling a microphone is placed at various sites along veins or arteries, and blood pressure is checked at several sites.
- Check with the vascular laboratory about special equipment or instructions.

After the Test
- Remove the conductive gel from the patient's skin.
- Assist the patient to a comfortable position.

Ductal Lavage of Breast Tissue

Normal Findings
- Absence of atypical or malignant cells

Abnormal Findings
- Increase in atypical cells, indicating a significant increase in the risk of developing breast cancer

Nursing Implications
- Anticipate the need for additional testing, and prepare the patient for follow-up treatment as indicated.
- Keep in mind that evidence of atypical cells doesn't positively indicate that cancer is present.
- Provide emotional support to the patient and her family.

Purpose
- To identify a woman's risk of developing breast cancer

Description
Ductal lavage of breast tissue is a minimally invasive method for assessing a woman's risk of developing breast cancer. This test permits the collection of cells from inside the milk ducts of the breast. Research has demonstrated that most breast cancers begin in the cells that line the breast ducts. These cells may take 8 to 10 years to develop into a tumor that's visible with a mammogram or palpated with a breast examination. This test helps to determine whether the woman has atypical cells in her milk ducts that have the potential for becoming malignant. The belief is that the earlier the abnormal cells are found, the more treatment options are available.

D

▶ Quality and Safety Nursing Alert

Fluid production suggests a higher risk of breast cancer development. If no fluid is aspirated, the lavage isn't performed.

Sometimes referred to as the "Pap test" for the breasts, this test is commonly performed in a health care provider's office as follows:

• The health care provider places a syringe-like aspirator device on the breast at the nipple area and gently pulls back on the syringe to expel fluid from the ducts. Typically, only one or two ducts produce extremely minute amounts (drops) of fluid.

(See the *Understanding Breast Ductal Lavage* box.)

• After the fluid-producing ducts have been identified, the health care provider inserts a microcatheter into these ducts and instills an anesthetic followed by saline solution to rinse the ducts.
• The breasts are massaged gently to move the fluid toward the nipple.
• The health care provider aspirates the fluid into the syringe and then transfers the fluid to specialized vials, which are sent to the laboratory for analysis. The procedure is repeated for other ducts that produced fluid. Although rare, malignant cells may be found.

Understanding Breast Ductal Lavage

1. A syringelike aspirator is placed over the breast at the nipple area. Suction is applied to the aspirator to draw out small amounts of fluid from the ducts to the nipple surface. Usually only one or two ducts produce fluid.

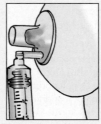

2. A microcatheter is then inserted into the ducts from which fluid was obtained.

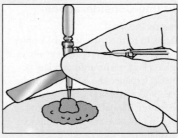

3. A small of amount of anesthetic may be instilled followed by a small amount of saline. The breast is massaged and then fluid is withdrawn into the catheter, which is attached to a syringe. The sample is then placed in a preservative and sent to the laboratory for analysis.

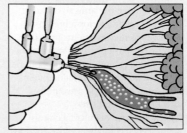

Interfering Factors
- Insufficient amount of sample ductal fluid

Precautions
- This test is indicated only for women considered to be at high risk for developing breast cancer based on personal and family factors.

Nursing Considerations
Before the Test
- Describe the procedure to the patient and explain that ductal lavage of breast tissue helps to identify cells that have the potential to become cancerous.
- Offer her emotional support and assure her that evidence of atypical cells doesn't necessarily indicate cancer.
- Tell the patient that she doesn't need to restrict food, fluids, and medication for the test.
- Tell her who will perform the test and when and where it will be done.
- Warn the patient that she may feel a sensation of breast fullness similar to lactation, tingling, or pinching. Also inform her that the discomfort is similar to that of a mammogram.
- Check the patient's history for hypersensitivity to local anesthetics.
- Apply a topical anesthetic agent, if appropriate, about 30 minutes to 1 hour before the test.
- Have the patient apply warmth to the breast and massage, if indicated.

After the Test
- Inspect the dressing over the test site; reinforce any instructions related to site care as appropriate.
- Provide emotional support to the patient while awaiting the results.

D-Xylose Absorption

Reference Values
Adults: Blood concentration 25 to 40 mg/dL in 2 hours; urine, 3.5 g excreted in 5 hours (Patients age 65 or older may have urine levels greater than 5 g in 24 hours.)
Children: Blood concentration greater than 30 mg/dL in 1 hour; urine, 16% to 33% of ingested D-xylose excreted in 5 hours

Abnormal Findings
Decreased Levels
- Malabsorption disorders that affect the proximal small intestine, such as sprue and celiac disease
- Regional enteritis involving the jejunum, Whipple's disease, multiple jejunal diverticula, myxedema, diabetic neuropathic diarrhea, rheumatoid arthritis, alcoholism, severe heart failure, and ascites

Nursing Implications
- Anticipate the need for additional testing and prepare the patient for follow-up treatment.
- Continue to monitor the patient's weight and nutritional status.

Purpose
- To aid in the differential diagnosis of malabsorption
- To determine the cause of malabsorption syndrome

Description
D-xylose is a pentose sugar that's absorbed in the small intestine without the aid of pancreatic enzymes; it passes through the liver without being metabolized and is excreted in the urine. Because of its absorption in the small intestine without digestion, a measurement of D-xylose in the urine and blood indicates the absorptive capacity of the small intestine. This test evaluates the patient with symptoms of malabsorption, such as weight loss and generalized malnutrition, weakness, and diarrhea.

Interfering Factors
- Failure to observe pretest restrictions and not fasting
- Aspirin (decreased D-xylose excretion by the kidneys)

- Indomethacin (Indocin) (decreased intestinal D-xylose absorption)
- Failure to obtain a complete urine specimen or to collect blood samples at designated times
- Intestinal overgrowth of bacteria, renal insufficiency, or renal retention of urine (possible drop in urine levels)
- Foods rich in pentose (fruits and preservatives)

Precautions
- Handle the sample gently to prevent hemolysis.

Nursing Considerations

Before the Test
- Confirm the patient's identity using two patient identifiers and confirmation of the patient's identification bracelet according to facility policy.
- Explain to the patient that the D-xylose absorption test helps evaluate digestive function by analyzing blood samples and urine specimens after ingestion of a sugar solution. Explain that the patient must fast overnight before the test and will have to fast and remain in bed during the test.
- Inform the patient that the test requires several blood samples and that slight discomfort from the tourniquet and needle punctures may be experienced.
- Inform the patient that all the urine will be collected for either a 5-hour or a 24-hour period. Advise the patient to avoid contaminating the urine specimens with toilet tissue or feces.
- Withhold drugs that alter test results, such as aspirin and indomethacin. Record any drugs the patient is taking on the laboratory request.

During the Test
- Perform a venipuncture to obtain a fasting blood sample and collect the sample in a 10-mL tube without additives. Also collect a first-voided morning urine specimen. Label these specimens and send them to the laboratory immediately to serve as a baseline.
- Give the patient 25 g of D-xylose dissolved in 3 oz (100 mL) of water, followed by an additional 8 oz (240 mL) of water.
- Record the time of D-xylose ingestion.
- For an adult, draw a blood sample at intervals of 30 minutes, 1 hour, and 2 hours after D-xylose ingestion. Collect the sample in a 10-mL tube without additives.

▶ *Quality and Safety Nursing Alert*

If the patient is younger than age 12, give 5 g of D-xylose. Collect the sample for a child 1 hour after ingestion.

- If ordered, obtain a blood sample after 5 hours to support the findings of the 1- or 2-hour sample.
- Collect and pool all urine during the 5 hours or 24 hours after D-xylose ingestion. Refrigerate the specimen during the collection period.

▶ *Quality and Safety Nursing Alert*

Because patients age 65 and older and those with borderline or elevated creatinine levels tend to have low 5-hour urine levels but normal 24-hour levels, the health care provider must establish the length of the collection period.

- Maintain the patient on bed rest and withhold food and fluids (other than D-xylose) throughout the test period.

After the Test
- Apply direct pressure to the venipuncture site until bleeding stops and to prevent hematoma formation.
- Observe the patient for abdominal discomfort or mild diarrhea caused by D-xylose ingestion.
- Instruct the patient to resume usual diet and medications.

Echocardiography

Normal Findings

- Anterior and posterior mitral valve leaflets normally separating in early diastole, with the anterior leaflet moving toward the chest wall and the posterior leaflet moving away from it
- Leaflets attaining maximum excursion rapidly and then moving toward each other during ventricular diastole; after atrial contraction, leaflets coming together and remaining so during ventricular systole
- Leaflets appearing as two fine lines within the echo-free, blood-filled left ventricular cavity (M-mode echocardiogram)
- Aortic valve cusps lying between the parallel walls of the aortic root, which move anteriorly during systole and posteriorly during diastole
- Cusps separating, appearing as a box-like configuration during ventricular systole; remaining open throughout systole and normally demonstrating a characteristic fine fluttering motion; then coming together and appearing as a single or double line within the aortic root during diastole (M-mode echocardiogram)
- Motion of the tricuspid valve resembling that of the mitral valve
- Motion of the pulmonic valve's posterior cusp (gradually moving posteriorly during diastole; during atrial systole, displacing posteriorly; during ventricular systole, quick movement posteriorly; during right ventricular ejection, movement anteriorly,

attaining its most anterior position during diastole)
- The left ventricular cavity appearing as an echo-free space between the interventricular septum and the posterior left ventricular wall; echoes produced by the chordae tendineae and the mitral leaflet appearing within this cavity
- The right ventricular cavity appearing as an echo-free space between the anterior chest wall and the interventricular septum

Abnormal Findings

- Narrowing that results from the leaflets' thickening and disordered motion, indicating mitral stenosis; instead of moving in opposite directions during diastole, mitral valve leaflets move anteriorly (See the *Real-Time Echocardiograms* box.)
- One or both leaflets ballooning into the left atrium during systole, indicating mitral valve prolapse
- Flutter seen in M-mode echocardiography, indicating aortic valve abnormalities, especially aortic insufficiency
- Thickening, with more echoes generated, indicating aortic stenosis caused by such conditions as rheumatic fever or bacterial endocarditis (In rheumatic fever, the valve may thicken slightly and allow normal motion during systole or thicken severely and curtail motion.)
- Disrupted valve motion, shaggy or fuzzy echoes usually appearing on or near the valve, indicating bacterial endocarditis

(text continues on page 232)

229

Real-Time Echocardiograms

The real-time (showing motion) echocardiograms shown below are short-axis, cross-sectional views of the mitral valve from a normal patient (top) and a patient with mitral stenosis (bottom). In the latter, note the greatly reduced mitral valve orifice caused by stenotic, calcified valve leaflets.

Normal

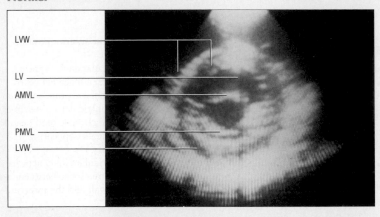

Mitral Stenosis

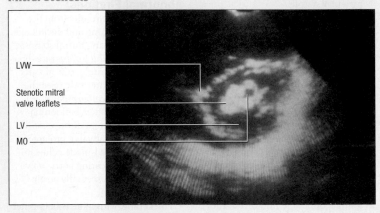

KEY:
AMVL = Anterior mitral valve leaflet
LV = Left ventricle
LVW = Left ventricular wall
MO = Mitral orifice
PMVL = Posterior mitral valve leaflet

The echocardiograms shown below are long-axis, cross-sectional views of the mitral valve from a normal patient (top) and a patient with hypertrophic cardiomyopathy, also known as *idiopathic hypertrophic stenosis* (bottom). Note the markedly thickened left ventricular wall in the latter.

Normal

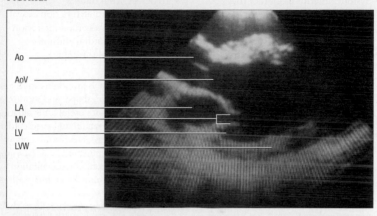

Hypertrophic Cardiomyopathy

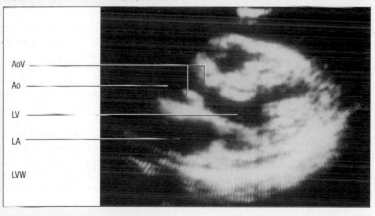

KEY:
Ao = Aorta
AoV = Aortic valve
LA = Left atrium
LV = Left ventricle
LVW = Left ventricular wall
MV = Mitral valve

- Congenital heart disorder such as aortic stenosis
- Small chamber size, indicating cardiomyopathy, valvular disorders, or heart failure; large chamber size, indicating restrictive pericarditis
- Systolic anterior motion of the mitral valve and asymmetric septal hypertrophy, indicating hypertrophic obstructive cardiomyopathy
- Shifting in and out of the mitral opening (a mass of echoes against the anterior mitral valve leaflet during diastole) and echoes shifting back into the atrium during ventricular systole, indicating left atrial tumors
- Absent or paradoxical motion in ventricular walls that normally move together and thicken during systole, indicating coronary artery disease (CAD), ischemia, or infarction; areas may fail to thicken or may become thinner, particularly if scar tissue is present
- Abnormal echo-free space, indicating pericardial effusion

Nursing Implications
- Anticipate the need for additional testing.
- Keep in mind that an echocardiogram should be correlated with the patient's history, physical examination, and other tests and laboratory findings.
- For a patient with a suboptimal echocardiogram, expect an agent composed of human albumin microspheres filled with perfluorocarbon gas (Optison) to be used. This agent can enhance the contrast of the ultrasound scans to opacify the left ventricle and improve the delineation of the left ventricular endocardial borders.
- Prepare the patient for follow-up treatment as indicated.
- Provide emotional support to the patient and family.

Purpose
- To diagnose and evaluate valvular abnormalities

- To measure the size of the heart's chambers
- To evaluate chambers and valves in congenital heart disorders
- To help diagnose hypertrophic and related cardiomyopathies
- To detect atrial tumors
- To evaluate cardiac function or wall motion after myocardial infarction
- To detect pericardial effusion
- To detect mural thrombi

Description
Echocardiography is a noninvasive test that shows the size, shape, and motion of cardiac structures. It's useful for evaluating patients with chest pain, enlarged cardiac silhouettes on X-rays, electrocardiographic (ECG) changes unrelated to CAD, and abnormal heart sounds on auscultation.

In this test, a transducer directs ultra-high-frequency sound waves toward cardiac structures, which reflect these waves. The echoes are converted to images that are displayed on a monitor and recorded on a strip chart or videotape. Results are correlated with clinical history, physical examination, and findings from additional tests.

The techniques most commonly used in echocardiography are M-mode (motion-mode), for recording the motion and dimensions of intracardiac structures, and two-dimensional (cross-sectional), for recording lateral motion and providing the correct spatial relationship between cardiac structures. (See the *M-Mode Echocardiograms* box.)

The usual procedure for echocardiography is as follows:

- After the patient is placed in a supine position, conductive gel is applied to the third or fourth intercostal space to the left of the sternum and the transducer is placed directly over it. The transducer is systematically angled to direct ultrasonic waves at specific parts of the patient's heart.
- During the test, the oscilloscope screen, which displays the returning echoes, is observed.

M-Mode Echocardiograms

In the normal motion-mode (M-mode) echocardiogram of the mitral valve shown below (top), valve movement appears as a characteristic lopsided, M-shaped tracing. The anterior and posterior mitral valve leaflets separate (D) in early diastole, quickly reach maximum separation (E), and then close during rapid ventricular filling (E-F).

Leaflet separation varies during mid-diastole, and the valve opens widely again (A) following atrial contraction. The valve starts to close with atrial relaxation (A–B) and is completely closed during the start of ventricular systole (C). The steepness of the E–F slope indirectly shows the speed of ventricular filling, which is normally rapid.

Normal Echocardiogram

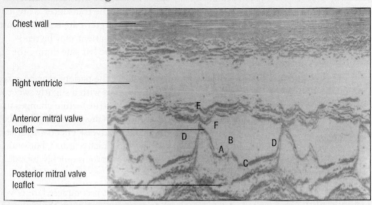

Abnormal Findings

Mitral stenosis is evident in the abnormal echocardiogram shown at right. The E-F slope (line) is very shallow, indicating slowed left ventricular filling.

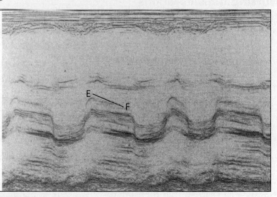

- Significant findings are recorded on a strip chart recorder (M-mode echocardiography) or on a videotape recorder (two-dimensional echocardiography).
- For a different view of the heart, the transducer is placed beneath the xiphoid process or directly above the sternum. For a left lateral view, the patient may be positioned on the left side.
- To record heart function under various conditions, the patient is asked to inhale and exhale slowly, to

hold the breath, or to inhale amyl nitrite.

• Doppler echocardiography may also be used to assess the speed and direction of blood flow. The sound of blood flow may be heard as the continuous-wave and pulsed-wave Doppler sampling of cardiac valves is performed. This technique is used primarily to assess heart sounds and murmurs as they relate to cardiac hemodynamics.

Interfering Factors

• Incorrect transducer placement and excessive movement
• Thick chest or chest wall abnormalities or chronic obstructive pulmonary disease (possible poor imaging)

Precautions

• Be aware that some laboratories require specific protocols for individualized preparation, including a signed informed consent. Check your facility's policy.

Nursing Considerations

Before the Test

• Confirm the patient's identity using two patient identifiers and confirmation of the patient's identification bracelet according to facility policy.
• Inform the patient that echocardiography is used to evaluate the size, shape, and motion of various cardiac structures.
• Explain who will perform the test, where and when it will take place, and that it's safe, painless, and noninvasive.
• Advise the patient that there are no food or fluid restrictions for this test.
• Describe the procedure, instructing the patient to remain still during the test because movement may distort results.
• Explain that the room may be darkened slightly to aid visualization on the monitor screen and that other procedures (ECG and phonocardiog-

raphy) may be performed simultaneously to time events in the cardiac cycle.

• Explain that conductive gel will be applied to the chest and that a quarter-sized transducer will be placed directly over it. Warn that the patient may feel minor discomfort, because pressure is exerted to keep the transducer in contact with the skin.
• Explain that the transducer is angled to observe different areas of the heart and that the patient may be repositioned on the left side during the procedure.
• Explain that the patient may be asked to inhale a gas with a slightly sweet odor (amyl nitrite) while changes in heart function are recorded; describe the possible adverse effects (dizziness, flushing, and tachycardia), but assure that such symptoms quickly subside.

After the Test

• When the test is completed, remove the conductive gel from the patient's skin.

Echocardiography, Dobutamine Stress

Normal Findings

• Increased ventricular wall contractility

Abnormal Findings

• Abnormal regional wall motion, indicating cardiac ischemia or infarction

Nursing Implications

• Anticipate the need for additional testing and prepare the patient for follow-up treatment as indicated.
• Monitor the patient for anginal symptoms; assess vital signs and cardiac status.
• Provide emotional support to the patient and family.

Purpose

• To identify causes of anginal symptoms

- To measure the size of the heart's chambers and determine functional capacity
- To help set limits for an exercise program
- To diagnose and evaluate valvular and wall motion abnormalities
- To detect atrial tumors, mural thrombi, vegetative growth on valve leaflets, and pericardial effusions
- To evaluate myocardial perfusion, coronary artery disease and obstruction, and the extent of myocardial damage following myocardial infarction

Description

Dobutamine stress echocardiography uses two-dimensional echocardiography combined with a dobutamine infusion to detect changes in regional cardiac wall motion. Dobutamine increases myocardial contractility and stroke volume and permits study of the heart under stress conditions without exercising the patient. Imaging is done during infusion of increasing amounts of dobutamine until the maximum predicted heart rate is achieved.

The usual procedure is as follows:

- The patient is placed in the supine position and an echocardiogram is obtained.
- An initial electrocardiogram (ECG) is obtained.
- ECG rhythm and blood pressure are monitored during the procedure.
- After IV access is obtained, a dobutamine infusion is given in increasing amounts. The infusion continues until the patient reaches the maximum predicted heart rate or becomes symptomatic. If the maximum predicted heart rate isn't reached with maximum dobutamine, IV atropine may be given.
- As the maximum predicted heart rate is achieved, a second (stress) echocardiogram is obtained.
- After the dobutamine infusion is completed, a third (recovery) echocardiogram is completed.

▶ Quality and Safety Nursing Alert

- Testing should be stopped for significant ECG changes, hypertension, hypotension, angina, dyspnea, syncope, or critical symptoms.
- This test should never be performed without a health care provider and emergency resuscitation equipment immediately available.

E

Precautions

- The test is contraindicated in patients who have had a myocardial infarction within the previous 10 days and in those with acute myocarditis or pericarditis, ventricular or atrial arrhythmias, or severe aortic or mitral stenosis.
- Other contraindications include hyperthyroidism or severe anemia, ventricular or dissecting aortic aneurysms, clinical heart failure, and acute severe infections.

Nursing Considerations

Before the Test

- Confirm the patient's identity using two patient identifiers and confirmation of the patient's identification bracelet according to facility policy.
- Make sure the patient has signed an appropriate consent form.
- Note and report all allergies and response to the allergens.
- Explain the need to refrain from eating, smoking, or drinking alcoholic or caffeine-containing beverages at least 4 hours before the test or as directed by the health care provider.
- Withhold all drugs the patient is currently taking before testing, as directed.
- Warn that the patient may feel palpitations, some mild shortness of breath, and some fatigue when the dobutamine infusion begins.
- Instruct the patient to report all symptoms experienced during the study.
- Explain that the test should take 60 to 90 minutes.

After the Test

- If the patient's heart rate doesn't return to baseline or if the patient becomes symptomatic, administer an IV beta-adrenergic blocker.
- Remove the electrodes and conductive gel from the patient's chest.
- Monitor the patient's vital signs, ECG, heart sounds, anginal symptoms, and respiratory status.

Echocardiography, Exercise

Normal Findings

- Increased contractility of the ventricular walls resulting in hyperkinesis linked to sympathetic and catecholamine stimulation
- Increase in heart rate that's directly proportional to the workload and metabolic oxygen demand; increase in systolic blood pressure as the workload increases
- Endurance level that's appropriate for the patient's age and exercise limits

Abnormal Findings

- Exercise-induced myocardial ischemia, indicating coronary artery disease (CAD)
- Myocardial hypokinesis or akinesis, indicating CAD
- Exercise-induced hypotension, ST-segment depression of 2 mm or more, or downsloping ST segments appearing within the first 3 minutes of exercise and lasting 8 minutes after the test ends, indicating multivessel or left CAD
- ST-segment elevation, indicating critical myocardial ischemia or injury

Nursing Implications

- Anticipate the need for additional testing, if indicated.
- Assess the patient's cardiopulmonary status closely; anticipate continuous cardiac monitoring.
- Prepare the patient for follow-up treatment as appropriate, including medication therapy.

Purpose

- To identify the causes of chest pain
- To determine the heart's chamber size and functional capacity
- To screen for asymptomatic cardiac disease
- To set limits for an exercise program
- To diagnose and evaluate valvular and wall motion abnormalities
- To detect atrial tumors, mural thrombi, vegetative growth on valve leaflets, and pericardial effusions
- To evaluate myocardial perfusion, CAD, and obstructions, and the extent of myocardial damage after myocardial infarction (MI)

Description

Exercise echocardiography, also called *stress echocardiography*, is two-dimensional echocardiography that uses exercise to detect changes in cardiac wall motion. The test collects images before and after exercise stress testing. The specificity and sensitivity of this test serve as an adjunct to results obtained in exercise electrocardiography.

> ### Quality and Safety Nursing Alert
> The procedure shouldn't be performed without a health care provider and emergency resuscitation equipment readily available.

The usual procedure is as follows:

- The patient is placed into the supine position and a baseline echocardiogram obtained.
- An initial baseline electrocardiogram (ECG) and an initial blood pressure reading are obtained.
- The patient is placed on the treadmill at slow speed.
- The work rate is increased every 3 minutes as tolerated (increasing the speed of the machine slightly and increasing the degree of incline by 3% each time).
- The cardiac monitor is observed continuously for changes, and blood

pressure is monitored at predetermined intervals.

- The rhythm strip is checked at preset intervals for arrhythmias, premature ventricular contractions, ST-segment changes, and T-wave changes.
- The test level and the amount of time it took to reach that level are marked on each strip.
- The patient is observed for common responses to maximal exercise, including dizziness, lightheadedness, leg fatigue, dyspnea, diaphoresis, and a slightly ataxic gait. If symptoms become severe, the test is stopped. (The test would also be stopped for significant ECG changes, arrhythmias, or symptoms of hypertension, hypotension, or angina.)
- After the patient has reached the maximum predicted heart rate, the treadmill is slowed.
- While the patient's heart rate is still elevated, he's helped off the treadmill and placed on a stretcher for a second echocardiogram.

Interfering Factors

- Wolff-Parkinson-white's syndrome, electrolyte imbalance, or the use of digoxin preparations (false-positive results)
- Conditions that cause left ventricular hypertrophy

Precautions

- This test is contraindicated in those with ventricular or dissecting aortic aneurysms, uncontrolled arrhythmias, pericarditis, myocarditis, severe anemia, uncontrolled hypertension, unstable angina, or heart failure.
- Possible complications include cardiac arrhythmias, myocardial ischemia or MI, cardiac arrest, and death.

Nursing Considerations

Before the Test

- Confirm the patient's identity using two patient identifiers and confirmation of the patient's identification bracelet according to facility policy.
- Make sure the patient has signed a consent form.
- Note and report all allergies and response to the allergen.
- Instruct the patient to refrain from eating, smoking, or drinking alcoholic or caffeine-containing beverages at least 3 to 4 hours before the test.
- Withhold all drugs the patient is currently taking before testing, as directed.
- Warn that the patient may feel tired, diaphoretic, and slightly short of breath during testing. Reassure that if symptoms become severe or if chest pain develops, the test will be stopped.
- Explain that the test takes approximately 60 minutes.

After the Test

- Remove electrodes and conductive gel from the patient.
- Monitor the patient's vital signs, ECG, and heart sounds.

Electrocardiography

Normal Findings (Lead II)

- P wave that doesn't exceed 2.5 mm (0.25 mV) in height or last longer than 0.12 second
- PR interval (includes the P wave plus the PR segment) persisting for 0.12 to 0.2 second for heart rates above 60 beats/minute
- QT interval that varies with the heart rate and lasts 0.4 to 0.52 second for heart rates above 60 beats/minute
- Voltage of the R wave in leads V_1 through V_6 that doesn't exceed 27 mm
- Total QRS complex lasting 0.06 to 0.1 second. (See the *Normal ECG Waveforms* box.)

Normal Electrocardiogram Waveforms

Because each lead takes a different view of heart activity, it generates its own characteristic tracing on an electrocardiogram (ECG). The traces shown here are representative of each of the 12 leads. Leads aV$_R$, V$_1$, V$_2$, V$_3$, and V$_4$ normally show strong negative deflections. Negative deflections indicate that the current is moving away from the positive electrode; positive deflections, that the current is moving toward the positive electrode.

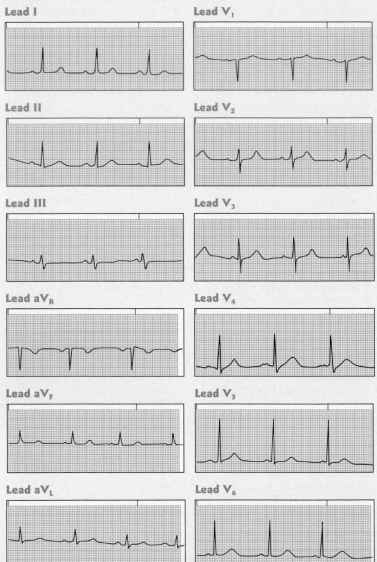

Lead I

Lead V$_1$

Lead II

Lead V$_2$

Lead III

Lead V$_3$

Lead aV$_R$

Lead V$_4$

Lead aV$_F$

Lead V$_5$

Lead aV$_L$

Lead V$_6$

Abnormal Findings

- Myocardial infarction (MI), right or left ventricular hypertrophy, arrhythmias, right or left bundle-branch block, ischemia, conduction defects or pericarditis, electrolyte abnormalities (such as hypokalemia and hyperkalemia), and abnormalities caused by cardioactive drugs
- Abnormal waveforms during angina episodes or during exercise (See the *Abnormal ECG Waveforms* box.)

Nursing Implications

- Anticipate the need for additional testing and prepare the patient for follow-up treatment as indicated.
- Assess the patient's cardiac status closely, including vital signs and heart rate and rhythm.
- Anticipate the need for continuous cardiac monitoring.
- Provide emotional support to the patient and family.

Purpose

- To help identify primary conduction abnormalities, cardiac arrhythmias, cardiac hypertrophy, pericarditis, electrolyte imbalances, myocardial ischemia, and the site and extent of MI
- To monitor recovery from an MI
- To evaluate the effectiveness of cardiac medication (cardiac glycosides, antiarrhythmics, antihypertensives, and vasodilators)
- To assess pacemaker performance
- To determine the effectiveness of thrombolytic therapy and the resolution of ST-segment depression or elevation and T-wave changes

Description

A common test for evaluating cardiac status, electrocardiography (ECG) graphically records the electric current (electrical potential) generated by the heart. This current radiates from the heart in all directions and, on reaching the skin, is measured by electrodes connected to an amplifier and strip chart recorder. The standard resting (scalar) ECG uses five electrodes to measure the electrical potential from 12 leads: the standard limb leads (I, II, III), the augmented limb leads (aV_R, aV_L, and aV_F), and the precordial, or chest, leads (V_1–V_6).

New computerized ECG machines don't routinely use gel and suction bulbs. The electrodes are small tabs that peel off a sheet and adhere to the patient's skin. The leads coming from the ECG machine are clearly marked and applied to the electrodes with alligator clamps. The entire tracing is displayed on a screen so that abnormalities (loose leads or artifact) can be corrected before the tracing is printed or transmitted to a central computer. The electrode tabs can remain on the patient's chest, arms, and legs to provide continuous lead placement for serial ECG studies.

Interfering Factors

- Improper placement of electrodes, patient movement or muscle tremors, strenuous exercise before the test, or medication reactions
- Mechanical difficulties, such as ECG machine malfunction, faulty adherence of electrode patches (e.g., because of diaphoresis), and electromagnetic interference (produces artifact)

Precautions

- The recording equipment and other nearby electrical equipment should be properly grounded to prevent electrical interference.
- Double-check color codes and lead markings to be sure connectors match.
- Make sure that the electrodes are firmly attached, and reattach them if loose skin contact is suspected. Don't use cables that are broken, frayed, or bare.
- Make sure that the patient is quiet and motionless during the test

Abnormal Electrocardiogram Waveforms

Premature ventricular contractions (PVCs) originate in an ectopic focus of the ventricular wall. They can be unifocal—having the same single focus—as shown in the electrocardiogram (ECG) tracing from lead V_1 (below), or multifocal—arising from more than one ectopic focus. In PVCs, the P wave is absent and the QRS complex shows considerable wide distortion, usually deflecting in the opposite direction from the patient's normal QRS complex. The T wave also deflects in the opposite direction from the QRS complex, and the PVC usually precedes a compensatory pause. Some examples of abnormalities causing PVCs include electrolyte imbalances (especially hypokalemia), myocardial infarction (MI), reperfusion of a new MI or injury, hypoxia, and drug toxicity (cardiac glycosides, beta-adrenergics).

PVC—Lead V_1

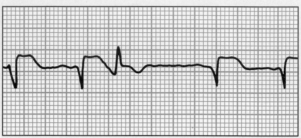

First-degree heart block, the most common conduction disturbance, occurs in healthy hearts, as well as diseased hearts, and usually is clinically insignificant. It's typically characteristic in elderly patients with chronic degeneration of the cardiac conduction system, and it occasionally occurs in patients receiving cardiac glycosides or antiarrhythmic drugs, such as procainamide and quinidine. In children, first-degree heart block may be the earliest sign of acute rheumatic fever. In the lead V_1 tracing (below), the interval between the P wave and the QRS complex (the PR interval) exceeds 0.20 second.

First-Degree Heart Block—Lead V_1

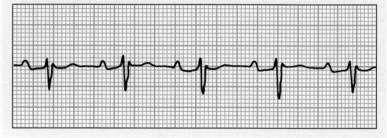

Abnormal Electrocardiogram Waveforms (continued)

Hypokalemia is a common electrolyte imbalance that's caused by low serum potassium levels, and it affects the electrical activity of the myocardium. Mild hypokalemia may cause only muscle weakness, fatigue, and, possibly, atrial or ventricular irritability; a severe imbalance causes pronounced muscle weakness, paralysis, atrial tachycardia with varying degrees of block, and PVCs that may progress to ventricular tachycardia and fibrillation.

Early signs of hypokalemia, as shown on this lead V₁ tracing, include prominent U waves, a prolonged QT interval, and flat or inverted T waves. Usually, T waves don't flatten or invert until potassium depletion becomes severe.

Hypokalemia—Lead V₁

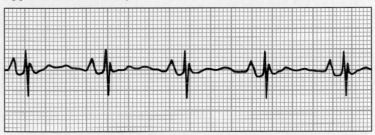

because talking and movement can distort the recordings.

- If the patient has a pacemaker in place, an ECG may be performed with or without a magnet. Indicate the presence of a pacemaker and whether a magnet is used. (Many pacemakers function only when the heartbeat falls below a preset rate; a magnet makes the pacemaker fire regularly, which permits evaluation of pacemaker performance.)

Nursing Considerations

Before the Test
- Confirm the patient's identity using two patient identifiers and confirmation of the patient's identification bracelet according to facility policy.
- Explain to the patient that an ECG evaluates the heart's electrical activity.
- Advise the patient that there are no food or fluid restrictions for this test.
- Describe the test, including who will perform it, when and where it will take place, and how long it will last.

- Tell the patient that electrodes will be attached to arms, legs, and chest and that the procedure is painless. Explain that, during the test, the patient will be asked to relax, lie still, and breathe normally.
- Advise the patient not to talk during the test because the sound of a voice may distort the ECG tracing.
- Check the patient's medication history for use of cardiac drugs and note the use of such drugs on the test request form.

During the Test
- Place the patient in a supine position. Help a patient who can't tolerate lying flat to assume semi-Fowler's position.
- Have the patient expose the chest, both ankles, and both wrists for electrode placement. If the patient is a woman, provide a chest drape until the chest leads are applied.
- Turn on the machine and check the paper supply.

Multichannel ECG

- Place electrodes on the inner aspect of the wrists, the medial aspect of the lower legs, and the chest. If using disposable electrodes, remove the paper backing before positioning.
- Connect the lead wires after all electrodes are in place.
- If frequent ECGs will be necessary, use a marking pen to indicate lead positions on the patient's chest to ensure consistent placement.
- Press the start button and record any required information (for example, the patient's name and room number).
- The machine produces a printout showing all 12 leads simultaneously. Check to make sure all leads are represented in the tracing. If not, determine which one has come loose, reattach it, and restart the tracing.
- Make sure the wave doesn't peak beyond the top edge of the recording grid. If it does, adjust the machine to bring the wave inside the boundaries.
- When the machine finishes the tracing, remove the electrodes and reposition the patient's gown and bed covers.

Single-Channel ECG

- Apply either disposable or standard electrodes to the inner aspect of the wrists and the medial aspect of the lower legs. Connect each leadwire to the corresponding electrode by inserting the wire prong into the terminal post and tightening the screw, if required.
- Set the paper speed, if required (usually 25 mm/second), and calibrate the machine by adjusting the sensitivity to normal. Recalibrate the machine after running each lead to provide a consistent test standard.

- Turn the lead selector to I. Then mark the lead by writing "I" on the paper strip or by depressing the marking button on the machine (some machines do this automatically). Record for 3 to 6 seconds and then return the machine to the standby mode. Repeat this procedure for leads II, III, aV_R, aV_L, and aV_F.
- Determine proper placement for the chest electrodes. (If frequent ECGs are necessary, mark these spots on the patient's chest to ensure consistent placement.)
- Connect the chest leadwire to the suction bulb, apply gel to each of the six chest positions, and then firmly press the suction bulb to attach the chest lead to the V_1 position. Mark the strips as before.
- Turn the lead selector to V_1 and record V_1 for 3 to 6 seconds. Return the lead selector to standby. Reposition the electrode and repeat the procedure for V_2 through V_6.
- After completing V_6, obtain a rhythm strip on lead II for at least 6 seconds. Assess the quality of the tracings and repeat any that are unclear.

After the Test

- Disconnect the equipment, remove the electrodes, and wipe the gel from the patient with a moist cloth towel. Wash the gel from the electrodes and dry them thoroughly. (If the patient is having recurrent chest pain or if serial ECGs are ordered, as with the use of thrombolytics, the electrodes are usually left in place.)
- Label each ECG strip with the patient's name and room number (if applicable), date and time of the procedure, and the health care provider's name. Note whether the ECG was performed during or on resolution of a chest pain episode.
- Report abnormal ECG findings to the health care provider.

Electrocardiography, Exercise

Normal Findings

- Minimal changes in P and T waves, QRS complexes, and ST segments
- Slight ST-segment depression (in some patients, especially women)
- Rise in heart rate in direct proportion to the workload and metabolic oxygen demand; rise in blood pressure with increased workload
- Attainment of endurance levels predicted by patient's age and the

appropriate exercise protocol (See the *Exercise ECG Tracings* box.)

Abnormal Findings

- Ischemia indicated by
  - flat or downsloping ST-segment depression of 1 mm or more for at least 0.08 second after the junction of the QRS and ST segments (J point) and a markedly depressed J point, with an upsloping but depressed ST segment of 1.5 mm below the baseline 0.08 second after the J point (Initial ST-segment

---

Exercise Electrocardiogram Tracings

These tracings are from an abnormal exercise electrocardiogram (ECG) obtained during a treadmill test performed on a patient who had just undergone a triple coronary artery bypass graft. The first tracing shows the heart at rest, with a blood pressure reading of 124/80 mm Hg. In the second tracing, the patient worked up to a 10% grade at 1.7 miles per hour before experiencing angina at 2 minutes, 25 seconds. The tracing shows a depressed ST segment; heart rate was 85 beats/minute, and blood pressure was 140/70 mm Hg. The third tracing shows the heart at rest 6 minutes after the test; blood pressure was 140/90 mm Hg.

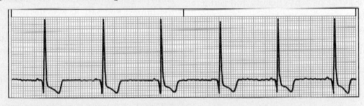

Resting Angina

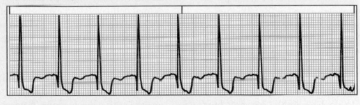

Recovery

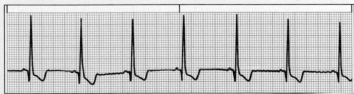

depression on the resting ECG must be further depressed by 1 mm during exercise to be considered abnormal.)
- T-wave inversion
- Multivessel or left coronary artery disease (CAD) indicated by
  - hypotension resulting from exercise
  - ST-segment depression of 3 mm or more, downsloping ST segments, and ischemic ST segments appearing within the first 3 minutes of exercise and lasting 8 minutes into the posttest recovery period
- Dyskinetic left ventricular wall motion or severe transmural ischemia (ST-segment elevation)

Nursing Implications
- Anticipate the need for additional testing.
- Keep in mind that the predictive value of this test for CAD varies with the patient's history and gender; false-negative and false-positive test results are common. This discrepancy is usually related to the effects of drugs, such as digoxin, or caffeine ingestion before testing. To detect CAD accurately, nuclear imaging and stress testing, exercise multiple-gated acquisition scanning, or coronary angiography may be necessary.
- Prepare the patient for follow-up treatment as indicated.
- Assess the patient's cardiopulmonary status closely, including vital signs, for changes.

Purpose
- To help diagnose the cause of chest pain or other possible cardiac pain
- To determine the functional capacity of the heart after surgery or a myocardial infarction (MI)
- To screen for asymptomatic CAD, particularly in men older than age 35
- To help set limitations for an exercise program

- To identify arrhythmias that develop during physical exercise
- To evaluate the effectiveness of antiarrhythmic or antianginal therapy
- To evaluate myocardial perfusion

Description

Also referred to as a *stress test*, an exercise electrocardiogram (ECG) evaluates the heart's response to physical stress, providing important diagnostic information that can't be obtained from a resting ECG alone.

An ECG and blood pressure readings are taken while the patient walks on a treadmill or pedals a stationary bicycle, and the response to a constant or an increasing workload is observed. Unless complications develop, the test continues until the patient reaches the target heart rate (determined by an established protocol) or experiences chest pain, fatigue, or sustained ventricular arrhythmias. The patient who has recently had an MI or coronary artery surgery may walk the treadmill at a slow pace to determine activity tolerance before discharge.

The usual procedure for exercise ECG is as follows:

- The electrode sites are cleaned with an alcohol swab and superficial epidermal cell layers and excess skin oils are removed with a gauze pad or fine sandpaper. After thorough cleaning and abrading, adequately prepared sites will appear slightly red.
- Chest electrodes are placed according to the lead system selected and are secured with adhesive tape, if necessary. The leadwire cable is placed over the patient's shoulder, and the leadwire box is placed on the chest. The cable is secured by pinning it to the patient's clothing or taping it to the shoulder or back. Then the leadwires are connected to the chest electrodes.

- The monitor is started, and a stable baseline tracing is obtained and checked for arrhythmias. A blood pressure reading is taken, and the patient is auscultated for the presence of third or fourth heart sounds (S₃ or S₄ gallops) and crackles.

- With a treadmill test, the treadmill is turned on to a slow speed, and the patient is shown how to step onto it and how to use the support railings to maintain balance but not support weight. Then the treadmill is turned off. The patient is instructed to step onto the treadmill; it will be turned on to slow speed until the patient gets used to walking on it. Exercise intensity is then increased every 3 minutes by slightly increasing the speed of the machine and, at the same time, increasing the incline by 3%.

- For a bicycle ergometer test, the patient is instructed to sit on the bicycle while the seat and handlebars are adjusted to comfortable positions. Instruct the patient not to grip the handlebars tightly, but to use them only for maintaining balance and to pedal until the desired speed is reached, as shown on the speedometer.

- In both tests, a monitor is observed continuously for changes in the heart's electrical activity. The rhythm strip is checked at preset intervals for arrhythmias, premature ventricular contractions (PVCs), and ST-segment and T-wave changes. The test level and the time elapsed in the test level are marked on each strip. Blood pressure is monitored at predetermined intervals, usually at the end of each test level, and changes in systolic readings are noted. Some common responses to maximal exercise include dizziness, lightheadedness, leg fatigue, dyspnea, diaphoresis, and a slightly ataxic gait. If symptoms become severe, the test is stopped.

▶ *Quality and Safety Nursing Alert*

The test is stopped if the ECG shows frequent PVCs or a significant increase in ectopy, if the systolic blood pressure falls below resting level, if the heart rate falls to 10 beats/minute below resting level, or if the patient becomes exhausted. Depending on the patient's condition, the test may also be stopped if the ECG shows evidence of bundle-branch block, ST-segment depression that exceeds 1.5 mm, persistent ST-segment elevation, or frequent or complicated PVCs; if blood pressure fails to rise above the resting level; if systolic pressure exceeds 220 mm Hg; or if the patient experiences angina.

- Usually, testing stops when the patient reaches the target heart rate. As the treadmill speed slows, the patient may be instructed to continue walking for several minutes to cool down. Then the treadmill is turned off, the patient is helped to a chair, and the blood pressure and ECG are monitored for 5 to 10 minutes or until the ECG returns to baseline.

Interfering Factors

- The patient's inability to exercise to the target heart rate because of fatigue or failure to cooperate
- Wolff-Parkinson-White's syndrome (anomalous atrioventricular excitation), electrolyte imbalance, or use of a cardiac glycoside (possible false positive)
- Conditions that affect left ventricular hypertrophy, such as congenital abnormalities and hypertension (possible interference with testing for ischemia)
- Beta-adrenergic blockers (may make test results difficult to interpret)

Precautions

- Keep in mind that because an exercise ECG places considerable stress on the heart, it may be contraindicated in the patient with ventricular aneurysm, dissecting aortic aneurysm, uncontrolled arrhythmias, pericarditis, myocarditis, severe anemia, uncontrolled hypertension, unstable angina, or heart failure.

Nursing Considerations

Before the Test

- Confirm the patient's identity using two patient identifiers and confirmation of the patient's identification bracelet according to facility policy.
- Explain to the patient that the exercise ECG records the heart's electrical activity and performance under stress.
- Instruct the patient not to eat, smoke, or drink alcoholic or caffeinated beverages for 3 hours before the test, but to continue taking the prescribed drug regimen unless directed otherwise.
- Describe to the patient who will perform the test, when and where it will take place, and how long it will last.
- Explain that the test will cause fatigue and that the patient will be slightly breathless and sweaty, but that the test poses few risks. The patient may, in fact, stop the test if fatigue or chest pain is experienced.
- Advise the patient to wear comfortable socks and shoes and loose, lightweight shorts or slacks. (Men usually don't wear a shirt during the test, and women generally wear a bra and a lightweight short-sleeved blouse or a patient gown with a front closure.)
- Explain to the patient that electrodes will be attached to several areas on the chest and, possibly, the back after the skin areas are cleaned and abraded. Explain that the patient won't feel current from the electrodes; however, they may itch slightly.
- Tell the patient that blood pressure will be checked periodically throughout the procedure and that the heart rate and ECG will be monitored continuously.

- If the patient is scheduled for a multistage treadmill test, explain that the speed and incline of the treadmill will increase at predetermined intervals and that the patient will be informed of each adjustment.
- If the patient is scheduled for a bicycle ergometer test, explain that the resistance experienced in pedaling increases gradually as a specific speed is maintained.
- Encourage the patient to report any feelings during the test. Explain that blood pressure and ECG will be monitored for 5 to 10 minutes after the test.
- Check the patient's history for a recent physical examination (within 1 week) and for baseline 12-lead ECG results.
- Make sure that the patient or a responsible family member has signed an informed consent form.

After the Test

- Remove the electrodes and clean the electrode sites before the patient leaves.
- Auscultate for the presence of an S_3 or S_4 gallop. An S_4 gallop commonly develops after exercise because of increased blood flow volume and turbulence. An S_3 gallop is more significant than an S_4 gallop, indicating transient left ventricular dysfunction.
- Instruct the patient to resume any activities and medications discontinued before the test, as ordered.

Electrocardiography, Signal-Averaged

Normal Findings

- QRS complexes lacking low potentials

Abnormal Findings

- Late potentials after the QRS complex, indicating ventricular arrhythmias

Nursing Implications

- Anticipate the need for additional testing, and prepare the patient for follow-up treatment as indicated.
- Assess the patient's cardiopulmonary status closely, including vital signs, for changes.

Purpose

- To detect destructive signals (late potentials) that may represent delayed, disorganized activity in patients who have survived an acute myocardial infarction
- To evaluate the risk of life-threatening arrhythmias

Description

Signal-averaged electrocardiography (ECG) amplifies, averages, and filters an ECG signal recorded on the body surface. It detects high-frequency, low-amplitude cardiac electrical signals in the last part of the QRS complex and in the ST segment. During this computerized procedure, each electrode lead's input is amplified, its voltage is measured or sampled at intervals of 1 msec or less, and each sample is converted into a digital number. Essentially, the ECG is a computer-readable ECG of 100 or more QRS complexes.

The usual procedure for this test is as follows:

- The patient is placed in the supine position (or the semi-Fowler's position, if the patient can't tolerate lying supine).
- Electrodes are attached to the patient's chest, ankles, and wrists.
- Multiple inputs are obtained from standard orthogonal bipolar X, Y, and Z leads over a series of ECG cycles.
- The average is taken over a large number of beats, typically 100 or more.

Interfering Factors

- Antiarrhythmic use
- Poor tissue–electrode contact (produces an artifact)
- Electromagnetic interferences

Precautions

- Recording equipment and other nearby electrical equipment should be properly grounded to prevent electrical interference.

Nursing Considerations

Before the Test

- Confirm the patient's identity using two patient identifiers and confirmation of the patient's identification bracelet according to facility policy.
- Make sure the patient has signed an appropriate consent form.
- Note and report all allergies and response to allergens.
- Record the use of antiarrhythmics on the patient's chart.
- Advise the patient that electrodes will be attached to the arms, legs, and chest and that the procedure is painless.
- Instruct the patient to lie still and breathe normally during the procedure.
- Explain that the test takes about 30 minutes and that there's no need to restrict food and fluids before the test.

After the Test

- Wash the conductive gel from the patient's skin and be sure that all electrodes have been removed.

Electroencephalography

Normal Findings

- Alpha waves occurring at a frequency of 8 to 11 cycles/second in a regular rhythm and present only in the waking state when the patient's eyes are closed, but mentally alert; usually disappearing with visual activity or mental concentration
- Beta waves (13–30 cycles/second), generally associated with anxiety, depression, and use of sedatives; seen most readily in the frontal and central regions of the brain

Comparing Electrocardiogram Tracings

The following tracings are examples of regular and irregular brain electrical activity as recorded by an EEG.

Normal (top, right temporal; bottom, parietal-occipital)

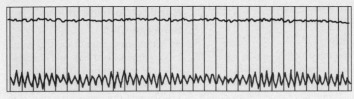

Absence Seizures (spikes and waves, 3/second)

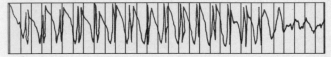

Generalized Tonic-Clonic Seizures (multiple high-voltage spiked waves)

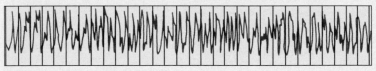

Right Temporal Lobe Epilepsy (focal spiked waves)

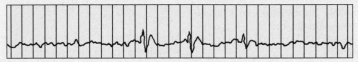

- Theta waves (4–7 cycles/second); most commonly found in children and young adults and appearing in the frontal and temporal regions
- Delta waves (0.5–3.5 cycles/second); normally occurring only in young children and during sleep (See the *Comparing EEG Tracings* box.)

Abnormal Findings
- Spikes and waves at a frequency of 3 cycles/second, indicating absence seizures
- Multiple, high-voltage, spiked waves in both hemispheres, indicating generalized tonic–clonic seizures

- Spiked waves in the affected temporal region, indicating temporal lobe epilepsy
- Localized, spiked discharges, indicating focal seizures
- Delta waves, but possibly unilateral beta waves, indicating intracranial lesions, such as a tumor or an abscess
- Focal abnormalities in the injured area, indicating vascular lesions, such as cerebral infarcts and intracranial hemorrhages
- Absence of electroencephalogram (EEG) pattern—a "flat" tracing, except for artifact, indicating brain death

Nursing Implications

- Anticipate the need for additional testing.
- Be aware that any condition that causes a diminishing level of consciousness alters the EEG pattern in proportion to the degree of consciousness lost. For example, in a patient with a metabolic disorder, an inflammatory process (such as meningitis or encephalitis), or increased intracranial pressure, the EEG shows generalized, diffuse, and slow brain waves.
- Assess the patient's neurologic status and report any changes.
- Prepare the patient for follow-up treatment as indicated.
- Provide emotional support to the patient and family.

Purpose

- To determine the presence and type of seizure disorder
- To help diagnose intracranial lesions, such as abscesses and tumors
- To evaluate the brain's electrical activity in metabolic disease, cerebral ischemia, head injury, meningitis, encephalitis, mental retardation, psychological disorders, and drugs
- To evaluate altered states of consciousness or brain death

Description

In EEG, electrodes attached to the patient's scalp record the brain's electrical activity and transmit this information to an EEG, which records the resulting brain waves on recording paper. The procedure may be performed in a special laboratory or by a portable unit at the bedside. Ambulatory recording EEGs are available for the patient to wear at home or the workplace to record the patient performing normal daily activities. Continuous-video EEG recording is available on an inpatient basis for identifying epileptic discharges during clinical events or for localization of a seizure focus during surgical evaluation of epi-

lepsy. Intracranial electrodes are surgically implanted to record EEG changes for localization of the seizure focus.

The usual procedure for conducting an EEG is as follows:

- After the patient is positioned, electrodes are attached to the scalp.
- During the recording, the patient is observed carefully; blinking, swallowing, talking, or other movements are noted and recorded on the tracing. (These activities may cause artifact on the tracing and be misinterpreted as an abnormal tracing.) The recording may be stopped at intervals to let the patient rest or reposition. (This is important because restlessness and fatigue can alter brain wave patterns.)
- After an initial baseline recording, the patient may be tested under various stress-producing conditions to elicit patterns not observable while at rest. For example, the patient may be asked to breathe deeply and rapidly for 3 minutes (hyperventilation), which may elicit brain wave patterns typical of seizure disorders or other abnormalities. This technique is commonly used to detect absence seizures. Also, photic stimulation tests may elicit central cerebral activity in response to bright light, accentuating abnormal activity in absence or myoclonic seizures. In this procedure, a strobe light placed in front of the patient is flashed 1 to 20 times/second; recordings are made with the patient's eyes opened and closed.

Interfering Factors

- Interference from extraneous electrical activity; head, body, eye, or tongue movement; or muscle contractions (possible production of excessive artifact)
- Anticonvulsants, barbiturates, tranquilizers, and other sedatives (possible masking of seizure activity)
- Acute drug intoxication or severe hypothermia, resulting in loss of consciousness (flat EEG)

E

Nursing Considerations

Before the Test

- Explain to the patient that the EEG records the brain's electrical activity and measures how well and how fast a nerve carries a stimulus. Explain that the test takes approximately 15 minutes.
- Describe the procedure to the patient and family members, and answer all their questions.
- Instruct the patient to avoid caffeine before the test; other than this, there are no food or fluid restrictions. Tell the patient to eat before the test, because skipping a meal before the test can cause relative hypoglycemia and alter the brain wave pattern.
- Inform the patient that smoking is prohibited for at least 8 hours before the test.
- Thoroughly wash and dry the patient's hair to remove hair sprays, creams, and oils.
- Explain that, during the test, the patient will relax in a reclining chair or lie on a bed and that electrodes will be attached to the scalp with a special paste. Assure the patient that the electrodes won't cause a shock.

► *Quality and Safety Nursing Alert*

Check the patient for a history of asthma. The electrode paste has a distinctive odor that may precipitate an asthmatic reaction.

- If needle electrodes are used, explain that the patient will feel a pricking sensation as they're inserted; however, flat electrodes are more commonly used.
- Do your best to allay the patient's fears because nervousness can affect brain wave patterns.
- Check the patient's medication history for drugs that may interfere with test results. Anticonvulsants,

tranquilizers, barbiturates, and other sedatives should be withheld for 24 to 48 hours before the test, as ordered by the health care provider.

► *Quality and Safety Nursing Alert*

Infants and very young children occasionally require sedation to prevent crying and restlessness during the test, but sedation itself may alter test results.

- If a patient with a seizure disorder requires a "sleep EEG," keep the patient awake the night before the test and administer a sedative (such as chloral hydrate) to help the patient sleep during the test.
- Before the recording procedure begins, instruct the patient to close the eyes, relax, and remain still.
- If the test is performed to confirm brain death, provide the patient's family members with emotional support.

After the Test

- Help the patient remove the electrode paste from the hair.
- If the patient received a sedative before the test, take safety precautions, such as raising the bed's side rails.

► *Quality and Safety Nursing Alert*

Observe the patient carefully for seizure activity. If seizure activity occurs, record seizure patterns and be prepared to provide assistance. Have suction equipment readily available.

- Carefully review the reinstatement of anticonvulsant medication or other drugs withheld before the test.
- If brain death is confirmed, provide the patient's family members with emotional support.
- If clinical events are found to be nonepileptic, a psychological evaluation may be needed.

Electromyography

Normal Findings

- At rest, a normal muscle exhibiting minimal electrical activity
- During voluntary contraction, markedly increased electrical activity
- Sustained contraction or one of increasing strength causing a rapid "train" of motor unit potentials (heard as a crescendo of sounds over the audio amplifier)
- Sequence of waveforms that vary in amplitude (height) and frequency (waveforms close together indicating a high frequency; waveforms far apart signifying a low frequency)

Abnormal Findings

- Short (low-amplitude) motor unit potentials with frequent, irregular discharges, indicating primary muscle diseases such as muscular dystrophy
- Isolated and irregular motor unit potentials with increased amplitude and duration, indicating amyotrophic lateral sclerosis (ALS) and peripheral nerve disorders
- Normal motor unit potentials that diminish in amplitude with continuing contractions, indicating myasthenia gravis

Nursing Implications

- Anticipate the need for additional testing.
- Be aware of the need to distinguish between waveforms that indicate a muscle disorder and those that indicate denervation. Findings must be correlated with the patient's history, clinical features, and the results of other neurodiagnostic testing.
- Assess the patient's neurologic and neuromuscular functioning.
- Prepare the patient for follow-up treatment as indicated.
- Provide emotional support to the patient and family.

Purpose

- To aid in differentiating between primary muscle disorders, such as the muscular dystrophies, and secondary disorders
- To help assess diseases characterized by central neuronal degeneration such as ALS
- To help diagnose neuromuscular disorders such as myasthenia gravis
- To help diagnose radiculopathies

Description

Electromyography (EMG) records the electrical activity of selected skeletal muscle groups at rest and during voluntary contraction. It involves percutaneous insertion of a needle electrode into a muscle. The electrical discharge of the muscle is then measured by an oscilloscope. Nerve conduction time is typically measured simultaneously.

The usual procedure for EMG is as follows:

- The patient is positioned in a manner that relaxes the muscles to be tested.
- The skin is cleaned with alcohol, the needle electrodes are quickly inserted, and a metal plate is placed under the patient to serve as a reference electrode. Then the muscle's electrical signal (motor unit potential), recorded during rest and contraction, is amplified 1 million times and displayed on an oscilloscope or a computer screen.
- The recorder leadwires are attached to an audio amplifier so that the fluctuation of voltage within the muscle can be heard.

Interfering Factors

- The patient's inability to comply with instructions
- Drugs affecting myoneural junctions, such as anticholinergics, cholinergics, and skeletal muscle relaxants

Precautions

- EMG is contraindicated in the patient with a bleeding disorder.

Nursing Considerations
Before the Test
- Confirm the patient's identity using two patient identifiers and confirmation of the patient's identification bracelet according to facilitya policy.
- Explain to the patient that EMG measures the electrical activity of the muscles. Describe the test, including who will perform it and when and where it will take place.
- Inform the patient that there are usually no restrictions on food and fluids. (In some cases, cigarettes, coffee, tea, and cola may be restricted for 2 to 3 hours before the test.)
- Explain that the patient may wear a gown or comfortable clothing that permits access to the muscles to be tested.
- Advise the patient that a needle will be inserted into selected muscles and discomfort may be experienced. Reassure that adverse effects and complications are rare.
- Make sure that the patient or a responsible family member has signed an informed consent form, if required.
- Check the patient's history for medications that may interfere with the test results—for example, cholinergics, anticholinergics, and skeletal muscle relaxants. If the patient is receiving such medications, note this on the chart and withhold medications as ordered.

After the Test
- Assess the patient's pain level. If the patient experiences residual pain, apply warm compresses and administer prescribed analgesics.
- Tell the patient to resume usual medications as ordered.
- Monitor the patient for signs and symptoms of infection at the needle electrode sites.

Electroneurography
Normal Findings
- Conduction velocity of approximately 50 to 60 m/second

Abnormal Findings
- Slowed conduction time, indicating peripheral nerve disorders or injuries

Nursing Implications
- Anticipate the need for additional testing; keep in mind that electroneurography is commonly performed with electromyography (EMG).
- Prepare the patient for follow-up treatment as indicated.
- Provide emotional support to the patient and family.

Purpose
- To identify peripheral nerve injury or peripheral nerve disorders

Description
Electroneurography, also called *nerve conduction studies*, helps diagnose peripheral nerve injuries and diseases affecting the peripheral nervous system, such as peripheral neuropathies. During testing, a nerve is electrically stimulated through the skin and underlying tissues. The patient experiences a mild electric shock with each stimulation. At a known distance from the point of stimulation, a recording electrode detects the response from the stimulated nerve. The time is measured, and the speed of conduction is calculated.

Testing usually occurs as follows:

- The patient is positioned to allow relaxation of the area being tested.
- Paste or a gel is applied to the surface of the electrode, and the electrode is then placed firmly in the area over the specified nerve. A reference electrode is applied to a nearby area.
- An electrical current is passed through to the area, causing a mild electrical shock, such as that from static electricity.
- At a known distance from the point of stimulation, a recording electrode

detects the response from the stimulated nerve. The time between stimulation of the nerve and the detected response is measured on an oscilloscope. The speed of conduction along the nerve is then calculated by dividing the distance between the point of stimulation and the recording electrode by the time between stimulus and response.

Interfering Factors
- Primary muscle disorders (false-positive results, slowed conduction velocity)

 Quality and Safety Nursing Alert

Conduction velocity commonly decreases with increasing age. It also varies from one person to another and from one nerve to another.

- Pain (false-positive results)
- Patient movement (false-positive results)
- Edema, hemorrhage, or thick subcutaneous fat (ineffective results)
- Drugs that affect myoneural junctions, such as cholinergics, anticholinergics, and skeletal muscle relaxants

Precautions
- When performed with EMG, this test is contraindicated in the patient with a bleeding disorder.

Nursing Considerations
Before the Test
- Confirm the patient's identity using two patient identifiers and confirmation of the patient's identification bracelet according to facility policy.
- Explain to the patient that the test measures how well and how fast a nerve carries a stimulus and that it takes approximately 15 minutes.
- Describe the test, including who will perform it and when and where it will take place.

- Inform the patient that there are usually no food or fluid restrictions for this test.
- Explain that the patient may wear a gown or comfortable clothing that permits access to the area to be tested.
- Advise the patient that the test involves the use of an electrical stimulus and that some discomfort may be experienced. Describe the sensation as that of a static electricity shock.
- Make sure that the patient or a responsible family member has signed an informed consent form, if required.
- Check the patient's history for medications that may interfere with the results of the test—for example, cholinergics, anticholinergics, and skeletal muscle relaxants. If the patient is receiving such medications, note this on the chart and withhold medications as ordered.

After the Test
- Help the patient remove any electrode paste or gel used.
- Assess the patient's pain level. If the patient experiences residual pain, apply warm compresses and administer prescribed analgesics.
- Instruct the patient to resume usual medications as ordered.

Electronystagmography and Video Nystagmography

Normal Findings
- See the *Results of Electronystagmography and Video Nystagmography* table.

Abnormal Findings
- Prolonged nystagmus after a head turn or nystagmus occurring when the patient isn't turning the head
- A peripheral lesion involving the end organ or the vestibular branch of the eighth cranial nerve, such as from Ménière's disease, multiple sclerosis, ischemic damage to the cochlea, autoimmune disease, and vestibular ototoxicity and eighth-nerve tumors.

(text continues on page 256)

Results of Electronystagmography and Video Nystagmography

Test and Abnormal Findings	Abnormal Findings	Unusual Underlying Conditions
Saccadic Pursuit Testing		
Square-wave patterns of differing amplitudes mimicking the target; minimal latency and good accuracy of eye movements	*Ocular dysmetria:* significant undershoots, overshoots, glissades, or pulsion; reduced eye velocity, accuracy, prolonged latency	Central nervous system (CNS) pathology: possible involvement of brainstem, cerebellum, or cortex Nonlocalizing: possible spontaneous or gaze nystagmus
Gaze Testing		
No nystagmus with eyes open; weak or no nystagmus with eyes closed	Spontaneous nystagmus: significant amount noted when eyes are closed or when tested in complete darkness under goggles while gazing forward	Nonlocalizing abnormality of the vestibular system: in acute peripheral disorders, it's horizontal and initially beats away from the affected ear; if present with eyes open, viewing a target, or if it changes direction, it's consistent with CNS involvement
	Gaze nystagmus: presence of nystagmus only when the eyes are deviated from midline	Generally consistent with CNS involvement: the patient with spontaneous nystagmus caused by peripheral lesions has stronger nystagmus when looking in the direction of the nystagmus fast phase
	Upbeating nystagmus: upward deviation of eye movement	Cerebellar or brain stem involvement
	Down-beating nystagmus: downward deviation of eye movement	Cerebellar or cervicomedullary junction involvement
	Rotary nystagmus: not classic benign paroxysmal positional vertigo (BPPV)	Brainstem or vestibular nuclei
Positional Testing (head in position)		
Eyes open, no nystagmus; eyes closed or wearing light-excluding goggles, no more than weak nystagmus in one or more positions	*Nystagmus:* either changes direction across positions or positioning or remains in the same direction, but isn't spontaneous	Nonlocalizing: suppression with visual fixation suggests peripheral involvement; enhancement of nystagmus or failure to suppress with visual fixation suggesting central etiology

E

Test and Abnormal Findings	Abnormal Findings	Unusual Underlying Conditions
Positioning Testing (head in movement toward the position)		
Eyes open, no nystagmus; eyes closed or wearing light-excluding goggles, no more than weak nystagmus in one or more positions	*Transient, fatigable torsional Dix-Hallpike procedure eye movement:* during Dix-Hallpike procedure, occurring in concert with subjective dizziness	BPPV: responding well to repositioning maneuvers
Smooth Pursuit Tracking		
Volitional smooth tracking of the target, accuracy within age norms	*Sinusoidal tracking:* with superimposed nystagmus	Nonlocalizing: possible spontaneous or gaze nystagmus
	Break-up in tracings or saccades: jerking rather than smooth movements; reduced velocity, accuracy, prolonged latency that isn't accounted for by advanced age or poor cooperation	CNS involvement if peripheral vision problems ruled out
Optokinetic Testing		
Eye movement follows stimulus at speeds up to 30 degrees per second; clear triangular wave pattern; similar pattern for stimuli traveling in both directions	*Significant asymmetry:* not explained by spontaneous or gaze nystagmus	CNS involvement
	Reduced eye velocity: when compared to age-appropriate norms	CNS involvement if peripheral vision problems ruled out
Caloric Testing		
Eyes closed, nystagmus occurring in all conditions; suppressed by visual fixation with cold stimuli, nystagmus beats to opposite ear; with warm stimuli, it beats to same ear (To help recall this phenomenon, use the acronym COWS—Cold, Opposite, Warm, Same.)	*Unilateral weakness:* greater than 20% to 30% difference in maximum low-phase velocities (averaged across temperatures) between ears	Peripheral lesion of weaker side
	Bilateral weakness: slow-phase velocity of the sum of the four caloric irrigations is reduced, typically below 20 degrees (average of each irrigation ≤5 degrees/second)	Bilateral peripheral or CNS involvement
	Directional preponderance: more than 30% difference in maximum slow-phase velocities for right- versus left-beating nystagmus	Nonlocalizing, usually resulting from underlying spontaneous nystagmus
	Failure to suppress fixation: visual fixation fails to reduce nystagmus by at least 40%	CNS involvement

- A central lesion involving the brain stem, cerebellum, cerebrum, or any of the connecting structures, such as from demyelinating diseases, tumors, or circulatory disorders

Nursing Implications
- Anticipate the need for additional testing and prepare the patient for follow-up treatment as indicated.
- Monitor the patient for complaints of dizziness or imbalance. Institute safety precautions as necessary.
- Provide emotional support to the patient and family.

Purpose
- To help identify the cause of dizziness and vertigo
- To confirm the presence and location (central or oculomotor, peripheral, or both) of a lesion
- To assess neurologic disorders

Description
In electronystagmography (ENG) testing and video nystagmography (VNG) testing, eye movements in response to specific stimuli are recorded and used to evaluate the interactions of the vestibular system and the muscles controlling eye movement in what's known as the *vestibulo-ocular reflex*. Nystagmus, the involuntary back-and-forth eye movements caused by this reflex, results from the vestibular system's attempts to maintain visual function during head movement. When the patient turns the head in one direction, the eyes deviate slowly in the opposite direction; on reaching their deviation limit, they quickly return to the center. If the head continues to turn, the pattern of eye movement continues.

Traditional ENG records nystagmus through electrodes that pick up corneoretinal potential and chart it. VNG records eye movements with an infrared camera. Both tests are performed by an audiologist and help determine whether the disorder originates in the peripheral or central nervous system. (See the *ENG Eye Movements* box.)

Electronystagmography Eye Movements

Traditional electronystagmography (ENG) involves the placement of electrodes above and below (vertical channel), and at the inner and outer canthi (horizontal channel), of one or both of the patient's eyes. Video nystagmography records the patient's eye movements optically. Both systems trace eye movement over time. The horizontal and vertical eye movements over time are shown separately here. The top illustration depicts a right-beating nystagmus, and the bottom illustration shows an upbeating nystagmus. The direction of the more rapid portion of the nystagmus determines the labeled direction.

Horizontal Channel

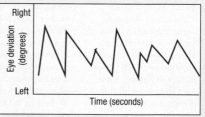

Vertical Channel

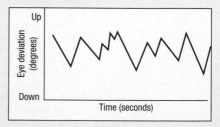

Testing involves setting up the device and connecting light bars to the equipment. The patient is positioned a calibrated distance from the light source and is asked to follow the movement of the lights using eye movement only. The eye movements are recorded and graphed. Procedures for specific tests are as follows:

Saccade Testing

- The patient is asked to watch the movement of a dot on the light bar. The dot position will move varying amounts, which correspond to eye deviations in degrees.
- The accuracy and velocity of the eye tracking the rapidly moving light are measured. The traces are analyzed to determine whether there's symmetrical (right versus left and up versus down) eye movement or dysmetria, such as excessive overshoot or undershoot. Glissades, a slowing of the eye movement as it approaches a target, is also ruled out.

Gaze Nystagmus Testing

- The patient is asked to look at the light on the light bar and hold a steady gaze. Gaze is directed left, right, up, and down.
- The patient is also asked to close the eyes and retain the gaze direction in traditional ENG testing.
- When VNG recordings are made, the goggles exclude light and the recordings are made with the eyes open. Nystagmus shouldn't occur with the patient's eyes open while the patient fixates on the target and should be minimal with eyes closed or when goggles exclude light.

Smooth Pursuit (Sinusoidal) Tracking Testing

- The patient watches the dot on the light bar as it moves smoothly back and forth at varying rates.
- The eye movement is observed to determine whether the patient can track the target accurately.

- Tracings are analyzed for left-right symmetry and "smoothness" of the eye's tracking (pursuit) of the target.

Optokinetics Testing

- The patient is instructed to look at the light bar as a series of dots move across the screen, first in one direction (for example, right to left) and then in the other.
- The patient's eyes rapidly move back to center and track another dot. This movement creates a tracing that looks like nystagmus: The patient follows a dot for a brief period; the eyes rapidly move back to center and track another moving dot. This test assesses the ability of the central nervous system (CNS) to control rapid eye movement and is affected by an existing nystagmus.

Positional and Positioning Testing

- The patient's eye movements are recorded as he's moved into various body positions and asked to remain in these positions. Recordings note whether nystagmus is present; if so, the positions eliciting the nystagmus are noted as having diagnostic significance.
- In the Dix-Hallpike test, diagnostic for benign paroxysmal positional vertigo (BPPV), the patient is initially seated. He's then rapidly moved into a supine, head-hanging position, with the head deviated to the side and then returned to a sitting position.
- If torsional eye movements are observed, time-locked to the subjective report of dizziness, the findings are positive for BPPV. The test is repeated to establish fatigability, also classic in BPPV. The direction of the rotational eye movement helps diagnose which semicircular canal is involved and helps establish the appropriate BPPV repositioning treatment.

Caloric Testing

- The patient lies supine with the head elevated 30 degrees so that the horizontal semicircular canals are perpendicular to the floor.

- The patient's ear is irrigated with water or air (depending on the system used) for about 60 seconds per irrigation. Four irrigations are completed (both warm and cold irrigations are used for each ear).

- Heating and cooling the outer ear causes a change in temperature of the middle ear. The horizontal semicircular canal is located behind the medial wall of the middle ear. The fluid in the semicircular canal moves when the temperature of the fluid is changed, eliciting nystagmus. Thus, for caloric testing, nystagmus is normal.

- The patient is instructed to open the eyes during one portion of each recording. Visual fixation reduces nystagmus if the CNS is normal.

- The symmetry of the nystagmus elicited by irrigation of each ear is assessed. The different temperatures produce different directions of nystagmus. The symmetry of the left-beating nystagmus and the right-beating nystagmus is analyzed.

- If the patient fails to respond to standard caloric stimulation, ice calorics may be used. A small quantity of ice water or very cold air is introduced into the ear canal to determine whether there's residual functioning of that ear's vestibular system.

Interfering Factors

- Alcoholic beverages, antihistamines, antivertigo agents, opioids, sleep medications, tranquilizers, and other medications that can create dizziness (including certain aminoglycoside antibiotics, antidepressants, diuretics, salicylates, and stimulants)
- Poor eyesight or extraocular muscle weakness
- Drowsiness and reduced alertness
- Poor patient cooperation

Precautions

- If the patient has a back or neck condition that could be aggravated by rapid changes in position, check with the health care provider to determine whether any of the positional tests should be omitted.

- Be aware that water caloric testing can't be safely used if the patient has a perforated tympanic membrane. Also, air caloric test results won't be accurate.

- The patient will be closely monitored by the audiologist and advised to remain in a position that reduces dizziness if it occurs after the procedure.

Nursing Considerations

Before the Test

- Confirm the patient's identity using two patient identifiers and confirmation of the patient's identification bracelet according to facility policy.

- Make sure that the patient's ear canals are free from cerumen before referring for ENG testing. The caloric testing portion of the ENG can't be conducted safely or accurately if there is cerumen accumulation or a tympanic membrane perforation.

- Inform the patient that tympanometry will be conducted before caloric testing to ensure tympanic membrane integrity.

- Explain to the patient the dizziness problems will be assessed by recording eye movements and that testing will take about 40 to 45 minutes to complete.

- Reassure the patient that the test isn't painful, but some portions may cause dizziness, so someone will be present to ensure that the patient doesn't fall. Because of the risk of dizziness, advise the patient not to eat or drink for 3 to 4 hours before the test.

- Suggest that someone accompany the patient to the evaluation because some patients don't feel well enough to drive after the appointment. Avoid overemphasizing the risk of discomfort because patient anxiety increases the risk of nausea and vomiting during the procedure.

• Encourage the patient to wear comfortable clothing.

• If testing involves traditional ENG with attachment of recording electrodes, inform the patient that the skin will need to be cleaned, so ideally makeup or facial creams shouldn't be used on the day of the test. VNG testing is compromised by mascara, so a woman should refrain from wearing makeup on the day of the test.

• Instruct the patient to refrain from smoking or drinking caffeinated beverages the day of the test and to avoid taking nonessential medications for 48 hours before the test, as ordered.

• Ask the patient to bring a list of medications to the evaluation. Warn the patient not take these agents for 48 hours before the test, as ordered, because they prevent accurate collection and interpretation of the results.

• Alert the health care facility performing the test if the patient has a history of back or neck problems that could be exacerbated by head or neck movement.

• The patient who wears glasses should bring them to the test. The patient who wears contact lenses should bring eyeglasses to the examination, if possible.

• Tell the patient that the audiologist will ask for a description of the dizziness, including when it began. Advise the patient to think about what situations create the dizziness or make it worse. Also, determine the progression of the patient's symptoms by asking the patient to think about words other than dizzy that might describe the dizziness.

After the Test
• Instruct the patient not to drive until all symptoms of imbalance have subsided.

• Instruct the patient to resume a usual diet.

Electrophysiology Studies
Normal Findings
• HV interval (conduction time from the bundle of His to the Purkinje fibers), 35 to 55 msec
• AH (atrioventricular nodal) interval, 45 to 150 msec
• PA (intra-atrial) interval, 20 to 40 msec

Abnormal Findings
• Prolonged HV interval, indicating acute or chronic disease
• AH interval delays, indicating atrial pacing, chronic conduction system disease, carotid sinus pressure, recent myocardial infarction, or drug use
• PA interval delays, indicating acquired, surgically induced, or congenital atrial disease and atrial pacing

Nursing Implications
• Anticipate the need for additional testing.
• Prepare the patient for follow-up treatment, such as antiarrhythmic therapy, as indicated.
• Continue to monitor the patient's cardiac status, including heart rate and rhythm; institute continuous cardiac monitoring, if ordered.
• Provide emotional support to the patient and family.

Purpose
• To diagnose arrhythmias and conduction anomalies
• To determine the need for an implanted pacemaker, an internal cardioverter–defibrillator, and cardioactive drugs and to evaluate their effects on the conduction system and ectopic rhythms
• To locate the site of a bundle-branch block, especially in an asymptomatic patient with conduction disturbances
• To determine the presence and location of accessory conducting structures

Description

Electrophysiology studies (also known as *bundle of His electrography*) permit measurement of discrete conduction intervals by recording electrical conduction during the slow withdrawal of a bipolar or tripolar electrode catheter from the right ventricle through the bundle of His to the sinoatrial node. The catheter is introduced into the femoral vein, passing through the right atrium and across the septal leaflet of the tricuspid valve.

Testing usually proceeds as follows:

- The patient is positioned supine on a special table and limb electrodes and precordial leads are applied for continuous monitoring. If not already in place, an IV line is started and dextrose 5% in water or normal saline solution is administered at a keep-vein-open rate.
- After a local anesthetic is injected at the catheterization site or the patient is placed under moderate sedation, a small incision or percutaneous puncture is made and a J-tip electrode is introduced IV into the femoral vein (or into the antecubital fossa). The catheter is guided to the cardiac chambers using fluoroscopy. It's advanced until it crosses the tricuspid valve and enters the right ventricle. Then the catheter is slowly withdrawn from the tricuspid area and recordings of conduction intervals are made from each pole of the catheter, either simultaneously or sequentially.
- The patient's vital signs are monitored frequently during the test, and any drop in blood pressure during an arrhythmia is noted.
- The catheter is removed, and a pressure dressing is applied after completion of the procedure.

Interfering Factors

- Malfunctioning recording equipment
- Improper catheter positioning

Precautions

- Electrophysiology studies are contraindicated in the patient with severe coagulopathy, recent thrombophlebitis, or acute pulmonary embolism.

Nursing Considerations

Before the Test

- Confirm the patient's identity using two patient identifiers and confirmation of the patient's identification bracelet according to facility policy.
- Explain to the patient that electrophysiology studies help to evaluate the heart's conduction system.
- Instruct the patient not to eat or drink anything for 3 to 6 hours before the test.
- Describe the test, including who will perform it and when and where it will take place.
- Inform the patient that after the hair in the groin area is clipped, a catheter will be inserted into the femoral vein and an IV line may be started. Assure that the electrocardiography electrodes attached to the chest during the test will cause no discomfort.
- Explain to the patient that a stinging sensation when a local anesthetic is injected to numb the incision site for catheter insertion may be felt and that pressure on catheter insertion may be experienced.
- Explain that the patient will be conscious but sedated during the test and should report any discomfort or pain.
- Make sure that the patient or a responsible family member has signed an informed consent form.
- Check the patient's history, and inform the health care provider of any ongoing drug therapy or the use of aspirin or other anticoagulants.
- Just before the procedure, ask the patient to void and to put on a gown.

After the Test

- Monitor the patient's vital signs every 15 minutes for 1 hour after the procedure and then every hour for 4 hours until he's stable. If he's unstable, check every 15 minutes and notify the health care provider.

> ### Quality and Safety Nursing Alert

Have emergency medication and resuscitation equipment available in case the patient develops arrhythmias.

- Observe the patient for shortness of breath, chest pain, pallor, or changes in pulse or blood pressure.
- Enforce bed rest for 4 to 8 hours.
- Ensure patient does not bend or flex the extremity.
- Check the catheter insertion site for bleeding, as ordered, usually every 30 minutes for 8 hours. If bleeding occurs, notify the health care provider and apply a pressure bandage until the bleeding stops.
- Instruct the patient to resume a usual diet.
- Make sure a 12-lead resting electrocardiogram is scheduled to assess for changes.

Endoscopic Retrograde Cholangiopancreatography
Normal Findings
- Duodenal papilla appearing as a small, red (or sometimes pale) erosion protruding into the lumen; orifice commonly bordered by a fringe of white mucosa, and a longitudinal fold running perpendicular to the deep circular folds of the duodenum marking its location
- Possible appearance of separate orifices for the pancreatic and hepatobiliary ducts, which usually unite in the ampulla of Vater and empty through the duodenal papilla
- Uniform filling of pancreatic duct, hepatobiliary tree, and gallbladder with contrast medium

Abnormal Findings
- Abnormalities of the hepatobiliary tree and pancreatic duct, such as stones, strictures, or irregular deviations, possibly suggesting biliary cirrhosis, primary sclerosing cholangitis, or carcinoma of the bile ducts (See the *Abnormal ERCP* box.)
- Stones, strictures, and irregular deviations possibly indicating pancreatic cysts and pseudocysts, a pancreatic tumor, carcinoma of the head of the pancreas, chronic pancreatitis, pancreatic fibrosis, carcinoma of the duodenal papilla, or papillary stenosis

Nursing Implications
- Anticipate the need for additional testing based on test findings; a definitive diagnosis may require further studies.
- Prepare the patient for follow-up treatment as indicated. Certain interventions, such as stent placement to allow drainage or a papillotomy to decrease scar tissue and allow light drainage, may be indicated.
- Provide emotional support to the patient and family.

Purpose
- To evaluate the cause of obstructive jaundice
- To diagnose cancer of the duodenal papilla, pancreas, and biliary ducts
- To locate calculi and stenosis in the pancreatic ducts and hepatobiliary tree
- To identify leaks from trauma or surgery
- To evaluate abdominal pain of unknown etiology

Description
Endoscopic retrograde cholangiopancreatography (ERCP) is the radiographic examination of the pancreatic ducts and hepatobiliary tree after injection of a contrast medium into the duodenal papilla. Complications may include cholangitis, pancreatitis, acute infection,

Abnormal Endoscopic Retrograde Cholangiopancreatographic

This endoscopic retrograde cholangiopancreatographic (ERCP) view shows a dilated pancreatic duct secondary to stenosis. Stenosis was caused by carcinoma at the head of the pancreas.

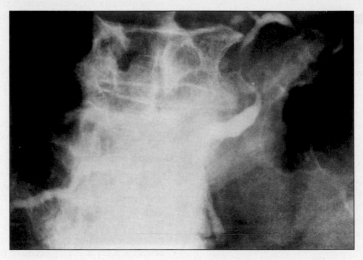

severe cardiopulmonary disease, or coagulopathy.

The usual procedure for ERCP is as follows:

- An IV infusion of 150 mL normal saline solution is started and a local anesthetic is administered, usually taking effect in about 10 minutes. If an anesthetic spray is used, the patient is asked to hold the breath while the mouth and throat are sprayed.
- The patient is placed in a left lateral position and given an emesis basin and tissues. Because the anesthetic causes the patient to lose some control of secretions, thus increasing the risk of aspiration, encourage the patient to allow saliva to drain from the side of the mouth. The patient is required to remove dentures or partial plates.
- A mouthguard is inserted.
- While the patient remains in the left lateral position, 5 to 20 mg IV

diazepam (Valium) or midazolam (Versed) is administered, as well as an opioid analgesic, if needed.

▶ Quality and Safety Nursing Alert

Continuous electrocardiographic monitoring, vital signs, and pulse oximetry monitoring should be instituted.

- When ptosis or dysarthria develops, the patient's head is bent forward and the patient is asked to open the mouth.
- The health care provider inserts the left index finger into the patient's mouth and guides the tip of the endoscope along the finger to the back of the patient's throat. The scope is then deflected downward with the left index finger and advanced. As the endoscope passes through the posterior pharynx and cricopharyngeal sphincter, the patient's head is slowly extended to help advance the

endoscope. The patient's chin must be kept midline. When the endoscope has passed the cricopharyngeal sphincter, the scope is advanced under direct vision. When it's well into the esophagus, the patient's chin is moved toward the table so saliva can drain from the mouth. The endoscope is advanced through the remainder of the esophagus and into the stomach under direct vision.

- When the pylorus is located, a small amount of air is insufflated and the tip of the endoscope is angled upward and passed into the duodenal bulb.
- After the endoscope is rotated clockwise to enter the descending duodenum, the patient is assisted to a prone position.
- An anticholinergic or IV glucagon is administered to induce duodenal atony and to relax the ampullary sphincter.
- Simethicone may be instilled in order to control the bubbles from the bile secretions.
- A small amount of air is insufflated, and the endoscope is manipulated until the optic lies opposite the duodenal papilla. Then the cannula filled with contrast medium is passed through the biopsy channel of the endoscope, the duodenal papilla, and into the ampulla of Vater.
- The pancreatic duct is visualized first under fluoroscopic guidance with injection of contrast medium.
- The cannula is repositioned at a more cephalad angle, and the hepatobiliary tree is visualized with injection of contrast medium.
- After each injection, rapid-sequence X-ray films are taken.
- The patient is told to remain prone while the films are developed and reviewed. If necessary, additional films may be taken.
- When the required radiographs have been obtained, the cannula is removed. Before the endoscope is

withdrawn, a tissue specimen may be obtained or fluid may be aspirated for histologic or cytologic examination, respectively.

Interfering Factors
- Barium in the GI tract from previous studies (possible poor imaging)

 Quality and Safety Nursing Alert

The patient's vital signs and airway patency should be monitored throughout the procedure for signs of respiratory depression, apnea, hypotension, excessive diaphoresis, bradycardia, and laryngospasm. Emergency resuscitation equipment and an opioid antagonist, such as naloxone (Narcan), must be readily available.

Precautions
- ERCP is contraindicated during pregnancy because of the risk of fetal harm secondary to radiation exposure.
- ERCP is contraindicated in the patient with infectious disease, pancreatic pseudocysts, stricture or obstruction of the esophagus or duodenum, or acute pancreatitis, cholangitis, or cardiorespiratory disease.
- Use of anticoagulants while undergoing this test increases the risk of bleeding.

Nursing Considerations
Before the Test
- Confirm the patient's identity using two patient identifiers and confirmation of the patient's identification bracelet according to facility policy.
- Explain to the patient that ERCP permits examination of the liver, gallbladder, and pancreas through X-ray films taken after injection of a contrast medium. Describe the test, including who will perform it and when and where it will take place.
- Instruct the patient to fast after midnight before the test.

- Explain that a local anesthetic will be sprayed into the patient's mouth to calm the gag reflex. Warn the patient that the spray has an unpleasant taste and makes the tongue and throat feel swollen, causing difficulty swallowing.
- Instruct the patient to let saliva drain from the side of the mouth, and warn the patient that suction may be used to remove saliva. A mouthguard will be inserted to protect the patient's teeth and the endoscope; assure the patient that it won't obstruct breathing.
- Explain that the patient will receive a sedative before insertion of the endoscope to assist with relaxation while the patient remains conscious.
- Explain that the patient will also receive an anticholinergic or IV glucagon after endoscope insertion. Describe the possible adverse effects of anticholinergics (dry mouth, thirst, tachycardia, urine retention, and blurred vision) or of glucagon (nausea, vomiting, urticaria, and flushing).
- Warn that the patient may experience transient flushing on injection of the contrast medium. Advise that the patient may have a sore throat for 3 or 4 days after the examination.
- Make sure that the patient or a responsible family member has signed an informed consent form.
- Check the patient's history for hypersensitivity to iodine, seafood, or contrast media used for other diagnostic procedures, and inform the health care provider of sensitivities.
- Just before the procedure, obtain the patient's baseline vital signs. Instruct the patient to remove all metallic or other radiopaque objects and constricting undergarments. Then tell the patient to void to minimize the discomfort of urine retention that may follow the procedure.

After the Test
- Observe the patient closely for signs of cholangitis and pancreatitis. (Hyperbilirubinemia, fever, and chills are the immediate signs of cholangitis; hypotension associated with gram-negative septicemia may develop later. Left upper quadrant pain and tenderness, elevated serum amylase levels, and transient hyperbilirubinemia are the usual signs of pancreatitis.) Draw blood samples for amylase and bilirubin determinations, if necessary, but remember that these levels usually rise after ERCP.
- Observe the patient for signs of perforation, such as abdominal pain, bleeding, rigid abdomen, and fever.
- Tell the patient that a feeling of fullness, some cramping, and passage of flatus several hours after the test may be experienced.
- Continue to watch the patient for signs of respiratory depression, apnea, hypotension, excessive diaphoresis, bradycardia, and laryngospasm. Check the patient's vital signs every 15 minutes for 1 hour, every 30 minutes for the next 2 hours, every hour for the next 4 hours, and then every 4 hours for 48 hours.

▶ *Quality and Safety Nursing Alert*

Withhold food and fluids until the patient's gag reflex returns. Test the gag reflex by touching the back of the throat with a tongue blade.

- When the gag reflex returns, allow fluids and a light meal.
- Discontinue or maintain the IV infusion as ordered.
- Check for signs of urine retention. Notify the health care provider if the patient hasn't voided within 8 hours.
- If the patient has a sore throat, provide soothing lozenges and warm saline gargles to ease discomfort.
- If a tissue biopsy or polypectomy occurred, expect a small amount of blood in the patient's first stool; this is normal.
- Inform the patient that abdominal pain may persist for several hours.

🚩 *Quality and Safety Nursing Alert*

Immediately report excessive amounts of blood in the stool to the health care provider.

• If this test is performed on an outpatient basis, be sure that transportation is available. The patient who has undergone anesthesia or sedation shouldn't operate an automobile for at least 12 hours postprocedure. Alcohol should be avoided for 24 hours.

Endoscopic Ultrasound

Normal Findings
• Normal anatomy without evidence of a tumor

Abnormal Findings
• Acute or chronic ulcers
• Benign or malignant tumors
• Inflammatory disease

Nursing Implications
• Anticipate the need for additional testing and prepare the patient for follow-up treatment as indicated.
• Assess the patient's GI status, including bowel sounds and abdominal distention or tenderness.
• Provide emotional support to the patient and family.

Purpose
• To evaluate or stage lesions of the esophagus, stomach, duodenum, pancreas, ampulla, biliary ducts, and rectum
• To evaluate submucosal tumors

Description
Endoscopic ultrasound (EUS) combines ultrasonography and endoscopy to show high-resolution images of the GI wall and adjacent structures. The procedure involves obtaining baseline vital signs and monitoring the patient during testing. It may be done with esophagogastroduodenoscopy or a sigmoidoscopy.

Interfering Factors
• Anticoagulants (increased risk of bleeding)
• Patient's inability to cooperate with the test
• Barium in the intestine from a previous study (poor visualization)
• Large amounts of stool in the intestine (poor visualization with sigmoid EUS)
• Esophageal stricture (hinders passage of the endoscope)

Precautions
• The procedure is usually safe but can lead to perforation.
• Esophagogastroduodenoscopy EUS is usually contraindicated in the patient with Zenker's diverticulum, a large aortic aneurysm, recent ulcer perforation, or an unstable cardiac or pulmonary condition.

Nursing Considerations

Before the Test
• Confirm the patient's identity using two patient identifiers and confirmation of the patient's identification bracelet according to facility policy.
• Make sure the patient has signed an appropriate consent form.
• Note and report all allergies and response to allergens.
• Explain to the patient that fasting is necessary for 6 to 8 hours before the test.
• For a sigmoid EUS, inform the patient that the scope will be inserted through the anus. The patient may have to take a laxative the evening before and may feel an urge to defecate during the study.
• Advise the patient that an IV sedative may be given to assist with relaxation before the endoscope is inserted.
• Explain that the test takes 30 to 90 minutes.

After the Test
• Instruct the patient to resume a usual diet and activity.

E

- Monitor the patient's vital signs, level of consciousness, and cardiac rhythm. Also monitor for bleeding and signs and symptoms of perforation.
- Advise the patient who received IV sedation to avoid alcohol and driving for 24 hours after the test.

Epstein-Barr Virus Antibodies

Reference Values
No detectable antibodies to the virus as measured by either the monospot test or the indirect immunofluorescence test.

Abnormal Findings
- Positive monospot test or an indirect immunofluorescence test that's either immunoglobulin (Ig) M positive or Epstein-Barr nuclear antigen (EBNA) negative, indicating acute Epstein-Barr virus (EBV) infection

Nursing Implications
- Anticipate the need for additional testing.
- Keep in mind that the monospot test is positive only during the acute phase of infection with EBV; the indirect immunofluorescence test detects and discriminates between acute and past infection with the virus.
- Be aware that a monospot-negative result doesn't necessarily rule out acute or past infection with EBV. Conversely, IgG class antibody to viral capsid antigen and EBNA antigens (IgM negative) indicates remote (more than 2 months) infection with EBV. Recognize that most cases of monospot-negative infectious mononucleosis are caused by cytomegalovirus infections.
- Prepare the patient for follow-up treatment as indicated.

Purpose
- To provide a laboratory diagnosis of heterophil-negative (or monospot-negative) cases of infectious mononucleosis

- To determine the antibody status to EBV of immunosuppressed patients with lymphoproliferative processes

Description
EBV, a member of the herpesvirus group, is the causative agent of heterophil-positive infectious mononucleosis, Burkitt's lymphoma, and nasopharyngeal carcinoma. Although the virus doesn't replicate in standard cell cultures, most EBV infections can be recognized by testing the patient's serum for heterophil antibodies (monospot test), which usually appear within the first 3 weeks of illness and then decline rapidly within a few weeks.

In about 10% of adults and a larger percentage of children, the monospot test is negative despite primary infection with EBV. Furthermore, EBV has been associated with lymphoproliferative processes in immunosuppressed patients. These disorders occur with reactivated, rather than primary, EBV infections and, therefore, are also monospot negative.

Alternatively, EBV-specific antibodies, which develop in response to several antigens of the virus during active infection, can be measured with a high level of sensitivity and specificity by indirect immunofluorescence.

Precautions
- Handle the sample gently to prevent hemolysis.

Nursing Considerations
Before the Test
- Confirm the patient's identity using two patient identifiers and confirmation of the patient's identification bracelet according to facility policy.
- Explain the purpose of the EBV antibodies test to the patient and inform the patient that it requires a blood sample.
- Advise the patient that slight discomfort from the tourniquet and the needle puncture may be experienced.

During the Test

• Perform a venipuncture and collect 5 mL of sterile blood in a clot activator tube.

After the Test

• Transfer the serum to a sterile tube or vial and send it to the laboratory immediately.

• If transfer must be delayed, store the serum at 39.2°F (4°C) for 1 to 2 days or at –4°F (–20°C) for longer periods to prevent contamination.

• Allow the blood to clot for at least 1 hour at room temperature.

• Apply direct pressure to the venipuncture site until bleeding stops and to prevent hematoma formation.

Erythrocyte Sedimentation Rate (ESR)

Reference Values

Newborns: 0 to 2 mm/hour
Children: 0 to 10 mm/hour
Females: Younger than 50 years, 0 to 25 mm/hour; older than 50 years, 0 to 30 mm/hour
Males: Younger than 50 years, 0 to 15 mm/hour; older than 50 years, 0 to 20 mm/hour

Rates increase gradually with age and are gender- and test method-dependent.

Abnormal Findings

Elevated Levels

• Pregnancy
• Anemia
• Acute or chronic inflammation
• Tuberculosis
• Paraproteinemias (especially multiple myeloma and Waldenström's macroglobulinemia)
• Rheumatic fever
• Rheumatoid arthritis
• Some cancers
• Advanced age
• Temporal arteritis
• Polymyalgia rheumatic
• Infection

• Menstruation
• Macrocytosis
• Hyperfibrinogenemia
• Heparin
• High-molecular-weight dextran
• Fever
• Extreme obesity
• High serum cholesterol

Decreased Levels

• Polycythemia
• Sickle cell anemia
• Hyperviscosity
• Low plasma fibrinogen or globulin levels
• Extreme leukocytosis
• Red blood cell abnormalities
• DIC
• Hypothermia
• Cachexia
• Congestive heart failure
• Valproic acid, steroids, anti-inflammatory agents

Nursing Implications

• Anticipate the need for additional testing and prepare the patient for follow-up treatment as indicated.

• Explain the underlying condition associated with the elevated erythrocyte sedimentation rate (ESR) or with the decreased levels of ESR.

• Assess the patient with decreased levels for signs and symptoms of possible thrombi.

• In patients with elevated levels, remember that conditions that elevate fibrinogen may also elevate ESR.

• Increased ESR rates in patients with rheumatoid arthritis may indicate impending heart failure.

• Provide emotional support to the patient and family.

Purpose

• To monitor inflammatory or malignant disease

• To help detect and diagnose occult disease, such as tuberculosis, tissue necrosis, or connective tissue disease

E

- To assist in the diagnosis of conditions associated with acute or chronic inflammation
- To monitor response to therapy in temporal arteritis and polymyalgia rheumatica

Description

Also known as *sedimentation rate* or *sed rate*, the ESR measures the degree of erythrocyte settling in a blood sample during a specified period. The ESR is a sensitive but nonspecific test that's commonly the earliest indicator of disease when other chemical or physical signs are normal. ESR levels usually increase significantly in widespread inflammatory disorders; elevations may be prolonged in localized inflammation and malignant disease. ESR alone is not an indicator of specific diseases; rather it assists in the diagnosis of certain conditions along with significant clinical findings. ESR may need to be repeated several weeks or months after the initial test to examine disease progression or effectiveness of therapy.

Interfering Factors

- Failure to use the proper anticoagulant, to adequately mix the sample and the anticoagulant, or to send the sample to the laboratory immediately
- Hemoconcentration caused by prolonged tourniquet constriction
- Delay in testing
- Refrigeration of specimen
- Drug interactions causing increased rate: anticonvulsants, aspirin, carbamazepine, cephalothin, cephapirin, clozapine, cyclosporin A, dexamethasone, dextran, etretinate, fluvastatin, hydralazine, indomethacin, isotretinoin, lomefloxacin, methyldopa, misoprostol, ofloxacin, oral contraceptives, procainamide, propafenone, quinidine, sulfamethoxazole, theophylline, vitamin A, zolpidem
- Drug interactions causing decreased rate: aspirin, corticotropin, cortisone, cyclophosphamide, dexamethasone,

gold, hydroxychloroquine, leflunomide, methotrexate, minocycline, NSAIDs, penicillamine, prednisolone, prednisone, quinine, sulfasalazine, tamoxifen, trimethoprim

Nursing Considerations

Before the Test

- Confirm the patient's identity using two patient identifiers and confirmation of the patient's identification bracelet according to facility policy.
- Explain to the patient that the ESR test is used to evaluate the condition of red blood cells.
- Inform the patient that a blood sample will be taken. Advise that slight discomfort from the tourniquet and the needle puncture may be felt.
- Inform the patient that there are no food or fluid restrictions for this test.

During the Test

- Perform a venipuncture and collect the sample in a 4.5-mL tube with EDTA added or a tube with sodium citrate added. (Check with the laboratory to determine its preference.)
- Completely fill the collection tube and invert it gently several times to thoroughly mix the sample and the anticoagulant.
- Handle the sample gently to prevent hemolysis.

After the Test

- Because prolonged standing decreases the ESR, examine the sample for clots or clumps and send it to the laboratory immediately. It must be tested within 2 hours.
- Apply direct pressure to the venipuncture site; ensure that subdermal bleeding has stopped before removing pressure.
- Assess the venipuncture site for hematoma development; if one develops, apply direct pressure to the site. If the hematoma is large, monitor pulses distal to the phlebotomy site.

Erythropoietin (EPO)

Reference Values
5 to 36 milliunits/mL (SI, 5–36 units/L)

Abnormal Findings

Elevated Levels
- Anemia as a compensatory mechanism in the reestablishment of homeostasis
- Polycythemia and erythropoietin (EPO)-secreting tumors (inappropriate elevations when the hematocrit is normal to high)
- Abuse of EPO, such as with athletic performance enhancement
- Hypoxia, as an adaptive response associated with conditions that produce tissue hypoxia, such as living at a high altitude, smoking, COPD, and sleep apnea
- Secondary polycythemia (increased RBCs in response to hypoxemia)

Decreased Levels
- Anemia with inadequate or absent hormone production
- Severe renal disease
- Polycythemia rubra vera, with an elevated hematocrit
- HIV treated with zidovudine (AZT), along with a decreased hematocrit

Nursing Implications
- Anticipate the need for additional testing and prepare the patient for follow-up treatment as indicated.
- If performance enhancement is suspected in patients with increased levels, watch for adverse reactions, including clotting abnormalities, headache, seizures, hypertension, nausea, vomiting, diarrhea, and rash.
- Increased EPO can lead to blood viscosity, increased circulating blood volume, and hypertension.
- Assess the patient with decreased levels for signs and symptoms associated with anemia, such as fatigue, pallor, lack of appetite, shortness of breath, and activity intolerance.

Purpose
- To help diagnose anemia and polycythemia
- To differentiate types of anemia
- To help diagnose renal tumors
- To detect EPO abuse by athletes
- To evaluate the kidney's ability to produce erythropoietin in patient's chronic kidney disease
- To determine an underlying condition leading to excess production of EPO

Description
The EPO test of renal hormone production measures EPO by immunoassay. Commonly used to evaluate anemia, polycythemia, and kidney tumors, it's also used to evaluate abuse of commercially prepared EPO by athletes who believe that the drug enhances performance.

A glycoprotein hormone, EPO is secreted by the liver of fetuses and by the kidneys in adults. The hormone acts on stem cells in the bone marrow to stimulate production of red blood cells (RBCs). It's regulated by a feedback loop involving red cell volume and oxygen saturation of the blood, especially in the brain. This ensures a stable number of RBCs. In hypoxic states, the kidneys will increase production and release of EPO.

Interfering Factors
- Failure to obtain the sample in a fasting state
- Drug interactions causing increased rate: anabolic steroids, daunorubicin, erythropoietin, fluoxymesterone, hydroxyurea, theophylline, AZT
- Drug interactions causing decreased rate: acetazolamide, amphotericin B, cisplatin, enalapril, furosemide, theophylline

Precautions
- Handle the sample gently to prevent hemolysis.

Nursing Considerations

Before the Test

- Confirm the patient's identity using two patient identifiers and confirmation of the patient's identification bracelet according to facility policy.
- Explain to the patient that the EPO test determines whether hormonal secretion is causing changes in RBCs.
- Instruct the patient to fast for 8 to 10 hours before the test.
- The test requires a blood sample. Explain that the patient may experience slight discomfort from the tourniquet and the needle puncture.
- Keep the patient relaxed and recumbent for 30 minutes before the test.

During the Test

- Perform a venipuncture and collect the sample in a 5-mL clot activator tube. If requested, a hematocrit may be drawn at the same time by collecting an additional sample in a 2-mL EDTA tube.

After the Test

- Apply direct pressure to the venipuncture site until bleeding stops and to prevent hematoma formation.
- Instruct the patient to resume a usual diet and activities.

Esophageal Acidity Test (Esophageal pH Testing)

Normal Findings

- pH of the esophagus exceeding 5.0

Abnormal Findings

- Intraesophageal pH of 1.5 to 2.0, indicating gastric acid reflux

Nursing Implications

- Anticipate the need for additional testing, such as barium swallow and esophagogastroduodenoscopy, as needed to diagnose and determine the extent of esophagitis.

- Prepare the patient for follow-up treatment as indicated.
- Assess the patient for complaints of reflux.
- Provide emotional support to the patient and family.

Purpose

- To evaluate the competence of the lower esophageal sphincter

Description

The esophageal acidity test evaluates the competence of the lower esophageal sphincter—the major barrier to reflux—by measuring intraesophageal pH with an electrode attached to a manometric catheter. This test monitors how much acid enters into the esophagus and how well it is cleared. *Bravo pH,* a newer method for measuring esophageal pH, uses a small capsule that's inserted endoscopically to monitor a patient's pH levels. (See the *Monitoring pH with the Bravo System* box.)

The traditional procedure for esophageal acidity testing is as follows:

- After the patient is placed in high Fowler's position, the catheter with the electrode is introduced into the mouth.

> ▶ *Quality and Safety Nursing Alert*
>
> During insertion, be aware that the catheter may enter the trachea instead of the esophagus. If the patient develops cyanosis or paroxysmal coughing, the catheter must be removed immediately. The patient also is observed closely during insertion because arrhythmias may develop.

- The patient is instructed to swallow when the electrode reaches the back of the throat.
- Using a manometer, the health care provider locates the lower esophageal sphincter. The catheter is then raised ¾-inch (1.9 cm). The patient is told to perform Valsalva's maneuver or

Monitoring pH with the Bravo System

Traditional testing for esophageal acid levels typically uses an esophageal catheter that's inserted for a 24-hour period. Recently, a new technique called the *Bravo pH monitoring system* was developed to measure acid levels in the esophagus via a capsule (about the size of a gel cap). The capsule is temporarily attached to the patient's esophageal wall using an endoscope and collects pH data, which are transmitted to a pager-sized receiver that the patient wears. Data are collected for 48 hours, downloaded from the receiver, and analyzed with special software.

The Bravo method is more accurate than catheter methods because the patient can eat normally and maintain regular activities during testing. The additional 24 hours also provides more information for diagnosing certain esophageal disorders.

In 7 to 10 days, the capsule spontaneously detaches from the esophageal wall and is passed through the patient's digestive system.

E

to lift the legs to stimulate reflux. After doing so, intraesophageal pH is measured.

- If the pH is normal, the catheter is passed into the patient's stomach. A prescribed acid solution (300 mL of 0.1 sodium hydrochloride) is instilled over 3 minutes (100 mL/minute). Then the catheter is raised ¾-inch above the sphincter. Again, the patient is asked to perform Valsalva's maneuver or to lift the legs and intraesophageal pH is measured.
- The catheter is clamped before removal to prevent fluid aspiration into the lungs.

Interfering Factors

- Antacids, histamine-2 blockers, anticholinergics, and proton pump inhibitors (possible lowering of intraesophageal pH because of a decrease in gastric secretions or acidity)
- Alcohol, cholinergics, corticosteroids, and reserpine (possible elevation of intraesophageal pH because of reflux from a relaxed lower esophageal sphincter or an increase in gastric secretions)
- Smoking (possible elevation of gastric secretions)

Nursing Considerations

Before the Test

- Confirm the patient's identity using two patient identifiers and confirma-

tion of the patient's identification bracelet according to facility policy.
- Explain to the patient that the esophageal acidity test evaluates the function of the sphincter between the esophagus and the stomach. Tell the patient to fast 8 to 12 hours and to avoid smoking after midnight before the test.
- Describe the test, including who will perform it and when and where it will take place.
- Advise the patient that a tube will be passed through the mouth into the stomach and there may be slight discomfort, a desire to cough, or a gagging sensation.
- Just before the test, check the patient's pulse rate and blood pressure and instruct the patient to void.
- Withhold antacids, anticholinergics, cholinergics, beta-adrenergic blockers, alcohol, corticosteroids, cimetidine, and reserpine for 24 hours before the test. If they must be continued, note this on the laboratory request.
- Make sure that the patient or a responsible family member has signed an informed consent form.

After the Test

- Tell the patient to resume usual diet and medications as ordered.
- Provide lozenges if the patient complains of a sore throat.

Esophagogastroduodenoscopy (EGD; Upper Endoscopy)

Normal Findings

- Esophageal mucosa that's smooth, yellow-pink, and marked by a fine vascular network
- Pulsation on the anterior wall of the esophagus between 8 and 10 inches (20.5 and 25.5 cm) from the incisor teeth, representing the aortic arch
- Orange-red mucosa of the stomach beginning at the "Z" line, an irregular transition line slightly above the esophagogastric junction
- Stomach with moist rugal folds and nonvisible blood vessels beneath the gastric mucosa
- Reddish mucosa of the duodenal bulb marked by a few shallow longitudinal folds
- Mucosa of the distal duodenum with prominent circular folds, lined with villi and appearing velvety and moist

Abnormal Findings

- Acute or chronic ulcers
- Benign or malignant tumors
- Inflammatory disease, including esophagitis, gastritis, and duodenitis
- Diverticula, varices, Mallory-Weiss' syndrome, esophageal rings, esophageal and pyloric stenoses, esophageal hiatal hernia, and polyps

Nursing Implications

- Anticipate the need for additional testing.
- Keep in mind that although esophagogastroduodenoscopy (EGD) can evaluate gross abnormalities of esophageal motility (as occur in achalasia), manometric studies are more accurate.
- Prepare the patient for follow-up treatment as indicated.
- Assess the patient's GI status, including complaints of nausea or vomiting, acid reflux, hematemesis, tarry bowel movements, bleeding, or abdominal pain or tenderness.

- The esophagus may not be able to be intubated in patients with anatomical abnormalities such as an abnormal cervical spine, Zenker's diverticulum, or certain tumors and may need alternative diagnostic testing.
- Provide emotional support to the patient and family.

Purpose

- To diagnose inflammatory disease, malignant and benign tumors, ulcers, Mallory-Weiss' syndrome, and structural abnormalities
- To evaluate the stomach and duodenum postoperatively
- To obtain an emergency diagnosis of duodenal ulcer or esophageal injury, such as that caused by chemical ingestion
- To evaluate various GI symptoms such as bleeding, upper abdominal pain, nausea, vomiting, or swallowing abnormalities
- To provide intervention such as gastric banding of varices, instillation of sclerosing agents for varices
- To remove esophageal polyps

Description

Also known as *upper GI* (UGI) *study, endoscopy,* and *gastroscopy,* EGD permits visual examination of the lining of the esophagus, stomach, and upper duodenum using a flexible fiberoptic or video endoscope. It's indicated for patients with GI bleeding, hematemesis, melena, substernal or epigastric pain, gastroesophageal reflux disease, dysphagia, anemia, strictures, or peptic ulcer disease; patients requiring foreign body retrieval; and postoperative patients with recurrent or new symptoms.

EGD eliminates the need for extensive exploratory surgery and can be used to detect small or surface lesions missed by radiography. Because the scope provides a channel for biopsy forceps or a cytology brush, it permits laboratory evaluation of abnormalities detected by radiography. Similarly, it allows for the removal of foreign bodies by suction (for small, soft objects) or by electrocautery snare or forceps (for large, hard objects). The scope may also be used to cauterize bleeding vessels within an ulcer.

The usual procedure for EGD is as follows:

- The patient's baseline vital signs are obtained, and the blood pressure cuff is left in place for monitoring throughout the procedure.
- Continuous electrocardiographic monitoring, heart rate, and respiratory rate should be instituted. Continuous pulse oximetry is also advisable, particularly in the patient with pulmonary compromise.
- The patient is asked to hold the breath while the mouth and throat are sprayed with a local anesthetic, if requested by the health care provider. Remind the patient to let saliva drain from the side of the mouth. (An emesis basis is provided to spit out saliva, and tissues are given to wipe saliva from the mouth; oropharyngeal suction can be used as needed.)
- The patient is then placed in a left lateral position, with head bent forward, and is asked to open the mouth.
- The health care provider guides the tip of the endoscope to the back of the patient's throat and downward. As the endoscope passes through the posterior pharynx and the cricopharyngeal sphincter, the patient's neck is slowly extended while the chin is kept at midline. The endoscope is then passed along the esophagus under direct vision. When the endoscope is well into the esophagus (about 12 inches [30.5 cm]), the patient's head is positioned with chin toward the table so that saliva can drain out of the mouth.
- After examination of the esophagus and the cardiac sphincter, the endoscope is rotated clockwise and advanced to allow examination of the stomach and duodenum. During

the examination, air or water may be introduced through the endoscope to aid visualization, and suction may be applied to remove insufflated air and secretions.

- Either a camera attached to the endoscope or an electronic video endoscope attached directly to a video processor may be used to photograph areas for later study or a measuring tube may be passed through the endoscope to determine the size of a lesion.
- Biopsy forceps or a cytology brush may be passed through the scope to obtain specimens for histologic or cytologic study.
- The endoscope is slowly withdrawn and suspicious-looking areas of the gastric and esophageal lining are reexamined.
- Specimens should be collected in accordance with laboratory and pathology guidelines. Tissue specimens are placed immediately in a specimen bottle containing 10% formalin solution; cell specimens are smeared on glass slides and placed in a Coplin jar containing 95% ethyl alcohol.

Interfering Factors

- Anticoagulants (increased risk of bleeding)
- Patient's inability to cooperate, preventing optimal visualization
- Failure to fast before the test
- Bleeding, which decreases optimal visualization

Precautions

- This procedure is generally safe, but it can cause perforation of the esophagus, stomach, or duodenum, especially if the patient is restless or uncooperative.
- EGD is usually contraindicated in the patient with Zenker's diverticulum, a large aortic aneurysm, recent ulcer perforation (known as *suspected viscus perforation*), or an unstable cardiac or pulmonary condition.

- EGD shouldn't be performed within 2 days after an upper GI series.
- A patient requiring dental prophylaxis may also require antibiotics before this procedure.

Nursing Considerations

Before the Test

- Confirm the patient's identity using two patient identifiers and confirmation of the patient's identification bracelet according to facility policy.
- Explain to the patient that EGD permits visual examination of the lining of the esophagus, stomach, and upper duodenum.
- Check the patient's medical history for allergies, medications, and information pertinent to the current complaint. Check for hypersensitivity to the medications and anesthetics ordered for the test.
- Instruct the patient to fast for solids and nonclear liquids for 6 to 8 hours prior to the procedure or starting at midnight and for 2 to 3 hours prior to the procedure for clear liquids.
- Inform the patient that a flexible instrument with a camera on the end will be passed through the mouth. Explain who will perform this procedure, where and when it will take place, and that it takes about 30 minutes.
- If emergency EGD is to be performed, tell the patient that stomach contents may be aspirated through a nasogastric tube.
- Inform the patient that a bitter-tasting local anesthetic will be sprayed into the mouth and throat to calm the gag reflex and that the tongue and throat may feel swollen, making swallowing seem difficult. Advise the patient to let the saliva drain from the side of the mouth; a suction machine may be used to remove saliva, if necessary.
- Explain that a mouthguard will be inserted to protect the teeth and the endoscope; assure that the mouthguard won't obstruct breathing.
- Inform the patient that an IV line will be started and that a sedative will be administered before the endoscope is inserted to assist with relaxation. If the procedure is being done on an outpatient basis, advise that the patient may feel drowsy from the sedative and should arrange for a ride home. Drugs that retard peristalsis of the upper GI tract may also be administered in some circumstances.
- Tell the patient that pressure in the stomach as the endoscope is moved about, as well as a feeling of fullness when air or carbon dioxide is insufflated may be experienced. If the patient is apprehensive, administer analgesic/sedative about 30 minutes before the test, as ordered.
- Make sure that the patient or a responsible family member has signed an informed consent form before administration of narcotics.
- Just before the procedure, instruct the patient to remove dentures, eyeglasses, and constricting garments.

After the Test

- Assess the patient for evidence of aspiration of gastric contents, which could precipitate aspiration pneumonia.
- Monitor the patient's vital signs and document them according to facility policy.
- Test the patient's gag reflex by touching the back of the throat with a tongue blade. Withhold food and fluids until the patient is awake and the gag reflex returns (usually within 1 hour), and then allow fluids and a light meal.
- Explain that the patient may burp some insufflated air and have a sore throat for 3 to 4 days. Throat lozenges and warm saline gargles may ease the discomfort.

- If the patient experiences soreness at the IV site, apply warm packs.
- Because of sedation, advise the outpatient to avoid alcohol for 24 hours and driving for 12 hours. Make sure the patient has transportation home.
- Instruct the patient to notify the health care provider immediately if persistent difficulty with swallowing, pain, fever, black stools, or bloody vomitus is experienced.
- Remove the IV access immediately before discharge.

> ### Quality and Safety Nursing Alert

Observe the patient for possible perforation. Perforation in the cervical area of the esophagus produces pain on swallowing. With neck movement, thoracic perforation causes substernal or epigastric pain that increases with breathing or movement of the trunk; diaphragmatic perforation produces shoulder pain and dyspnea. Gastric perforation causes abdominal or back pain, cyanosis, fever, and pleural effusion.

Also observe the patient closely for adverse effects of the sedative: respiratory depression, apnea, hypotension, excessive diaphoresis, bradycardia, and laryngospasm. Have emergency resuscitation equipment and an opioid antagonist, such as naloxone (Narcan), available. Be prepared to intervene as needed.

Estrogens (Serum) (E1)

Reference Values

Children: Prepuberty, less than 25 pg/mL, less than 25 ng/mL; puberty: 30 to 280 pg/mL, 30 to 280 ng/mL

Males: 20 to 80 pg/mL (SI, 40–125 pmol/L)

Premenopausal females: Variation during the menstrual cycle, ranging from 60 to 400 pg/mL or 60 to 400 ng/mL

Postmenopausal females: Less than 130 pg/mL or less than 130 ng/mL

Abnormal Findings

Elevated Levels

- Estrogen-producing tumors
- Precocious puberty
- Severe hepatic disease (such as cirrhosis)
- Congenital adrenal hyperplasia
- Tumors of the ovary, testes, or adrenal glands

Decreased Levels

- Primary hypogonadism or ovarian failure (as in Turner's syndrome or ovarian agenesis)
- Secondary hypogonadism (such as in hypopituitarism) or menopause
- Failing pregnancy (estriol)
- Stein-Leventhal's syndrome (PCOS)
- Anorexia nervosa
- Extreme endurance exercise

Nursing Implications

- Anticipate the need for additional testing and prepare the patient for follow-up treatment as indicated.
- Provide emotional support to the patient and family.

Purpose

- To determine sexual maturation and fertility
- To help diagnose gonadal dysfunction, such as precocious or delayed puberty, menstrual disorders (especially amenorrhea), and infertility
- To help diagnose tumors known to secrete estrogen

Description

Estrogens (and progesterone) are secreted by the ovaries under the influence of the pituitary gonadotropins—follicle-stimulating hormone (FSH) and luteinizing hormone (LH). Estrogens—in particular, estradiol, the most potent estrogen—interact with the hypothalamic-pituitary axis through negative and positive feedback mechanisms. Slowly rising or sustained high levels inhibit secretion of FSH and LH (negative feedback), but a rapid rise in estrogen just before ovulation seems to stimulate LH secretion (positive feedback).

Estrogens are responsible for the development of secondary female sexual characteristics and for normal menstruation; levels are usually undetectable in children. These hormones are secreted by ovarian follicular cells during the first half of the menstrual cycle and by the corpus luteum during the luteal phase and during pregnancy. In menopause, estrogen secretion drops to a constantly low level.

This radioimmunoassay measures serum levels of estradiol, estrone, and estriol (the only estrogens that appear in serum in measurable amounts) and has diagnostic significance in evaluating female gonadal dysfunction. Tests of hypothalamic-pituitary function may be required to confirm the diagnosis.

Interfering Factors

- Pregnancy and pretest use of estrogens, such as hormonal contraceptives (possible increase)
- Drug interactions causing increased levels: glucocorticosteroids, ampicillin, estrogen-containing drugs, phenothiazines, pituitary-based hormones such as dexamethasone (Decadron), and tetracyclines
- Drug interactions causing decreased levels: clomiphene

Nursing Considerations

Before the Test

- Confirm the patient's identity using two patient identifiers and confirmation of the patient's identification bracelet according to facility policy.
- Explain to the patient that the estrogens radioimmunoassay helps determine whether secretion of female hormones is normal and that the test may be repeated during the various phases of the menstrual cycle.
- Tell the patient that she doesn't need to restrict food and fluids before the test.

- Inform the patient that the test requires a blood sample, and explain that she may experience slight discomfort from the tourniquet and the needle puncture.
- Withhold all steroid and pituitary-based hormones as ordered. If they must be continued, note this information on the laboratory request slip.
- Care may vary slightly, depending on whether plasma or serum is being measured.

During the Test

- Perform a venipuncture and collect the sample in a 10-mL clot activator tube.
- If the patient is premenopausal, indicate the phase of her menstrual cycle on the laboratory request slip.
- Handle the sample gently to prevent hemolysis.

After the Test

- Send the sample to the laboratory immediately.
- Apply direct pressure to the venipuncture site until bleeding stops and to prevent hematoma formation.
- Instruct the patient that she may resume medications that were discontinued before the test, as ordered.

Estrogens (Urine)

Reference Values

Males: 15 to 40 mcg/24 hours (SI, 55–147 nmol/day)

Menstruating women: 15 to 80 mcg/24 hours (SI, 55–294 nmol/day)

Pregnant females: First trimester, 0 to 800 mcg/24 hours (SI, 0–2,900 nmol/day); second trimester, 800 to 5,000 mcg/24 hours (SI, 2,900–18,350 nmol/day); third trimester, 5,000 to 50,000 mcg/24 hours (SI, 2,900–183,000 nmol/day)

Postmenopausal females: Less than 20 mcg/24 hours (SI, less than 73 nmol/day)

Abnormal Findings

Elevated Levels

- Glucose in the urine and urinary tract infections
- Hyperthyroidism
- Feminization in children (testicular feminization syndrome)
- Precocious puberty secondary to adrenal tumor
- *Males:* testicular tumors
- *Females:* tumors of ovarian or adrenocortical origin, adrenocortical hyperplasia, or a metabolic or hepatic disorder

Decreased Levels

- Ovarian agenesis, primary ovarian insufficiency (caused by Stein-Leventhal's syndrome, for example), or secondary ovarian insufficiency (caused by pituitary or adrenal hypofunction or metabolic disturbances)
- Primary and secondary hypogonadism
- Kallmann's syndrome

Nursing Implications

- Anticipate the need for additional testing, and prepare the patient for follow-up treatment as indicated.
- If the patient is pregnant, expect to obtain serial levels indicating a rising titer.
- Provide emotional support to the patient and family.

Purpose

- To evaluate ovarian activity and help determine the cause of amenorrhea and female hyperestrogenism
- To help diagnose tumors of ovarian, adrenocortical, or testicular origin
- To assess fetoplacental status

Description

A total urine estrogens test is a quantitative analysis of total urine levels of estradiol, estrone, and estriol—the major estrogens present in significant amounts. A common method for measuring urine estrogen levels involves putrification by gel filtration, followed by spectrophotofluorimetry. Supplementary tests that may provide further information about ovarian function include cytologic examination of vaginal smears, measurement of urine levels of pregnanediol and follicle-stimulating hormone, and evaluation of response to a progesterone injection.

Interfering Factors

- Steroid hormones, methenamine mandelate (Mandelamine), phenazopyridine hydrochloride (Pyridium), phenothiazines, tetracyclines, phenolphthalein, ampicillin, meprobamate (Miltown), senna, cascara sagrada, and hydrochlorothiazide (HydroDIURIL) (possible increase or decrease)
- Drug interactions causing increased levels: glucocorticosteroids, ampicillin, estrogen-containing drugs, phenothiazines, pituitary-based hormones such as dexamethasone (Decadron), and tetracyclines
- Drug interactions causing decreased levels: clomiphene, estrogen therapy, oral contraceptives, progesterone therapy

Nursing Considerations

Before the Test

- Confirm the patient's identity using two patient identifiers and confirmation of the patient's identification bracelet according to facility policy.
- Explain to the female patient that the total urine estrogens test helps evaluate ovarian function or, if pregnant, that this test helps evaluate fetal development and placental function. Explain to the male patient that this test helps evaluate testicular function.
- Inform the patient that the test requires collection of urine over a 24-hour period.
- Advise the patient that it isn't necessary to restrict food and fluids for this test.
- If the 24-hour specimen is to be collected at home, teach the patient the proper collection technique.

E

- Notify the laboratory and health care provider of any medications the patient is taking that may affect test results; they may need to be restricted.

During the Test
- Collect the patient's urine over a 24-hour period, discarding the first specimen and retaining the last. Use a bottle containing a preservative to keep the specimen at a pH of 3 to 5.
- If the patient is pregnant, note the approximate week of gestation on the laboratory request slip. If not pregnant, note the stage of her menstrual cycle.
- Refrigerate the specimen or keep it on ice during the collection period.

After the Test
- Instruct the patient to resume any usual medications as ordered.

Ethyl Alcohol Levels (Blood, Urine, Breath, Saliva) (Alcohol, EtOH)

Reference Values
Less than 10 mg/dL or less than 2 mmol/L considered negative
Less than 20 mg/dL or less than 4.34 mmol/L considered negative by the U.S. Department of Transportation (USDOT)

Critical Values
Greater than 300 mg/dL (SI, greater than 64.8 mmol/L)

Abnormal Findings
Elevated Levels
- Alcohol intoxication (greater than 40 mg/dL [SI, greater than 8.68 mmol/L]) considered positive by the U.S. Department of Transportation; greater than 80 mg/dL [SI, greater than 17.4 mmol/L] considered positive by most state laws for driving under the influence)

Nursing Implications
- Assess the patient closely for changes in level of consciousness and behavior.

- Keep in mind that alcohol intoxication can produce signs and symptoms similar to those for diabetic ketoacidosis, head injury, or drug overdose.
- Remember that urine alcohol levels are similar to blood alcohol levels, but that saliva samples typically reveal results 1.2 times those for blood.
- Prepare to initiate overdose protocols if critical values are detected.

Purpose
- To identify a quantitative level of alcohol in the body
- To diagnose alcohol intoxication
- To screen for alcoholism

Description
Ethyl alcohol (ethanol) is a central nervous system depressant that, if ingested in sufficient quantity, can lead to coma and death. The sample can be obtained from the patient's blood, urine, gastric contents, or breath.

Interfering Factors
- Increase in blood ketones (false elevation of blood or breath alcohol levels)
- Intake of other alcohols
- Drug interactions causing increased levels: aspirin, chloral hydrate, cimetidine, metoclopramide, ranitidine
- Drug interactions causing decreased levels: ascorbic acid, atropine, phenobarbital, propantheline
- Dehydration

Nursing Considerations
Before the Test
- Confirm the patient's identity using two patient identifiers and confirmation of the patient's identification bracelet according to facility policy.
- Inform the patient that the test is done to identify the amount of alcohol in the body.
- Explain that the test requires a blood, urine, or breath sample, and that restricting food and fluids isn't necessary for testing. Warn that slight

discomfort from the tourniquet and the needle puncture if a blood sample is used may be experienced.

- Advise the patient of legal rights related to samples.
- Ensure that an informed consent is obtained if required by facility policy.

During the Test

- Follow facility protocol for collecting any blood sample or urine specimen that may be used for legal purposes.
- Obtain the appropriate sample:
  - If taking a blood sample, clean the venipuncture site with a non–alcohol-based solution. Perform the venipuncture and collect the sample in the appropriate tube.
  - If obtaining a urine specimen, collect approximately 20 to 50 mL of the patient's urine.
  - If a breath sample is needed, have the patient inhale deeply and then exhale into the tubelike mouthpiece attached to the collection device.
- Mark the exact time of collection on the laboratory request form.
- If required by facility policy, sign the form and have it witnessed.

After the Test

- Send the sample or specimen to the laboratory immediately.
- If a venipuncture was performed, apply direct pressure to the venipuncture site until bleeding stops. Assess the site for hematoma development; if a hematoma develops, apply direct pressure to the site.
- Continue to monitor the patient's neurologic status for changes.
- Carbohydrate deficient transferring (CDT) may be ordered to assess for chronic alcohol use.

Euglobulin Lysis Time

Reference Values

No lysis of a clot in 60 to 120 minutes (at 37°C).
Lysis normally occurring within 2 to 4 hours (SI, 2–4 hours)

Abnormal Findings

- Increased plasminogen activator activity (clot lysis within 1 hour [SI, 1 hour])
- Less than 1 hour indicates abnormal fibrinolysis
- Pathologic fibrinolysis (5–10 minutes [SI, 5–10 minutes])

Nursing Implications

- Anticipate the need for additional testing and prepare the patient for follow-up treatment as indicated.
- Assess the patient for evidence of bruising or bleeding, such as oozing from IV or injection sites.
- Institute bleeding precautions to reduce the risk of bleeding.
- Provide emotional support to the patient and family.

Purpose

- To assess the fibrinolytic system
- To help detect abnormal fibrinolytic states
- May be used to assess fibrinolytic therapy (urokinase, streptokinase)

Description

Also known as *fibrinolysis* and *diluted whole blood clot lysis*, euglobulin lysis time measures the interval between clot formation and clot dissolution in plasma. A precipitated plasma extract is clotted with thrombin, and the time required for the clot to lyse is measured.

Interfering Factors

- Prolonged tourniquet constriction, vigorous vein preparation, or excessive pumping of the fist (decreased levels)
- Hemolysis caused by excessive probing at the venipuncture site or rough handling of the sample
- Failure to place the collection tube and sample on ice
- Drug interactions causing increased levels: cyclosporine A
- Drug interactions causing decreased levels: asparaginase, clofibrate, dextran, gemfibrozil
- Thrombolytic therapy

Nursing Considerations

Before the Test
- Confirm the patient's identity using two patient identifiers and confirmation of the patient's identification bracelet according to facility policy.
- Explain to the patient that the euglobulin lysis time test is used to evaluate the blood clotting mechanism.
- Inform the patient that a blood sample will be taken and explain that there may be slight discomfort from the tourniquet and the needle puncture.
- Inform the patient that there are no food or fluid restrictions for this test.

During the Test
- Perform a venipuncture. Collect a 5-mL sample in a tube with sodium citrate or in a chilled tube with 0.5 mL sodium oxalate.

> ▶ Quality and Safety Nursing Alert
>
> When drawing the sample, don't rub the area over the vein too vigorously, pump the fist excessively, or leave the tourniquet in place too long. Also avoid excessive probing during the venipuncture and handle the sample gently.

- If a tube with sodium citrate is used, mix the sample and anticoagulant thoroughly. If a chilled tube containing 0.5 mL sodium oxalate is used, mix the sample and preservative thoroughly.
- Pack the sample in ice and send it to the laboratory immediately.

After the Test
- Apply direct pressure to the venipuncture site until bleeding stops and to prevent hematoma formation.

Evoked Potential Studies

Normal Findings

Visual Evoked Potentials
- P100 (a positive wave appearing about 100 msec after the pattern-shift stimulus is applied)

- Absolute P100 latency (the time between stimulus application and peaking of the P100 wave) and the difference between the P100 latencies of each eye; variable among laboratories and patients

Somatosensory Evoked Potentials
- Variable waveforms obtained, depending on locations of the stimulating and recording electrodes
- Positive and negative peaks labeled in sequence, based on normal time of appearance

Abnormal Findings

Visual Evoked Potentials
- Extended P100 latencies confined to one eye, indicating a visual pathway lesion anterior to the optic chiasm
- Bilateral abnormal P100 latencies, indicating multiple sclerosis, optic neuritis, retinopathies, amblyopia (although abnormal latencies don't correlate well with impaired visual acuity)m spinocerebellar degeneration, adrenoleukodystrophy, sarcoidosis, Parkinson's disease, and Huntington's disease

Somatosensory Evoked Potentials
- Abnormal interwave latency, indicating a neurologic lesion
- Abnormal upper limb interwave latencies, indicating cervical spondylosis, intracerebral lesions, or sensorimotor neuropathies
- Abnormalities in the lower limb interwave latencies, indicating peripheral nerve and root lesions, such as those in Guillain-Barré's syndrome, compressive myelopathies, multiple sclerosis, transverse myelitis, and traumatic spinal cord injury

Nursing Implications
- Anticipate the need for additional testing. Information from evoked potential studies is useful but is insufficient to confirm a specific diagnosis.

Test data must be interpreted in light of clinical information.

- Prepare the patient for follow-up treatment, as indicated.
- Assess the patient's neurologic status for changes.
- Provide emotional support to the patient and family.

Purpose

- To help diagnose nervous system lesions and abnormalities
- To assess the patient's neurologic function
- Monitoring for injury prevention during neurologic and orthopedic surgeries

Description

Also known as *evoked responses/potentials* (visual evoked response [VER] and somatosensory evoked response [SSER]), evoked potential studies evaluate the integrity of visual, somatosensory, and auditory nerve pathways by measuring evoked potentials—the brain's electrical response to stimulation of the sensory organs or peripheral nerves. Evoked potentials are recorded as electronic impulses by surface electrodes attached to the scalp and skin over various peripheral sensory nerves. A computer extracts these low-amplitude impulses from background brain wave activity and averages the signals from repeated stimuli. (See the *Visual Evoked Potentials* box.)

Three types of responses are measured:

- Visual evoked potentials, produced by exposing the eye to a rapidly reversing checkerboard pattern, help evaluate demyelinating diseases, traumatic injury, and puzzling visual complaints.
- Somatosensory evoked potentials, produced by electrically stimulating a peripheral sensory nerve, help diagnose peripheral nerve disease and locate brain and spinal cord lesions.
- Auditory brainstem-evoked potentials, produced by delivering clicks to

the ear, help locate auditory lesions and evaluate brain stem integrity.

The usual procedures for visual evoked potentials and somatosensory evoked potentials are discussed here. (For information on auditory brain stem–evoked potentials, see the entry "Auditory Evoked Potentials" on page 70.)

Visual Evoked Potentials

- After the patient is positioned in a reclining chair or on a bed and asked to relax, electrodes are attached to the scalp at occipital, parietal, and vertex sites; a reference electrode is placed on the midfrontal area or ear.
- The patient is positioned 3 feet (0.9 m) from the pattern-shift stimulator.
- One eye is occluded, and the patient is instructed to fix the gaze on a dot in the center of the screen.
- A checkerboard pattern is projected and then rapidly reversed or shifted 100 times, once or twice per second.
- A computer amplifies and averages the brain's response to each stimulus, and the results are plotted as a waveform.
- The procedure is repeated for the other eye.

Somatosensory Evoked Potentials

- After positioning the patient in a reclining chair or on a bed, electrodes are attached to the patient's skin over somatosensory pathways—typically, the wrist, knee, and ankle—to stimulate peripheral nerves. Recording electrodes are placed on the scalp over the sensory cortex of the hemisphere opposite the limb to be stimulated. Additional electrodes may be placed at Erb's point (above the clavicle overlying the brachial plexus), at the second cervical vertebra, and over the lower lumbar vertebrae. Midfrontal or noncephalic electrodes are placed for reference.
- Painless electrical stimulation is delivered at a rapid rate to the

E

Visual Evoked Potentials

Visual (Pattern-Shift) Evoked Potentials

In the visual (pattern-shift) evoked potentials test, visual neural impulses are recorded as they travel along the pathway from the eye to the occipital cortex. Wave P100 is the most significant component of the resultant waveform. Normal P100 latency is about 100 msec after the application of a visual stimulus, as shown in the top diagram. Increased P100 latency, shown in the bottom diagram, is an abnormal finding, indicating a lesion along the visual pathway.

Normal Tracing

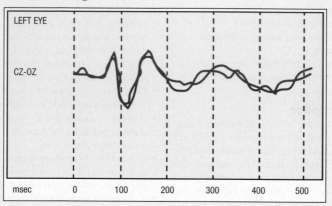

Tracing in Multiple Sclerosis

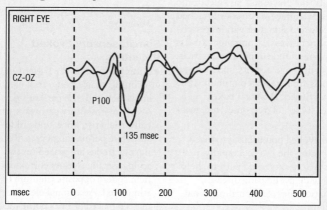

KEY:
CZ = vertex
OZ = mid occiput

peripheral nerve through the electrode. The intensity is adjusted to produce a minor muscle response, such as a thumb twitch on median nerve stimulation at the wrist.

- Electrical stimuli are delivered 500 or more times at a rate of 5 per second.
- A computer measures and averages the time it takes for the electric current to reach the cortex; the results, expressed in milliseconds (msec), are recorded as waveforms.
- The test is repeated once to verify results, and then the electrodes are repositioned and the entire procedure is repeated for the other side.

Interfering Factors

- Incorrect electrode placement or equipment failure
- Patient tension, inability to relax, or failure to cooperate
- Poor patient vision
- Obesity, edema
- Inadequate calibration of equipment

Nursing Considerations

Before the Test

- Confirm the patient's identity using two patient identifiers and confirmation of the patient's identification bracelet according to facility policy.
- Inform the patient that evoked potential studies measure the electrical activity of the nervous system.
- Explain who will perform the test and when and where it will take place.
- Explain that the patient will sit in a reclining chair or lie on a bed. If visual evoked potentials will be measured, electrodes will be attached to the scalp; if somatosensory evoked potentials will be measured, electrodes will be placed on the scalp, neck, lower back, wrist, knee, and ankle.
- Assure the patient that the electrodes won't hurt. Encourage relaxation; tension can affect neurologic function and interfere with test results.
- Have the patient remove all jewelry and other metal objects.

- Instruct the patient to wash and rinse the hair before testing. Tell the patient not to apply any other hair products after the hair is clean.

After the Test

- Assess the patient's response to testing.

Excretory Urography (Intravenous Pyelogram)

Normal Findings

- Kidneys, ureters, and bladder without gross evidence of soft- or hard-tissue lesions
- Prompt visualization of the contrast medium in the kidneys demonstrating bilateral renal parenchyma and pelvicaliceal systems of normal conformity
- Outline of ureters and bladder
- Postvoiding radiograph showing no mucosal abnormalities and minimal residual urine

Abnormal Findings

- Renal or ureteral calculi; abnormal size, shape, or structure of kidneys, ureters, or bladder; a supernumerary or an absent kidney; polycystic kidney disease associated with renal hypertrophy; a redundant pelvis or ureter; a space-occupying lesion; pyelonephrosis; renal tuberculosis; hydronephrosis; and renovascular hypertension (See the *Abnormal Excretory Urogram* box.)

Purpose

- To evaluate the structure and excretory function of the kidneys, ureters, and bladder
- To support a suspected differential diagnosis of renovascular hypertension

Description

The cornerstone of a urologic workup, excretory urography (also called *IV pyelography* [IVP] or *IV urography* [IVU]) requires IV administration of a contrast medium and allows visualization of the renal parenchyma, calyces, and pelvis, as well as of the ureters, the bladder, and, in some cases, the urethra. In some

Abnormal Excretory Urogram

In a patient with suspected renal hypertension, an excretory urogram taken 8 minutes after injection of a contrast medium shows normal filling of the right kidney but delayed filling of the left kidney and ureter (shown here). This impaired excretion of the contrast material commonly results from narrowing of the renal artery feeding the subject kidney. Constriction hinders blood flow to the glomerulus and leads to increased renal absorption of water and decreased urine output. Demonstration of delayed filling can distinguish unilateral renal hypertension from essential hypertension.

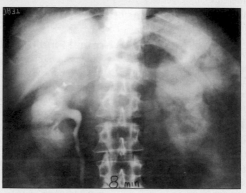

facilities, a nonenhanced computed tomographic scan of the urinary tract is commonly performed instead of this test if urinary tract stones are suspected.

The usual procedure for excretory urography is as follows:

- The patient is placed in a supine position on the X-ray table.
- A kidney–ureter–bladder X-ray is exposed, developed, and studied for gross abnormalities of the urinary system. Contrast medium is injected (dosage varies according to age), and the patient is observed for signs of hypersensitivity (flushing, nausea, vomiting, hives, or dyspnea).
- The first X-ray, visualizing the renal parenchyma, is obtained about 1 minute after the injection, possibly supplemented by tomography if small space-occupying masses, such as cysts or tumors, are suspected.
- Films are then exposed at regular intervals—usually 5, 10, and 15 or 20 minutes after the injection.
- Ureteral compression is performed after the 5-minute film is exposed.

This compression can be accomplished through inflation of two small rubber bladders placed on the abdomen on both sides of the midline, secured by a fastener wrapped around the patient's torso. The inflated bladders occlude the ureters without causing the patient discomfort and facilitate retention of the contrast medium by the upper urinary tract. (Ureteral compression is contraindicated by ureteral calculi, aortic aneurysm, pregnancy, or a recent abdominal trauma or surgical procedure.)

- After the 10-minute film is exposed, ureteral compression is released. As the contrast flows into the lower urinary tract, another film is taken of the lower halves of both ureters and then, finally, one is taken of the bladder.
- At the end of the procedure, the patient voids and another film is made immediately to visualize residual bladder contents or mucosal abnormalities of the bladder or urethra.

Interfering Factors

- End-stage kidney disease or stool or gas in the colon (possible poor imaging)
- Insufficient injection of contrast medium, a recent barium enema, or a recent GI or gallbladder series (possible poor imaging)
- Failure to maintain NPO status before test
- Feces or intestinal gas, which may obstruct visualization

Precautions

- Premedication with corticosteroids may be indicated for the patient with severe asthma or a history of sensitivity to the contrast medium.
- This test may be contraindicated in the patient with abnormal renal function (as evidenced by increased creatinine and blood urea nitrogen [BUN] levels) and in a child or an elderly patient with actual or potential dehydration.

Nursing Considerations

Before the Test

- Confirm the patient's identity using two patient identifiers and confirmation of the patient's identification bracelet according to facility policy.
- Explain to the patient that excretory urography helps to evaluate the structure and function of the urinary tract. Tell the patient who will perform the test and when and where it will take place.
- Make sure that the patient is well hydrated. Instruct the patient to fast for 12 hours before the test (all food, liquids, and medications). Obtain BUN and creatinine levels as ordered.
- Inform the patient that there may be a transient burning sensation and metallic taste when the contrast medium is injected. Tell the patient to report other sensations that may be experienced.
- Warn the patient that the X-ray machine may make loud clacking sounds during the test.

- Make sure that the patient or a responsible family member has signed an informed consent form.
- Check the patient's history for hypersensitivity to iodine, iodine-containing foods, or contrast media containing iodine. Mark sensitivities on the chart and notify the health care provider.
- Administer a laxative, if necessary, the night before the test, to minimize poor resolution of X-ray films as a result of stool and gas in the GI tract.
- Explain that an enema may be necessary the morning of the test.

After the Test

- Assess the IV site used for injection of the contrast medium. If a hematoma develops at the injection site, apply direct pressure.
- Continue IV fluids or provide oral fluid to increase hydration.
- Observe the patient for delayed reactions to the contrast medium.
- Administer medications as ordered.

Extractable Nuclear Antigen Antibodies (ENAs)

Reference Values

Negative for antiribonucleoprotein (RNP), anti-Smith (Sm), and anti-Sjögren's syndrome B (SS-B) antibodies

Abnormal Findings

Elevated Levels

- Systemic lupus erythematosus (SLE) (indicated by presence of anti-Sm antibodies specific for SLE [in 35% to 40% of cases], anti-Sjögren's syndrome A [SS-A] antibodies, and anti-SS-B antibodies) and mixed connective tissue disease
- Sjögren's syndrome (indicated by presence of anti-SS-A in 40% to 45% of cases and anti-SS-B antibodies in up to 60% of cases)
- Scleroderma (anti-Scl-70)
- Polymyositis (anti-Jo-1)

E

Nursing Implications

• Anticipate the need for additional testing and prepare the patient for follow-up treatment as indicated.
• Explain the underlying mechanism associated with autoimmune disorders.
• Provide emotional support to the patient and family.

Purpose

• To aid in the differential diagnosis of autoimmune disease
• To distinguish between anti-RNP and anti-Sm antibodies
• To screen for anti-RNP antibodies (common in mixed connective tissue disease)
• To screen for anti-Sm antibodies (common in SLE)
• To support the diagnosis of collagen vascular autoimmune diseases
• To monitor the patient's response to therapy

Description

Extractable nuclear antigen (ENA) is a group of nuclear antigens. One of them—ribonucleoprotein (RNP)—is susceptible to degradation by ribonuclease. The Smith (Sm) antigen is an acidic nuclear protein that resists ribonuclease degradation. The SS-A (Ro) antigen and SS-B (La) antigen form a precipitate when an antibody is present.

Antibodies to these antigens are associated with certain autoimmune disorders. Tests to detect ENA antibodies help differentiate autoimmune disorders with similar signs and symptoms.

The RNP antibody test detects RNP autoantibodies, which are associated with SLE, progressive systemic sclerosis, and other rheumatic disorders. This test aids in the differential diagnosis of systemic rheumatic disease and is a useful follow-up test for collagen vascular autoimmune disease.

The anti-Sm antibody test detects Sm autoantibodies, which are a specific marker for SLE; thus, positive results strongly suggest a diagnosis of SLE. This test, too, helps monitor collagen vascular autoimmune disease. The Sjögren's antibody test detects the SS-B autoantibodies produced by Sjögren's syndrome, an immunologic abnormality sometimes associated with rheumatic arthritis and SLE. However, this test doesn't confirm a diagnosis of Sjögren's syndrome.

The anti-Scl-70 is specific for scleroderma. The anti-Jo-1, antihistidyl transfer synthase, is present in about 20% of patients with myositis.

Nursing Considerations

Before the Test

• Confirm the patient's identity using two patient identifiers and confirmation of the patient's identification bracelet according to facility policy.
• Explain to the patient that the ENA antibody test detects certain antibodies and that the test results help determine diagnosis and treatment. It also assesses the effectiveness of treatment, when appropriate.
• Inform the patient that there are no food or fluid restrictions for this test.
• Inform the patient that the test requires a blood sample and advise that slight discomfort from the tourniquet and the needle puncture may be experienced.

During the Test

• Perform a venipuncture and collect the sample in a 7-mL tube without additives.

After the Test

• Send the sample to the laboratory immediately.
• Because a patient with an autoimmune disease has a compromised immune system, check the venipuncture site for infection and report changes promptly.
• Keep a clean, dry bandage over the site for at least 24 hours.
• Apply direct pressure to the venipuncture site until bleeding stops and to prevent hematoma formation.

Fasting Plasma Glucose

Reference Values

70 to 110 mg (SI, 3.9–6.1 mmol/L) of true glucose per deciliter of blood (after at least an 8-hour fast)

Critical Values

Females and children: Less than 40 mg/dL (SI, less than 2.22 mmol/L), possibly leading to brain damage

Males: Less than 50 mg/L (SI, less than 2.77 mmol/L), possibly leading to brain damage

All patients: Greater than 400 mg/dL (SI, greater than 22.2 mmol/L), possibly leading to coma

Abnormal Findings

Elevated Levels

- Diabetes (fasting plasma glucose levels of 126 mg/dL [SI, 7 mmol/L] or more obtained on two or more occasions)
- Impaired fasting glucose or impaired glucose tolerance (levels ranging from 110 to 125 mg/dL)
- Pancreatitis, recent acute illness (such as myocardial infarction), Cushing syndrome, acromegaly, and pheochromocytoma
- Acute stress
- Hyperthyroidism
- Pancreatic cancer
- Hyperlipoproteinemia (especially types III, IV, or V), chronic hepatic disease, nephrotic syndrome, brain tumor, sepsis, and gastrectomy with dumping syndrome; also typical in eclampsia, anoxia, and seizure disorders
- Use of corticosteroids
- Advanced liver and kidney disease

Decreased Levels

- Addison's disease, hyperinsulinism, insulinoma, von Gierke's disease, functional and reactive hypoglycemia, myxedema, adrenal insufficiency, congenital adrenal hyperplasia, hypopituitarism, malabsorption syndrome, some cases of hepatic insufficiency, insulin overdose, hypothyroidism, starvation, alcohol intake

Nursing Implications

- Anticipate the need for additional testing.
- Keep in mind that in the patient with borderline or transient elevated levels, a 2-hour postprandial plasma glucose test or oral glucose tolerance test may be performed to confirm the diagnosis.
- Prepare the patient for follow-up treatment as indicated.
- Assess the patient with increased levels for signs and symptoms of hyperglycemia.
- Assess the patient with decreased levels for signs and symptoms of hypoglycemia.
- Administer medications, as ordered, to control glucose levels.

Purpose

- To screen for diabetes and prediabetes
- To monitor drug or diet therapy in the patient with diabetes
- To monitor for hyperglycemia and hypoglycemia

Description

The fasting plasma glucose (or fasting blood sugar) test is used to measure plasma glucose levels after a fast of at least 8 hours. This test is commonly used to screen for diabetes and prediabetes, in which absence or deficiency of insulin allows persistently high glucose levels.

Interfering Factors
- Recent illness, infection, or pregnancy (possible increase)
- Glycolysis resulting from failure to refrigerate the sample or to send it to the laboratory immediately (possible false negative)
- Acetaminophen, if using the glucose oxidase or hexokinase method (possible false positive)
- Arginine, benzodiazepines, chlorthalidone (Hygroton), corticosteroids, dextrothyroxine, diazoxide (Proglycem), epinephrine (Adrenalin), furosemide (Lasix), hormonal contraceptives, phenothiazines, lithium (Eskalith), phenytoin (Dilantin), recent IV glucose infusions, large doses of nicotinic acid, thiazide diuretics, and triamterene (Dyrenium) (increase)
- Ethacrynic acid (may cause hyperglycemia); large doses in patients with uremia (can cause hypoglycemia)
- Alcohol, beta-adrenergic blockers, insulin, monoamine oxidase inhibitors, and oral antidiabetic agents (possible decrease)
- Strenuous exercise (decrease)
- Drug interactions: numerous medications may alter blood glucose levels

Nursing Considerations
Before the Test
- Confirm the patient's identity using two patient identifiers and confirmation of the patient's identification bracelet according to facility policy.
- Explain to the patient that the fasting plasma glucose test is used to detect disorders of glucose metabolism and helps diagnose diabetes.
- Inform the patient that the test requires a blood sample and explain that the patient may experience slight discomfort from the tourniquet and the needle puncture.

- Instruct the patient to fast for 12 to 14 hours before the test; however, water is allowed.
- Tell the patient to withhold use of insulin or oral antidiabetic agents until after the test is done, unless ordered otherwise.
- Notify the laboratory and health care provider about any medications the patient is taking that may affect test results; these may need to be restricted.

> ### ▶ Quality and Safety Nursing Alert
> Monitor the patient for signs and symptoms of hypoglycemia (weakness, restlessness, nervousness, hunger, and sweating), and report any symptoms immediately.

During the Test
- Perform a venipuncture and collect the sample in a 5-mL clot activator tube.

After the Test
- Send the sample to the laboratory immediately. If transport is delayed, refrigerate the sample.
- Note on the laboratory request slip when the patient last ate, the sample collection time, and when the last pretest dose of insulin or oral antidiabetic drug (if applicable) was given.
- Apply direct pressure to the venipuncture site until bleeding stops and to prevent the formation of a hematoma.
- Provide a balanced meal or a snack.
- Instruct the patient to resume his usual medications that were discontinued before the test, as ordered.

Febrile Agglutination Tests
Reference Values
Negative or positive (positive results are titered)

Normal dilutions: Salmonella antibody less than 1:80, brucellosis antibody less than 1:80, tularemia antibody less than 1:40, rickettsia antibody less than 1:40

Abnormal Findings

- Observed rise and fall of titers; for all febrile agglutinins, a fourfold increase in titers is strong evidence of active infection
- Weil-Felix test positive with antibodies to *Proteus* 6 to 12 days after infection; titers peaking in 1 month and usually dropping to negative in 5 to 6 months, indicating *Rickettsia*
- H and O agglutinins usually appearing in serum after 1 week, titers rising for 3 to 6 weeks, indicating *Salmonella* infection; O agglutinins usually falling to insignificant levels within 6 to 12 months; agglutinin titers possibly remaining elevated for years
- Titers usually rising after 2 to 3 weeks and reaching their highest levels between 4 and 8 weeks, indicating brucellosis; absence of *Brucella* agglutinins doesn't rule out brucellosis
- Titers usually becoming positive for tularemia during the second week of infection, exceeding 1:320 by the third week, peaking within 4 to 7 weeks, and usually declining gradually 1 year after recovery

Nursing Implications

- This test can't be used to diagnose rickettsialpox or Q fever because the antibodies of these diseases don't cross-react with *Proteus* antigens; the test shows positive titers in *Proteus* infections and, in such cases, is nonspecific for rickettsiae.
- Anticipate the need for additional testing and prepare the patient for follow-up treatment as indicated.
- Institute infection control precautions as appropriate.

Purpose

- To support clinical findings in the diagnosis of disorders caused by *Salmonella*, *Rickettsia*, *Francisella tularensis*, and *Brucella* organisms
- To identify the cause of fever or unknown origin

Description

Sometimes bacterial infections (such as tularemia, brucellosis, and the disorders caused by *Salmonella*) and rickettsial infections (such as Rocky Mountain spotted fever and typhus) cause puzzling fevers, called *fevers of undetermined origin* (FUO). In these infections and others in which microorganisms are difficult to isolate from blood or excreta, febrile agglutination tests can provide important diagnostic information. The Weil-Felix test for rickettsial disease, Widal's test for *Salmonella* infection, and tests for brucellosis and tularemia are essentially the same. In these tests, a serum sample is mixed with a few drops of prepared antigens in normal saline solution on a slide and the reaction is observed.

The Weil-Felix test establishes rickettsial antibody titers. It uses three forms of *Proteus* antigens (OX-19, OX-2, and OX-K) that cross-react with the various strains of rickettsiae. Antibodies to certain rickettsial strains react with more than one *Proteus* antigen, whereas antibodies to other strains fail to react with any *Proteus* antigens.

Widal's test establishes the titers for flagellar (H) and somatic (O) antigens, which may indicate salmonella gastroenteritis and extraintestinal focal infections, caused by *S. enteritidis*, or enteric (typhoid) fever, caused by *S. typhosa*. A third antigen, the Vi or envelope antigen, may indicate typhoid carrier status, which commonly tests negative for H and O antigens. Widal's test isn't recommended for diagnosing *Salmonella* gastroenteritis.

Slide agglutination and tube dilution tests, using killed suspensions of the disease organisms as antigens, establish titers for the gram-negative coccobacilli *Brucella* and *F. tularensis*, which cause brucellosis and tularemia, respectively.

Interfering Factors

- Vaccination or continuous exposure to bacterial or rickettsial infection, resulting in immunity (high titers)

- Antibody cross-reaction with bacteria causing other infectious diseases, such as tularemia antibodies cross-reacting with *Brucella* antigens
- Immunodeficiency (negative titers even during symptom-producing infection as a result of inability to form antibodies)
- Antibiotics (low titers early in the course of infection)
- Elevated immunoglobulin levels due to hepatic disease or excessive drug use (high *Salmonella* titers)
- Skin tests with *Brucella* antigen (possible high *Brucella* titers)
- *Proteus* infections (possible positive Weil-Felix titers for rickettsial disease)
- An inaccurate test result may occur if the tourniquet is left on the arm for longer than 1 minute. A new sample may be required.
- Drugs that may affect test results: antibiotics, cocaine, hallucinogens, marijuana, narcotics

Nursing Considerations

Before the Test

- Confirm the patient's identity using two patient identifiers and confirmation of the patient's identification bracelet according to facility policy.
- Explain to the patient that the febrile agglutination test detects and quantifies microorganisms that may cause fever and other symptoms.
- Inform the patient that there are no food, fluid, or medication restrictions for this test.
- Inform the patient that the test requires a blood sample and that slight discomfort from the tourniquet and the needle puncture may be experienced.
- Advise the patient that this test may require a series of blood samples to detect a pattern of titers characteristic of the suspected disorder, if appropriate. Reassure that a positive titer only suggests a disorder.

- Note on the laboratory request slip when antimicrobial therapy began, if appropriate.

During the Test

- Perform a venipuncture and collect the sample in a 7-mL clot activator tube.
- Use standard precautions when collecting and handling samples.

After the Test

- Send samples to the laboratory immediately.
- Apply direct pressure to the venipuncture site until bleeding stops and to prevent hematoma formation.
- In FUO and suspected infection, contact the facility's infection control department. Infection control measures may be necessary.

Fecal Lipids (Fecal Fat Stain)

Normal Findings

Adult: Fecal lipids comprising less than 20% of excreted solids, with excretion less than 7 g/24 hours
Child: Less than 2.0 g/24 hours
Infant: Less than 1.0 g/24 hours

Abnormal Findings

- Impaired lipid digestion, indicating pancreatic insufficiency
- Impaired release of lipase, indicating pancreatic resection, cystic fibrosis, chronic pancreatitis, or ductal obstruction by calculi or tumor
- Inadequate bile salt production and lipid digestion, indicating impaired hepatic function
- Abnormal release of bile salts, indicating biliary obstruction
- Abnormal enterohepatic bile salt circulation, indicating extensive small-bowel resection or bypass
- Regional ileitis and atrophy caused by malnutrition, causing gross structural changes in the intestinal wall
- Mucosal abnormalities, indicating celiac disease, Crohn's disease, or tropical sprue

- Steatorrhea, indicating scleroderma, radiation enteritis, fistulas, intestinal tuberculosis, small intestine diverticula, or altered intestinal flora
- Inhibited fat absorption, indicating Whipple's disease, or lymphomas

Nursing Implications
- Anticipate the need for additional testing, and prepare the patient for follow-up treatment as indicated.
- Provide emotional support to the patient and family.
- Assess the patient's nutritional status.

Purpose
- To confirm steatorrhea

Description
Lipids excreted in stools include monoglycerides, diglycerides, triglycerides, phospholipids, glycolipids, soaps (fatty acids and fatty acid salts), sterols, and cholesterol esters. When biliary and pancreatic secretions are adequate, emulsified dietary lipids are almost completely absorbed in the small intestine.

Excessive excretion of fecal lipids (steatorrhea) occurs in several malabsorption syndromes. Qualitative and quantitative tests are used to detect excessive excretion of lipids in patients exhibiting signs of malabsorption, such as weight loss, abdominal distention, and scaly skin.

Interfering Factors
- A contaminated or incomplete stool specimen (total weight less than 300 g)
- Alcohol, aluminum hydroxide, azathioprine (Imuran), bisacodyl, calcium carbonate (Caltrate), cholestyramine (Questran), colchicine, kanamycin (Kantrex), mineral oil, neomycin (Mycifradin), and potassium chloride (possible increase or decrease due to inhibited absorption or altered chemical digestion)
- Enemas, laxatives, rectal suppositories, and/or oily creams applied to the perineum.
- Ingestion of castor oil, mineral oil, low-calorie mayonnaise, oily salad dressings.

Nursing Considerations
Before the Test
- Confirm the patient's identity using two patient identifiers and confirmation of the patient's identification bracelet according to facility policy.
- Explain to the patient that the fecal lipid test evaluates fat digestion and that it requires a 72-hour stool collection.
- Instruct the patient to abstain from alcohol and to maintain a high-fat diet (100 g/day) for 3 days before the test and during the collection period.
- Notify the laboratory and health care provider about any medications the patient is taking that may affect test results; these may need to be restricted.
- Teach the patient how to collect a timed stool specimen and provide the necessary equipment. Tell the patient to be careful to avoid contaminating the stool specimen with toilet tissue or urine.
- Inform the patient that the laboratory requires 1 or 2 days to complete the analysis.

During the Test
- Don't use a waxed collection container because the wax may become incorporated in the stool and interfere with accurate testing.
- Collect a 72-hour stool specimen.
- Refrigerate the collection container and keep it tightly covered.

After the Test
- Instruct the patient to resume a usual diet and medications as ordered.

Fecal Occult Blood Test (FOBT)
Normal Findings
- Less than 2.5 mL of blood present in stools, resulting in a green reaction

Abnormal Findings
- Positive test, indicating GI bleeding, which may result from many

disorders, such as varices, a peptic ulcer, carcinoma, ulcerative colitis, dysentery, or hemorrhagic disease

Nursing Implications

- Anticipate the need for additional testing and prepare the patient for follow-up treatment as indicated.
- Keep in mind that this test is particularly important for the early diagnosis of colorectal cancer. Further tests, such as barium swallow, analyses of gastric contents, and endoscopic procedures, are necessary to define the site and extent of bleeding.
- The American Cancer Society recommends annual testing for those older than 50.
- Continue to assess the patient's stool for evidence of frank bleeding.
- Provide emotional support to the patient and family.

Purpose

- To detect GI bleeding
- To aid in the early diagnosis of colorectal cancer

Description

FOBT is also known as *stool occult blood test, Hemoccult test, guaiac smear test, gFOBT,* or *occult blood test.* Fecal occult blood is detected by microscopic analysis or by chemical tests for hemoglobin, such as the guaiac test. Normally, stools contain small amounts of blood (2–2.5 mL/day); therefore, tests for occult blood detect quantities larger than this. Testing is indicated when clinical symptoms and preliminary blood studies suggest GI bleeding. Additional tests are required to pinpoint the origin of the bleeding. (See the *Common Sites and Causes of GI Blood Loss* box.)

Interfering Factors

- Indomethacin (Indocin), phenylbutazone, rauwolfia derivatives, and steroids (possible increase due to association with GI blood loss)
- Drug interactions causing a false-positive result: boric acid, bromides, colchicine, iodine, Betadine

- Drug interactions causing a false-negative result: ascorbic acid (false normal, even with significant bleeding), iron supplements containing vitamin C
- Ingestion of 2 to 5 mL of blood, such as from bleeding gums
- Active bleeding from hemorrhoids (possible false-positive results)
- Foods that my interfere with results: meats that contain hemoglobin and myoglobin and contain certain enzymes (such as liver), vegetables and fruits with peroxidase activity (turnips, mushrooms, broccoli, radishes, cantaloupe, apples, bananas)
- Menstruation and hematuria
- Toilet bowl cleaners

Nursing Considerations

Before the Test

- Confirm the patient's identity using two patient identifiers and confirmation of the patient's identification bracelet according to facility policy.
- Explain to the patient that the fecal occult blood test helps detect abnormal GI bleeding.
- Instruct the patient to maintain a high-fiber diet and to refrain from eating red meats, turnips, and horseradish for 48 to 72 hours before the test, as well as throughout the collection period.
- Inform the patient that the test requires the collection of three stool specimens. Occasionally, only a random specimen is collected.
- Instruct the patient to avoid contaminating the stool specimen with toilet tissue or urine.
- Notify the laboratory and health care provider about any medications the patient is taking that may affect test results; these may need to be restricted. If these drugs must be continued, note this information on the laboratory request slip.

Common Sites and Causes of GI Blood Loss

Illustrated here are potential areas that can cause blood loss, resulting in positive fecal occult blood testing. Further clinical assessment and testing is necessary to determine the specific area involved.

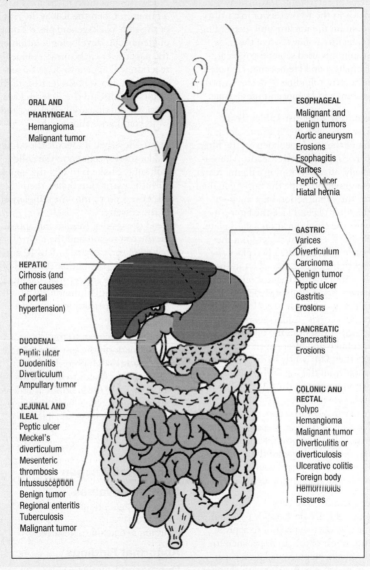

ORAL AND PHARYNGEAL
Hemangioma
Malignant tumor

HEPATIC
Cirhosis (and other causes of portal hypertension)

DUODENAL
Peptic ulcer
Duodenitis
Diverticulum
Ampullary tumor

JEJUNAL AND ILEAL
Peptic ulcer
Meckel's diverticulum
Mesenteric thrombosis
Intussusception
Benign tumor
Regional enteritis
Tuberculosis
Malignant tumor

ESOPHAGEAL
Malignant and benign tumors
Aortic aneurysm
Erosions
Esophagitis
Varices
Peptic ulcer
Hiatal hernia

GASTRIC
Varices
Diverticulum
Carcinoma
Benign tumor
Peptic ulcer
Gastritis
Erosions

PANCREATIC
Pancreatitis
Erosions

COLONIC AND RECTAL
Polyps
Hemangioma
Malignant tumor
Diverticulitis or diverticulosis
Ulcerative colitis
Foreign body
Hemorrhoids
Fissures

During the Test
- Collect three stool specimens or a random stool specimen, as ordered. Obtain specimens from two different areas of each stool. Testing may take place in the laboratory or in a utility room on the nursing unit, depending on facility policy. Two of the most commonly used screening tests are Hematest and Hemoccult. Hematest uses orthotoluidine to detect hemoglobin, and Hemoccult uses guaiac.

Hematest Reagent Tablet Test
- Use a wooden applicator to smear a bit of the stool specimen on the filter paper supplied with the kit. Alternatively, after performing a digital rectal examination, wipe the finger you used for the examination on a square of the filter paper. Place the filter paper with the stool smear on a glass plate.
- Remove a reagent tablet from the bottle and immediately replace the cap tightly. Place the tablet in the center of the stool smear on the filter paper. Add 1 drop of water to the tablet and allow it to soak in for 5 to 10 seconds. Add a second drop, letting it run from the tablet onto the specimen and filter paper. If necessary, tap the plate gently to dislodge any water from the top of the tablet.
- After 2 minutes, the filter paper will turn blue if the test is positive. Don't read the color that appears on the tablet itself or that develops on the filter paper after the 2-minute period. Note the results and discard the filter paper. Remove and discard your gloves and wash your hands thoroughly.

Hemoccult Slide Test
- Open the flap on the slide pack and use a wooden applicator to apply a thin smear of the stool specimen to the guaiac-impregnated filter paper exposed in box A. Alternatively, after performing a digital rectal examination, wipe the finger you used for the examination on a square of filter paper.

Apply a second smear from another part of the specimen to the filter paper exposed in box B because some parts of the specimen may not contain blood.
- Allow the specimen to dry for 3 to 5 minutes. Open the flap at the rear of the slide package and place 2 drops of Hemoccult developing solution on the paper over each smear. A blue reaction will appear in 30 to 60 seconds if the test is positive. Record the results and discard the slide package. Remove and discard your gloves and wash your hands thoroughly.

Instant-View Fecal Occult Blood Test
- Add a stool specimen to the collection tube. Shake it to mix the sample with the extraction buffer, then dispense 4 drops into the sample well of the cassette.
- Read the results. Results will appear on the test region and the control region of the cassette in 5 to 10 minutes, indicating whether the level of hemoglobin is greater than 0.05 mcg/mL. Results will also indicate whether the device is performing properly.

After the Test
- Send the specimen to the laboratory or perform the test immediately, depending on which test is used.
- Instruct the patient to resume his usual diet and medications as ordered.
- Single digital office-based tests may not be as accurate as serial home-collected tests.

Fecal Urobilinogen

Reference Values
50 to 300 mg/24 hours (SI, 100–400 EU/100 g)
Newborn to 6 months: Negative

Abnormal Findings

Decreased Levels
- Intrahepatic disorders (such as hepatocellular jaundice due to cirrhosis or hepatitis) or extrahepatic disorders

(such as choledocholithiasis or tumor of the head of the pancreas, ampulla of Vater, or bile duct (absent or low levels)
- Complete biliary obstruction
- Depressed erythropoiesis, such as in aplastic anemia (low levels)
- Oral antibiotic therapy
- Thalassemia
- Hemolytic anemia
- Sickle cell anemia
- Pernicious anemia

Nursing Implications
- Anticipate the need for additional testing and prepare the patient for follow-up treatment as indicated.
- Provide emotional support to the patient and family.

Purpose
- To help diagnose hepatobiliary and hemolytic disorders

Description
Urobilinogen, the end product of bilirubin metabolism, is a brown pigment formed by bacterial enzymes in the small intestine. It's excreted in stools or reabsorbed into portal blood, where it's returned to the liver and excreted in bile. A small amount is excreted in urine. Proper bilirubin metabolism depends on normal hepatobiliary system functioning and a normal erythrocyte life span.

Although measuring fecal urobilinogen is a useful indicator of hepatobiliary and hemolytic disorders, the test is rarely performed because it's easier to measure serum bilirubin and urine urobilinogen.

Interfering Factors
- Broad-spectrum antibiotics (possible decrease due to inhibition of bacterial growth in the colon)
- Sulfonamides, which react with the reagent used by the laboratory in this test, and large doses of salicylates (possible increase)
- Drug interactions causing increased levels: amyl nitrate

- Drug interactions causing decreased levels: acetazolamide, allopurinol, aspirin, azathioprine, butamide, chlorothiazide, chlorthalidone, chlordiazepoxide, chlorpromazine, erythromycin, methimazole, nalidixic acid, neomycin, oral contraceptives, oxymetholone, prochlorperazine, promazine, sulfamethoxazole, sulfisoxazole, tetracycline, thiabendazole, thiazides, tolbutamide, trifluoperazine

Nursing Considerations
Before the Test
- Confirm the patient's identity using two patient identifiers and confirmation of the patient's identification bracelet according to facility policy.
- Explain to the patient that the fecal urobilinogen test evaluates liver and bile duct function or detects red blood cell disorders.
- Inform the patient that there are no food or fluid restrictions for this test.
- Tell the patient that the test requires collection of a random stool specimen and to be careful to avoid contaminating the stool specimen with toilet tissue or urine.
- Notify the laboratory and health care provider about any medications the patient is taking that may affect test results; these may need to be restricted.

During the Test
- Collect a random stool specimen.
- Use a light-resistant collection container because urobilinogen breaks down to urobilin when exposed to light.

After the Test
- Send the specimen to the laboratory immediately after collection.
- Refrigerate the specimen if transport or testing is delayed more than 30 minutes; freeze the specimen if the test is to be performed by an outside laboratory.
- Instruct the patient to resume usual medications as ordered.

Ferritin, Serum

Reference Values
Adult females: 18 to 160 ng/mL
(SI, 18–160 mcg/L)
Adult males: 18 to 270 ng/mL
(SI, 18–270 mcg/L)
Neonates: 25 to 200 ng/mL
(SI, 25–200 mcg/L)
Infants age 1 month: 50 to 200 ng/mL
(SI, 50–200 mcg/L)
Infants ages 2 to 5 months: 50 to 200 ng/mL
(SI, 50–200 mcg/L)
Children ages 6 months to 15 years: 7 to
140 ng/mL (SI, 7–140 mcg/L)
Values increase with age.

Critical Values
Less than 10 ng/mL (SI, less than 10 mcg/L)

Abnormal Findings
Elevated Levels
• Acute or chronic hepatic disease, iron
overload, leukemia, acute or chronic
infection or inflammation, Hodgkin's
disease, or chronic hemolytic anemia
• Hemosiderosis
• Hemochromatosis
• Cancer
• History of multiple transfusions
• Hyperthyroidism
• End-stage kidney disease
• Renal cell carcinoma
• Thalassemia
• Chronic kidney disease

Decreased Levels
• Chronic iron deficiency
• Bleeding, including heavy menstrual
bleeding
• Iron deficiency anemia

Nursing Implications
• Anticipate the need for additional
testing and prepare the patient for
follow-up treatment as indicated.
• For the patient with decreased levels,
assess the color of the patient's skin
and mucous membranes; assess for
signs and symptoms associated with
iron deficiency, such as fatigue and
activity intolerance.

• Provide emotional support to the
patient and family.

Purpose
• To screen for iron deficiency and iron
overload
• To measure iron storage
• To distinguish between iron
deficiency (a condition of low iron
storage) and chronic inflammation
(a condition of normal storage)

Description
Ferritin, a major iron-storage protein,
normally appears in small quantities in
serum. In healthy adults, serum ferritin
levels are directly related to the amount
of available iron stored in the body and
can be measured accurately by radioimmunoassay.

Interfering Factors
• Recent blood transfusion (possible
false high) or blood donation
• Recently administered radioactive
medications
• Oral contraceptives
• Antithyroid therapy

Precautions
• Handle the sample gently to prevent
hemolysis.

Nursing Considerations
Before the Test
• Confirm the patient's identity using
two patient identifiers and confirmation of the patient's identification
bracelet according to facility policy.
• Explain to the patient that the serum
ferritin test is used to assess the available iron stored in the body.
• Inform the patient that a blood
sample will be taken and that slight
discomfort from the tourniquet and
the needle puncture may be experienced.
• Review the patient's history for blood
transfusion within the past 4 months.
• Inform the patient that there are no
food, fluid, or medication restrictions
for this test.

During the Test
- Perform a venipuncture.
- Collect the sample in a 10-mL tube without additives.

After the Test
- Send the sample to the laboratory immediately.
- Apply pressure at the venipuncture site until bleeding stops and to prevent hematoma formation.

Fetal Hemoglobin

Reference Values
Children (age 24 months and older) and adults: 0% to 2% (SI, 0–0.02)
Infants (age 1–23 months): 2% (SI, 0.02)
Neonates (age 0–30 days): 60% to 90% (SI, 0.60–0.90)

Abnormal Findings

Elevated Levels
- Beta-thalassemia major (fetal hemoglobin [Hb F] 30% or more of the total hemoglobin [Hb])
- Thalassemia major and minor
- Hereditary familial fetal hemoglobinemia
- Hyperthyroidism
- Juvenile myeloid leukemia with absence of Philadelphia chromosome
- Aplastic anemia, homozygous sickle cell disease, and myeloproliferative disorders (slight increases)
- Pregnancy (increase to as much as 5%)

Nursing Implications
- Anticipate the need for additional testing and prepare the patient for follow-up treatment as indicated.
- Assess the patient for signs and symptoms associated with anemia.
- Provide the patient and parents with access to counseling related to the underlying disorder.

Purpose
- To diagnose thalassemia

Description
Hb F is normally produced in the red blood cells of a fetus and, in smaller amounts, in infants. It constitutes 50% to 90% of the Hb in a neonate; the remaining Hb consists of Hb A_1 and Hb A_2, the Hb in adults.

Under normal conditions, the body ceases to manufacture Hb F during the first years of life and begins to manufacture adult Hb. If this changeover doesn't occur and Hb F continues to constitute more than 5% of the Hb after age 6 months, an abnormality—particularly thalassemia—should be suspected.

Fetal hemoglobin is also known as *hemoglobin F* or *alkali-resistant hemoglobin*.

Interfering Factors
- Delay in analyzing the sample for more than 2 to 3 hours (possible false high)
- Infants who are small for gestational age and those with chronic intrauterine anoxia (persistently elevated Hb F)
- Anticonvulsant therapy (increased Hb F)

Precautions
- Handle the sample gently to prevent hemolysis.

Nursing Considerations

Before the Test
- Confirm the patient's identity using two patient identifiers and confirmation of the patient's identification bracelet according to facility policy.
- Explain to the patient (or parents) that the Hb test is used to detect thalassemia.
- Inform the patient (or parents) that a blood sample will be taken from the finger or earlobe. Explain that the patient may feel slight discomfort from the tourniquet and the needle puncture. Offer reassurance that drawing the sample will take less than 3 minutes.
- Inform the patient (or parents) that there are no food or fluid restrictions for this test.

During the Test
- Perform a venipuncture and collect the sample in a 4.5-mL EDTA tube.
- Completely fill the collection tube and invert it gently several times to mix the sample and the anticoagulant thoroughly.

After the Test
- Apply pressure to the venipuncture site until bleeding stops and to prevent hematoma formation.

Fetal–Maternal Erythrocyte Distribution

Reference Values
No fetal red blood cells (RBCs)

Abnormal Findings
Elevated Levels
- Rh isoimmunization because no Rh immunization is present

Nursing Implications
- Prepare the patient for follow-up treatment as indicated.
- Keep in mind that an elevated fetal RBC volume in the maternal circulation necessitates administration of more than one dose of Rh_o (D) immune globulin.
- Determine the number of vials needed by dividing the calculated fetomaternal hemorrhage by 30. (A single vial of Rh_o (D) immune globulin provides protection against a 30-mL fetomaternal hemorrhage.)
- Administer Rh_o(D) immune globulin to an unsensitized Rh-negative mother as soon as possible (no later than 72 hours) after the birth of an Rh-positive infant or after a spontaneous or elective abortion, to prevent complications in subsequent pregnancies.
- Be aware that most clinicians are now administering Rh_o (D) immune globulin prophylactically at 28 weeks' gestation to women who are Rh negative but have no detectable Rh antibodies.

- Anticipate screening the following patients for Rh isoimmunization or irregular antibodies: all Rh-negative mothers during their first prenatal visit and at 28 weeks' gestation and all Rh-positive mothers with histories of transfusion, a jaundiced infant, stillbirth, cesarean delivery, or induced or spontaneous abortion.

Purpose
- To detect and measure fetal–maternal blood transfer
- To determine the amount of Rh_o (D) immune globulin needed to prevent maternal immunization to the D antigen

Description
Some transfer of RBCs from the fetal to the maternal circulation occurs during most spontaneous or elective abortions and most normal deliveries. Usually, the amount of blood transferred is minimal and has no clinical significance. However, transfer of significant amounts of blood from an Rh-positive fetus to an Rh-negative mother can result in maternal immunization to the D antigen and the development of anti-D antibodies in the maternal circulation.

During a subsequent pregnancy, the maternal immunization subjects an Rh-positive fetus to potentially fatal hemolysis and erythroblastosis. This test measures the number of fetal RBCs in the maternal circulation.

The fetal–maternal erythrocyte distribution is also known as *Kleihauer-Betke stain* and *fetal hemoglobin stain*.

Interfering Factors
- Delay of testing for more than 72 hours after sample collection

Nursing Considerations
Before the Test
- Confirm the patient's identity using two patient identifiers and confirmation of the patient's identification bracelet according to facility policy.

- Explain to the patient that this test determines the amount of fetal blood transferred to the maternal circulation and helps determine the appropriate treatment, if necessary.
- Tell the patient that she doesn't need to restrict food and fluids for the test.
- Advise the patient that the test requires a blood sample and explain that she may experience slight discomfort from the tourniquet and the needle puncture.
- Check the patient's history for recent administration of dextran, IV contrast media, or drugs that may alter results.

During the Test
- Perform a venipuncture and collect the sample in a 7-mL EDTA tube.
- Label the sample with the patient's name, the hospital or blood bank number, the date, and your initials.

After the Test
- Send the sample to the laboratory immediately with a properly completed laboratory request slip.
- Apply direct pressure to the venipuncture site until bleeding stops and to prevent hematoma formation.
- If unable to send to the lab immediately, place in refrigerator.
- Instruct the patient that she may resume her usual diet and medications as ordered.

Fibrinogen, Plasma

Reference Values
200 to 400 mg/dL (SI, 2–4 g/L)

Critical Values
Less than 100 mg/dL (SI, less than 2.9 mcmol/L)
Greater than 700 mg/dL (SI, greater than 20.6 mcmol/L)

Abnormal Findings
Elevated Levels
- Cancer of the stomach, breast, or kidney
- Inflammatory disorders, such as pneumonia or membranoproliferative glomerulonephritis

- Cerebral vascular accidents and cerebral diseases
- Acute myocardial infarction
- Pregnancy, eclampsia
- Nephrotic syndrome
- Multiple myeloma

Decreased Levels
- Congenital afibrinogenemia; hypofibrinogenemia or dysfibrinogenemia
- Disseminated intravascular coagulation
- Fibrinolysis
- Severe hepatic disease
- Cancer of the prostate, pancreas, or lung
- Bone marrow lesions
- Obstetric complications or trauma

Nursing Implications
- Anticipate the need for additional testing.
- In patients with decreased levels, prolonged partial thromboplastin time, prothrombin time, and thrombin time may also indicate a fibrinogen deficiency.
- Prepare the patient for follow-up treatment as indicated.
- Monitor the patient with increased levels for possible development of thrombi.
- Institute measures to prevent bleeding in the patient with decreased levels
- Keep in mind that markedly decreased fibrinogen levels impede the accurate interpretation of coagulation tests that have a fibrin clot as an end point.
- Provide emotional support to the patient and family.

Purpose
- To help diagnose suspected clotting or bleeding disorders caused by fibrinogen abnormalities

Description
Fibrinogen, an important coagulation protein, originates in the liver and is converted to fibrin by thrombin during clotting. Because fibrin is necessary for clot formation, fibrinogen deficiency

F

can produce mild to severe bleeding disorders. Fibrinogen is increased in diseases of tissue damage and inflammation.

Interfering Factors

- A diet rich in omega-3 fatty acids or omega-6 fatty acids (decreased levels)
- High levels of heparin
- Cigarette smoking (may elevate levels)
- Drug interactions causing increased levels: aspirin, bicalutamide, chemotherapy, estropipate, estrogens, fluvastatin, gemfibrozil, lovastatin, norethandrolone, oral contraceptives, oxandrolone, oxymethanolone, pyrazinamide, simvastatin
- Drug interactions causing decreased levels: anabolic steroids, asparaginase, atenolol, cefamandole, clofibrate, danazol, dextran, estrogen/progestin therapy, factor VIIa, fenofibrate, 5-fluorouracil, gemfibrozil, iron, kanamycin, lamotrigine, lovastatin, medroxyprogesterone, oral contraceptives, pegaspargase, pentoxifylline, phosphorous, pravastatin, prednisone, raloxifene, reteplase, simvastatin, streptokinase, sulfisoxazole, tetracycline, triamterene, trimethoprim

Precautions

- Be aware that the plasma fibrinogen test is contraindicated in the patient with active bleeding or acute infection or illness and in a patient who has had a blood transfusion within the past 4 weeks.

Nursing Considerations

Before the Test

- Confirm the patient's identity using two patient identifiers and confirmation of the patient's identification bracelet according to facility policy.
- Explain to the patient that the plasma fibrinogen test is used to determine whether the blood clots normally.
- Inform the patient that a blood sample will be taken and explain to the patient that slight discomfort

from the tourniquet and the needle puncture may be experienced.

- Notify the laboratory and health care provider about any medications the patient is taking that may affect test results; these may need to be restricted.
- Inform the patient that there are no food or fluid restrictions for this test.

During the Test

- Perform a venipuncture and collect the sample in a 3- or 4.5-mL tube with sodium citrate added.
- Avoid excessive probing during venipuncture and handle the sample gently.
- Completely fill the collection tube, invert it gently several times, and send it to the laboratory immediately or place it on ice.

After the Test

- Apply pressure to the venipuncture site; ensure that subdermal bleeding has stopped before releasing pressure.
- Instruct the patient to resume any medications that were discontinued before the test, as ordered.

Fibrin Split Products (FSPs)

Reference Values

Serum: Less than 10 mcg/mL (SI, less than 10 mg/L) of fibrin split products (FSP)

Quantitative assay: Less than 3 mcg/mL (SI, less than 3 mg/L)

Critical Values

Greater than 40 mcg/mL (SI, greater than 40 mg/L)

Abnormal Findings

Elevated Levels

- Primary fibrinolytic states (because of increased levels of circulating profibrinolysin)
- Secondary fibrinolytic states (because of disseminated intravascular coagulation [DIC] and subsequent fibrinolysis)

- Alcoholic cirrhosis, preeclampsia, abruptio placentae, intrauterine death, congenital heart disease, pulmonary embolus, deep vein thrombosis, sunstroke, or burns (transient increase)
- Myocardial infarction (after 1 or 2 days)
- Active renal disease or renal transplant rejection (levels usually exceeding 100 mcg/mL [SI, greater than 100 mg/L])
- Recent clot formation and breakdown

Nursing Implications
- Anticipate the need for additional testing and prepare the patient for follow-up treatment as indicated.
- Institute bleeding and safety precautions.
- Provide emotional support to the patient and family.

Purpose
- To detect FSP in the circulation
- To help determine the presence and severity of a hyperfibrinolytic state (such as DIC) that may result in primary fibrinogenolysis or hypercoagulability

Description
After a fibrin clot forms in response to vascular injury, the clot is eventually degraded by plasmin, a fibrin-dissolving enzyme. The resulting fragments are known as FSP. They are also called *fibrin degradation products (FDPs)* or *fibrin breakdown products*. This test detects FSP in the diluted serum left in a blood sample after clotting and is a reflection of clotting activity and breakdown.

Interfering Factors
- Pretest administration of heparin (false high)
- Failure to fill the collection tube completely, to adequately mix the sample and additive, or to send the sample to the laboratory immediately
- Hemolysis from rough handling of the sample

- Fibrinolytic drugs, such as urokinase, streptokinase, and tissue plasminogen activator, and large doses of barbiturates (increase)

Nursing Considerations
Before the Test
- Confirm the patient's identity using two patient identifiers and confirmation of the patient's identification bracelet according to facility policy.
- Explain to the patient that the FSP test determines whether blood clots normally.
- Inform the patient that the test requires a blood sample and that slight discomfort from the tourniquet and the needle puncture may be experienced.
- Notify the laboratory and health care provider about any drugs the patient is taking that may affect test results; it may be necessary to restrict these.
- Inform the patient that there are no food or fluid restrictions for this test.

During the Test
- Perform a venipuncture and draw 2 mL of blood into a plastic syringe.
- Draw the sample before giving heparin, to avoid false-positive test results.
- Transfer the sample to the tube provided by the laboratory, which contains a soybean trypsin inhibitor and bovine thrombin.
- Gently invert the collection tube several times to mix the contents thoroughly.

▶ *Quality and Safety Nursing Alert*

The blood clots within 2 seconds; after clotting, the sample must be sent immediately to the laboratory for incubation at 98.6°F (37°C) for 30 minutes before testing proceeds.

After the Test
- Apply pressure to the venipuncture site. Ensure that subdermal bleeding has stopped before releasing pressure.

- Assess the venipuncture site for bruising and hematoma formation. If a large hematoma develops at the site, monitor pulses distal to the site.
- Instruct the patient to resume any medications stopped before the test, as ordered.

Fluorescein Angiography (FA)

Normal Findings

- Sodium fluorescein reaching the retina in 12 to 15 seconds after rapid injection into the antecubital vein (filling phase)
- Choroidal flush (as the choroidal vessels and choriocapillaries fill, the background of the retina fluoresces, taking on an evenly mottled appearance)
- Dye filling the arteries (arterial phase)
- Complete filling of the arteries and capillaries until the earliest appearance of dye in the veins (arteriovenous phase)
- Emptying of arteries to the time the veins fill and empty (venous phase)
- Barely detectable amounts of fluorescein (if at all present) in the retinal vessels (recirculation phase, occurring 30–60 minutes after the injection)
- No leakage from the retinal vessels

Abnormal Findings

- Abnormalities detected in the early filling phase, indicating microaneurysms, arteriovenous shunts, and neovascularization
- Delayed or absent flow of the dye through the arteries; stenosis; and prolonged venous drainage, indicating arterial occlusion
- Vessel dilation and fluorescein leakage, indicating venous occlusion
- Recanalization and collateral circulation, indicating chronic obstruction
- Increased vascular tortuosity, microaneurysms around zones of capillary nonperfusion, and generalized suffusion of the dye in the retina, indicating hypertensive retinopathy

- Leakage of fluorescein and being surrounded by hard, yellow exudates, indicating aneurysms and capillary hemangiomas
- Variable fluorescein patterns, depending on the histologic type, indicating tumors
- Variable degrees of fluorescence, indicating retinal edema or inflammation and fibrous tissue
- Vascular leakage in the disk area, indicating papilledema

Nursing Implications

- Anticipate the need for additional testing and prepare the patient for follow-up treatment as indicated.
- Assess the patient's visual status as ordered, noting and reporting any changes.
- Provide emotional support to the patient and family.

Purpose

- To document retinal circulation when evaluating intraocular abnormalities, such as retinopathy, macular degeneration, tumors, and circulatory or inflammatory disorders

Description

In fluorescein angiography, a special camera takes rapid-sequence photographs of the fundus following IV injection of sodium fluorescein (a contrast medium), thereby recording the appearance of blood vessels within the eye. This technique provides enhanced visibility of the microvascular structures of the retina and choroid, which permits the evaluation of the entire retinal vascular bed, including retinal circulation. The varying and complex findings after fluorescein angiography require interpretation by a highly skilled ophthalmologist with extensive experience in diagnosing retinal disorders.

Testing, which may be done by the ophthalmologist or a technician, usually proceeds as follows:

- After the patient is seated in the examination chair, the antecubital vein is prepared and punctured; however, dye isn't injected yet. At this time, a few photographs may be taken. The patient must keep the arm extended; if necessary, an arm board may be used.

- The patient may experience nausea and a feeling of warmth and should be observed for hypersensitivity reactions (vomiting, dry mouth, metallic taste, suddenly increased salivation, sneezing, light-headedness, fainting, or hives). In rare instances, anaphylactic shock may occur.
- As the dye is injected, 25 to 30 photographs are taken in rapid sequence. Each photograph is taken 1 second after the other.
- The needle and syringe are removed carefully; pressure and a dressing are applied to the injection site.
- If late-phase photographs are needed, the patient is told to sit and relax for 20 minutes and then is repositioned for 5 to 10 photographs. If necessary, photographs may be taken up to 1 hour after the injection.

Interfering Factors

- Inadequate view of the fundus because of insufficient pupillary dilation (possible poor imaging)
- Cataract, media opacity, or inability to keep eyes open and to maintain fixation (possible poor imaging)

Nursing Considerations

Before the Test

- Confirm the patient's identity using two patient identifiers and confirmation of the patient's identification bracelet according to facility policy.
- Explain that fluorescein angiography takes about 30 minutes and evaluates the small blood vessels in the eyes.
- Make sure the patient or a responsible family member has signed an informed consent form.
- Check the patient's history for glaucoma and hypersensitivity reactions or allergies, especially to contrast

media and dilating eyedrops. If necessary, tell the patient with glaucoma not to use miotic eyedrops on the day of the test.

- Explain to the patient that eyedrops will be instilled to dilate the pupils. The drops may cause a stinging or burning sensation. A dye will be injected into the arm, which may cause nausea. The patient's eyes will be photographed with a special camera before and after the injection. Stress that these are photographs, not X-rays.
- Warn the patient that the skin may be discolored and that urine may appear orange for 24 to 48 hours after the procedure.

During the Test

- Administer mydriatic eyedrops. Usually, two instillations are necessary to achieve maximum mydriasis within 15 to 40 minutes.
- Following mydriasis, seat the patient comfortably in the examination chair facing the camera.
- Have the patient loosen or remove any restrictive clothing around the neck.
- Tell the patient to place the chin in the chin rest and the forehead against the bar. Tell the patient to open the eyes wide and stare straight ahead, while keeping the teeth together and maintaining normal breathing and blinking.
- Provide support and reassurance during the venipuncture for dye instillation. Keep in mind that the needle must be placed in the vein correctly; extravasation of dye around the injection site is painful.
- Warn the patient that the dye will be injected rapidly. Remind the patient to maintain the position and to continue to stare straight ahead while the dye is injected.
- Don't leave the patient unattended in case of a mild adverse reactions, such as nausea, vomiting, sneezing, paresthesia of the tongue, and dizziness.

- Monitor the patient for evidence of hypersensitivity reactions.

> ### ▶ Quality and Safety Nursing Alert
>
> **Have emergency resuscitation equipment on hand. Serious adverse effects (laryngeal edema, bronchospasm, and respiratory arrest) are possible. If a reaction occurs, note it on the patient's allergy history.**

After the Test

- Remind the patient that the skin and urine will be slightly discolored for 24 to 48 hours after the test. Encourage the patient to drink increased amounts of fluids to help excrete the dye.
- Explain to the patient that near vision will be blurred for up to 12 hours. Tell the patient to avoid direct sunlight and to refrain from driving during this time.

Fluorescent Treponemal Antibody Absorption (FTA-ABS)

Reference Values

Nonreactive and negative for syphilis
Sensitivity of FTA-ABS: Primary syphilis, 84%; secondary syphilis, 100%; latent syphilis, 100%; late syphilis, 96%

Abnormal Findings

Elevated Levels

- Primary and secondary syphilis (found in nearly all patients with secondary syphilis)
- Nonsyphilitic conditions (such as systemic lupus erythematosus, genital herpes, and increased or abnormal globulins) or pregnancy (minimally reactive levels)

Nursing Implications

- Anticipate the need for additional testing.
- Keep in mind that a nonreactive test doesn't necessarily rule out syphilis. *Treponema pallidum* causes no detectable

immunologic changes in the blood for 14 to 21 days after initial infection. Organisms may be detected earlier by examining suspicious lesions with a dark-field microscope. Low antibody levels and other nonspecific factors produce borderline findings. In such cases, repeated testing and a thorough review of the patient's history may be productive.

- Be aware that the fluorescent treponemal antibody absorption (FTA-ABS or FTA) test doesn't always distinguish between *T. pallidum* and certain other treponemals, such as those that cause pinta, yaws, and bejel.
- Prepare the patient for follow-up treatment as indicated; institute appropriate infection control measures.
- Provide emotional support to the patient and family, as well as information about syphilis and how it's spread. Emphasize the need for antibiotic therapy, if appropriate.
- Report positive results to state public health authorities and prepare the patient for mandatory inquiries.
- If the test is nonreactive or findings are borderline but syphilis hasn't been ruled out, instruct the patient to return for follow-up testing. Explain that inconclusive results don't necessarily indicate that he or she is free from the disease. False-negative results may occur early in the disease course or during inactive or later stages of the disease.

Purpose

- To confirm primary and secondary syphilis
- To screen for suspected false-positive results of Venereal Disease Research Laboratories tests

Description

The FTA-ABS test uses indirect immunofluorescence to detect antibodies to the spirochete *T. pallidum* in serum. This spirochete causes syphilis.

Two Tests for *Treponema pallidum*

The microhemagglutination assay for the *Treponema pallidum* antibody increases the specificity of syphilis testing by eliminating methodologic interference. In this assay, tagged sheep red blood cells are coated with *T. pallidum* antigen and combined with absorbed test serum. Hemagglutination occurs in the presence of specific anti–*T. pallidum* antibodies in the serum.

In the enzyme-linked immunosorbent assay, tubes coated with *T. pallidum* are washed and then treated with enzyme-labeled antihuman globulin. After the substrate for the enzymes is added to the tubes, the enzymatic activity is measured by quantitating the reaction product formed.

In this test, prepared T. *pallidum* is fixed on a slide, and the patient's serum is added after the addition of an absorbed preparation of Reiter treponema. This addition to the test serum prevents interference by antibodies from nonsyphilitic treponema; Reiter treponema combines with most nonsyphilitic antibodies, making the FTA-ABS test specific for T. *pallidum*.

If syphilitic antibodies are present in the test serum, they'll coat the treponemal organisms. The slide is then stained with fluorescein-labeled antiglobulin. This antiglobulin attaches to the coated spirochetes, which fluoresce when viewed under an ultraviolet microscope.

Although the FTA-ABS test is generally performed on a serum sample to detect primary or secondary syphilis, a cerebrospinal fluid (CSF) specimen is required to detect tertiary syphilis. Because antibody levels remain constant for long periods, the FTA-ABS test isn't recommended for monitoring the patient's response to therapy. (See the *Two Tests for* Treponema pallidum box.)

Precautions
• Handle the sample gently to prevent hemolysis.

Interfering Factors
• Hemolysis (false positive)
• Hepatitis (false positive)
• Testing too soon after exposure (false negative)

Nursing Considerations
Before the Test
• Confirm the patient's identity using two patient identifiers and confirmation of the patient's identification bracelet according to facility policy.
• Explain to the patient that the FTA-ABS test can confirm or rule out syphilis.
• Inform the patient that there are no food, fluid, or medication restrictions for this test.
• Inform the patient that the test requires a blood sample and explain that slight discomfort from the tourniquet and the needle puncture may be experienced.

During the Test
• Perform a venipuncture and collect the sample in a 7-mL clot activator tube.

After the Test
• Apply direct pressure to the venipuncture site until bleeding stops and to prevent hematoma formation.
• If the test is reactive, explain the nature of syphilis and stress the importance of proper treatment and the need to find and treat the patient's sexual contacts.

Folic Acid
Reference Values
Adults: 3 to 13 ng/mL (SI, 6.8–29.5 nmol/L)
Children: 5 to 21 ng/mL (SI, 11.3–47.6 nmol/L)
Infants: 14 to 51 ng/mL (SI, 31.7–115.5 nmol/L)

Abnormal Findings
Elevated Levels
• Excessive dietary intake of folic acid or folic acid supplements

- Pernicious anemia, vitamin B_{12} deficiency
- Blind loop syndrome

Decreased Levels

- Hematologic abnormalities, such as anemia (especially megaloblastic anemia), leukopenia, and thrombocytopenia
- Hypermetabolic states (such as hyperthyroidism), inadequate dietary intake, small-bowel malabsorption syndrome, hepatic or renal diseases, chronic alcoholism, or pregnancy

Nursing Implications

- Anticipate the need for additional testing. Be aware that the Schilling test is usually performed in patients with decreased levels to rule out vitamin B_{12} deficiency, which also causes megaloblastic anemia.
- Prepare the patient with decreased levels for follow-up treatment, including possible folic acid supplementation.
- Assess the patient's nutritional intake, including foods high in folic acid; teach the patient with decreased levels about foods containing this vitamin.
- Keep in mind that, even when taken in large doses, this vitamin is nontoxic.

Purpose

- To aid in the differential diagnosis of megaloblastic anemia, which may result from folic acid or vitamin B_{12} deficiency
- To assess folate stores during pregnancy

Description

The folic acid test is a quantitative analysis of serum folic acid levels (also called *pteroylglutamic acid*, *folacin*, or *folate*) by radioisotope assay of competitive binding. It's commonly performed concomitantly with measurement of serum vitamin B_{12} levels. Like vitamin B_{12}, folic acid is a water-soluble vitamin that influences hematopoiesis, deoxyribonucleic acid synthesis, and overall body growth.

Normally, diet supplies folic acid in organ meats, such as liver or kidneys, yeast, fruits, leafy vegetables, fortified breads and cereals, eggs, and milk. Inadequate dietary intake may cause a deficiency, especially during pregnancy. Because of folic acid's vital role in hematopoiesis, the usual indication for this test is a suspected hematologic abnormality.

Interfering Factors

- Alcohol, anticonvulsants such as primidone (Mysoline), antimalarials, antineoplastics, folic acid antagonists, hormonal contraceptives, and phenytoin (Dilantin) (possible decrease)
- Multiple medications, which may alter results

Precautions

- Handle the sample gently to prevent hemolysis.

Nursing Considerations

Before the Test

- Confirm the patient's identity using two patient identifiers and confirmation of the patient's identification bracelet according to facility policy.
- Explain to the patient that the folic acid test determines the folic acid level in the blood.
- Instruct the patient to fast overnight before the test.
- Inform the patient that the test requires a blood sample and explain that slight discomfort from the tourniquet and the needle puncture may be experienced.
- Notify the laboratory and health care provider about any medications the patient is taking that may affect test results; these may need to be restricted.

During the Test

- Perform a venipuncture and collect the sample in a 4.5-mL tube without additives.
- Protect the sample from light.

After the Test

- Send the sample to the laboratory immediately.
- Apply direct pressure to the venipuncture site until bleeding stops and to prevent hematoma formation.
- Instruct the patient to resume a usual diet and medications as ordered.

Follicle-Stimulating Hormone, Serum (FSH)

Reference Values

Menstruating females: Follicular phase, 1.68 to 15 milli-international units/L (SI, 1.68–15 international units/mL); ovulatory phase, 21.9 to 56.6 milli-international units/L (SI, 21.9–56.6 international units/mL); luteal phase, 0.61 to 16.3 milli-international units/L (SI, 0.61–16.3 international units/mL)

Menopausal females: 14.2 to 52.3 milli-international units/L (SI, 14.2–52.3 international units/mL)

Males: 1.25 to 7.8 milli-international units/L (SI, 1.24–7.8 international units/mL)

Abnormal Findings

Elevated Levels

- Ovarian failure associated with Turner's syndrome (primary hypogonadism) or Stein-Leventhal's syndrome (polycystic ovary syndrome)
- Precocious puberty (idiopathic or with central nervous system lesions) and postmenopause
- Destruction of the testes (from mumps orchitis or X-ray exposure), testicular failure, seminoma, or male climacteric
- Congenital absence of the gonads and early-stage acromegaly (both sexes)

Decreased Levels

- Male or female infertility (aspermatogenesis in males and anovulation in females)
- Secondary hypogonadotropic states, such as from anorexia nervosa, panhypopituitarism, or hypothalamic lesions

Nursing Implications

- Anticipate the need for additional testing and prepare the patient for follow-up treatment as indicated.
- For patients with increased levels, keep in mind that plasma levels fluctuate widely in *females;* to obtain a true baseline level, daily testing may be necessary (for 3–5 days) or multiple samples may be drawn on the same day.
- Provide emotional support to the patient and family.

Purpose

- To help diagnose and treat infertility and disorders of menstruation, such as amenorrhea
- To help diagnose precocious puberty in girls (before age 9) and in boys (before age 10)
- To aid in the differential diagnosis of hypogonadism
- To determine the cause of hypothyroidism in women

Description

The follicle-stimulating hormone (FSH) test of gonadal function, performed more commonly on females than on males, measures FSH levels and is vital in infertility studies. Its overall diagnostic significance typically depends on the results of related hormone tests (for luteinizing hormone, estrogen, or progesterone, for example).

A glycoprotein secreted by the anterior pituitary gland, FSH stimulates gonadal activity in both sexes. In females, it spurs development of primary ovarian follicles into graafian follicles for ovulation. Secretion varies diurnally and fluctuates during the menstrual cycle, peaking at ovulation. In males, continuous secretion of FSH (and testosterone) stimulates and maintains spermatogenesis. Reference values for the FSH test vary, depending on the patient's age, stage of sexual development, and (for females) phase of menstrual cycle.

F

Interfering Factors

• Ovarian steroid hormones, such as estrogen and progesterone, related compounds, and phenothiazines such as chlorpromazine (possible decrease through negative feedback by inhibiting FSH flow from the hypothalamus and pituitary gland)

• Radioactive scan performed within 1 week before the test

Precautions

• Handle the sample gently to prevent hemolysis.

Nursing Considerations

Before the Test

• Confirm the patient's identity using two patient identifiers and confirmation of the patient's identification bracelet according to facility policy.

• Explain to the patient (or to the parents of a minor) that the serum FSH test helps determine whether hormonal secretion is normal.

• Inform the patient that the test requires a blood sample, and explain that there may be slight discomfort from the tourniquet and the needle puncture.

• Tell the patient that there is no need to restrict food and fluids for the test.

• Withhold medications that may interfere with accurate determination of test results for 48 hours before the test, as ordered. If they must be continued (for example, for infertility treatment), note this on the laboratory request slip.

• Make sure the patient is relaxed and recumbent for 30 minutes before the test.

> ◤ *Quality and Safety Nursing Alert*
>
> If the patient is female, indicate the phase of her menstrual cycle on the laboratory request slip. If she's menopausal, also note this on the laboratory slip.

During the Test

• Perform a venipuncture, preferably between 6 AM and 8 AM and collect the sample in a 7-mL clot activator tube. Send the sample to the laboratory immediately.

After the Test

• Apply direct pressure to the venipuncture site until bleeding stops and to prevent hematoma formation.

• Instruct the patient to resume medications that were discontinued before the test, as ordered.

Fractionated Erythrocyte Porphyrins (FEP)

Reference Values

Total porphyrin levels: 16 to 60 mcg/dL (SI, 0.25–1.062 mcmol/L) of packed red blood cells (RBCs)

Protoporphyrin levels: 16 to 60 mcg/dL (SI, 0.25–1.062 mcmol/L)

Coproporphyrin and uroporphyrin levels: Less than 2 mcg/dL (SI, less than 0.035 mcmol/L)

Abnormal Results

Elevated Levels

• Erythropoietic protoporphyria, infection, increased erythropoiesis, thalassemia, sideroblastic anemia, iron deficiency anemia, halogenated solvents, or heavy metal and chemical poisoning (increased protoporphyrin levels)

• Congenital erythropoietic porphyria, erythropoietic protoporphyria or coproporphyria, or sideroblastic anemia (increased coproporphyrin levels)

• Congenital erythropoietic porphyria or erythropoietic protoporphyria (increased uroporphyrin levels)

Nursing Implications

• Anticipate the need for additional testing; keep in mind that increased total porphyrin levels suggest the need for further enzyme testing to identify the specific porphyria.

• Prepare the patient for follow-up treatment as indicated.

Purpose

- To help diagnose congenital and acquired erythropoietic porphyrias
- To help confirm the diagnosis of disorders affecting RBC activity
- To screen for iron deficiency and lead exposure in children 6 months to 5 years

Description

This test measures erythrocyte porphyrins (also called *erythropoietic porphyrins*): coproporphyrin, protoporphyrin, and uroporphyrin. Porphyrins are present in all protoplasm and are significant in energy storage and use; they're produced during heme biosynthesis and usually appear in small amounts in the blood, urine, and stools. Production and excretion of porphyrins or their precursors increase in porphyria.

Interfering Factors

- Exposure of the sample to direct sunlight or ultraviolet light

Precautions

- Handle the sample gently to prevent hemolysis.

Nursing Considerations

Before the Test

- Confirm the patient's identity using two patient identifiers and confirmation of the patient's identification bracelet according to facility policy.
- Explain to the patient that the fractionated erythrocyte porphyrin test detects RBC disorders.
- Advise the patient to abstain from alcohol for 24 hours before the test, because ethanol induces some enzyme activity and suppresses other enzymes along the hemebiosynthetic pathway.
- Inform the patient that the test requires a blood sample and explain that slight discomfort from the tourniquet and the needle puncture may be experienced.

During the Test

- Perform a venipuncture and collect the sample in a 5-mL or larger heparinized tube.

After the Test

- Label the sample, place it on ice, and send it to the laboratory immediately.
- Apply direct pressure to the venipuncture site until bleeding stops.
- Assess the venipuncture site for hematoma formation; if a hematoma develops, apply direct pressure to the site.

Free Thyroxine (FT$_4$) and Free Triiodothyronine (FT$_3$)

Reference Values

Free thyroxine (FT$_4$): 0.9 to 2.3 ng/dL (SI, 10–30 nmol/L)
Free triiodothyronine (FT$_3$): 0.2 to 0.6 ng/dL (SI, 0.003–0.009 nmol/L)

Abnormal Findings

Elevated Levels

- Hyperthyroidism, unless peripheral resistance to thyroid hormone is present (elevated FT$_4$ and FT$_3$)
- Triiodothyronine (T$_3$) toxicosis, a distinct form of hyperthyroidism (high FT$_3$ levels with normal or low FT$_4$ values)
- Graves' disease, euthyroid sick syndrome, hypothyroidism treatment with thyroxine (high FT$_4$ levels)

Decreased Levels

- Hypothyroidism, except in patients receiving replacement therapy with T$_3$ (low FT$_4$ levels) (Patients receiving thyroid therapy may have varying levels of FT$_4$ and FT$_3$, depending on the preparation used and the time of sample collection.)
- Third trimester of pregnancy (decreased FT$_3$ levels)

Nursing Implications

- Anticipate the need for additional testing and prepare the patient for follow-up treatment as indicated.
- Assess the patient with increased levels for signs and symptoms of hyperthyroidism, such as an enlarged thyroid gland, exophthalmos, nervousness, heat intolerance, weight loss, and excessive sweating.

- Instruct the patient with increased levels about hyperthyroidism and possible treatment measures.
- Assess the patient with decreased levels for signs and symptoms of hypothyroidism, such as fatigue, sensitivity to cold, weight gain, and constipation.
- Review the need for possible thyroid replacement hormone therapy in patients with decreased levels.

Purpose

- To measure the metabolically active form of the thyroid hormones
- To help diagnose hyperthyroidism and hypothyroidism when thyroxine-binding globulin (TBG) levels are abnormal

Description

The FT_4 and FT_3 tests, commonly done simultaneously, measure serum levels of FT_4 and FT_3, the minute portions of thyroxine (T_4) and T_3 not bound to TBG and other serum proteins. These unbound hormones are responsible for the thyroid's effects on cellular metabolism. Measuring free hormone levels is the best indicator of thyroid function.

Because of disagreement as to whether FT_4 or FT_3 is the better indicator, laboratories commonly measure both. The disadvantages of these tests include a cumbersome and difficult laboratory method, inaccessibility, and cost. This test may be useful in the 5% of patients in whom the standard T_3 or T_4 tests fail to produce diagnostic results.

Interfering Factors

- Thyroid therapy, depending on dosage (possible increase)
- High altitude and recently administered radioisotopes (elevates T_3)
- Heparin (falsely elevates T_4)

Precautions

- Handle the sample gently to prevent hemolysis.

Nursing Considerations

Before the Test

- Confirm the patient's identity using two patient identifiers and confirmation of the patient's identification bracelet according to facility policy.
- Explain to the patient that the FT_4 and FT_3 tests help to evaluate thyroid function.
- Inform the patient that the test requires a blood sample and explain that slight discomfort from the tourniquet and the needle puncture may be experienced.
- Advise the patient that there are no food or fluid restrictions for this test.
- Check the patient's medical history for use of any thyroid therapy and notify the health care provider accordingly; therapy may need to be restricted.

During the Test

- Perform a venipuncture and collect the sample in a 7-mL clot activator tube.

After the Test

- Apply direct pressure to the venipuncture site until bleeding stops and to prevent hematoma formation.

Fungal Serology

Normal Findings

- Negative finding or normal titer (depending on the test method)

Abnormal Findings

- See the *Serum Test Methods for Fungal Infections* table for information about specific organisms.

Nursing Implications

- Anticipate the need for additional testing and prepare the patient for follow-up treatment as indicated.
- Asses the patient for signs and symptoms of fungal infections.

Serum Test Methods for Fungal Infections

Disease and Normal Values	Clinical Significance of Abnormal Results
Blastomycosis	
Complement fixation: titers <1:8	Titers ranging from 1:8 to 1:16 suggest infection; titers >1:32 denote active disease. A rising titer in serial samples taken every 3 to 4 weeks indicates disease progression; a falling titer indicates regression. This test has limited diagnostic value because of a high percentage of false-negative results.
Immunodiffusion: negative	A more sensitive test for blastomycosis; detects 80% of infected people.
Coccidioidomycosis	
Complement fixation: titers <1:2	Most sensitive test for this fungus. Titers ranging from 1:2 to 1:4 suggest active infection; titers >1:16 usually denote active disease. Test may remain active in mild infections.
Immunodiffusion: negative	Most useful for screening, followed by complement fixation test for confirmation.
Precipitin: titers <1:16	Good screening test; titers >1:16 usually indicate infection. About 80% of infected people show positive titers by 2 weeks; most revert to negative by 6 months. Early primary disease is shown by positive precipitin and negative complement fixation test. A positive complement fixation and negative precipitin test indicate chronic disease.
Histoplasmosis	
Complement fixation (histoplasmin): titers <1:8	Titers ranging from 1:8 to 1:16 suggest infection; titers >1:32 indicate active disease. Antibodies generally appear 10 to 21 days after initial infection. Test is positive in 10% to 15% of cases.
Complement fixation: titers <1:18	Titers ranging from 1:8 to 1:16 suggest infection; titers >1:32 indicate active disease. More sensitive than histoplasmin complement fixation test; gives positive results in 75% to 80% of cases. (Histoplasmin and yeast antigens are positive in 10% of cases.) A rising titer in serial samples taken every 2 to 3 weeks indicates progressive infection; a decreasing titer indicates regression.
Immunodiffusion (histoplasmin): negative	Appearance of H and M bands indicates active infection. If the M band appears first and lasts longer than the H band, the infection may be regressing. The M band alone may indicate early infection, chronic disease, or a recent skin test.

(continued on page 312)

Serum Test Methods for Fungal Infections (continued)

Disease and Normal Values	Clinical Significance of Abnormal Results
Aspergillosis	
Complement fixation: titers <1:8	Titers >1:8 suggest infection; 70% to 90% of patients with known pulmonary aspergillosis or aspergillus allergy present antibodies. This test can't detect invasive aspergillosis because patients with this disease don't have antibodies; biopsy is required.
Immunodiffusion: negative	One or more precipitin bands suggests infection. The number of bands is related to complement fixation titers; the more precipitin bands, the higher the titer.
Sporotrichosis	
Agglutination: titers <1:40	Titers >1:80 usually indicate active infection. The test usually is negative in cutaneous infections and positive in extracutaneous infections.
Cryptococcosis	
Latex agglutination for cryptococcal antigen: negative	About 90% of patients with cryptococcal meningitis exhibit positive latex agglutination in cerebrospinal fluid. Culturing is definitive because false-positive results do occur. (Presence of rheumatoid factor may cause a positive reaction.) Serum antigen tests are positive in 33% of patients with pulmonary cryptococcosis; biopsy is usually required.

Purpose
- To rapidly detect the presence of antifungal antibodies, aiding in the diagnosis of mycoses
- To monitor the effectiveness of therapy for mycoses

Description
Most fungal organisms enter the body as spores inhaled into the lungs or infiltrated through wounds in the skin or mucosa. If the body's defenses can't destroy the organisms initially, the fungi multiply to form lesions; blood and lymph vessels may then spread the mycoses throughout the body. Most healthy people easily overcome initial mycotic infection, but elderly people and others with a deficient immune system are more susceptible to acute or chronic mycotic infection and to disorders secondary to such infection. Mycosis may be deep seated or superficial. Deep-seated mycosis occurs primarily in the lungs; superficial mycosis, in the skin or mucosal linings.

Although cultures are usually performed to diagnose mycoses by identifying the causative organism, serologic tests occasionally provide the sole evidence for mycosis. Such serologic tests use immunodiffusion, complement fixation, precipitin, latex agglutination, or agglutination methods to demonstrate the presence of specific mycotic antibodies.

Interfering Factors
- Cross-reaction of antibodies with other antigens, such as blastomycosis and histoplasmosis antigens (possible false positive or high titers)

- Recent skin testing with fungal antigens (possible high titers)
- Mycosis-caused immunosuppression (low titers or false negative)

Nursing Considerations

Before the Test

- Confirm the patient's identity using two patient identifiers and confirmation of the patient's identification bracelet according to facility policy.
- Explain to the patient that the fungal serology test helps diagnose certain fungal infections. If appropriate, tell the patient that this test monitors response to antimycotic therapy and that it may be necessary to repeat the test.
- Instruct the patient to restrict food and fluids for 12 to 24 hours before the test.

- Inform the patient that the test requires a blood sample and explain that slight discomfort from the tourniquet and the needle puncture may be experienced.

During the Test

- Perform a venipuncture and collect the sample in a 10-mL sterile clot activator tube.

After the Test

- Send the sample to the laboratory immediately.
- If transport to the laboratory is delayed, store the sample at 39.2°F (4°C).
- Apply direct pressure to the venipuncture site until bleeding stops and to prevent hematoma formation.
- Instruct the patient to resume a usual diet as ordered.

F

Gamma Glutamyl Transferase

Reference Values
Females: 5 to 25 units/L (SI, 0.08–0.42 mckat/L)
Males: 6 to 38 units/L (SI, 0.10–0.63 mckat/L)

Abnormal Findings

Elevated Levels
- Acute hepatic disease
- Acute pancreatitis
- Renal disease
- Prostatic metastasis
- Alcohol ingestion
- Obstructive jaundice
- Hepatic metastatic infiltrations
- Acute myocardial infarction (5–10 days after infarction occurred)

Nursing Implications
- Report abnormal findings to the health care provider. Observe for clinical manifestations of hepatic damage, such as restlessness, jaundice, hepatic flap, tremors, and spider angiomas.
- Prepare to educate the patient about the diagnosis, including instructions for appropriate dietary measures, including a well-balanced diet consisting of adequate protein and carbohydrates.

Purpose
- To provide information about hepatobiliary diseases, to assess liver function, and to detect alcohol ingestion
- To distinguish between skeletal and hepatic disease when the serum ALP level is elevated (A normal gamma glutamyl transferase [GGT] level suggests that such elevation stems from skeletal disease.)

Description
This test measures serum GGT levels. Also called *gamma glutamyl transpeptidase,* GGT participates in the transfer of amino acids across cellular membranes and, possibly, in glutathione metabolism. The highest GGT concentrations exist in the renal tubules, but the enzyme also appears in the liver, biliary tract, epithelium, pancreas, lymphocytes, brain, and testes.

Because GGT isn't elevated in bone growth or pregnancy, this test is a somewhat more sensitive indicator of hepatic necrosis than the aspartate aminotransferase assay and equally or more sensitive than the alkaline phosphatase (ALP) assay. However, the test is nonspecific, providing little data about the hepatic disease type, because increased levels also occur in renal, cardiac, and prostatic disease, and with use of certain medications. GGT is particularly sensitive to the effects of alcohol on the liver, and levels may be elevated after moderate alcohol intake and in chronic alcoholism, even without clinical evidence of hepatic injury. Moderate increases can also occur postoperatively.

Interfering Factors
- Hormonal contraceptives (decrease)
- Aminoglycosides, barbiturates, glutethimide (Doriden), phenytoin (Dilantin), warfarin (Coumadin) (increase)
- Moderate alcohol intake (increase for at least 60 hours)

Precautions
- Handle the sample gently to prevent hemolysis.
- GGT activity is stable in serum at room temperature for 2 days.

Nursing Considerations
Before the Test
- Confirm the patient's identity using two patient identifiers and confirmation of the patient's identification bracelet according to facility policy.
- Explain to the patient that the GGT test is used to evaluate liver function.
- Advise the patient that the test requires a blood sample. Explain that slight discomfort from the tourniquet and needle puncture may be experienced.
- Inform the patient that there are no food or fluid restrictions for this test.

During the Test
- Perform a venipuncture and collect the sample in a 4-mL red-topped tube without additives.

After the Test
- Apply direct pressure to the venipuncture site until bleeding stops and to prevent hematoma formation.

Gastroesophageal Reflux Scanning
Normal Findings
- Technetium 99m (^{99m}Tc) sulfur colloid descending through the esophagus in about 6 seconds
- Radioactivity only in the stomach and small bowel
- Typically, less than 4% gastric reflux

Abnormal Findings
- Prolonged transit time of ^{99m}Tc, indicating diffuse esophageal spasm or achalasia
- Radioactivity in the esophagus, indicating gastroesophageal reflux

Nursing Implications
- Report abnormal findings to the health care provider.

- Prepare to educate the patient about the diagnosis.
- Prepare to administer medications, as ordered.

Purpose
- To identify reflux
- To evaluate for esophageal disorders such as regurgitation
- To aid in identifying the cause of persistent nausea and vomiting
- To aid in differentiating reflux from vomiting in infants

Description
When barium swallow X-ray results are inconclusive, gastroesophageal reflux scanning may be done to test esophageal function and identify evidence of reflux. This test delivers less radiation than a barium swallow and is a much more sensitive indicator of reflux. It also allows reflux to be measured without insertion of an esophageal tube.

The procedure for gastroesophageal reflux scanning is as follows:

- The patient is placed in a supine or upright position and a binder is applied to the abdomen. The patient then is asked to swallow the solution containing a radiopharmaceutical such as ^{99m}Tc sulfur colloid. The radiopharmaceutical may be mixed with orange juice or with scrambled eggs.

> ▶ **Quality and Safety Nursing Alert**
>
> For an infant, the radiopharmaceutical is mixed with milk. A portion of the milk solution is given, and then the infant is burped. Then the remainder of the milk is given, followed by some radiopharmaceutical-free milk to clear the esophagus.

- The radiopharmaceutical may also be administered via a nasogastric (NG) tube.
- The binder may be inflated to exert abdominal pressure at specific intervals while a gamma counter is passed

over the patient's chest to record the passage of the radiopharmaceutical through the esophagus and into the stomach to determine transit time and evaluate esophageal function.

- The patient may be repositioned as the stomach distends, with continuous recordings to visualize events.
- A computer analysis is done to calculate the percentage of reflux (using a mathematical formula).

Interfering Factors

- Previous X-rays of the upper GI tract
- Presence of an NG tube (false-positive result)
- Presence of previous gastric banding

Precautions

- Endoscopic tube insertion is used with patients who have esophageal motor dysfunction, hiatal hernia, or difficulty swallowing.
- The patient needs to be able to tolerate abdominal compression. The binder must be applied below the ribs to avoid fractures.
- Gastroesophageal reflux scanning is contraindicated during pregnancy and lactation.

Nursing Considerations

Before the Test

- Explain the purpose of the gastroesophageal reflux scanning test in evaluating the patient's complaints of reflux and identifying possible causes.
- Tell the patient to fast beginning at midnight on the day before the test.
- Tell the patient that the test will be performed in the nuclear medicine department and that the test is painless and safe.
- Inform the patient that a binder with a balloonlike compression device will be applied to the abdomen. The binder will fit snugly, and the balloon may be inflated to apply pressure.
- Explain that the patient will be required to drink a solution such as orange juice or eat a small portion

of scrambled eggs that contains a radioisotope. Check for any patient allergies to eggs.

- Tell the patient that, after ingesting the solution or eggs, a machine will be passed over the patient's chest to monitor the radioisotope's passage.

> **Quality and Safety Nursing Alert**

Inform the parents of an infant that the radioisotope will be given with milk.

After the Test

- Explain that images usually will be obtained in approximately 2 hours.
- Instruct the patient to resume a usual diet after the procedure, as ordered.

Glucagon, Plasma

Reference Values

Less than 60 pg/mL (SI, less than 60 ng/L)

Abnormal Findings

Elevated Levels (900 to 7,800 pg/mL [SI, 900–7,800 ng/L])

- Glucagonoma
- Diabetes
- Acute pancreatitis
- Pheochromocytoma

Decreased Levels

- Idiopathic glucagon deficiency
- Hypoglycemia caused by chronic pancreatitis

Nursing Implications

- Report abnormal results to the health care provider.
- Prepare to educate the patient about the diagnosis.
- Prepare to administer any medications, as ordered.

Purpose

- To help diagnose glucagonoma and hypoglycemia caused by chronic pancreatitis or idiopathic glucagon deficiency

Description

Glucagon, a polypeptide hormone secreted in the pancreas by the alpha cells of the islets of Langerhans, acts primarily on the liver to promote glucose production and control glucose storage. Glucagon is secreted in response to hypoglycemia; secretion is inhibited by the other pancreatic hormones, insulin, and somatostatin. Normally, the coordinating release of glucagon, insulin, and somatostatin ensures an adequate and constant fuel supply while maintaining blood glucose levels within relatively stable limits.

This test, a quantitative analysis of plasma glucagon by radioimmunoassay, evaluates patients suspected of having glucagonoma (alpha cell tumor) or hypoglycemia due to idiopathic glucagon deficiency or pancreatic dysfunction. Glucagon is usually measured concomitantly with serum glucose and insulin because glucose and insulin levels influence glucagon secretion.

Interfering Factors

- Exercise, stress, prolonged fasting, insulin, or catecholamines (increase)
- Radioactive scans and tests performed within 48 hours of the test

Precautions

- Place the sample on ice and send it to the laboratory immediately.
- Handle the sample gently to prevent hemolysis.

Nursing Considerations

Before the Test

- Confirm the patient's identity using two patient identifiers and confirmation of the patient's identification bracelet according to facility policy.
- Explain to the patient that the plasma glucagon test helps to evaluate pancreatic function.
- Instruct the patient to fast for 8 to 12 hours before the test.
- Tell the patient that the test requires a blood sample. Explain that slight discomfort from the tourniquet and needle puncture may be experienced.
- Withhold insulin, catecholamines, and other drugs that could influence the test results, as ordered. If they must be continued, note this information on the laboratory request.
- Have the patient lie down and relax for 30 minutes before the test.

During the Test

- Perform a venipuncture and collect the sample in a chilled 10-mL EDTA tube.

After the Test

- Apply direct pressure to the venipuncture site until bleeding stops and to prevent hematoma formation.
- Instruct the patient to resume a usual diet and any medications that were discontinued before the test, as ordered.

Glucose Monitoring

Reference Values

Fasting: 60–110 mg/dL
After a meal (2 hours): 65–140 mg/dL

Critical Values

- A fasting glucose level of <40 mg/dL in children and in women or <50 mg/dL in men may cause brain damage

Abnormal Findings

Elevated Levels
- Diabetes

Nursing Implications
- Report abnormal findings to the health care provider.

Purpose

To help assess whether hematologic blood sugar levels are being controlled by treatment measures (i.e., oral medication, insulin)

Description

Blood sugar levels are measured clinically by drawing blood or by using an electronic measuring device in the patient's home.

Interfering Factors

- High humidity
- Ambient temperatures exceeding 104°F
- Test strips that are out of date or have been improperly stored
- Low ambient temperatures (may affect blood flow to the fingers)
- Improperly calibrated meters (affect accurate readings)
- Unclean hands (may contaminate the test strip and produce inaccurate readings)

Nursing Considerations

Before the Test

- Confirm the patient's identity using two patient identifiers and confirmation of the patient's identification bracelet according to facility policy.
- Be certain the patient's hands are washed thoroughly. Make sure the patient clearly understands the need to avoid anything that might cause an inaccurate reading. Explain the procedure carefully from hand-washing right through to reading the metered result and recording the reading accurately.

During the Test

- The blood should be drawn using a fresh sharp each time to avoid possible contamination.

After the Test

- The test result should be logged accurately and reported to the health care provider when asked.
- Instruct the fasting patient to resume a normal diet.

Growth Hormone Suppression Test

Reference Values

Undetectable to 3 ng/mL (SI, 3 mcg/L) in 30 minutes to 2 hours
In children: Rebound stimulation possible after 2 to 5 hours

Abnormal Findings

Elevated Levels

- Acromegaly
- Gigantism

Nursing Implications

- Report abnormal results to the health care provider.
- Prepare to educate the patient about the diagnosis.
- Prepare to administer any medications, as ordered.

Purpose

- To assess elevated baseline levels of human growth hormone (hGH)
- To confirm diagnosis of gigantism in children and acromegaly in adults and adolescents

Description

Also called *glucose loading,* the growth hormone suppression test evaluates excessive hGH baseline levels from the anterior pituitary gland. Normally, hGH raises plasma glucose and fatty acid concentrations; in response, insulin secretion increases to counteract these effects, causing a glucose load that should suppress hGH secretions. In a patient with excessive hGH levels, suppression failure indicates anterior pituitary dysfunction and confirms an acromegaly or a gigantism diagnosis.

Interfering Factors

- Corticosteroids and phenothiazines such as chlorpromazine (Thorazine) (possible decrease in hGH secretion)
- Amphetamines, arginine, estrogens, glucagon, levodopa, and niacin (possible increase in hGH secretion)
- Radioactive scan within 1 week before the test

Precautions

- Handle the samples gently to prevent hemolysis.
- Send each sample to the laboratory immediately because hGH has a half-life of only 20 to 25 minutes.

Nursing Considerations

Before the Test

- Confirm the patient's identity using two patient identifiers and confirmation of the patient's identification bracelet according to facility policy.
- Explain to the patient, or parents if the patient is a child, that this test helps determine the cause of abnormal growth.
- Instruct the patient to fast and limit physical activity for 10 to 12 hours before the test.
- Advise the patient that two blood samples will be drawn.
- Warn that nausea after drinking the glucose solution and some discomfort from the tourniquet and needle punctures may be experienced.
- Withhold all steroids and other pituitary-based hormones. If they or other medications must be continued, note this on the laboratory request.
- Tell the patient to lie down and relax for 30 minutes before the test.

During the Test

- Perform a venipuncture and collect 6 mL of blood (basal sample) in a 7-mL clot activator tube between 6 AM and 8 AM.
- Administer 100 g of glucose solution by mouth. To prevent nausea, advise the patient to drink the glucose slowly.
- About 1 hour later, draw venous blood into a 7-mL clot activator tube. Label the tubes appropriately and send them to the laboratory immediately.

After the Test

- Apply direct pressure to the venipuncture site until bleeding stops and to prevent hematoma formation.
- Instruct the patient to resume a usual diet and any activities and medications that were discontinued before the test, as ordered.

G

Helicobacter Pylori Antibodies

Reference Values
No antibodies to *Helicobacter pylori* bacterium

Abnormal Findings
• Antibodies to the *H. pylori* bacterium

Nursing Implications
• Report abnormal values to the health care provider.
• Prepare to educate the patient about the diagnosis, medication regimen, and possible dietary restriction or alterations.

Purpose
• To help diagnose *H. pylori* infection in patients with GI symptoms (used only for patients with GI symptoms because a large number of healthy people have *H. pylori* antibodies)

Description
H. pylori is a spiral, gram-negative bacterium linked to chronic gastritis and idiopathic chronic duodenal ulceration. Although a gastric specimen can be obtained by endoscopy and cultured for *H. pylori*, the antibody blood test is a more useful, noninvasive screening procedure, and it may be performed using the enzyme-linked immunosorbent assay. (See the *Additional Tests for Helicobacter pylori* box.) Test results are reported as negative or positive.

Nursing Considerations

Before the Test
• Confirm the patient's identity using two patient identifiers and confirmation of the patient's identification bracelet according to facility policy.
• Inform the patient that this test diagnoses the infection that may cause ulcers.
• Advise the patient that the test requires a blood sample. Explain that slight discomfort from the tourniquet and the needle puncture may be experienced.

During the Test
• Perform a venipuncture and collect the sample in a 7-mL clot activator tube.
• Send the sample to the laboratory immediately.

After the Test
• Apply direct pressure to the venipuncture site until bleeding stops and to prevent hematoma formation.

Hematocrit

Reference Values
Females: 36% to 48% (SI, 0.36–0.48)
Males: 42% to 52% (SI, 0.42–0.52)
Children age 1 year: 29% to 41% (SI, 0.29–0.41)
Children age 10 years: 36% to 40% (SI, 0.36–0.4)
Infants age 1 month: 37% to 49% (SI, 0.37–0.49)
Infants age 3 months: 30% to 36% (SI, 0.30–0.36)
Neonates age 1 week: 47% to 65% (SI, 0.47–0.65)
Neonates older than 1 week: 55% to 68% (SI, 0.55–0.68)

Critical Values
Less than 20% (SI, less than 0.20) or greater than 60% (SI, greater than 0.60)

Additional Tests for *Helicobacter pylori*

Helicobacter pylori is diagnosed through blood, breath, stool, and tissue tests. Blood tests are the most common. They detect antibodies to *H. pylori* bacteria.

Urea breath tests are an effective diagnostic tool for *H. pylori*. They're also used after treatment to see whether it has been effective. In the health care provider's office, the patient swallows a capsule or drinks a urea solution that contains a special carbon atom. If *H. pylori* is present, it breaks down the urea, releasing the carbon. The blood carries the carbon to the lungs, and the patient exhales it. The breath test is 96% to 98% accurate.

A stool antigen test detects substances that trigger the immune system to fight an *H. pylori* infection. Stool antigen

testing is less expensive, and results can be obtained in about 3 hours.

Tissue tests are usually done using a biopsy specimen taken with an endoscope. There are three types:
• The rapid urease test detects the enzyme disease produced by *H. pylori*.
• A histology test allows the health care provider to find and examine the actual bacteria.
• A culture test involves allowing *H. pylori* to grow in the tissue specimen.

In diagnosing *H. pylori*, blood, breath, and stool tests are commonly done before tissue tests because they're less invasive. However, blood tests aren't used to detect *H. pylori* following treatment because a patient's blood can show positive results even after *H. pylori* has been eliminated.

Abnormal Findings

Elevated Levels
• Polycythemia
• Hemoconcentration caused by blood loss and dehydration
• Pathological conditions such as emphysema in the late stages, transient cerebral ischemia (TIA), eclampsia, trauma surgery, and burns

Decreased Levels
• Anemia
• Hemodilution
• Massive blood loss
• Leukemias, lymphomas, Hodgkin's disease
• Adrenal insufficiency

Nursing Implications
• Report abnormal values to the health care provider.
• Prepare to educate the patient about the diagnosis.
• Administer IV fluids or blood replacement, as ordered.

Purpose
• To aid diagnosis of polycythemia, anemia, or abnormal states of hydration
• To aid in the calculation of erythrocyte indices

Description

A hematocrit (HCT) test, which may be performed separately or as part of a complete blood count, measures percentage by volume of packed red blood cells (RBCs) in a whole blood sample. For example, a 40% HCT indicates that a 100-mL sample of blood contains 40 mL of packed RBCs. Packing is achieved by centrifuging anticoagulated whole blood in a capillary tube so that RBCs pack tightly without hemolysis. Test results may be used to calculate two RBC indices: mean corpuscular volume and mean corpuscular hemoglobin concentration.

Interfering Factors
• Failure to fill the tube properly, to use the proper anticoagulant, or to adequately mix the sample and the anticoagulant
• Hemolysis from rough handling of the sample or drawing the blood through a small-gauge needle for venipuncture
• Hemoconcentration caused by tourniquet constriction for longer than 1 minute (increase, typically 2.5–5%)
• Hemodilution from drawing the blood from the arm above an IV infusion

Nursing Considerations

Before the Test
- Confirm the patient's identity using two patient identifiers and confirmation of the patient's identification bracelet according to facility policy.
- Explain to the patient that the HCT test detects anemia and other abnormal blood conditions.
- Advise the patient that the test requires a blood sample. Explain that slight discomfort from the tourniquet and the needle puncture may be experienced.
- Inform the patient that there are no food or fluid restrictions for this test.
- If the patient is a child, explain to the patient (if old enough) and the parents that a small amount of blood will be taken from the finger or earlobe.

During the Test
- Perform a finger stick using a heparinized capillary tube with a red band on the anticoagulant end. Fill the tube from the red-banded end to about two-thirds capacity; seal this end with clay. Alternatively, perform a venipuncture by filling a 3- or 4.5-mL EDTA tube.
- Invert the tube gently several times to mix the sample.
- Send the sample to the laboratory immediately.

After the Test
- Place the tube in the centrifuge with the red end pointing outward.
- Ensure subdermal bleeding has stopped before removing pressure from the finger stick or venipuncture site.
- If large hematoma develops at the venipuncture site, monitor pulses distal to the site.

Hemoglobin

Reference Values
Females up to middle age: 12 to 16 g/dL (SI, 120–160 g/L)
Females after middle age: 11.7 to 13.8 g/dL (SI, 117–138 g/L)
Males up to middle age: 14 to 17.4 g/dL (SI, 140–174 g/L)
Males after middle age: 12.4 to 14.9 g/dL (SI, 124–149 g/L)
Children: 11 to 13 g/dL (SI, 110–130 g/L)
Infants age 1 month: 11 to 15 g/dL (SI, 110–150 g/L)
Neonates age 1 week: 15 to 20 g/dL (SI, 150–200 g/L)
Neonates older than age 1 week: 17 to 22 g/dL (SI, 170–220 g/L)

Critical Values
Less than 7 g/dL (SI, less than 70 g/L) or greater than 20 g/dL (SI, greater than 200 g/L)

Abnormal Findings

Elevated Levels
- Hemoconcentration from polycythemia or dehydration

Decreased Levels
- Anemia
- Acute or chronic hemorrhage
- Fluid retention
- Liver disease, hypothyroidism
- A variety of systemic diseases

Nursing Implications
- Report abnormal values to the health care provider.
- Prepare to educate the patient about the diagnosis.
- With elevated levels, administer IV fluids as ordered.

Purpose
- To measure the severity of anemia or polycythemia and to monitor the patient's response to therapy
- To obtain data for calculating the mean corpuscular hemoglobin (MCH) and mean corpuscular hemoglobin concentration (MCHC)

Description
Total hemoglobin (Hb) measures the amount of Hb present in a deciliter (dL, or 100 mL) of whole blood. The Hb level correlates closely with the red blood cell (RBC) count and affects the Hb-to-RBC ratio (MCH and MCHC).

Interfering Factors
- Failure to use the proper anticoagulant or to adequately mix the sample and the anticoagulant
- Hemolysis from rough handling of the sample
- Hemoconcentration resulting from prolonged tourniquet constriction
- Very high white blood cell counts, lipemia, or RBCs that are resistant to lysis (false high)
- Living in high altitudes (may increase Hb levels)
- Pregnancy
- Extreme physical exercise

Precautions
- Handle the sample gently to prevent hemolysis.

Nursing Considerations
Before the Test
- Confirm the patient's identity using two patient identifiers and confirmation of the patient's identification bracelet according to facility policy.
- Explain to the patient that the Hb test detects anemia or polycythemia or assesses response to treatment.
- Tell the patient that the test requires a blood sample. Explain that slight discomfort from the tourniquet and the needle puncture may be experienced.
- If the patient is an infant or child, explain to the parents that a small amount of blood will be taken from the finger or earlobe.
- Inform the patient that there are no food or fluid restrictions for this test.

During the Test
- For adults and older children, perform a venipuncture and collect the sample in a 3- or 4.5-mL EDTA tube.
- For younger children and infants, collect the sample by finger stick or heel stick in a microcollection device with EDTA.

- Completely fill the collection tube and invert it gently several times to thoroughly mix the sample and the anticoagulant.

After the Test
- Apply direct pressure to the venipuncture site until bleeding stops and to prevent hematoma formation.
- If a large hematoma develops at the venipuncture site, monitor pulses distal to the site.

Hemoglobin Electrophoresis
Reference Values
Hemoglobin (Hb) A: 95% (SI, 0.95) of all Hb
Hb A$_2$: 1.5% to 3% (SI, 0.015–0.030)
Hb F: Less than 2% (SI, less than 0.02)
Neonates: Hb F normally half the total; Hb S and Hb C normally absent

Abnormal Findings
- Hemolytic disease (See the *Variations of Hemoglobin Type and Distribution* table.)

Nursing Implications
- Report abnormal values to the health care provider.
- Prepare to educate the patient about the diagnosis.

Purpose
- To measure the amount of Hb A and to detect abnormal Hb
- To help diagnose thalassemia

Description
Hb electrophoresis is probably the most useful laboratory method for separating and measuring normal and abnormal Hb. Through electrophoresis, different types of Hb are separated to form a series of distinctly pigmented bands in a medium. Results are compared with those of a normal sample.

Interfering Factors
- Failure to fill the tube completely, to use the proper anticoagulant, or to adequately mix the sample and the anticoagulant

Variations of Hemoglobin Type and Distribution

Use this table to identify the clinical implications of hemoglobin (Hb) type and distribution.

Hemoglobin	Percentage of Total Hemoglobin	Clinical Implications
Hb A	95% to 100% (SI, 0.95–1.0)	Normal
Hb A₂	4% to 5.8% (SI, 0.04–0.058)	β-thalassemia minor
	1.5% to 3% (SI, 0.015–0.03)	Normal
	Under 1.5% (SI, <0.015)	Hb H disease
Hb F	Under 1% (SI, <0.01)	Normal
	2% to 5% (SI, 0.02–0.05)	β-thalassemia minor
	10% to 90% (SI, 0.1–0.9)	β-thalassemia major
	5% to 15% (SI, 0.05–0.15)	β-thalassemia minor
	5% to 35% (SI, 0.05–0.35)	Heterozygous hereditary persistence of fetal Hb (HPFH)
	100% (SI, 1.0)	Homozygous HPFH
	15% (SI, 0.15)	Homozygous Hb S
Homozygous Hb S	70% to 98% (SI, 0.7–0.98)	Sickle cell disease
Homozygous Hb C	90% to 98% (SI, 0.9–0.98)	Hb C disease
Heterozygous Hb C	24% to 44% (SI, 0.24–0.44)	Hb C trait

- Hemolysis from rough handling of the sample
- Blood transfusion within the past 4 months

Nursing Considerations

Before the Test

- Confirm the patient's identity using two patient identifiers and confirmation of the patient's identification bracelet according to facility policy.
- Explain that Hb electrophoresis evaluates Hb.
- Tell the patient that the test requires a blood sample. Explain that slight discomfort from the tourniquet and the needle puncture may be experienced.
- If the patient is an infant or a child, explain to the parents that a small amount of blood will be taken from a finger.
- Inform the patient that there are no food or fluid restrictions for this test.
- Ask if the patient has received a blood transfusion within the past 4 months.

During the Test

- Perform a venipuncture and collect the sample in a 3- or 4.5-mL EDTA tube.

- For young children, collect capillary blood in a microcollection device.
- Completely fill the collection tube and invert it gently several times; don't shake the tube vigorously.

After the Test

- Apply pressure to the venipuncture site until bleeding stops.

Hemoglobin, Urine

Reference Values

No hemoglobin (Hb)

Abnormal Findings

- Severe intravascular hemolysis caused by a blood transfusion reaction, burns, or a crush injury
- Acquired hemolytic anemias caused by chemical or drug intoxication or malaria
- Congenital hemolytic anemias, such as hemoglobinopathies or enzyme defects
- Cystitis
- Ureteral calculi
- Urethritis
- Acute glomerulonephritis or pyelonephritis

• Renal tumor
• Tuberculosis

Nursing Implications
• Report abnormal findings to the health care provider.
• Prepare to educate the patient about the diagnosis.
• Administer medication, as prescribed.
• Prepare the patient for possible surgery, as indicated.

Purpose
• To help diagnose hemolytic anemias, infection, or severe intravascular hemolysis from a transfusion reaction

Description
Free Hb in the urine may occur in hemolytic anemias, infection, strenuous exercise, or severe intravascular hemolysis from a transfusion reaction. Contained in red blood cells (RBCs), Hb consists of an iron–protoporphyrin complex (heme) and a polypeptide (globin). Usually, RBCs are destroyed in the reticuloendothelial system, but when they're destroyed in the circulation, free Hb enters the plasma and binds with haptoglobin. If the plasma level of Hb exceeds that of haptoglobin, the excess free Hb is excreted in the urine (hemoglobinuria). Heme proteins act like enzymes that catalyze oxidation of organic substances. This reaction produces a blue coloration; the intensity of color depends on the amount of Hb present. Microscopic examination is necessary to identify intact RBCs in urine (hematuria), which can occur in the presence of free Hb.

Interfering Factors
• Nephrotoxic drugs and anticoagulants (positive results)
• Large doses of vitamin C or drugs that contain vitamin C as a preservative (false negative)
• Lysis of RBCs in stale or alkaline urine and contamination of the specimen by menstrual blood
• Bacterial peroxidases in highly infected specimens (false positive)

Nursing Considerations
Before the Test
• Confirm the patient's identity using two patient identifiers and confirmation of the patient's identification bracelet according to facility policy.
• Explain to the patient that the urine hemoglobin test detects excessive RBC destruction.
• Inform the patient that there are no food or fluid restrictions for this test.
• Advise the patient that the test requires a random urine specimen and teach him the proper collection technique.
• If a female patient is menstruating, reschedule the test because menstrual blood can interfere with the result.
• Notify the laboratory and health care provider of drugs the patient is taking that may affect test results; it may be necessary to restrict them.

During the Test
• Collect a random urine specimen.

Dipstik, Multistix, or Chemstrip Method
• Dip the stick into the urine specimen and withdraw it.
• After 30 seconds, read the results using the chart provided by the manufacturer.

Occult Tablet Test
• Put one drop of urine onto the filter paper, place a test tablet on the urine, and apply 2 drops of water to the tablet.
• After 2 minutes, inspect the filter paper. Blue indicates a positive test result.

Occult Solution
• Place a drop of urine on the filter paper, close the package, and turn it over.
• Apply 2 drops of solution to the site indicated.
• Read the test results after 30 seconds. Blue indicates a positive reaction.

After the Test
- Explain that the patient may resume usual medications.

Hepatitis A Antibodies

Reference Values
Negative for hepatitis A (HAV) antibodies

Abnormal Findings
- Rising anti-HAV titers confirming recent or current infection

Nursing Implications
- Report abnormal findings to the health care provider.
- Prepare to educate the patient about the diagnosis.
- Administer medication, as ordered.
- Advise the patient that confirmed viral hepatitis is reported to public health authorities in most states.

Purpose
- To aid in the differential diagnosis of viral hepatitis

Description
This test identifies HAV antibodies that appear in the serum or body fluid of patients. These antibodies are present in blood and feces only briefly before symptoms appear.

Interfering Factors
- Hepatitis vaccine (possible false positive)

Nursing Considerations
Before the Test
- Confirm the patient's identity using two patient identifiers and confirmation of the patient's identification bracelet according to facility policy.
- Check the patient's history for administration of hepatitis vaccine.
- Explain to the patient that this test helps identify a type of viral hepatitis.
- Inform the patient that there are no food or fluid restrictions for this test.
- Advise the patient that the test requires a blood sample. Explain that

discomfort from the tourniquet and the needle puncture may be experienced.

During the Test
- Perform a venipuncture and collect the sample in two 3- or 4.5-mL EDTA tubes.

After the Test
- Apply direct pressure to the venipuncture site until bleeding stops.

Hepatitis B Core Antibodies

Reference Values
Negative for hepatitis B core antibodies

Abnormal Findings
- Positive for hepatitis B core antibodies, indicating recovery from an acute hepatitis B virus (HBV) infection

Nursing Implications
- Report abnormal findings to the health care provider.
- Prepare to educate the patient about the diagnosis.

Purpose
- To screen blood donors for hepatitis B
- To screen those at high risk for contracting hepatitis B, such as hemodialysis nurses
- To aid in the differential diagnosis of viral hepatitis

Description
This test identifies HBV core antibodies, which are produced during or after an acute HBV infection. The core antigen is part of HBV, and the antibodies to the core antigen usually are present in chronic carriers. HBV is identified by the presence of hepatitis B antibodies, protein molecules (immunoglobulins) in serum or body fluid that either neutralize antigens or tag them for attack by other cells or chemicals.

Interfering Factors
- Hepatitis vaccine (possible false positive)
- Undetectable level of hepatitis B surface antigens (false negative)

Nursing Considerations

Before the Test
- Confirm the patient's identity using two patient identifiers and confirmation of the patient's identification bracelet according to facility policy.
- Explain to the patient that this test helps identify a type of viral hepatitis.
- Inform the patient that there are no food or fluid restrictions for this test.
- Tell the patient that the test requires a blood sample. Explain that discomfort from the tourniquet and the needle puncture may be experienced.
- Check the patient's history for administration of hepatitis vaccine.

During the Test
- Perform a venipuncture and collect the sample in two 3- or 4.5-mL EDTA tubes.

After the Test
- Apply direct pressure to the venipuncture site until bleeding stops.
- Advise the patient that confirmed viral hepatitis is reported to public health authorities in most states.

Hepatitis B Surface Antibodies

Reference Values
Negative for hepatitis B core surface antigens

Abnormal Findings
- Positive, indicating immunity to hepatitis B virus (HBV) infection

Nursing Implications
- Report abnormal findings to the health care provider.
- Prepare to educate the patient about the diagnosis.

Purpose
- To screen blood donors
- To screen those at high risk for contracting hepatitis B, such as hemodialysis nurses and other health care workers who are at risk for blood exposure

- To aid in the differential diagnosis of viral hepatitis

Description
HBV is identified by the presence of hepatitis B antibodies, protein molecules (immunoglobulins) in serum or body fluids that either neutralize antigens or tag them for attack by other cells or chemicals. The presence of hepatitis B surface antigens indicates that a patient who has been exposed to HBV is no longer contagious and is protected from future HBV infection.

Interfering Factors
- Hepatitis vaccine (possible false positive)

Nursing Considerations

Before the Test
- Confirm the patient's identity using two patient identifiers and confirmation of the patient's identification bracelet according to facility policy.
- Explain to the patient that this test helps identify a type of viral hepatitis.
- Inform the patient that there are no food or fluid restrictions for this test.
- Advise the patient that the test requires a blood sample. Explain that discomfort from the needle and the tourniquet may be experienced.
- Check the patient's history for administration of hepatitis vaccine.

During the Test
- Perform a venipuncture and collect the sample in two 3- or 4.5-mL EDTA tubes.

After the Test
- Apply direct pressure to the venipuncture site until bleeding stops.
- Advise the patient that confirmed viral hepatitis is reported to public health authorities in most states.

Hepatitis B Surface Antigen

Reference Values
Negative for hepatitis B surface antigen (HBsAg)

Abnormal Findings
- Positive for HBsAg, indicating hepatitis B, possible hemophilia, Hodgkin's disease, or leukemia

Nursing Implications
- Donor blood containing HBsAg must be discarded to avoid the risk of transmitting hepatitis.
- Positive blood samples should be retested to ensure accuracy.

Purpose
- To screen blood donors for hepatitis B
- To screen those at high risk for contracting hepatitis B, such as hemodialysis nurses and other health care workers who are at risk for blood exposure
- To aid in the differential diagnosis of viral hepatitis

Description
HBsAg, also called *hepatitis-associated antigen* or *Australia antigen*, appears in the serum of the patient with hepatitis B virus. HBsAg is detectable by radioimmunoassay or, less commonly, reverse passive hemagglutination during the extended incubation period, usually during the first 3 weeks of acute infection, or when the patient is a carrier.

Because hepatitis transmission is one of the gravest complications associated with blood transfusion, all donors must be screened for hepatitis B before their blood is stored. This screening, required by the Food and Drug Administration's Bureau of Biologics, has helped reduce the incidence of hepatitis. This test doesn't screen for hepatitis A virus (infectious hepatitis).

Interfering Factors
- Hepatitis B vaccine (possible false positive)

Nursing Considerations
Before the Test
- Confirm the patient's identity using two patient identifiers and confirmation of the patient's identification bracelet according to facility policy.

- Explain to the patient that this test helps identify a type of viral hepatitis.
- Inform the patient that there are no food or fluid restrictions for this test.
- Advise the patient that the test requires a blood sample. Explain that slight discomfort from the tourniquet and the needle puncture may be experienced.
- Check the patient's history for administration of hepatitis B vaccine.
- If the patient is giving blood, explain the donation procedure.

During the Test
- While wearing gloves, perform a venipuncture, and collect the sample in a 10-mL clot activator tube.
- Wash your hands carefully after the procedure.
- Dispose of the needle properly in a biohazard sharps container.

After the Test
- Apply direct pressure to the venipuncture site until bleeding stops.
- Advise the patient that confirmed viral hepatitis is reported to public health authorities in most states.

Hepatitis C Virus Antibodies

Reference Values
Negative for hepatitis C virus (HCV) antibodies

Abnormal Findings
- Positive for antibodies (further testing needed to determine if infection is current or past)
- False positive (test needs to be repeated)
- Negative (may indicate antibodies haven't developed yet)

Nursing Implications
- Report abnormal findings to the health care provider.
- Prepare to educate the patient about the diagnosis.
- Report abnormal findings to the public health authorities, according to facility policy.

Purpose

- To test for the presence of HCV antibodies

Description

This test detects HCV by checking for antibodies in the blood. Patients with risk factors for the disease and those who exhibit symptoms may be tested. Antibodies may indicate an infection or past infection.

Interfering Factors

- Patients with weakened immune systems, such as those with HIV, end-stage kidney disease, and organ transplants, may be unable to produce HCV antibodies, even if infected.

Nursing Considerations

Before the Test

- Confirm the patient's identity using two patient identifiers and confirmation of the patient's identification bracelet according to facility policy.
- Explain to the patient that the test can't distinguish between an acute or chronic infection and doesn't indicate whether the HCV infection is cured.
- Advise the patient that the test requires a blood sample. Explain that discomfort from the tourniquet and the needle puncture may be experienced.

During the Test

- Perform a venipuncture and collect the sample in two 3- or 4.5-mL EDTA tubes.

After the Test

- Apply direct pressure to the venipuncture site.
- Offer appropriate referrals after testing is completed.
- Tell the patient that confirmed viral hepatitis is reported to public health authorities in most states.

Hepatitis D Antibodies

Reference Values

Negative for hepatitis D virus (HDV) antibodies

Abnormal Findings

- Positive for hepatitis D antibodies

Nursing Implications

- Report abnormal findings to the health care provider.
- Prepare to educate the patient about the diagnosis.

Purpose

- To aid in the differential diagnosis of viral hepatitis

Description

Hepatitis D occurs primarily in patients with acute or chronic episodes of hepatitis B. Infection requires the presence of the hepatitis B surface antigen, whereas HDV depends on the double-shelled type B virus to replicate. Type D infection can't outlast a type B infection.

Interfering Factors

- Lipemia (possible false positive)
- High titer rheumatoid factor (possible false positive)

Nursing Considerations

Before the Test

- Confirm the patient's identity using two patient identifiers and confirmation of the patient's identification bracelet according to facility policy.
- Explain to the patient that the test can't distinguish between an acute and a chronic infection and doesn't indicate whether the HCV infection is cured.
- Advise the patient that the test requires a blood sample. Explain that discomfort from the tourniquet and the needle puncture may be experienced.

During the Test

- Perform a venipuncture and collect the sample in two 3- or 4.5-mL EDTA tubes.

After the Test

- Apply direct pressure to the venipuncture site.

- Advise the patient that confirmed viral hepatitis is reported to public health authorities in most states.

Herpes Simplex Antibodies

Reference Values
No detectable antibodies (less than 1:5)

Abnormal Findings
- Active herpes simplex virus (HSV) infection

Nursing Implications
- Report abnormal findings to the health care provider.
- Prepare to educate the patient about diagnosis.

Purpose
- To confirm infections caused by HSV
- To detect recent or past HSV infection

Description
HSV, a member of the herpes virus group, causes various clinically severe manifestations, including genital lesions, keratitis or conjunctivitis, generalized dermal lesions, and pneumonia. Severe involvement is associated with intrauterine or neonatal infections and encephalitis, the most serious occurring in immunosuppressed patients. Type 1 usually causes infections above the waistline, and type 2 mostly involves the external genitalia. Primary viral contact occurs in early childhood as acute stomatitis or, more commonly, as an inapparent infection. More than 50% of adults have antibodies to HSV. Sensitive assays, such as indirect immunofluorescence and enzyme immunoassay, demonstrate immunoglobulin (Ig) M class antibodies to HSV or detect a fourfold or greater increase in IgG class antibodies between acute- and convalescent-phase sera.

Interfering Factors
- Hemolysis from rough handling of the sample

Precautions
- Handle the sample gently to prevent hemolysis.

Nursing Considerations

Before the Test
- Confirm the patient's identity using two patient identifiers and confirmation of the patient's identification bracelet according to facility policy.
- Explain the purpose of the test to the patient.
- Advise the patient that the test requires a blood sample. Explain slight discomfort from the tourniquet and the needle puncture may be experienced.

During the Test
- Perform a venipuncture and collect the sample in a 7-mL clot activator tube.
- Allow the blood to clot for at least 1 hour at room temperature.
- Transfer the serum to a sterile tube or vial and send it to the laboratory promptly.
- If not transferred immediately, store the serum at 39.2°F (4°C) for 1 to 2 days or at −47°F (−43.9°C) for longer periods to avoid contamination.

After the Test
- Apply direct pressure to the venipuncture site until bleeding stops.
- If the patient's immune system is compromised, check the venipuncture site for signs and symptoms of infection and report them immediately.

Heterophile Antibodies

Reference Values
Titer less than 1:28 (possibly higher in elderly patients)
Negative or no reaction (as reported by some laboratories)

Abnormal Findings

Elevated Levels
- Infectious mononucleosis (titer greater than 1:56 with gradual increase during week 3 or 4 followed by a gradual decrease during weeks 4 to 8; reactive titer 2 weeks after symptoms' onset)

- Systemic lupus erythematosus, syphilis, cryoglobulinemia, or the presence of antibodies to nonsyphilitic treponematosis (yaws, pinta, bejel)

Nursing Implications
- Report abnormal findings to the health care provider.
- Prepare to educate the patient about the diagnosis.
- If the titer is positive but infectious mononucleosis isn't confirmed, or if the titer is negative but symptoms persist, explain that additional testing will be necessary in a few days or weeks to confirm the diagnosis and plan effective treatment.

Purpose
- To aid in the differential diagnosis of infectious mononucleosis

Description
There are two ways to identify immunoglobulin (Ig) M antibodies in human serum that react against foreign red blood cells (RBCs): the Paul-Bunnell and Davidsohn differential absorption antibodies tests. In the Paul-Bunnell test—also called the *presumptive test*—Epstein-Barr virus (EBV) antibodies, found in the sera of patients with infectious mononucleosis, agglutinate with sheep RBCs in a test tube. Forssman antibodies, present in the sera of some normal persons, as well as in the sera of patients with such conditions as serum sickness, also agglutinate with sheep RBCs, rendering test results inconclusive for infectious mononucleosis. If the Paul-Bunnell test establishes a presumptive titer, the Davidsohn differential absorption test can then distinguish between EBV and Forssman antibodies.

Interfering Factors
- Hemolysis from rough handling of the sample
- Hepatitis, leukemia, lymphomas, opioid use, and phenytoin therapy (false positive)

Nursing Considerations
Before the Test
- Confirm the patient's identity using two patient identifiers and confirmation of the patient's identification bracelet according to facility policy.
- Explain to the patient that this test helps detect infectious mononucleosis.
- Advise the patient that the test requires a blood sample. Explain that slight discomfort from the tourniquet and the needle puncture may be experienced.

During the Test
- Perform a venipuncture and collect the sample in a 7-mL clot activator tube.

After the Test
- Apply direct pressure to the venipuncture site until bleeding stops.
- If the titer is positive and infectious mononucleosis is confirmed, explain the treatment plan to the patient.

Hexosaminidase A and B, Serum
Reference Values
Total hexosaminidase serum levels: 5 to 12.9 units/L (hexosaminidase A accounting for 55% to 76% of the total)

Abnormal Findings
- Absence of hexosaminidase A, indicating Tay-Sachs' disease; total hexosaminidase levels can be normal
- Absence of hexosaminidase A and B, indicating Sandhoff's disease, an uncommon, virulent variant of Tay-Sachs' disease causing rapid deterioration

Nursing Implications
- Report abnormal findings to the health care provider.
- Prepare to educate the patient about the diagnosis.
- Refer the patient and family to community resources, as appropriate.

Purpose
- To confirm or rule out Tay-Sachs' disease in the neonate
- To screen for a Tay-Sachs' carrier
- To establish prenatal diagnosis of hexosaminidase A deficiency

Description
Hexosaminidase is a group of enzymes necessary for metabolism of gangliosides, the water-soluble glycolipids found primarily in brain tissue. This fluorometric test measures the hexosaminidase A and B content of serum samples drawn by venipuncture, collected from a neonate's umbilical cord or obtained by amniocentesis from amniotic fluid. Testing cultured skin fibroblasts also can identify a hexosaminidase deficiency, but it's costly and technically complex.

Hexosaminidase A deficiency indicates Tay-Sachs' disease, which affects people of Eastern European Jewish ancestry about 100 times more often than the general population. Both parents must carry the defective gene to transmit Tay-Sachs' disease to their children. Sandhoff's disease, which results from a deficiency of hexosaminidase A and B, is uncommon and not prevalent in any ethnic group.

Interfering Factors
- Hemolysis from rough handling of the sample
- Hormonal contraceptives (false-high levels)
- Rifampin and isoniazid (increase in levels)

Precautions
- Handle the sample gently to prevent hemolysis.

Nursing Considerations
Before the Test
- Confirm the patient's identity using two patient identifiers and confirmation of the patient's identification bracelet according to facility policy.

- Explain to the patient that this test identifies carriers of Tay-Sachs' disease.
- Advise the patient that the test requires a blood sample. Explain that slight discomfort from the tourniquet and the needle puncture may be experienced.
- Inform the patient that there are no food or fluid restrictions for this test.
- If the test is prenatal, advise the patient of preparations for amniocentesis.
- When testing a neonate, explain to the parents that this test detects Tay-Sachs' disease.
- Advise them that blood will be drawn from the neonate's arm, neck, or umbilical cord; that the procedure is safe and quickly performed; and that the neonate will have a small bandage on the venipuncture site.
- Inform the parents that no pretest restrictions of food or fluid are needed for the test.

During the Test
- Perform a venipuncture, collect cord blood, or assist with amniocentesis, as appropriate.
- Collect the sample in a 7-mL clot activator tube.
- The serum of a pregnant woman can't be tested, but her leukocytes or amniotic fluid can be, if necessary; if the father's blood test result is negative, the child won't inherit Tay-Sachs' disease.

After the Test
- Apply direct pressure to the venipuncture site until bleeding stops.
- If the test can't occur immediately, freeze the sample.

Holter Monitoring
Normal Findings
- No significant arrhythmias or ST-segment changes in the electrocardiogram (ECG) during various activities or at rest
- Heart rate changes during various activities

Abnormal Findings
- Symptomatic or asymptomatic arrhythmias
- ST-T wave changes coinciding with patient symptoms or increased patient activity (possible myocardial ischemia)

Nursing Implications
- Report abnormal findings to the health care provider.
- Prepare to educate the patient about the diagnosis.

Purpose
- To detect cardiac arrhythmias
- To evaluate chest pain
- To evaluate the effectiveness of antiarrhythmic drug therapy
- To monitor pacemaker function
- To correlate symptoms and palpitations with actual cardiac events and patient activities
- To detect sporadic arrhythmias missed by an exercise or resting ECG

Description
Holter monitoring provides continuous recording of heart activity as the patient follows a normal routine, usually for 24 hours. The patient-activated monitor, also known as *ambulatory electrocardiography* or *dynamic monitoring*, is worn for 5 to 7 days, allowing the patient to manually initiate heart activity recording when symptoms are experienced.

The procedure for Holter monitoring is as follows:

- Electrodes are applied to the chest wall and securely attached to the leadwires and monitor.
- Placing electrodes over large muscles masses, such as the pectorals, is avoided to limit artifact.
- A new or fully charged battery is inserted in the recorder.
- A tape is inserted and the recorder is started.
- The electrode attachment circuit is tested by connecting the recorder to a standard ECG machine, noting artifact during normal patient movement.

Nursing Considerations

Before the Test
- Confirm the patient's identity using two patient identifiers and confirmation of the patient's identification bracelet according to facility policy.
- Make sure the patient has signed an appropriate consent form.
- Note and report all allergies.
- Provide bathing instructions, because some equipment must not get wet.
- Instruct the patient to avoid magnets, metal detectors, high-voltage areas, and electric blankets.
- Explain the importance of maintaining a diary to log activities, as well as emotional upsets, physical symptoms, and ingestion of medication.
- Explain how to mark the tape at the onset of symptoms, if applicable.
- Explain how to check the recorder to make sure it's working properly.

After the Test
- Remove all chest electrodes.
- Clean the electrode sites.

Homocysteine, Total, Plasma

Reference Values
4 to 17 mcmol/L

Abnormal Findings

Elevated Levels
- Atherosclerotic vascular disease
- Modest deterioration in renal function in patients with type 2 diabetes

Decreased Levels
- Inborn or acquired folate or cobalamin deficiency and inborn B_6 or B_{12} deficiency

Nursing Implications
- Report abnormal findings to the health care provider.
- Prepare to educate the patient about the diagnosis.

Purpose
- To make a biochemical diagnosis of inborn errors of methionine, folate, and vitamins B_6 and B_{12} metabolism

- To indicate acquired folate or cobalamin deficiency
- To evaluate the risk factors for atherosclerotic vascular disease
- To evaluate as a contributing factor in the pathogenesis of neural tube defects
- To evaluate the cause of recurrent spontaneous abortions
- To evaluate delayed child development or failure to thrive in infants

Description

Homocysteine (tHcy), a sulfur-containing amino acid, is a transmethylation product of methionine. It's an intermediate in the synthesis of cysteine, which is produced by the enzymatic or acid hydrolysis of proteins. This test is useful for the biochemical diagnosis of inborn errors of methionine, folate, and vitamins B_6 and B_{12} metabolism.

Interfering Factors

- Failure to adhere to dietary restrictions
- Failure to immediately freeze the specimen
- Penicillamine (reduces the plasma levels of tHcy)
- Azauridine, nitrous oxide, and a methotrexate deficiency (causes increased plasma tHcy levels)

Precautions

- Handle the sample gently to prevent hemolysis.

Nursing Considerations

Before the Test

- Confirm the patient's identity using two patient identifiers and confirmation of the patient's identification bracelet according to facility policy.
- Inform the patient that this test detects tHcy levels in plasma.
- Instruct the patient to fast for 12 to 14 hours before the test.
- Advise the patient that this test requires a blood sample. Explain that slight discomfort from the tourniquet and the needle puncture may be experienced.

During the Test

- Perform a venipuncture and collect the sample in a 5-mL tube with EDTA added.
- Immediately put the sample on ice and send it to the laboratory.

After the Test

- Apply direct pressure to the venipuncture site until bleeding stops.

Human Chorionic Gonadotropin, Blood

Reference Values

Less than 4 international units/L (varies widely during pregnancy, depending partly on days since last normal menses)

Abnormal Findings

Elevated Levels

- Pregnancy
- Hydatidiform mole, trophoblastic neoplasms of the placenta, and nontrophoblastic carcinomas that secrete hCG (including gastric, pancreatic, and ovarian adenocarcinomas)

Decreased Levels

- Ectopic pregnancy or a pregnancy of less than 9 days

Nursing Implications

- Report abnormal findings to the health care provider.
- Prepare to educate the patient about the diagnosis.
- Prepare the patient for further testing, as indicated.

Purpose

- To detect early pregnancy
- To determine adequacy of hormonal production in high-risk pregnancies (for example, habitual abortion)
- To help diagnose trophoblastic tumors, such as hydatidiform mole and choriocarcinoma, and tumors that ectopically secrete hCG
- To monitor treatment for induction of ovulation and conception

Description

Produced in the placenta, hCG is a glycoprotein hormone that can be detected by using the beta-subunit assay in the blood 9 days after ovulation if conception has occurred. This interval coincides with the implantation of the fertilized ovum into the uterine wall.

Although the precise function of hCG is still unclear, it appears that hCG, with progesterone, maintains the corpus luteum during early pregnancy. Production of hCG increases steadily during the first trimester, peaking at around 10 weeks' gestation. Levels then fall to less than 10% of first-trimester peak levels during the remainder of the pregnancy. About 2 weeks after delivery, the hormone may no longer be detectable. This serum immunoassay, a quantitative analysis of hCG beta-subunit level, is more sensitive (and costlier) than the routine pregnancy test using a urine sample.

Interfering Factors

- Hemolysis from rough handling of the sample
- Heparin anticoagulants and EDTA (decreased levels)
- Anticonvulsants, hypnotics, drugs to treat Parkinson's disease (increased levels)

Precautions

- Handle the sample gently to prevent hemolysis.

Nursing Considerations

Before the Test

- Confirm the patient's identity using two patient identifiers and confirmation of the patient's identification bracelet according to facility policy.
- Explain to the patient that this test determines if she's pregnant.
- If pregnancy detection isn't the diagnostic objective, offer the appropriate explanation.
- Inform the patient that she doesn't need to restrict food and fluids for the test.

- Advise the patient that the test requires a blood sample. Explain that she may experience slight discomfort from the tourniquet and the needle puncture.

During the Test

- Perform a venipuncture and collect the sample in a 7-mL clot activator tube.
- Send the sample to the laboratory immediately.

After the Test

- Apply direct pressure to the venipuncture site until bleeding stops.

Human Chorionic Gonadotropin, Urine

Reference Values

Nonpregnant females and males: Negative for human chorionic gonadotropin (hCG)

Pregnant females: Positive for hCG; first trimester, up to 500,000 international units/24 hours; second trimester, 10,000 to 25,000 international units/24 hours; third trimester, 5,000 to 15,000 international units/24 hours

Abnormal Findings

Elevated Levels
During Pregnancy
- Multiple pregnancy
- Erythroblastosis fetalis

For Nonpregnant Females or for Males
- Choriocarcinoma
- Ovarian or testicular tumors
- Melanoma
- Multiple myeloma
- Gastric, hepatic, pancreatic, or breast cancer

Decreased Levels (During Pregnancy)
- Threatened abortion
- Ectopic pregnancy

Nursing Implications
- Report abnormal findings to the health care provider.
- Prepare to educate the patient about the diagnosis.
- Prepare the patient for further diagnostic testing, as indicated.
- Refer the pregnant patient for community resources, as indicated.

Purpose
- To detect and confirm pregnancy
- To help diagnose hydatidiform mole or hCG-secreting tumors, threatened abortion, or dead fetus

Description
Qualitative hCG urine level analysis detects pregnancy as early as 14 days after ovulation. A glycoprotein that is produced after conception, hCG prevents degeneration of the corpus luteum at the end of a normal menstrual cycle. During the first trimester, hCG levels rise steadily and rapidly, peaking around 10 weeks' gestation, and subsequently taper off to less than 10% of peak levels. The most common and inexpensive method of evaluating qualitative and quantitative hCG levels is through hemagglutination inhibition of a urine sample. The serum hCG test (beta-subunit assay) is a more expensive alternative.

Interfering Factors
- Gross proteinuria (greater than 1 g/24 hours), hematuria, or an elevated erythrocyte sedimentation rate (possible false positive, depending on the laboratory method)
- Early pregnancy, ectopic pregnancy, or threatened abortion (possible false negative)
- Phenothiazine (possible false negative or false positive)

Nursing Considerations

Before the Test
- Confirm the patient's identity using two patient identifiers and confirmation of the patient's identification bracelet according to facility policy.
- If appropriate, explain to the patient that the urine hCG test determines whether she's pregnant or determines the status of her pregnancy. Alternatively, explain how the test functions as a screen for some types of cancer.
- Explain that the patient doesn't need to restrict food but should restrict fluids for 8 hours before the test.
- Inform the patient that the test requires a first-voided morning specimen or urine collection over a 24-hour period, depending on whether the test is qualitative or quantitative.
- Notify the laboratory and health care provider of drugs the patient is taking that may affect test results; it may be necessary to restrict them.

During the Test
- For verification of pregnancy (qualitative analysis), collect a first-voided morning specimen. If this isn't possible, collect a random specimen.
- For quantitative analysis, collect the patient's urine over a 24-hour period in the appropriate container, discarding the first specimen and retaining the last.
- Specify the date of the patient's last menstrual period on the laboratory request. Be sure the test occurs at least 5 days after a missed period to avoid a false-negative result.
- Refrigerate the 24-hour specimen or keep it on ice during the collection period.

After the Test
- Instruct the patient to resume her usual diet and medications.

Human Growth Hormone, Serum

Reference Values
Females: Less than 10 ng/mL (SI, 10 mcg/L)
Males: Less than 5 ng/mL (SI, 5 mcg/L)
Children: 0 to 20 ng/mL (SI, 16 mcg/L)

Abnormal Findings

Elevated Levels

- Pituitary or hypothalamic tumor (gigantism in children, acromegaly in adults and adolescents)
- Diabetes without acromegaly

Decreased Levels

- Pituitary infarction
- Metastatic disease
- Pituitary tumor
- Dwarfism

Nursing Implications

- Prepare the patient with elevated levels for suppression testing to confirm diagnosis.
- Prepare the patient with decreased levels for stimulation testing with arginine or insulin to confirm the diagnosis.
- Report abnormal findings to the health care provider.
- Prepare to educate the patient about the diagnosis.

Purpose

- To differentiate between pituitary or thyroid hypofunction in the diagnosis of dwarfism
- To confirm the diagnosis of acromegaly and gigantism in the adult
- To help diagnose pituitary and hypothalamic tumors
- To help evaluate human growth hormone (hGH) therapy

Description

The hGH protein, also known as *somatotropin*, is secreted by the pituitary gland and is the primary regulator of human growth. It affects many body tissues and has no easily defined feedback mechanism or single target gland. Like insulin, hGH promotes protein synthesis and stimulates amino acid uptake by cells, raises plasma glucose levels by inhibiting glucose uptake and use by cells, and increases free fatty acid levels by enhancing lipolysis. Its secretion is diurnal and varies with exercise, sleep, stress, and nutrition, and is regulated by the hypothalamus through a growth hormone-releasing factor and a growth hormone release–inhibiting factor (somatostatin). Hyposecretion or hypersecretion may induce pathologic states (such as dwarfism or gigantism); altered levels are common in pituitary dysfunction. Quantitative analysis of plasma hGH levels is done as part of an anterior pituitary stimulation or suppression test and is crucial because hGH deficiency clinical manifestations are rarely reversible by therapy.

Interfering Factors

- Failure to observe pretest restrictions
- Hemolysis from rough handling of the sample
- Arginine, beta-adrenergic blockers such as propranolol, and estrogens (increase)
- Amphetamines, bromocriptine, levodopa, dopamine, pituitary-based steroids, methyldopa, and histamine (increase)
- Insulin (induced hypoglycemia), glucagon, and nicotinic acid (increase)
- Phenothiazines (such as chlorpromazine) and corticosteroids (decrease)
- Radioactive scan performed within 1 week before the test

Precautions

- Handle the sample gently to prevent hemolysis.

Nursing Considerations

Before the Test

- Confirm the patient's identity using two patient identifiers and confirmation of the patient's identification bracelet according to facility policy.
- Explain to the patient, or parents if the patient is a child, that this test measures hormone levels and helps determine the cause of abnormal growth.
- Instruct the patient to fast and limit activity for 10 to 12 hours before the test.
- Advise the patient that the test requires a blood sample and that

another sample may be necessary the next day for comparison. Explain that slight discomfort from the tourniquet and the needle puncture may be experienced.

- Withhold all drugs that affect hGH levels, such as pituitary-based steroids. If the patient must continue them, note this on the laboratory request.
- Make sure that the patient is relaxed and recumbent for 30 minutes before the test; stress and activity elevate hGH levels.

During the Test

- Between 6 AM and 8 AM on two consecutive days, perform a venipuncture and collect at least 7 mL of blood in a clot activator tube.
- Send the sample to the laboratory immediately, because hGH has a half-life of only 20 to 25 minutes.

After the Test

- Apply direct pressure to the venipuncture site until bleeding stops.
- Advise the patient to resume a usual diet, activities, and medications.

Human Immunodeficiency Virus Antibodies

Reference Values

Negative for human immunodeficiency virus (HIV) antibodies

Abnormal Findings

- Positive for HIV antibody, indicating previous exposure to HIV (even in apparently healthy patients) or acquired immune deficiency syndrome (AIDS)
- No antibodies (in late-stage AIDS patients because of inability to mount antibody response)

Nursing Implications

- Report abnormal findings to the health care provider.
- Prepare to educate the patient about the diagnosis.
- Reassure the patient that test results will be kept confidential.

- If the patient has questions about the condition, be sure to provide full and accurate information.
- Refer the patient to counseling or community resources, as appropriate.
- When the patient receives the results, give him or her another opportunity to ask questions.
- Encourage the patient with positive screening tests to seek medical follow-up care, even if asymptomatic.
- Tell the patient to report early signs of AIDS, such as fever, weight loss, axillary or inguinal lymphadenopathy, rash, and persistent cough or diarrhea. Female patients should also report gynecologic symptoms.
- To prevent possible virus transmission, advise the patient about safer sex practices. The patient should assume that the virus can be transmitted from the patient to others until conclusively proved otherwise.
- Instruct the patient not to share razors, toothbrushes, or utensils (which may be contaminated with blood) and to clean such items with household bleach diluted 1:10 in water.
- Advise the patient against donating blood, tissues, or an organ.
- Warn the patient to inform the health care provider and dentist about the condition so that they can take proper precautions.

Purpose

- To screen for HIV
- To screen donated blood for HIV

Description

HIV is the virus that causes AIDS. It's transmitted by direct exposure of a person's blood to body fluids containing the virus—through the exchange of contaminated blood and blood products, during sexual intercourse with an infected partner, when IV drugs are shared, or from an infected mother to her child during pregnancy or breastfeeding.

Initial HIV identification usually occurs through serum enzyme-linked immunosorbent assay. The Western blot test and immunofluorescence confirm positive findings; other available tests may detect antibodies.

Nursing Considerations

Before the Test
- Confirm the patient's identity using two patient identifiers and confirmation of the patient's identification bracelet according to facility policy.
- Explain to the patient that this test detects HIV infection.
- Provide adequate counseling about the reasons for performing the test; usually, a patient's health care provider requests it.
- Advise the patient that the test requires a blood sample. Explain that slight discomfort from the tourniquet and the needle puncture may be experienced.

During the Test
- Perform a venipuncture and collect the sample in a 10-mL barrier tube.
- Barrier tubes help prevent contamination when pouring the serum in the laboratory.
- Observe standard precautions when drawing a blood sample.
- Use gloves, properly dispose of needles, and use blood–fluid precaution labels on tubes, as necessary.

After the Test
- Apply direct pressure to the venipuncture site until bleeding stops.
- Keep the venipuncture site clean and dry because the patient may have a compromised immune system.
- Keep the test results confidential.

Human Leukocyte Antigens

Reference Values
Human leukocyte antigen (HLA)-A, -B, and -C testing: No lymphocytes reaction
HLA-D testing: No leukocytes reaction

Abnormal Findings
- Presence of specific HLAs, indicating such diseases as ankylosing spondylosis (HLA-B27), multiple sclerosis (HLA-B27, Dw2, A3, B18), sarcoidosis (HLA-B8), type 1 diabetes (B15, B8), Reiter's syndrome or acute anterior uveitis (B27), psoriasis (HLA-A13, B17), Graves' disease or juvenile rheumatoid arthritis (B27), or celiac disease (B8)
- Positive or negative paternity

Nursing Implications
- Report abnormal findings to the health care provider.
- Prepare to educate the patient about the diagnosis.
- Refer the patient to appropriate community resources, as appropriate.

Purpose
- To provide histocompatibility typing of transplant recipients and donors
- To aid in genetic counseling
- To aid in paternity testing

Description
HLA testing identifies a group of antigens present on the surface of all nucleated cells but most easily detected on lymphocytes: HLA-A, HLA-B, HLA-C, and HLA-D. These antigens are essential to immunity and determine the degree of histocompatibility between transplant recipients and donors. There are numerous antigenic determinants (more than 60, for instance, at the HLA-B locus) present for each site; one set of each antigen is inherited from each parent. A high incidence of specific HLA types is linked to specific diseases, such as rheumatoid arthritis and multiple sclerosis, but these findings have little diagnostic significance.

Interfering Factors
- Hemolysis from rough handling of the sample
- HLA from blood transfusion within 72 hours before sample collection

Precautions
• Handle the sample gently to prevent hemolysis.

Nursing Considerations
Before the Test
• Confirm the patient's identity using two patient identifiers and confirmation of the patient's identification bracelet according to facility policy.
• Explain that this test detects antigens on white blood cells.
• Inform the patient that there are no food or fluid restrictions.
• Advise the patient that the test requires a blood sample. Explain that slight discomfort from the tourniquet and the needle puncture may be experienced.
• Check the patient's history for recent blood transfusions. It may be necessary to postpone HLA testing if the patient has recently undergone a transfusion.

During the Test
• Perform a venipuncture and collect the sample in a tube containing anticoagulant acid citrate dextrose solution.

After the Test
• Apply direct pressure to the venipuncture site until bleeding stops.
• Refer the patient and family to appropriate counseling services.

Hysterosalpingography
Normal Findings
• Symmetrical uterine cavity
• Fallopian tubes of normal caliber
• Freely spilling contrast medium into the peritoneal cavity
• No contrast medium leakage from the uterus

Abnormal Findings
• Asymmetrical uterus, suggesting intrauterine adhesions or masses
• Impaired contrast flow, suggesting partial or complete blockage of the fallopian tubes

• Leakage of contrast medium through the uterine wall, indicating fistulas

Nursing Implications
• Report abnormal findings to the health care provider.
• Prepare to educate the patient about her diagnosis.
• Prepare the patient for further testing or surgery, as appropriate.

Purpose
• To confirm tubal abnormalities, such as adhesions
• To confirm uterine abnormalities, such as congenital malformations
• To confirm the presence of fistulas or peritubal adhesions
• To evaluate the cause of repeated miscarriage

Description
Hysterosalpingography is a radiologic examination during which contrast medium flows through the uterus and the fallopian tubes and fluoroscopic X-rays are taken. Performed as part of an infertility study, it shows the uterine cavity, fallopian tubes, and peritubal area.

The procedure for hysterosalpingography is as follows:
• The patient is assisted into the lithotomy position and a scout film is taken.
• A bimanual examination determines uterine size and position.
• A speculum is inserted in the vagina, and the vagina and cervix are cleaned.
• A cannula is inserted into the cervix and anchored to a tenaculum.
• Contrast medium is injected through the cannula.
• The uterus and fallopian tubes are viewed fluoroscopically and X-rays are taken.
• For oblique views, the table is tilted or the patient is asked to change position.
• Films may be taken later to evaluate the spillage of contrast medium into the peritoneal cavity.

Nursing Considerations

Before the Test
- Confirm the patient's identity using two patient identifiers and confirmation of the patient's identification bracelet according to facility policy.
- Make sure the patient has signed an appropriate consent form.
- Note and report all allergies, including any to iodinated contrast media.
- Check the patient's history for recent pelvic infection. A test for pelvic infections may be necessary before the study, and antibiotics may be prescribed before the test.
- Explain that the procedure should take place 2 to 5 days after menstruation ends.
- Warn the patient that she might experience moderate cramping.
- Explain that she may receive a mild sedative or a nonprescription prostaglandin inhibitor 30 minutes before the procedure.
- Explain that the test takes about 15 minutes.
- Explain that a small amount of vaginal bleeding and pelvic cramping is normal for a few days after the study.

After the Test
- Instruct the patient to return to normal activities gradually.
- Tell the patient that additional tests and studies may be necessary to establish a precise diagnosis.
- Monitor the patient's vital signs.
- Monitor for signs and symptoms of infection and uterine perforation.
- Monitor for bleeding.
- Watch for an adverse reaction to the contrast medium.

Hysteroscopy

Normal Findings
- Uterus interior that's of normal size and shape and free from adhesions and lesions

Abnormal Findings
- Uterine polyps
- Uterine wall tumors
- Adhesions

Nursing Implications
- Prepare to educate the patient about her diagnosis.
- Prepare the patient for further testing or possible surgery, as indicated.

Purpose
- To investigate abnormal uterine bleeding
- To remove polyps
- To evaluate infertility
- To direct the removal of intrauterine devices
- To aid in the diagnosis and treatment of intrauterine adhesions
- To diagnose uterine fibroids

Description
A hysteroscopy is done with a small-diameter endoscope to see the interior of the uterus. It's usually performed within the first week after the end of a patient's menstrual cycle in the physician's office after giving the patient a local anesthetic or mild sedative.

The procedure for hysteroscopy is as follows:
- The patient is assisted into a modified dorsal lithotomy position with her legs in stirrups.
- A local anesthetic is given.
- The vagina is cleaned and the hysteroscope is inserted.
- The physician performs a complete pelvic examination. Visualization begins at the level of the internal os.
- In contact hysteroscopy, the uterus isn't distended; only the area in direct contact with the hysteroscope is visible.
- In panoramic hysteroscopy, an external illumination source and media (such as carbon dioxide) for distention are used to make the tissue visible from a distance.
- Cultures of the vagina and cervix may be taken.

Interfering Factors
Heavy bleeding or a distended bladder

Nursing Considerations

Before the Test
- Confirm the patient's identity using two patient identifiers and confirmation of the patient's identification bracelet according to facility policy.
- Make sure the patient has signed an appropriate consent form.
- Note and report all allergies.
- Check the patient's history for hypersensitivity to the anesthetic.
- Obtain the results of the patient's last Pap test.
- Instruct the patient to restrict food and fluids before the test.
- Instruct the patient to empty her bladder before the test.

- Warn the patient that the physician may inflate her uterus with carbon dioxide. Tell her that her body will absorb it but that it may cause upper abdominal or shoulder pain lasting 24 to 36 hours after the test.
- Explain that some vaginal bleeding and mild abdominal cramping may occur after the test.
- Recommend that the patient have a friend or relative drive her home after the procedure.

After the Test
- Provide the patient with a sanitary pad, if needed.
- Provide analgesics as needed.
- Monitor vital signs.
- Monitor for bleeding.
- Watch for adverse reactions to analgesics.
- Watch for signs and symptoms of infection, such as fever and pain.

Immune Complex Assays

Reference Values
None in serum

Abnormal Findings
- Detectable immune complexes, indicating immune complex (type III) glomerulonephritis, bacterial endocarditis, hepatitis C, Hodgkin's disease, or systemic lupus erythematosus (SLE)

Nursing Implications
- For a definitive diagnosis, the presence of these complexes must be considered with the results of other studies.
- Be aware that, in SLE, immune complexes are associated with high titers of antinuclear antibodies and circulating antinative deoxyribonucleic acid antibodies.
- Know that renal biopsy can detect immune complexes and provide conclusive evidence for immune complex (type III) glomerulonephritis, differentiating it from other types of glomerulonephritis.
- Report abnormal findings to the health care provider.
- Prepare to educate the patient about the diagnosis and the need for further testing, as appropriate.

Purpose
- To demonstrate circulating immune complexes in serum
- To monitor the patient's response to therapy
- To estimate disease severity

Description
Histologic examination of tissue obtained by biopsy and the use of fluorescence or peroxidase staining with antibodies specific for immunologic types generally detect immune complexes. However, tissue biopsies can't provide information about titers of complexes still in circulation; therefore, serum assays, which detect circulating immune complexes indirectly, may be required. Because of the inherent variability of these complexes, several serum test methods may be appropriate using C1, rheumatoid factor (RF), or cellular substrates, such as Raji cells, as reagents.

Most immune complex assays haven't been standardized, so more than one test may be required to achieve accurate results.

Interfering Factors
- Presence of cryoglobulins in the serum
- Inability to standardize RF inhibition tests and platelet aggregation assays

Precautions
- Send the sample to the laboratory immediately to prevent deterioration of immune complexes.

Nursing Considerations

Before the Test
- Confirm the patient's identity using two patient identifiers and confirmation of the patient's identification bracelet according to facility policy.
- Explain to the patient that the immune complex assay tests help evaluate the immune system.
- Inform the patient that the test will be repeated to monitor the response to therapy, if appropriate.
- Inform the patient that there are no food or fluid restrictions for this test.

- Advise the patient that the test requires a blood sample. Explain that slight discomfort from the tourniquet and needle puncture may be experienced.
- If the patient is scheduled for C1q assay (a component of C1), check the patient's history for recent heparin therapy and report such therapy to the laboratory.

During the Test
- Perform a venipuncture and collect the sample in a 7-mL clot activator tube.

After the Test
- Because many patients with immune complexes have a compromised immune system, keep the venipuncture site clean and dry.
- Apply direct pressure to the venipuncture site until bleeding stops and to prevent hematoma formation.

Insulin

Reference Values
0 to 35 microunits/mL (SI, 144–243 pmol/L)

Abnormal Findings
- Insulin levels interpreted in light of prevailing glucose concentration
- Normal insulin level inappropriate for glucose results
- High insulin and low glucose levels after a significant fast, indicating insulinoma

Elevated Levels
- Type 2 diabetes

Decreased Levels
- Type 1 diabetes

Nursing Implications
- Report abnormal findings to the health care provider.
- Prepare to educate the patient about the diagnosis.
- Prolonged fasting or stimulation testing may be required to confirm the diagnosis

Purpose
- To help diagnose hyperinsulinemia and hypoglycemia resulting from a tumor or hyperplasia of pancreatic islet cells, glucocorticoid deficiency, or severe hepatic disease
- To help diagnose diabetes and insulin-resistant states

Description
The insulin test, a radioimmunoassay, is a quantitative analysis of serum insulin levels. Insulin is usually measured concomitantly with glucose levels because glucose is the primary stimulus for insulin release from pancreatic islet cells.

Insulin regulates the metabolism and transport or mobilization of carbohydrates, amino acids, proteins, and lipids. Stimulated by increased plasma levels of glucose, insulin secretion reaches peak levels after meals, when metabolism and food storage are greatest.

Interfering Factors
- Agitation and stress
- Corticotropin, corticosteroids (including hormonal contraceptives), thyroid hormones, and epinephrine (possible increase)
- Use of insulin by the patient with type 2 diabetes (possible increase)
- High levels of insulin antibodies in the patient with type 1 diabetes

Precautions
- Pack the insulin sample in ice and send it, along with the glucose sample, to the laboratory immediately.
- In the patient with an insulinoma, fasting for this test may precipitate dangerously severe hypoglycemia. Keep an ampule of dextrose 50% available to counteract possible hypoglycemia.
- Handle the samples gently to prevent hemolysis.

Nursing Considerations
Before the Test
- Confirm the patient's identity using two patient identifiers and confirmation

of the patient's identification bracelet according to facility policy.

- Explain to the patient that the insulin test helps determine if the pancreas is functioning normally.
- Instruct the patient to fast for 10 to 12 hours before the test.
- Advise the patient that the test requires a blood sample. Explain that slight discomfort from the tourniquet and needle puncture may be experienced.
- Explain that questionable results may require a repeat test or a simultaneous glucose tolerance test, which requires that the patient drink a glucose solution.
- Withhold corticotropin, corticosteroids (including hormonal contraceptives), thyroid supplements, epinephrine, and other medications that may interfere with test results, as ordered. If they must be continued, note this information on the laboratory request.
- Make sure the patient is relaxed and recumbent for 30 minutes before the test.

During the Test

- Perform a venipuncture and collect one sample for the insulin level in a 7-mL EDTA tube.
- Collect another sample for the glucose level in a tube with sodium fluoride and potassium oxalate.

After the Test

- Apply direct pressure to the venipuncture site until bleeding stops and to prevent hematoma formation.
- Instruct the patient to resume usual activities, diet, and medications that were discontinued before the test, as ordered.

Insulin Tolerance Test

Reference Values

Blood glucose 50% of fasting level 20 to 30 minutes after insulin administration 10- to 20-ng/dL (SI, 10–20 mcg/L) increase. In human growth hormone (hGH) and corticotropin

baseline values; peak levels 60 to 90 minutes after insulin administration.

Abnormal Findings

- Failure of stimulation or blunted response, suggesting hypothalamic pituitary adrenal axis dysfunction
- hGH increase of less than 10 ng/dL (SI, less than 10 mcg/L) above baseline, indicating hGH deficiency
- Increase in corticotropin levels less than 10 ng/dL, indicating adrenal insufficiency

Nursing Implications

- Be aware that a definitive diagnosis of hGH deficiency requires a supplementary stimulation test, such as the arginine test.
- Prepare the patient for further testing, as appropriate.

Purpose

- To help diagnose hGH and corticotropin deficiency
- To identify pituitary dysfunction
- To aid differential diagnosis of primary and secondary adrenal hypofunction

Description

The insulin tolerance test measures hGH and corticotropin serum levels after a loading dose of insulin is administered. It's more reliable than direct measurement of hGH and corticotropin because many healthy people have undetectable fasting levels of these hormones. Insulin-induced hypoglycemia stimulates hGH and corticotropin secretion in persons with an intact hypothalamic–pituitary–adrenal axis. Stimulation failure indicates anterior pituitary or adrenal hypofunction and helps confirm an hGH or a corticotropin deficiency.

Because the insulin tolerance test stimulates an adrenergic response, it isn't recommended for patients with cardiovascular or cerebrovascular disorders, epilepsy, or low basal plasma cortisol levels.

Interfering Factors

- Corticosteroids and pituitary-based drugs (increase in hGH)
- Beta-adrenergic blockers and gluco-corticoids (decrease in hGH)
- Alcohol, amphetamines, calcium gluconate, estrogens, glucocorticoids, methamphetamines, and spirono-lactone (Aldactone) (decrease in corticotropin)

Precautions

- Have concentrated glucose solution readily available in the event that the patient has a severe hypoglycemic reaction to insulin.
- Handle the samples gently to prevent hemolysis.

Nursing Considerations

Before the Test

- Confirm the patient's identity using two patient identifiers and confirmation of the patient's identification bracelet according to facility policy.
- Explain to the patient or parents, if the patient is a child, that the insulin tolerance test evaluates hormonal secretion.
- Instruct the patient to fast and restrict physical activity for 10 to 12 hours before the test.
- Explain that the test involves IV infusion of insulin and the collection of multiple blood samples.
- Warn the patient that an increased heart rate, diaphoresis, hunger, and anxiety after administration of insulin may be experienced. Reassure the patient that these symptoms are transient and that, if they become severe, the test will be discontinued.
- Instruct the patient to lie down and relax for 90 minutes before the test.

During the Test

- Between 6 AM and 8 AM, perform a venipuncture and collect three 5-mL samples of blood for basal levels: one in a gray-topped tube (for blood glucose) and two in green-topped tubes (for hGH and corticotropin).
- Administer an IV bolus of 100 units regular insulin (0.15 unit/kg, or as ordered) over 1 to 2 minutes.
- Use an indwelling venous catheter to avoid repeated venipunctures. Collect additional blood samples 15, 30, 45, 60, 90, and 120 minutes after insulin administration. At each interval, collect three samples: one in a tube with sodium fluoride and potassium oxidate and two in heparinized tubes.
- Label the tubes appropriately, including the collection times on the laboratory request, and send all samples to the laboratory immediately.

After the Test

- Apply direct pressure to the veni-puncture site until bleeding stops.
- If a hematoma develops at the IV or venipuncture site, apply direct pressure.
- Instruct the patient to resume a usual diet, activities, and medications that were discontinued before the test, as ordered.

International Normalized Ratio

Reference Values

Warfarin (Coumadin) therapy: 2.0 to 3.0 (SI, 2.0–3.0)
Mechanical prosthetic heart valves: 3.0 to 4.5 (SI, 2.5–3.5)

Abnormal Findings

Elevated Levels

- Disseminated intravascular coagulation (DIC)
- Cirrhosis
- Hepatitis
- Vitamin K deficiency
- Salicylate intoxication
- Uncontrolled oral anticoagulation
- Massive blood transfusion

Nursing Implications

- Report abnormal findings to the health care provider.
- Prepare to administer vitamin K, as indicated.

- Advise the patient that the warfarin dose may need to be adjusted, as ordered.
- Prepare to educate the patient about the diagnosis.

Purpose
- To evaluate the effectiveness of oral anticoagulant therapy

Description
The International Normalized Ratio (INR) system is viewed as the best means of standardizing measurement of prothrombin time to monitor oral anticoagulant therapy. It isn't used as a screening test for coagulopathies.

Precautions
- Completely fill the collection tube; otherwise, an excess of citrate appears in the sample.
- Gently invert the tube several times to thoroughly mix the sample and the anticoagulant.
- To prevent hemolysis, avoid excessive probing during venipuncture and handle the sample gently.
- Put the sample on ice and send it to the laboratory promptly.

Nursing Considerations
Before the Test
- Confirm the patient's identity using two patient identifiers and confirmation of the patient's identification bracelet according to facility policy.
- Explain to the patient that the INR test is used to determine the effectiveness of oral anticoagulant therapy.
- Advise the patient that a blood sample will be taken. Explain that slight discomfort from the tourniquet and needle puncture may be experienced.

During the Test
- Perform a venipuncture and collect the sample in a 4.5-mL tube with sodium citrate added.

After the Test
- If a hematoma develops at the venipuncture site, apply direct pressure.

Iron and Total Iron-Binding Capacity

Reference Values
Serum Iron
Females: 50 to 130 mcg/dL (SI, 9–23.3 mcmol/L)
Males: 60 to 170 mcg/dL (SI, 10.7–30.4 mcmol/L)

Total Iron-Binding Capacity
Males and females: 300 to 360 mcg/dL (SI, 54–64 mcmol/L)

Saturation
Males and females: 20% to 50% (SI, 0.2–0.5)

Abnormal Findings
Elevated Levels
- Hemochromatosis

Decreased Levels
- Iron deficiency (serum iron levels decrease and total iron-binding capacity [TIBC] increases, decreasing saturation)
- Chronic inflammation, such as in rheumatoid arthritis (serum iron may be low but TIBC may remain unchanged or may decrease)

Nursing Implications
- Report abnormal findings to the health care provider.
- Prepare to educate the patient about the diagnosis.
- Prepare the patient with elevated levels for phlebotomy, as indicated.
- Advise the patient with elevated levels not to take iron supplements or to ingest iron-rich foods.
- Prepare the patient with decreased levels for blood transfusions, as indicated.
- Administer iron supplements as ordered to patients with decreased levels.
- Educate the patient with decreased levels about eating iron-rich foods.

Purpose
- To estimate total iron storage
- To help diagnose hemochromatosis

I
J

Siderocyte Stain

Siderocytes are red blood cells (RBCs) containing particles of nonhemoglobin iron known as *siderocytic granules.* In neonates, siderocytic granules are normally present in normoblasts and reticulocytes during hemoglobin synthesis. However, the spleen removes most of these granules from normal RBCs, and they disappear rapidly with age.

In adults, an elevated siderocyte level usually indicates abnormal erythropoiesis, which may occur in congenital spherocytic anemia, chronic hemolytic anemias (such as the thalassemias), pernicious anemia, hemochromatosis, toxicities (such as lead poisoning), infection, or severe burns. Elevated levels may also follow splenectomy because the spleen normally removes siderocytic granules.

Performing the Test

The siderocyte stain test measures the number of circulating siderocytes. Venous blood is drawn into a 3- or 4.5-mL EDTA tube or, for infants and children, collected in a Microtainer or pipette and smeared directly on a 3 × 5 glass slide. When the blood smear is stained, siderocytic granules appear as purple-blue specks clustered around the periphery of mature erythrocytes. Cells containing these granules are counted as a percentage of total RBCs. The results aid differential diagnosis of the anemias and hemochromatosis and help detect toxicities.

Interpreting Results

Normally, neonates have a slightly elevated siderocyte level that reaches the normal adult value of 0.5% (SI, 0.05) of total RBCs in 7 to 10 days. In patients with pernicious anemia, the siderocyte level is 8% to 14% (SI, 0.08 to 0.14); in chronic hemolytic anemia, 20% to 100% (SI, 0.2 to 1.0); in lead poisoning, 10% to 30% (SI, 0.1 to 0.3); and in hemochromatosis, 3% to 7% (SI, 0.03 to 0.07). A high siderocyte level calls for additional testing (including bone marrow examination) to determine the cause of abnormal erythropoiesis.

- To help distinguish iron deficiency anemia from anemia of chronic disease (For information on another test used to differentiate anemias, see the *Siderocyte Stain* box.)
- To help evaluate nutritional status

Description

Iron is essential to the formation and function of hemoglobin, as well as of many other heme and nonheme compounds. After iron is absorbed by the intestine, it's distributed to various body compartments for synthesis, storage, and transport.

An iron assay is used to measure the amount of iron bound to transferrin in blood plasma. TIBC measures the amount of iron that would appear in plasma if all the transferrin were saturated with iron.

Serum iron and TIBC are of greater diagnostic usefulness when performed with the serum ferritin assay, but together these tests may not accurately reflect the state of other iron compartments,

such as myoglobin iron and the labile iron pool. Bone marrow or liver biopsy and iron absorption or excretion studies may yield more information.

Interfering Factors

- Chloramphenicol and hormonal contraceptives (possible false positive)
- Corticotropin (ACTH) (possible false negative)
- Iron supplements (possible false-positive serum iron values, but false-negative TIBC)

Precautions

- Serum iron concentration is normally highest in the morning; therefore, the sample should be drawn in the morning.
- Handle the sample gently to prevent hemolysis.
- Send the sample to the laboratory immediately.

Nursing Considerations

Before the Test

- Confirm the patient's identity using two patient identifiers and confirmation

of the patient's identification bracelet according to facility policy.

- Explain to the patient that this test evaluates the body's capacity to store iron.
- Advise the patient that a blood sample will be taken. Explain that slight discomfort from the tourniquet and needle puncture may be experienced.
- Notify the laboratory and health care provider of medications the patient is taking that may affect test results; these may need to be restricted.

- Tell the patient that there are no food or fluid restrictions for this test.

During the Test
- Perform a venipuncture and collect the sample in a 4.5-mL clot activator tube.

After the Test
- If a hematoma develops at the venipuncture site, apply pressure.
- Explain that the patient may resume medications that were discontinued before the test, as ordered.

I

J

17-Ketogenic Steroids, Urine

Reference Values

Females: 2 to 12 mg/24 hours (SI, 7–42 mcmol/day)

Males: 4 to 14 mg/24 hours (SI, 13–49 mcmol/day)

Children ages 11 to 14: 2 to 9 mg/24 hours (SI, 7–31 mcmol/day)

Infants and children younger than age 11: 0.1 to 4 mg/24 hours (SI, 0.3–14 mcmol/day)

Abnormal Findings

Elevated Levels

- Hyperadrenalism
- Cushing syndrome
- Adrenogenital syndrome (congenital adrenal hyperplasia)
- Adrenal carcinoma or adenoma
- Severe physical stress (such as that caused by burns, infections, or surgery)
- Emotional stress

Decreased Levels

- Addison's disease
- Panhypopituitarism
- Cachexia

Nursing Implications

- Report abnormal findings to the health care provider.
- Prepare to educate the patient about the diagnosis.
- Prepare the patient for further testing, as appropriate.
- Refer the patient for counseling or community resources, as appropriate.

Purpose

- To evaluate adrenocortical and testicular function

- To help diagnose Cushing syndrome and Addison's disease

Description

Using spectrophotofluorimetry, this test determines urine levels of the 17-ketogenic steroids (17-KGS), which consists of the 17-hydroxycorticosteroids (cortisol and its metabolites, for example) and other adrenocortical steroids, such as pregnanetriol, that can be oxidized in the laboratory to 17-ketosteroids. The results provide an excellent overall assessment of adrenocortical function. For accurate diagnosis of a specific disease, results must be compared with those of other tests, including plasma corticotropin, plasma cortisol, corticotropin stimulation, single-dose metyrapone, and dexamethasone suppression.

Nursing Considerations

Before the Test

- Confirm the patient's identity using two patient identifiers and confirmation of the patient's identification bracelet according to facility policy.
- Explain to the patient that the urine 17-KGS test evaluates adrenal function.
- Inform the patient that there are no food or fluids restrictions but that excessive physical exercise and stressful situations should be avoided during the collection period.
- Advise the patient that the test requires urine collection over a 24-hour period, and teach the patient how to collect the specimen correctly.
- Notify the laboratory and physician of drugs the patient is taking that may affect test results; it may be necessary to restrict these.

During the Test
- Collect the patient's urine over a 24-hour period, discarding the first specimen and retaining the last.
- Label the specimen and laboratory requests with the patient's name and gender.

After the Test
- Instruct the patient to resume usual activities and medications, as ordered.
- Inform the health care provider of abnormal results.

Ketones, Urine

Reference Values
Negative for ketones

Abnormal Findings
- Positive for ketones, indicating carbohydrate dehydration (diabetic ketoacidosis [DKA], starvation, or a metabolic complication of total parenteral nutrition)

Nursing Implications
- Report abnormal findings to the health care provider.
- Prepare to educate the patient about the diagnosis.
- For DKA, prepare to administer isotonic saline solution and potassium replacement, as ordered.

Purpose
- To screen for ketonuria
- To identify DKA and carbohydrate deprivation
- To distinguish between a diabetic and nondiabetic coma
- To check for a metabolic complication of total parenteral nutrition
- To monitor control of diabetes, ketogenic weight reduction, and treatment of DKA

Description
Ketones are by-products of fat metabolism and include acetoacetic acid, acetone, and beta-hydroxybutyric acid. Testing for the urine level of ketones is a routine and semiquantitative screening done with a commercially prepared product, such as Acetest tablet, Ketostix, or Keto-Diastix, each of which measures a specific ketone body.

Interfering Factors
- Failure to keep the reagent container tightly closed to prevent absorption of light or moisture or bacterial contamination of the specimen (false negative)
- Levodopa and phenazopyridine (Pyridium) (false-positive results when Ketostix or Keto-Diastix is used instead of Acetest)

Precautions
- If the patient is taking levodopa or phenazopyridine or has recently received sulfobromophthalein, use Acetest tablets because reagent strips may produce inaccurate results.

Nursing Considerations

Before the Test
- Confirm the patient's identity using two patient identifiers and confirmation of the patient's identification bracelet according to facility policy.
- Inform the patient that there is no need to restrict food and fluids for the test.
- Explain to the patient that the ketone test evaluates fat metabolism.
- If the patient is newly diagnosed with diabetes, explain how to perform the test.

During the Test
- Instruct the patient to void, then give the patient a drink of water.
- Collect a second-voided midstream specimen about 30 minutes later.

Acetest
- Lay the tablet on a piece of white paper and place 1 drop of urine on the tablet.
- After 30 seconds, compare the tablet color (white, lavender, or purple) with the color chart.

Ketostix
- Dip the reagent stick into the specimen and remove it immediately.

• After 15 seconds, compare the stick color (buff or purple) with the color chart. Record the results as negative, small, moderate, or large amounts of ketones.

Keto-Diastix

• Dip the reagent strip into the specimen and remove it immediately. Tap the edge of the strip against the container or a clean, dry surface to remove excess urine.

• Hold the Keto-Diastix strip horizontally to prevent mixing the chemicals from the two areas. Interpret each area of the strip separately. Compare the color of the ketone section (buff or purple) with the appropriate color chart after exactly 15 seconds; compare the color of the glucose section after 30 seconds.

All Tests

• Don't use tablets or strips that have become discolored or darkened.

• Ignore color changes that occur after the specified waiting periods. Record the results as negative or positive for small, moderate, or large amounts of ketones.

• Test the specimen within 1 hour after it's obtained or refrigerate it until ready to test.

• Let refrigerated specimens return to room temperature before testing.

After the Test

• Record the results as negative or positive for small, moderate, or large amounts of ketones.

Kidney–Ureter–Bladder Radiography

Normal Findings

• Bilateral kidney shadows, with the right kidney appearing slightly lower than the left

• Both kidneys about the same size, superior poles tilted slightly toward the vertebral column, paralleling the shadows of the psoas muscles

• Bladder shadow less clearly visible than kidney shadows

Abnormal Findings

• Bilateral renal enlargement, suggesting polycystic kidney disease, multiple myeloma, lymphoma, amyloidosis, hydronephrosis, or compensatory renal hypertrophy

• Abnormally small kidneys, indicating end-stage glomerulonephritis or bilateral atrophic pyelonephritis

• Decrease in size of one kidney, indicating congenital hypoplasia or atrophic pyelonephritis

• Renal displacement, indicating retroperitoneal tumor

• Opaque bodies, suggesting calculi, vascular calcification, fecaliths, foreign bodies, or abnormal fluid or gas collection

Nursing Implications

• Report abnormal findings to the health care provider.

• Prepare to educate the patient about the diagnosis.

• Prepare the patient for further testing or surgery, as indicated.

• Administer medications, as prescribed.

Purpose

• To evaluate the size, structure, and position of the kidneys and bladder

• To screen for abnormalities, such as calcifications, in the area of the kidneys, ureters, and bladder

Description

Usually, the first step in diagnostic testing of the urinary system, kidney–ureter–bladder (KUB) radiography surveys the abdomen to determine the position of the kidneys, ureters, and bladder and to detect gross abnormalities.

This test doesn't require intact renal function and may aid differential diagnosis of urologic and GI diseases, which commonly produce similar signs and symptoms. However, KUB radiography has many limitations and usually must be followed by more elaborate tests, such as excretory urography or renal computed tomography. KUB radiography shouldn't follow recent instillation of barium.

The procedure for KUB radiography is as follows:

- The patient is placed in a supine position in correct body alignment on an X-ray table. The arms are extended overhead, and the iliac crests are checked for symmetrical positioning.
- The patient may lie on the left side with the right arm up if unable to extend arms or stand.
- A single X-ray is taken.

Interfering Factors

- Contrast medium, foreign bodies, gas, or stools in the intestine (possible poor imaging)
- Calcified uterine fibromas or ovarian lesions
- Ascites or obesity (possible poor imaging)

Precautions

- A male patient should have gonadal shielding to prevent irradiation of the testes. A female patient's ovaries can't be shielded because they're too close to the kidneys, ureters, and bladder.

Nursing Considerations

Before the Test

- Confirm the patient's identity using two patient identifiers and confirmation of the patient's identification bracelet according to facility policy.
- Explain to the patient that KUB radiography helps detect urinary system abnormalities.
- Inform the patient that there is no need to restrict food and fluids for the test.
- Advise the patient who will perform the test, where and when it will take place, and that it takes only a few minutes.

After the Test

- Answer the patient's questions about the test.

K

Lactate Dehydrogenase

Reference Values
Total lactate dehydrogenase (LD): 71 to
207 units/L (SI, 1.2–3.52 mckat/L);
levels may be slightly increased in
older adults because of declining
muscle mass and liver function

LD_1: 14% to 26% (SI, 0.14–0.26) of total
LD_2: 29% to 39% (SI, 0.29–0.39) of total
LD_3: 20% to 26% (SI, 0.20–0.26) of total
LD_4: 8% to 16% (SI, 0.08–0.16) of total
LD_5: 6% to 16% (SI, 0.06–0.16) of total

Abnormal Findings
- Total LD within normal limits,
  but abnormal proportions of each
  enzyme, indicating specific organ
  tissue damage
- Increased midzone fractions (LD_2,
  LD_3, LD_4), indicating granulocytic
  leukemia, lymphomas, and platelet
  disorders

Nursing Implications
- Report abnormal findings to the
  health care provider.
- Prepare to educate the patient about
  the diagnosis.
- Because many common diseases
  increase total LD levels, isoenzyme
  electrophoresis is usually needed to
  pinpoint a diagnosis.
- Prepare the patient for further testing,
  as appropriate.

Purpose
- To aid in diagnosis of myocardial
  infarction (MI)
- To aid differential diagnosis of pulmonary infarction, anemias, hepatic
  disease, and malignant neoplasms

- To monitor the patient's response to
  some forms of chemotherapy

Description
The specificity of LD isoenzymes and
their distribution pattern is useful in
diagnosing hepatic, pulmonary, and
erythrocyte damage. (See the *LD Isoenzyme Variations in Disease* box.)

Interfering Factors
- Recent surgery or pregnancy (possible
  increase)
- Prosthetic heart valve (possible
  increase caused by chronic hemolysis)
- Alcohol, anabolic steroids, anes-
  thetics, opioids, and procainamide
  (Procanbid) (increase)

Precautions
- Draw the samples on schedule to
  avoid missing peak levels and mark
  the collection time on the laboratory
  request.
- Handle the sample gently to prevent
  artifactual blood sample hemolysis
  because red blood cells contain LD_1.

Nursing Considerations
Before the Test
- Confirm the patient's identity using
  two patient identifiers and confirmation of the patient's identification bracelet according to facility
  policy.
- Explain to the patient that the LD
  test is used primarily to detect tissue
  alterations.
- Advise the patient that the test
  requires a blood sample. Explain that
  slight discomfort from the tourniquet
  and needle puncture may be experienced.

LD Isoenzyme Variations in Disease

This chart shows lactate dehydrogenase (LD) variations in various cardiovascular, pulmonary, hematologic, and hepatobiliary diseases.

Disease	LD$_1$	LD$_2$	LD$_3$	LD$_4$	LD$_5$
Cardiovascular					
Rheumatic carditis	▨	▨			
Myocarditis	▨	▨			
Heart failure (decompensated)					▨
Shock	▨	▨			
Angina pectoris	■				
Pulmonary					
Pulmonary embolism	■				
Pulmonary infarction			▨		
Hematologic					
Pernicious anemia	▨	▨			
Hemolytic anemia	▨	▨			
Sickle cell anemia	▨	▨			
Hepatobiliary					
Hepatitis					▨
Active cirrhosis					▨
Hepatic congestion					▨

KEY: ■ Normal   ▨ Diagnostic   ☐ Not diagnostic

- Inform the patient that there are no food or fluid restrictions for this test.
- If an MI is suspected, tell the patient that the test will be repeated on the next two mornings to monitor progressive changes.

During the Test
- Perform a venipuncture and collect the sample in a 4-mL clot activator tube.
- Send the sample to the laboratory immediately or, if transport is delayed, keep the sample at room temperature. Changes in temperature reportedly inactivate LD$_5$, thus altering isoenzyme patterns.

After the Test
- Apply direct pressure to the venipuncture site until bleeding stops and to prevent hematoma formation.

Laryngoscopy, Direct

Normal Findings
- No evidence of inflammation, lesions, strictures, or foreign bodies

Abnormal Findings
- Laryngeal carcinoma (combined with biopsy and radiography)
- Benign lesions
- Strictures
- Foreign bodies
- Vocal cord dysfunction

Nursing Implications
- Report abnormal findings to the health care provider.
- Prepare to educate the patient about the diagnosis.
- Prepare the patient for further testing or surgery, as appropriate.

Purpose

- To detect lesions, strictures, or foreign bodies
- To remove benign lesions or foreign bodies from the larynx
- To help diagnose laryngeal or upper airway abnormalities
- To examine the larynx when indirect laryngoscopy is inadequate

Description

Direct laryngoscopy allows visualization of the larynx by the use of a fiberoptic endoscope or laryngoscope passed through the mouth or nose and pharynx to the larynx. It's indicated for any condition requiring direct visualization or specimen samples for diagnosis, such as in patients with strong gag reflexes resulting from anatomic abnormalities and in those who have had no response to short-term therapy for symptoms of pharyngeal or laryngeal disease, such as chronic hoarseness, stridor, and hemoptysis. Secretions or tissue may be removed during this procedure for further study. The test is usually contraindicated in patients with epiglottitis, but it may be performed on them in an operating room with resuscitative equipment.

The procedure for direct laryngoscopy is as follows:

- The patient is placed in the supine position and encouraged to breathe through the nose and relax with the arms at the sides.
- A general anesthetic may be administered, or the patient's mouth and throat may be sprayed with a local anesthetic.
- A laryngoscope is introduced through the patient's mouth or nostril, the larynx is examined for abnormalities, and a specimen or secretions may be removed for further study; minor surgery, such as removal of polyps or nodules, may be performed at this time.
- Specimens are collected and placed in their respective containers in accordance with laboratory and pathology guidelines.

Interfering Factors

- Inability to pass the scope

Nursing Considerations

Before the Test

- Confirm the patient's identity using two patient identifiers and confirmation of the patient's identification bracelet according to facility policy.
- Explain to the patient that direct laryngoscopy is used to detect laryngeal abnormalities.
- Instruct the patient to fast for 6 to 8 hours before the test.
- Inform the patient who will perform the procedure and when and where it will be done.
- Advise the patient that a relaxing sedative, medication to reduce secretions, and, during the procedure, a general or local anesthetic will be given. Reassure the patient that this procedure won't obstruct the airway.
- Make sure that the patient or a responsible family member has signed an informed consent form.
- Check the patient's history for hypersensitivity to the anesthetic.
- Obtain the patient's baseline vital signs.
- Administer the sedative and other medication (usually 30 minutes to 1 hour before the test), as ordered.
- Instruct the patient to remove dentures, contact lenses, and jewelry and to void before receiving the sedative.

After the Test

- Place the conscious patient in semi-Fowler's position. Place the sedated patient on the side with the head slightly elevated to prevent aspiration.
- Check the patient's vital signs, pulse oximetry, and cardiac monitor rhythm according to facility protocol, or every 15 minutes until the patient is stable and then every 30 minutes for 2 hours, every hour for the next

4 hours, and then every 4 hours for 24 hours. Immediately report to the health care provider any adverse reaction to the anesthetic or sedative (tachycardia, palpitations, hypertension, euphoria, excitation, and rapid, deep respirations).

• Apply an ice collar per institution protocol to minimize laryngeal edema.

• Provide an emesis basin and instruct the patient to spit out saliva rather than swallow it. Observe sputum for blood and report excessive bleeding immediately.

• Instruct the patient to refrain from clearing the throat and coughing to prevent hemorrhaging at the biopsy site.

• Advise the patient to avoid smoking until vital signs are stable and there's no evidence of complications.

• Immediately report subcutaneous crepitus around the patient's face and neck, which may indicate tracheal perforation.

• Listen to the patient's neck with a stethoscope for signs of stridor and airway obstruction.

> **Quality and Safety Nursing Alert**
>
> Observe the patient with epiglottitis for signs of airway obstruction. Immediately report signs of respiratory difficulty. Keep emergency resuscitation equipment available; keep a tracheotomy tray nearby for 24 hours.

• Restrict food and fluids to avoid aspiration until the gag reflex returns (usually within 2 hours). The patient may then resume a usual diet, beginning with sips of water and ice chips.

• Assure the patient that voice loss, hoarseness, and sore throat are temporary. Provide throat lozenges or a soothing liquid gargle when the gag reflex returns.

Leucine Aminopeptidase

Reference Values
Females: 75 to 185 units/mL (SI, 75–185 kilounits/L)
Males: 80 to 200 units/mL (SI, 80 to 200 kilounits/L)

Abnormal Findings
Elevated Levels
• Biliary obstruction
• Tumors
• Liver damage (cirrhosis, hepatitis, cancer)
• Strictures
• Atresia
• Advanced pregnancy (severe preeclampsia)
• Therapy with drugs containing estrogen or progesterone

Nursing Implications
• Report abnormal findings to the health care provider.
• Prepare to educate the patient about the diagnosis.
• Prepare the patient for further testing or surgery, as indicated.

Purpose
• To provide information about suspected liver, pancreatic, and biliary diseases
• To differentiate skeletal disease from hepatobiliary or pancreatic disease
• To evaluate neonatal jaundice

Description
The leucine aminopeptidase (LAP) test is used to measure serum levels of LAP, an isoenzyme of alkaline phosphatase (ALP) that's widely distributed in body tissues. The greatest concentrations appear in the hepatobiliary tissues, pancreas, and small intestine. Serum LAP levels parallel serum ALP levels in hepatic disease.

Interfering Factors
• Advanced pregnancy (false high)
• Estrogen or progesterone (false high)

Precautions
- Handle the sample gently to avoid hemolysis.
- Transport the sample to the laboratory immediately.

Nursing Considerations
Before the Test
- Confirm the patient's identity using two patient identifiers and confirmation of the patient's identification bracelet according to facility policy.
- Explain to the patient that the LAP test is used to evaluate liver and pancreatic function.
- Advise the patient that the test requires a blood sample. Explain that slight discomfort from the tourniquet and needle puncture may be experienced.
- Instruct the patient to fast for at least 8 hours before the test.
- Notify the laboratory and health care provider of medications the patient is taking that may affect test results; these may need to be restricted.

During the Test
- Perform a venipuncture and collect the sample in a 4-mL clot activator tube.
- Apply direct pressure to the venipuncture site until bleeding stops.

After the Test
- Instruct the patient to resume a usual diet and medications that were discontinued before the test, as ordered.

Lipase, Serum
Reference Values
Less than 160 units/L (SI, less than 2.72 mckat/L)

Abnormal Findings
Elevated Levels
- Acute pancreatitis
- Pancreatic duct obstruction
- Perforated peptic ulcer with chemical pancreatitis caused by gastric juices
- High intestinal obstruction (bowel infarction)

- Pancreatic cancer
- Renal disease with impaired excretion

Nursing Implications
- Report abnormal findings to the health care provider.
- Prepare to educate the patient about the diagnosis.
- Prepare the patient for further testing or surgery, as indicated.

Purpose
- To help diagnose acute pancreatitis or other pancreatic disorders

Description
Lipase is produced in the pancreas and secreted into the duodenum, where it converts triglycerides and other fats into fatty acids and glycerol. The destruction of pancreatic cells, which occurs in acute pancreatitis, causes large amounts of lipase to be released into the blood. The lipase test is used to measure serum lipase levels and is most useful when performed with a serum or urine amylase test.

Interfering Factors
- Cholinergics, codeine, and morphine (false high due to spasm of the sphincter of Oddi)
- Acetaminophen, cimetidine, NSAIDs
- Hemodialysis
- EDTA anticoagulant

Precautions
- Handle the sample gently to prevent hemolysis.

Nursing Considerations
Before the Test
- Confirm the patient's identity using two patient identifiers and confirmation of the patient's identification bracelet according to facility policy.
- Explain to the patient that the serum lipase test is used to evaluate pancreatic function.
- Advise the patient that the test requires a blood sample. Explain that slight discomfort from the tourniquet and needle puncture may be experienced.

- Instruct the patient to fast after midnight before the test.
- Notify the laboratory and health care provider of medications the patient is taking that may affect test results; these may need to be restricted.

During the Test

- Perform a venipuncture and collect the sample in a 4-mL clot activator tube.

After the Test

- Apply direct pressure to the venipuncture site until bleeding stops and to prevent hematoma formation.
- Instruct the patient to resume a usual diet and medications that were discontinued before the test, as ordered.

Lipoprotein Electrophoresis

Reference Values

High-Density Lipoprotein (HDL) Levels

Females: 40 to 85 mg/dL (SI, 1.03–2.2 mmol/L)

Males: 37 to 70 mg/dL (SI, 0.96–1.8 mmol/L)

Low-Density Lipoprotein (LDL) Levels

Ideally, 60 mg/dL or lower

Abnormal Findings

Elevated LDL Levels

- Increased coronary artery disease (CAD) risk

Elevated HDL Levels

- Chronic hepatitis
- Early stage of primary biliary cirrhosis
- Alcohol consumption
- Long-term aerobic and vigorous exercise
- CAD (indicated by a sharp rise in a second type of HDL [alpha$_2$ HDL] to as high as 100 mg/dL [SI, 2.58 mmol/L]) (See the *PLAC Test* box.)
- Hyperlipoproteinemias (I, IIa, IIb, III, IV, and V)

- Hypolipoproteinemias (hypobetalipoproteinemia, beta-lipoproteinemia, and alpha-lipoprotein deficiency)
- Uncontrolled diabetes
- Hypothyroidism

Nursing Implications

- Report abnormal findings to the health care provider.
- Prepare to educate the patient about the diagnosis.
- Prepare the patient for further testing, as indicated.
- Advise the patient about lifestyle changes to reduce the risk of further CAD damage.

Purpose

- To assess the risk of CAD
- To assess the efficacy of lipid-lowering drug therapy
- To determine the classification of hyperlipoproteinemia and hypolipoproteinemia (phenotyping)

Description

Lipoprotein electrophoresis involves fractionation and phenotyping tests. Fractionation tests are used to isolate and measure the types of cholesterol in

 PLAC Test

The PLAC test can help determine who might be at risk for coronary artery disease (CAD). It works by measuring lipoprotein-associated phospholipase A$_2$, an enzyme produced by macrophages, a type of white blood cell. When heart disease is present, macrophages increase production of the enzyme.

A multicenter study sponsored by the National Heart, Lung, and Blood Institute showed that an elevated PLAC test result, in conjunction with a low-density lipoprotein (LDL) cholesterol level of less than 130 mg/dL, generally indicates that a patient has two to three times the risk of CAD compared with similar patients with lower PLAC test results. The study also found that those people with the highest PLAC test results and LDL cholesterol levels lower than 130 mg/dL had the greatest risk of heart disease.

serum: LDLs and HDLs. The HDL level is inversely related to the risk of CAD; the higher the HDL level, the lower the incidence of CAD. Conversely, the higher the LDL level, the higher the incidence of CAD.

Lipoprotein phenotyping is used to determine levels of the four major lipoproteins: chylomicrons, very-low-density (pre-beta) lipoproteins, low-density (beta) lipoproteins, and high-density (alpha) lipoproteins.

(See the *Familial Hyperlipoproteinemias* table.) Detecting altered lipoprotein patterns is essential in identifying hyperlipoproteinemia and hypolipoproteinemia.

Interfering Factors

- Concurrent illness, especially if accompanied by fever, recent surgery, or MI
- Heparin administration (which activates the enzyme lipase, producing

Familial Hyperlipoproteinemias

Type	Causes and Incidence	Clinical Signs	Laboratory Findings
I	• Deficient lipoprotein lipase, resulting in increased chylomicrons • May be induced by alcoholism • Incidence: rare	• Eruptive xanthomas • Lipemia retinalis • Abdominal pain	• Increased chylomicron, total cholesterol, and triglyceride levels • Normal or slightly increased VLDLs • Normal or decreased LDLs and high-density lipoproteins • Cholesterol triglyceride ratio <0.2
IIa	• Deficient cell receptor, resulting in increased low-density lipoproteins (LDLs) and excessive cholesterol synthesis • May be induced by hypothyroidism • Incidence: common	• Premature coronary artery disease (CAD) • Arcus cornealis • Xanthelasma • Tendinous and tuberous xanthomas	• Increased LDL • Normal VLDL • Cholesterol-triglyceride ratio >2.0
IIb	• Deficient cell receptor, resulting in increased LDL and excessive cholesterol synthesis • May be induced by dysgammaglobulinemia, hypothyroidism, uncontrolled diabetes, and nephritic syndrome • Incidence: common	• Premature CAD • Obesity • Possible xanthelasma	• Increased LDL, VLDL, total cholesterol, and triglycerides
III	• Unknown cause, resulting in deficient very-low-density lipoproteins (VLDL)-to-LDL conversion • May be induced by hypothyroidism, uncontrolled diabetes, and paraproteinemia • Incidence: rare	• Premature CAD • Arcus cornealis • Eruptive tuberous xanthomas	• Increased total cholesterol, VLDL, and triglycerides • Normal or decreased LDL • Cholesterol-triglyceride ratio >0.4 • Broad beta band observed on electrophoresis

Familial Hyperlipoproteinemias (continued)

Type	Causes and Incidence	Clinical Signs	Laboratory Findings
IV	• Unknown cause, resulting in decreased levels of lipase • May be induced by uncontrolled diabetes, alcoholism, pregnancy, steroid or estrogen therapy, dysgammaglobulinemia, and hyperthyroidism • Incidence: common	• Possible premature CAD • Obesity • Hypertension • Peripheral neuropathy	• Increased VLDL and triglycerides • Normal LDL • Cholesterol-triglyceride ratio <0.25
V	• Unknown cause, resulting in defective triglyceride clearance • May be induced by alcoholism, uncontrolled diabetes, nephrotic syndrome, pancreatitis, and steroid therapy • Incidence: rare	• Premature CAD • Abdominal pain • Lipemia retinalis • Eruptive xanthomas • Hepatosplenomegaly	• Increased VLDL, total cholesterol, and triglyceride levels • Chylomicrons present • Cholesterol-triglyceride ratio <0.6

L

fatty acids from triglycerides) or sample collection in a heparinized tube (possible false high due to activation of the enzyme lipase, which causes release of fatty acids from triglycerides)
• Antilipemic medications, such as cholestyramine (Questran), gemfibrozil, and niacin (decrease)
• Alcohol, disulfiram, hormonal contraceptives, miconazole, and high doses of phenothiazines (possible increase in fractionation)
• Estrogens (possible increase or decrease in fractionation)
• Presence of bilirubin, hemoglobin, iodine, salicylates, and vitamins A and D (altered fractionation results)
• Not fasting prior to test (possible false elevation)

Precautions
• When drawing multiple samples, collect the sample for lipoprotein phenotyping first, because venous obstruction for 2 minutes can affect test results.

• Fill the collection tube completely, and invert it gently several times to mix the sample and the anticoagulant thoroughly.
• Handle the sample gently to prevent hemolysis.

Nursing Considerations
Before the Test
• Confirm the patient's identity using two patient identifiers and confirmation of the patient's identification bracelet according to facility policy.
• Explain to the patient that the fractionation test is used to determine the risk of CAD and that lipoprotein typing is used to determine how the body metabolizes fats.
• Advise the patient that the test requires a blood sample. Explain that slight discomfort from the tourniquet and needle puncture may be experienced.
• Instruct the patient to maintain a normal diet for 2 weeks before the test, to abstain from alcohol for 24 hours before the test, and to fast

and avoid exercise for 12 to 14 hours before the test.

- Notify the laboratory and health care provider of medications the patient is taking that may affect test results; these may need to be restricted.
- For the patient undergoing the phenotyping test:
  - Check the patient's drug history for heparin use.
  - Withhold antilipemics, such as cholestyramine, about 2 weeks before the test, as ordered.
  - Instruct the patient to eat a low-fat meal the night before the test.
  - Notify the laboratory if the patient is receiving treatment for another condition that might significantly alter lipoprotein metabolism, such as diabetes, nephrosis, or hypothyroidism.

During the Test
- Perform a venipuncture and collect the sample. Use a 7-mL EDTA tube for the fractionation test and a 4-mL EDTA tube for the phenotyping test.
- Send the sample to the laboratory immediately to avoid spontaneous redistribution among the lipoproteins.
- If the sample can't be transported immediately, refrigerate it but don't freeze it.

After the Test
- Apply direct pressure to the venipuncture site until bleeding stops and to prevent hematoma formation.
- Instruct the patient to resume a usual diet and medications discontinued before the test, as ordered.

Loop Electrosurgical Excision Procedure

Normal Findings
- Normal cervix squamous cells (flatten with growth)

Abnormal Findings
- Abnormal tissue growth, indicating cervical dysplasia or cervical cancer

Nursing Implications
- Report abnormal findings to the health care provider.
- Prepare to educate the patient about her diagnosis.
- Prepare the patient for further testing or surgery, as indicated.

Purpose
- To confirm results of colposcopy and Pap smear
- To identify lesions as benign or cancerous, invasive or noninvasive
- To remove cervical dysplasia and noninvasive cervical cancers

Description
Loop electrosurgical excision procedure (LEEP) is a method for obtaining cervical tissue specimens for biopsy and removing abnormal tissue from the cervix and high in the endocervical canal. This procedure usually is done after a Papanicolaou smear and colposcopy to ensure the accuracy of results, to exclude an invasive cancer diagnosis, and to determine the extent of noninvasive lesions. LEEP complications include heavy bleeding, severe cramping, infection, and accidental cutting or burning of normal tissue. Cervical stenosis is also a possible risk.

The procedure for LEEP is as follows:

- The patient is placed in the lithotomy position and encouraged to relax.
- A vaginal speculum is inserted and a local anesthetic is applied to the area.
- The cervix is cleaned with a mild vinegar solution (3% acetic acid solution) or iodine to remove any debris or mucus. The solution also aids in identifying normal and abnormal tissues.
- A thin wire loop attached to a high-frequency current is then inserted, and the loop is used to remove the suspected tissue. The tissue is sent to the laboratory.

- A cervical paste is applied to the area where tissue was removed to reduce bleeding.

Interfering Factors
- Inability to obtain a full specimen for removal

Precautions
- LEEP is contraindicated in patients with active menstrual bleeding or who are pregnant.

Nursing Considerations

Before the Test
- Confirm the patient's identity using two patient identifiers and confirmation of the patient's identification bracelet according to facility policy.
- Describe the procedure to the patient and explain that it provides a cervical tissue specimen for microscopic study and treats abnormal tissue growth.
- Help allay the patient's anxiety about a possible diagnosis of cervical cancer.
- Advise the patient who will perform the procedure and when and where it will be done.
- Explain to the patient that she may experience mild discomfort during and after the procedure and that she may have some vaginal drainage afterward.
- Advise the patient to have someone drive her home after the procedure.
- Make sure the patient or a responsible family member has signed an informed consent form.

After the Test
- Inform the patient that she may experience some vaginal bleeding and mild cramping immediately after the procedure, a brown-black vaginal discharge or a white watery discharge for about 1 week, and possible spotting for up to 4 weeks. Encourage her to wear a perineal pad and change it frequently.

- Instruct the patient to notify her health care provider if she experiences fever, bleeding greater than normal menstrual flow, increasing pelvic pain or severe abdominal pain, or a foul-smelling or malodorous vaginal discharge.
- Advise the patient not to douche, use tampons or bubble baths, or engage in sexual intercourse for approximately 3 to 4 weeks.
- Urge the patient to return for follow-up with her health care provider, as indicated, for information about results.

Lumbar Puncture

Normal Findings
- *Pressure:* 50 to 180 mm H_2O
- *Appearance:* Clear, colorless
- *Protein:* 15 to 45 mg/dL
- *Gamma globulin:* 3% to 12% of total protein
- *Glucose:* 50 to 80 mg/dL
- *Cell count:* 0 to 5 white blood cells (WBCs), no red blood cells (RBCs)
- *Venereal Disease Research Laboratory (VDRL)* test: nonreactive
- *Chloride:* 118 to 130 mEq/L
- *Gram stain:* No organisms

Abnormal Findings
- Tumor, hemorrhage, or trauma-induced edema, indicating increased intracranial pressure (ICP)
- Spinal subarachnoid obstruction, indicating decreased ICP
- Cloudy appearance, indicating infection
- Yellow or bloody appearance, indicating intracranial hemorrhage or spinal cord obstruction
- Brown or orange appearance, indicating increased protein levels or RBC breakdown
- Increased protein, indicating tumor, trauma, diabetes, or blood in cerebrospinal fluid (CSF)

L

...ed protein, indicating rapid
...roduction
...eased gamma globulin, indicating
...myelinating disease or Guillain-
...arré syndrome
Increased glucose, indicating hyperglycemia
• Decreased glucose, indicating hypoglycemia, infection, or meningitis
• Increased cell count, suggesting meningitis, tumor, abscess, demyelinating
disease
• RBCs, indicating hemorrhage
• Positive VDRL test result, indicating
neurosyphilis
• Decreased chloride, indicating
infected meninges
• Gram-positive or gram-negative
organisms, indicating bacterial
meningitis

Nursing Implications
• Report abnormal findings to the
health care provider.
• Prepare to educate the patient about
the diagnosis.
• Administer antibiotics, as indicated.
• Prepare the patient for further testing
or surgery, as indicated.
• Institute isolation precautions, as
indicated.

Purpose
• To measure CSF pressure
• To aid in the diagnoses of viral or
bacterial meningitis, subarachnoid
or intracranial hemorrhage, tumors
and brain abscesses, neurosyphilis,
and chronic central nervous system
(CNS) infections

Description
The lumbar puncture, also known as
a *spinal tap*, permits CSF sampling for
qualitative analysis and is more common
than a cisternal or ventricular puncture.
    The procedure for lumbar puncture
is as follows:

• The patient is positioned on the
side at the edge of the bed with the
knees drawn up to the abdomen and
chin tucked against chest (the fetal
position) or sitting while leaning over
a bedside table. When the patient
is positioned supine, pillows are
provided to support the spine on a
horizontal plane.
• The skin site is prepared and draped
and a local anesthetic is injected.
• The spinal needle is inserted in
the midline between the spinous
processes of the vertebrae (usually
between the third and fourth or the
fourth and fifth lumbar vertebrae).
• The stylet is removed from the
needle. If the stylet is properly
positioned, CSF will drip out of the
needle. A stopcock and manometer
are attached to the needle to measure
the initial (opening) CSF pressure.
• Specimens are collected and placed in
the appropriate containers.

▶ **Quality and Safety Nursing Alert**

During the procedure, the patient
is observed closely for signs of an
adverse reaction (elevated pulse
rate, pallor, or clammy skin). In a patient with increased ICP, CSF should
be removed with extreme caution
because cerebellar herniation and
medullary compression can result.

• The needle is removed and a small
sterile dressing applied.

Precautions
• Lumbar puncture is contraindicated
in patients with skin infection at the
puncture site.
• In cases of increased ICP, anatomic
changes, or previous spinal surgery,
weigh risks of lumbar puncture
against the benefits.
• In the case of a "bloody tap" (blood in
the CSF), remove the needle, apply
pressure, and begin again.

Nursing Considerations
Before the Test
• Confirm the patient's identity using
two patient identifiers and confirmation

of the patient's identification bracelet according to facility policy.

- Explain to the patient the purpose of the test, how it's done, and who will perform the procedure and when and where.
- Advise the patient that the test takes at least 15 minutes and that there are no food or fluid restrictions for this test.
- Note and report all allergies.
- Explain to the patient that headache is the most common adverse effect.
- Make sure the patient has signed a consent form.

After the Test

- Keep the patient lying flat for 4 to 6 hours. Inform the patient that he or she can turn from side to side, but that remaining prone will help avoid postprocedure headache.
- Encourage the patient to drink fluids and assist as needed.
- Administer analgesics, as ordered.
- Monitor the patient's vital signs, neurologic status, and intake and output.
- Monitor the puncture site for redness, swelling, and drainage.

Lung Biopsy

Normal Findings

- Uniform texture of the alveolar ducts, alveolar walls, bronchioles, and small vessels

Abnormal Findings

- Squamous cell or oat cell carcinoma and adenocarcinoma
- Parenchymal pulmonary disease

Nursing Implications

- Report abnormal findings to the health care provider.
- Prepare to educate the patient about his diagnosis.
- Prepare the patient for further testing or surgery, as indicated.
- Make sure a chest X-ray is repeated as soon as the biopsy has been completed.

Purpose

- To confirm a diagnosis of diffuse parenchymal pulmonary disease and pulmonary lesions

Description

In lung biopsy, a pulmonary tissue specimen is excised by closed or open technique for histologic examination. Transbronchial biopsy, the removal of multiple tissue specimens through a fiberoptic bronchoscope, may be used in patients with diffuse infiltrative pulmonary disease or tumors, or when severe debilitation contraindicates open biopsy. Open biopsy is appropriate for the study of a well-circumscribed lesion that may require resection.

Generally, a lung biopsy is recommended after chest X-rays, computed tomographic (CT) scan, and bronchoscopy have failed to identify the cause of diffuse parenchymal pulmonary disease or a pulmonary lesion. Complications of lung biopsy include bleeding, infection, and pneumothorax.

The procedure for lung biopsy is as follows:

- After the biopsy site is selected, lead markers are placed on the patient's skin and X-rays are ordered to verify their correct placement.
- The patient is positioned sitting, with arms folded on a table in front of him or her. Instruct the patient to maintain this position, remaining as still as possible, and to refrain from coughing.
- The skin is prepared over the biopsy site and the appropriate area is draped.
- A local anesthetic is injected just above the rib, below the selected site, to prevent damage to the intercostal nerves and vessels.
- Using a 22G needle, the physician anesthetizes the intercostal muscles and parietal pleura, makes a small incision (2–3 mm) with a scalpel, and introduces the biopsy needle through the incision, chest wall, and pleura into the tumor or pulmonary tissue.

L

- If the intercostal space at the incision site is wide, the needle is inserted at a 90-degree angle; if the ribs overlap and the intercostal space is narrow, the needle is inserted at a 45-degree angle. When the needle is in the tumor or pulmonary tissue, the specimen is obtained and the needle is withdrawn.
- The specimen is divided immediately: The tissue for histology is placed in a properly labeled bottle containing 10% neutral buffered formalin solution; the tissue for microbiology is placed in a sterile container.
- Immediately following the procedure, pressure is applied to the biopsy site to stop bleeding and a small bandage is applied.

Interfering Factors
- Inability to obtain a representative tissue specimen

Precautions
- Needle biopsy is contraindicated in the patient with a lesion that's separated from the chest wall or accompanied by emphysematous bullae, cysts, or gross emphysema and in the patient with coagulopathy, hypoxia, pulmonary hypertension, or cardiac disease with cor pulmonale.
- During biopsy, observe for signs of respiratory distress—shortness of breath, elevated pulse rate, change in mentation, increasing restlessness, and cyanosis (late sign). If such signs develop, report them immediately.
- Because coughing and movement during biopsy can cause lung tearing by the biopsy needle, keep the patient calm and still.

Nursing Considerations
Before the Test
- Confirm the patient's identity using two patient identifiers and confirmation of the patient's identification bracelet according to facility policy.

- Explain to the patient that the lung biopsy is used to confirm or rule out a diagnostic finding in the lung.
- Describe the procedure to the patient and answer any questions. Inform the patient who will perform the biopsy and when and where it will be done.
- Advise the patient that a chest X-ray and blood studies (prothrombin time, partial thromboplastin time, and platelet count) will be performed before the biopsy.
- Instruct the patient to fast after midnight before the procedure. (Sometimes the patient is permitted to have clear liquids the morning of the test.)
- Check the patient's history for hypersensitivity to the local anesthetic.
- Administer a mild sedative, as ordered, 30 minutes before the biopsy to help the patient relax. Tell the patient that a local anesthetic will be administered, but that a sharp, transient pain may be experienced when the biopsy needle touches the lung.
- Reinforce that the patient needs to hold still during the procedure because any movement or coughing can result in laceration of lung tissue by the biopsy needle.
- Make sure the patient or a responsible family member has signed an informed consent form.

After the Test
- Check the patient's vital signs every 15 minutes for 1 hour, every 30 minutes for 2 hours, every hour for 4 hours, and then every 4 hours until the patient is stable or until discharge. Watch for bleeding, dyspnea, elevated pulse rate, diminished breath sounds on the biopsy side, and, eventually, cyanosis. Complications include pneumothorax and bleeding.
- Instruct the patient to resume a usual diet, as ordered.

Lung Perfusion and Ventilation Scan

Normal Findings
- *Lung perfusion scan:* Uniform uptake pattern of the radioactive substance
- *Lung ventilation scan:* Gas distribution in both lungs and normal wash-in and wash-out phases

Abnormal Findings
- Low radioactive uptake, suggesting embolism
- Decreased regional blood flow, indicating pneumonitis
- Unequal gas distribution in the lungs

Nursing Implications
- Report abnormal findings to the health care provider.
- Prepare to educate the patient about the diagnosis.
- Prepare the patient for further testing or surgery, as indicated.

Purpose
- To assess arterial perfusion of the lungs
- To detect pulmonary emboli
- To evaluate pulmonary function before lung resection
- To identify areas of the lung capable of ventilation, evaluate regional respiratory function, and locate regional hypoventilation, which may indicate atelectasis, obstructing tumors, or chronic obstructive pulmonary disease (COPD) (ventilation scan)

Description
Sometimes called a V/Q scan, a lung perfusion scan produces an image of pulmonary blood flow after IV injection of a radiopharmaceutical, either human serum albumin microspheres or macro aggregated albumin bonded to technetium.

The lung ventilation scan is performed after the patient inhales a mixture of air and radioactive gas that delineates areas of the lung ventilated during respiration. The scan records gas distribution during three phase... active gas (wash-in p... rebreathing when rad... a steady level (equilibri... after removal of the radioac... the lungs (wash-out phase). T... are performed to determine if t... ventilatory problem or vascular... mality causing the decreased lung ca... ity and oxygenation.

The procedures for lung perfusion and lung ventilation scans are as follows:

Lung Perfusion Scan
- With the patient supine and taking moderately deep breaths, the radiopharmaceutical is injected IV slowly over 5 to 10 seconds to allow more even distribution of pulmonary blood flow.
- After the injection, the gamma camera takes a series of single stationary images in the anterior, posterior, oblique, and both lateral chest views.
- Images, which are projected on an oscilloscope screen, show the distribution of radioactive particles.

Lung Ventilation Scan
- After the patient inhales air mixed with a small amount of radioactive gas through a mask, its distribution in the lungs is monitored on a nuclear scanner.
- The patient's chest is scanned as he or she exhales.

Interfering Factors
- Scheduling more than one radionuclide test per day, especially if using different tracing substances (may hinder diffusion of tracer isotope in a second test)
- Administering all the radiopharmaceutical while the patient is sitting (possible poor imaging resulting from settling of tracer isotope in lung bases)
- Conditions such as COPD, vasculitis, pulmonary edema, tumor, sickle cell disease, sarcoidosis, and parasitic disease (possible poor imaging)

L

...welry and other
... the scanning field
...aging)

...s
...usion scanning is con-
...ated in the patient who's
...sensitive to the radiopharma-
...tical.
...ith a ventilation scan, watch for
radioactive gas leaks, such as through
the mask, which can contaminate the
surrounding atmosphere.

Nursing Considerations

Before the Test

- Confirm the patient's identity using
  two patient identifiers and confirmation of the patient's identification
  bracelet according to facility policy.
- Explain to the patient that the lung
  perfusion and ventilation scan helps
  evaluate respiratory function.
- Describe the test to the patient,
  including who will perform it and
  when and where it will take place.
- Advise the patient that there are no
  food or fluid restrictions for this test.
- On the test request, note if the
  patient has COPD, vasculitis, pulmonary edema, tumor, sickle cell disease,
  or parasitic disease, which may affect
  test results.
- Ensure that the patient or a responsible family member has signed an
  informed consent form.

Lung Perfusion Scan

- Advise the patient that a radiopharmaceutical will be injected into an
  arm vein and that the patient will
  be seated in front of a camera or lie
  under it. Explain that neither the
  camera nor the uptake probe emits
  radiation and that the amount of
  radioactivity in the radiopharmaceutical is minimal.
- Assure the patient that he or she
  will be comfortable during the test
  and that there is no need to remain
  perfectly still.

Lung Ventilation Scan

- Ask the patient to remove all jewelry
  and metal objects from the scanning
  field.
- Explain to the patient that he or she
  will be asked to hold the breath for
  a short time after inhaling a gas and
  to remain still while a machine scans
  the chest.
- Reassure the patient that a minimal
  amount of radioactive gas is used.

After the Test

- If a hematoma develops at the injection site from the perfusion scan,
  apply pressure.

Lupus Erythematosus Cell Preparation

Reference Values

Absence of lupus erythematosus (LE)
cells

Abnormal Findings

- Presence of at least two LE cells,
  indicating systemic lupus erythematosus (SLE) or possible active hepatitis,
  rheumatoid arthritis, or scleroderma

Nursing Implications

- Report abnormal findings to the
  health care provider.
- Prepare to educate the patient about
  the diagnosis.
- Prepare the patient for further testing
  or surgery, as indicated.

Purpose

- To help diagnose SLE
- To monitor SLE treatment (About
  60% of successfully treated patients
  fail to show LE cells after 4 to 6 weeks
  of therapy.)

Description

LE cell preparation is an in vitro procedure
used in diagnosing SLE. Although this test
is less sensitive and reliable than either the
antinuclear antibody (ANA) or the anti-
deoxyribonucleic acid (DNA) antibody
test, it's commonly used because it requires
minimal equipment and reagents.

In this test, a blood sample is mixed with laboratory-treated nucleoprotein (the antigen). If the sample contains ANAs, they react with the nucleoprotein, causing swelling and rupture. Phagocytes from the serum then engulf the extruded nuclei, forming LE cells, which are then detected by microscopic examination of the sample.

Interfering Factors
- Hydralazine, isoniazid, and procainamide (may produce a syndrome resembling SLE)
- Chlorpromazine (Thorazine), ethosuximide (Zarontin), gold salts, hormonal contraceptives, methyldopa (Aldomet), penicillin, phenytoin (Dilantin), primidone (Mysoline), propylthiouracil, quinidine, streptomycin, sulfonamides, and tetracyclines

Precautions
- Handle the sample gently to prevent hemolysis.

Nursing Considerations

Before the Test
- Confirm the patient's identity using two patient identifiers and confirmation of the patient's identification bracelet according to facility policy.
- Explain to the patient that the LE cell preparation test helps detect antibodies to one's own tissue.
- If appropriate, inform the patient that the test will be repeated to monitor response to therapy.
- Inform the patient that there are no food or fluid restrictions for this test.
- Advise the patient that the test requires a blood sample. Explain that slight discomfort from the tourniquet and needle puncture may be experienced.
- Check the patient's medication history for drugs that may affect test results, such as isoniazid, hydralazine, and procainamide. If such drugs must be continued, note this information on the laboratory request.

During the Test
- Perform a venipuncture and collect the sample in a 7-mL red-topped tube.

After the Test
- Because the patient with SLE may have a compromised immune system, keep a clean, dry bandage over the venipuncture site for at least 24 hours and check for infection.
- Apply direct pressure to the venipuncture site until bleeding stops and to prevent hematoma formation.
- If test results indicate SLE, advise the patient that further tests may be required to monitor treatment.

Lyme Disease Serology

Reference Values
Nonreactive normal serum values

Abnormal Findings
- Positive result (not definitive)
- High rheumatoid factor titers, indicating other treponemal diseases (false positive)

Nursing Implications
- Report abnormal findings to the health care provider.
- Prepare to educate the patient about the diagnosis.
- Prepare the patient for further testing, as indicated.

Purpose
- To confirm diagnosis of Lyme disease

Description
Epidemiologic and serologic studies implicate a common tick-borne spirochete, *Borrelia burgdorferi*, as the causative agent. Serologic tests for Lyme disease, both indirect immunofluorescent and enzyme-linked immunosorbent assays, measure antibody response to this spirochete and indicate current infection or past exposure. Serologic tests can identify 50% of patients with early-stage Lyme disease and all patients with later complications of carditis, neuritis, and arthritis or patients in remission.

In an indirect immunofluorescent assay, *B. burgdorferi* is grown in culture, fixed to a microscope slide, and then incubated with a human serum sample. A fluorescein-labeled antiglobulin is then introduced into the antigen–antibody complex. Any human antibody that binds to the spirochete is detected by viewing (under an ultraviolet microscope) the fluorescent antiglobulin that attaches to it.

Interfering Factors

- High serum lipid levels (possible inaccurate results, requiring a repeat test after a period of restricted fat intake)
- Samples contaminated with other bacteria (possible false positive)
- Measurement too early in disease
- Antibiotic treatment
- Failure to develop antibodies (occurs in more than 15% of patients with Lyme disease)

Precautions

- Handle the specimen carefully to prevent hemolysis.

Nursing Considerations

Before the Test

- Confirm the patient's identity using two patient identifiers and confirmation of the patient's identification bracelet according to facility policy.
- Explain to the patient that the Lyme disease serology test helps determine whether symptoms are caused by Lyme disease.
- Instruct the patient to fast for 12 hours before the sample is drawn, but to drink fluids as usual.
- Advise the patient that the test requires a blood sample. Explain that slight discomfort from the tourniquet and needle puncture may be experienced.

During the Test

- Perform a venipuncture and collect the sample in a 7-mL clot activator tube.
- Send the specimen to the laboratory immediately.

After the Test

- Apply direct pressure to the venipuncture site until bleeding stops and to prevent hematoma formation.
- Instruct the patient to resume a usual diet, as ordered.

Lymph Node Biopsy

Normal Findings

- Lymph node encapsulated by collagenous connective tissue and divided into smaller lobes by tissue strands (trabeculae)
- Outer cortex composed of lymphoid cells and nodules or follicles containing lymphocytes
- Inner medulla composed of reticular phagocytic cells that collect and drain fluid

Abnormal Findings

- Lymphatic cancer
- Sarcoidosis
- Fungal disease
- Tuberculosis
- Hodgkin's disease

Nursing Implications

- Report abnormal findings to the health care provider.
- Prepare to educate the patient about the diagnosis.
- Prepare the patient for further testing or surgery, as indicated.

Purpose

- To determine the cause of lymph node enlargement
- To distinguish between benign and malignant lymph node processes
- To stage metastatic cancer

Description

Lymph node biopsy is the surgical excision of an active lymph node or the needle aspiration of a nodal specimen for histologic examination. Both techniques usually use a local anesthetic and sample the superficial nodes in the cervical, supraclavicular, axillary, or inguinal region. Excision is preferred because it yields a larger specimen.

Although lymph nodes swell during infection, biopsy is indicated when nodal enlargement is prolonged and accompanied by backache, leg edema, breathing and swallowing difficulties, and, later, weight loss, weakness, severe itching, fever, night sweats, cough, hemoptysis, and hoarseness. Generalized or localized lymph node enlargement is typical of such diseases as chronic lymphatic leukemia, Hodgkin's disease, infectious mononucleosis, and rheumatoid arthritis.

Complete blood count, liver function studies, liver and spleen scans, and X-rays should precede this test.

The procedure for lymph node biopsy is as follows:

Excisional Biopsy

- After the skin over the biopsy site is prepared and draped, the local anesthetic is administered.
- The physician makes an incision, removes an entire node, and places it in a properly labeled bottle containing normal saline solution.
- The wound is sutured and a sterile dressing is applied.

Needle Biopsy

- After preparing the biopsy site and administering a local anesthetic, the physician grasps the node with thumb and forefinger, inserts the needle directly into the node, and obtains a small core specimen.
- The needle is removed, and the specimen is placed in a properly labeled bottle containing normal saline solution.
- Pressure is exerted at the biopsy site to control bleeding, and an adhesive bandage is applied.

Interfering Factors

- Inability to obtain a representative tissue specimen
- Inability to differentiate nodal disorder

Precautions

- Storing the tissue specime_ normal saline solution inst_ formalin solution allows par_ specimen to be used for cytolo_ impression smears, which are st_ along with the biopsy specimen.

Nursing Considerations

Before the Test

- Confirm the patient's identity using two patient identifiers and confirmation of the patient's identification bracelet according to facility policy.
- Explain to the patient that the lymph node biopsy allows microscopic study of lymph node tissue.
- Describe the procedure to the patient, answer any questions, and inform the patient when and where the procedure will be done.
- For excisional biopsy, instruct the patient to restrict food after midnight and to drink only clear liquids on the morning of the test. (If general anesthesia is needed for deeper nodes, the patient also must restrict fluids.)
- For needle biopsy, inform the patient that there are no food or fluid restrictions for this test.
- If the patient is to receive a local anesthetic, explain that slight discomfort may be experienced during the injection. Check the patient's history for hypersensitivity to the anesthetic.
- Record the patient's baseline vital signs just before the biopsy.
- Make sure the patient or a responsible family member has signed an informed consent form.

After the Test

- Check the patient's vital signs and watch for bleeding, tenderness, and redness at the biopsy site.
- Instruct the patient to resume a usual diet, as ordered.

L

Magnesium, Serum

Reference Values

Adults: 1.8 to 2.6 mg/dL (SI, 0.74–1.07 mmol/L)

Children: 1.7 to 2.1 mg/dL (SI, 0.70–0.86 mmol/L)

Newborns: 1.5 to 2.2 mg/dL (SI, 0.62–0.91 mmol/L)

Abnormal Findings

Elevated Levels

- Renal failure
- Magnesium administration or ingestion
- Adrenocortical insufficiency (Addison's disease)
- Diabetic acidosis
- Hypercalcemia
- Chronic pancreatitis
- Pregnancy
- Excessive loss of body fluids

Decreased Levels

- Chronic alcoholism
- Malabsorption syndrome
- Diarrhea
- Faulty absorption after bowel resection
- Prolonged bowel or gastric aspiration
- Acute pancreatitis
- Primary aldosteronism
- Severe burns
- Hypercalcemic conditions (including hyperparathyroidism)
- Malnutrition
- Certain diuretic therapy

Nursing Implications

- Observe the patient with elevated levels for lethargy; flushing; diaphoresis; decreased blood pressure; slow, weak pulse; muscle weakness; diminished deep tendon reflexes; and slow, shallow respiration.
- Report electrocardiogram (ECG) changes (such as prolonged PR interval, wide QRS complex, elevated T waves, atrioventricular block, premature ventricular contractions [PVCs]) in patients with elevated levels.
- In patients with decreased levels, watch for leg and foot cramps, hyperactive deep tendon reflexes, arrhythmias, muscle weakness, seizures, twitching, tetany, tremors, and ECG changes (PVCs and ventricular fibrillation). In cases of refractive ventricular tachycardia, consider torsade de pointe and administer magnesium, as ordered.

Purpose

- To evaluate electrolyte status
- To assess neuromuscular and renal function
- To assess therapeutics levels with magnesium drip

Description

The magnesium test measures serum levels of magnesium, an electrolyte that's vital to neuromuscular function, helps in intracellular metabolism, activates many essential enzymes, and affects nucleic acid and protein metabolism. Magnesium also helps transport sodium and potassium across cell membranes and influences intracellular calcium levels. Most magnesium is found in bone and intracellular fluid; a small amount is found in extracellular fluid. Magnesium is absorbed by the small intestine and excreted in urine and stools.

Interfering Factors

- Venous stasis caused by tourniquet use
- Obtaining a sample above an IV site that's receiving a solution containing magnesium
- Excessive antacid or cathartic use or excessive magnesium sulfate infusion (increase)
- Prolonged IV infusions without magnesium; excessive diuretic use (decrease)
- IV administration of calcium gluconate (possible false-low finding if measured using the Titan yellow method)
- Lithium (increase)
- Alcohol, aminoglycosides, amphotericin B, calcium salts, cardiac glycosides, cisplatin (Platinol-AQ), and loop and thiazide diuretics (decrease)

Precautions

- Handle the sample gently to prevent hemolysis.

Nursing Considerations

Before the Test

- Confirm the patient's identity using two patient identifiers and confirmation of the patient's identification bracelet according to facility policy.
- Explain to the patient that the serum magnesium test is used to determine the magnesium content of the blood.
- Instruct the patient not to use magnesium salts (such as milk of magnesia or Epsom salt) for at least 3 days before the test, but explain that the patient doesn't need to restrict food and fluids.
- Advise the patient that the test requires a blood sample. Explain that slight discomfort from the tourniquet and needle puncture may be experienced.

During the Test

- Perform a venipuncture without a tourniquet, if possible, and collect the sample in a 3- or 4-mL clot activator tube.

After the Test

- Apply pressure to the venipuncture site until bleeding stops and to prevent hematoma formation.

Magnetic Resonance Imaging

Normal Findings

- See the MRI Findings table.

Abnormal Findings

- See the MRI Findings table.

Nursing Implications

- Report abnormal findings to the health care provider.
- Anticipate the need for additional testing.
- Prepare to educate the patient about the diagnosis.
- Prepare the patient for follow-up and treatment, as indicated.
- Provide emotional support to the patient and family.

Purpose

- See the MRI Findings table.

Description

Magnetic resonance imaging (MRI) has the ability to "see through" bone and to delineate fluid-filled soft tissue in great detail and produce images of organs and vessels in motion. In this noninvasive procedure, the patient is placed in a magnetic field into which a radiofrequency beam is introduced. Resulting energy changes are measured and used by the MRI computer to generate images on a monitor. Cross-sectional images of the anatomy are viewed in multiple planes and recorded for the permanent record.

Because the magnetic fields and radiofrequency waves used are imperceptible by the patient, no harmful effects have been documented. Research continues on the optimal magnetic fields and radiofrequency waves for various tissue types. (See the New Methods of Monitoring Cerebral Function and the Intracranial MRI Techniques boxes.)

M

MRI Findings

This table outlines normal and abnormal findings for various types of magnetic resonance imaging (MRI).

Area	Test Purpose	Normal Findings	Abnormal Findings
Cardiac	• Evaluate cardiac wall motion • Visualize cardiac structures, valves, and coronary arteries	• No anatomic or structural dysfunctions in cardiac tissue	• Cardiomyopathy and pericardial disease • Atrial or ventricular septal defects or other congenital defects • Paracardiac or intracardiac masses • Pericardial or vascular disease
Intracranial	• Help diagnose intracranial and spinal lesions and soft-tissue abnormalities	• Normal anatomic details of the central nervous system • Distinct and sharply defined brain and spinal cord structures • Varying tissue color and shading, depending on the radiofrequency energy, magnetic strength, and degree of computer enhancement	• Cloudy, gray, or dark areas, indicating cerebral edema • Changes in normal anatomy, indicating pontine and cerebellar tumors • Curdlike, gray, or gray-white areas of demyelination, indicating multiple sclerosis
Skeletal	• Evaluate bony and soft-tissue tumors • Identify changes in bone marrow composition • Identify spinal disorders	• No disease in bones, muscles, or joints	• Diseases of the spinal canal and cord • Primary and metastatic bone tumors
Urinary	• Evaluate genitourinary tract tumors and abdominal or pelvic masses • Detect prostate stones and cysts • Detect cancer invasion into seminal vesicles and pelvic lymph nodes	• Expected blood vessel size and anatomy	• Tumors, abscess, malformations • Strictures • Stenosis • Thrombosis • Inflammation • Edema, fluid collection • Bleeding, hemorrhage • Organ atrophy

New Methods of Monitoring Cerebral Function

Optical Imaging

Optical imaging uses fiberoptic light and a camera to produce visual images of the brain as it responds to stimulation. This technique produces higher resolution pictures of the brain than magnetic resonance imaging (MRI) or positron emission tomography scans. Researchers believe optical imaging may be valuable during neurosurgery to minimize damage to crucial areas of the brain that control speech, movement, and other activities. Because the procedure scans only the brain's surface, it's meant to be used in combination with other diagnostic techniques.

Fast MRI

Fast MRI produces pictures less than a second apart. These images display blood flow through the brain and the changes that occur in blood flow when the patient performs different tasks. Neuroscientists believe that active areas of the brain must consume more oxygen and that areas of the brain that are currently working become laden with oxygen. Fast MRI can distinguish between oxygen-laden and oxygen-depleted blood. Thus, this test may be used to help identify which areas of the normal brain are involved in certain activities and emotions. Possible applications for fast MRI include guiding neurosurgeons during surgery and helping researchers better understand epilepsy, brain tumors, and even psychiatric illnesses.

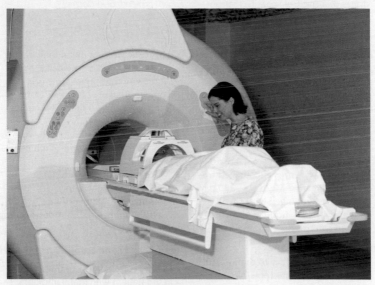

M

Photo from Timby, B. K. *Introductory Medical-Surgical Nursing*, 10th ed. Philadelphia: Lippincott Williams & Wilkins, 2010, Figure 36-8, page 512.

The procedure for MRI is as follows:
- If indicated, an IV line is started to administer a contrast medium before the procedure begins.
- The patient is placed in a supine position on a narrow, padded, non-

metallic bed that slides to the desired position inside the scanner.
- The patient is asked to remain still.
- Radiofrequency energy is directed at the area being tested. The radiologist may vary the waves and use the

Intracranial MRI Techniques

Magnetic resonance imaging (MRI) can be used to provide clear images of parts of the brain, such as the brainstem and cerebellum, that are difficult to image by other methods. These four MRI techniques are used to visualize other aspects of the brain.

Magnetic Resonance Angiography

Magnetic resonance angiography allows the visualization of blood flowing through the cerebral vessels. Images of blood vessels done with magnetic resonance angiography aren't as clear as those obtained by angiography, but this technique is less invasive.

Magnetic Resonance Spectroscopy

Magnetic resonance spectroscopy creates images over time that show the metabo-

lism of certain chemical markers in a specific area of the brain. Some researchers have dubbed this test a "metabolic biopsy" because it reveals pathologic neurochemistry over time.

Diffusion-Perfusion Imaging

Diffusion-perfusion imaging uses a stronger-than-normal magnetic gradient to reveal areas of focal cerebral ischemia within minutes. Currently used in stroke research, this MRI technique may be used by diagnosticians to distinguish permanent from reversible ischemia.

Neurography

Neurograms provide a three-dimensional image of nerves. They may be used to find the exact location of nerves that are damaged, crimped, or in disarray.

computer to manipulate and enhance the images.
- The resulting images are displayed on a monitor and recorded on film or magnetic tape for permanent storage.
- Advise the patient to keep the eyes closed to promote relaxation and prevent a closed-in feeling.
- If nausea occurs because of claustrophobia, the patient is encouraged to take deep breaths.
- If the test is prolonged with the patient lying flat, monitor for orthostatic hypotension.

Interfering Factors
- The patient's inability to remain still during the procedure (possible poor imaging)
- The patient's inability to fit into the scanner

Precautions
- The claustrophobic patient may experience anxiety.
- Because MRI works through a powerful magnetic field, it can't be performed on the patient with a pacemaker, an intracranial aneurysm

clip, other ferrous metal implants, or gunshot wounds to the head.
- Make sure that no metallic or computer-based equipment (for example, ventilators and IV pumps) enter the MRI area.
- Keep in mind that an anesthesiologist may be needed to monitor a heavily sedated patient.
- Make sure that the technician maintains verbal contact with the conscious patient.
- MRI should be used cautiously during pregnancy.

 Quality and Safety Nursing Alert

Urinary tract MRI is contraindicated in the patient with metal implants, rods, screws, or prosthetic devices. It's also contraindicated during pregnancy unless its benefits greatly outweigh the possible risks to the fetus.

Nursing Considerations
Before the Test
- Confirm the patient's identity using two patient identifiers and confirmation

of the patient's identification bracelet according to facility policy.

- Explain to the patient the purpose of the test, as well as who will perform the test and when and where it will take place.
- Explain that the patient will need to lie flat on a narrow bed, which slides into a large cylinder that houses the MRI magnets. Tell the patient that the scanner will make clicking, whirring, and thumping noises as it moves inside its housing and that the patient may receive earplugs.
- Explain to the patient that MRI is painless and involves no exposure to radiation from the scanner. A radioactive contrast dye may be used, depending on the tissue being studied.
- For MRI of the urinary tract, advise the patient to avoid alcohol, caffeine-containing beverages, and smoking for at least 2 hours and food for at least 1 hour before the test. Explain that the patient can continue taking medications, except for iron, which interferes with the imaging.
- Advise the patient that he or she will have to remain still for the entire procedure.
- Explain that the patient who's claustrophobic or anxious about the test's duration will receive a mild sedative to reduce anxiety or may need to be scanned in an open MRI scanner, which may take longer but is less confining. Explain that the patient will be able to communicate with the technician at all times and that the procedure will be stopped if the patient feels claustrophobic.
- If contrast media will be used, obtain a history of allergies or hypersensitivity to these agents. Mark any sensitivities on the chart and notify the health care provider.
- Instruct the patient to remove all metallic objects, including jewelry, hairpins, and watches.

- Ask if the patient has any implanted metal devices or prostheses, such as vascular clips, shrapnel, pacemakers, joint implants, filters, and intrauterine devices. If so, the test may not be able to be performed.
- Make sure that the patient or a responsible family member has signed an informed consent form.
- Administer the prescribed sedative if ordered.
- At the scanner room door, recheck the patient one last time for metal objects.
- Just before the procedure, have the patient urinate.

During the Test
- Remind the patient to remain still throughout the procedure.
- Assess how the patient responds to the enclosed environment. Provide reassurance if necessary.
- Monitor the cardiac patient for signs of ischemia (chest pressure, shortness of breath, or changes in hemodynamic status).
- If the patient is unstable, make sure an IV line with no metal components is in place and that all equipment is compatible with MRI. If necessary, monitor the patient's oxygen saturation, cardiac rhythm, and respiratory status during the test. An anesthesiologist may be needed to monitor a heavily sedated patient.

After the Test
- Tell the patient to resume usual activities as ordered.

▶ *Quality and Safety Nursing Alert*

If the patient is sedated, monitor hemodynamic, cardiac, respiratory, and mental status until the effects of the sedative have worn off.

- If the test took a long time and the patient was lying flat for an extended period, observe for orthostatic hypotension.

M

- Provide comfort measures and pain medication as needed and ordered because of prolonged positioning in the scanner.
- Monitor the patient for adverse reactions to the contrast medium (flushing, nausea, urticaria, and sneezing).

Mammography

Normal Findings
- Normal duct, glandular tissue, and fat architecture
- No abnormal masses or calcifications

Abnormal Findings
- Benign cysts
- Malignant tumor

Nursing Implications
- Report abnormal findings to the health care provider.
- Prepare to educate the patient about the diagnosis.
- Prepare the patient for further testing or surgery, as indicated.

Purpose
- To screen for malignant breast tumors
- To investigate palpable and impalpable breast masses, breast pain, or nipple discharge
- To help differentiate between benign breast disease and breast cancer
- To monitor the patient with breast cancer who has been treated with breast-conserving surgery and radiation

Description
Mammography is used as a screening test for breast cancer. It helps to detect breast cysts or tumors, especially those not palpable on physical examination. Biopsy of suspicious areas may be required to confirm malignancy. Mammography may follow screening procedures, such as ultrasonography or thermography. (See the *Using Ultrasonography to Detect Breast Cancer* box.)

Although mammography can detect 90% to 95% of breast cancers, this test produces many false-positive results. The American College of Radiologists and the American Cancer Society have established separate guidelines for the use and potential risks of mammography. Both groups agree that despite low radiation levels, the test is contraindicated during pregnancy. Magnetic resonance imaging, which is highly sensitive, is becoming a more popular method of breast imaging; however, it isn't very specific and leads to biopsies of many benign lesions. Mammography may also be done with a new digital imaging scan approved by the U.S. Food and Drug Administration. (See the *Digital Mammography* box.)

For the patient at high risk for breast cancer, a newer test, ductal lavage, may identify abnormal cells before they're large enough to form a tumor.

The mammography procedure is as follows:

- The patient stands and is asked to rest one breast on a table above an X-ray cassette.
- The compression plate is placed on the breast and the patient is told to hold the breath. A radiograph is taken of the craniocaudal view.

Using Ultrasonography to Detect Breast Cancer

Ultrasonography is especially useful for diagnosing tumors less than 0.6 cm in diameter and in distinguishing cysts from solid tumors in dense breast tissue. As in other ultrasound techniques, a transducer sends a beam of high-frequency sound waves through the patient's skin and into the breast. The sound waves are then processed and displayed for interpretation.

A benefit to ultrasonography is that it can show all areas of the breast, including the area close to the chest wall, which is difficult to study with X-rays. When used as an adjunct to mammography, ultrasound increases diagnostic accuracy; when used alone, it's more accurate than mammography in examining the denser breast tissue of a young patient.

Digital Mammography

Digital mammography produces pictures of the breast using X-rays. Instead of film, this process uses detectors that change the X-rays into electrical signals, which are then converted to an image. Digital mammography is used for screening and diagnosis and has been shown to be effective in the detection of breast cancer and other abnormalities. For the patient, the procedure is the same as with ordinary mammography.

Digital mammography may offer the following advantages over conventional mammography:

• The images can be stored and retrieved electronically, which makes long-distance consultations with other mammography specialists easier.
• Because the images can be adjusted by the radiologist, subtle differences between tissues may be noted.
• The number of follow-up procedures that are necessary may be reduced.
• The need for fewer exposures with digital mammography can reduce the already low levels of radiation.

The U.S. Food and Drug Administration has recently approved the Lorad Digital Breast Imager to be used in conjunction with the Lorad M-IV Mammography X-ray System for this digital procedure.

The machine is rotated, the breast is compressed again, and a radiograph of the lateral view is taken.
• The procedure is repeated on the other breast.
• After the films are developed, they're checked to make sure they're readable.

Interfering Factors

• Powders, deodorants, or salves on the breasts and axilla (possible false-positive results)
• Failure to remove jewelry and clothing (possible false-positive results or poor imaging)
• Glandular breasts (common in patients younger than age 30), active lactation, and previous breast surgery (possible poor imaging)
• Breast implants (possible hindrance in detecting masses)

Nursing Considerations

Before the Test
• Confirm the patient's identity using two patient identifiers and confirmation of the patient's identification bracelet according to facility policy.
• Assess the patient's understanding of mammography, answer any questions, and correct any misconceptions.

• Tell the patient who will perform the test and where and when it will take place.
• Instruct the patient to avoid using underarm deodorant or powder on the day of the examination.
• Explain that patients who have breast implants must inform the staff when scheduling the mammogram so that a technologist familiar with imaging implants is on duty.
• Inform the patient that although the test takes only about 15 minutes to perform, the patient may be asked to wait while the films are checked to make sure they're readable. Advise that there's a high rate of false-positive results.
• Just before the test, give the patient a gown to wear that opens in the front and ask the patient to remove all jewelry and clothing above the waist.

Mediastinoscopy

Normal Findings
• Normal tissue without malignancies

Abnormal Findings
• Tissue that's positive for malignancy, such as lung or esophageal cancer or lymphomas

M

Nursing Implications
- Report abnormal findings to the health care provider.
- Prepare to educate the patient about the diagnosis.
- Prepare the patient for further testing or surgery, as indicated.

Purpose
- To diagnose bronchogenic carcinoma, lymphoma (including Hodgkin's disease), and sarcoidosis
- To determine stages of lung cancer

Description
Using an exploring speculum with built-in fiber light and side slit, mediastinoscopy allows direct mediastinal structure viewing and permits palpation and biopsy of paratracheal and carinal lymph nodes. This surgical procedure is indicated when other tests, such as sputum cytology, lung scans, radiography, and bronchoscopic biopsy, fail to confirm the diagnosis.

The procedure for mediastinoscopy is as follows:

- After the endotracheal tube is in place, a small transverse suprasternal incision is made.
- Using finger dissection, the surgeon forms a channel and palpates the lymph nodes.
- The mediastinoscope is inserted and tissue specimens are collected and sent to the laboratory for frozen section examination.
- If analysis confirms malignancy of a resectable tumor, thoracotomy and pneumonectomy may follow immediately.

Precautions
- Scarring of the area from previous mediastinoscopy may interfere with test results and is a contraindication for this procedure.

Nursing Considerations
Before the Test
- Confirm the patient's identity using two patient identifiers and confirmation of the patient's identification bracelet according to facility policy.
- Explain to the patient that mediastinoscopy is used to evaluate the lymph nodes and other structures in the chest. Review the patient's history for previous mediastinoscopy (scarring from a previous procedure contraindicates the test).
- Describe the procedure to the patient and answer any questions.
- Instruct the patient to fast after midnight before the test.
- Inform the patient who will perform the procedure, where it will be done, that a general anesthesia will be administered, and that the procedure takes about 1 hour, followed by a recovery period in the post anesthesia care unit.
- Advise the patient that temporary chest pain, tenderness at the incision site, or a sore throat (from intubation) may be experienced. Assure that complications are rare.
- Make sure that the patient or a responsible family member has signed an informed consent form.
- Check the patient's history for hypersensitivity to the anesthetic and family or patient complications from anesthesia.
- Give a sedative the night before the test and again before the procedure, as ordered.

After the Test
- Send the collected specimens to the laboratory immediately.
- Monitor the patient's postoperative vital signs and check dressings for bleeding and fluid drainage.

> ▶ *Quality and Safety Nursing Alert*
>
> Observe the patient for fever (a sign of mediastinitis); crepitus (a sign of subcutaneous emphysema); dyspnea, cyanosis, and diminished breath sounds on the affected side (signs of pneumothorax); and tachycardia and hypotension (signs of hemorrhage).

- Administer the prescribed analgesic as needed.

Myelography

Normal Findings
- Contrast medium flowing freely through the subarachnoid space
- No obstruction or structural abnormalities

Abnormal Findings
Areas of altered contrast flow, suggesting any of these conditions:
- Herniated intervertebral disks
- Metastatic tumors, tumors in the posterior fossa of the skull, neurofibromas, meningiomas, ependymomas, astrocytomas
- Spinal stenosis or abscess
- Syringomyelia (a congenital abnormality marked by fluid-filled cavities within the spinal cord and widening of the cord itself)
- Arachnoiditis
- Spinal nerve root injury
- Fractures or dislocations
- Osteoporosis
- Deformities in the curvature of the spine
- Bone spurs
- Vertebral degeneration

Nursing Implications
- Report abnormal findings to the health care provider.
- Prepare to educate the patient about the diagnosis.
- Prepare the patient for further testing or surgery, as indicated.

Purpose
- To evaluate and determine the cause of neurologic symptoms (numbness, pain, weakness)
- To identify lesions, such as tumors and herniated intervertebral disks, that partially or totally block the flow of cerebrospinal fluid (CSF) in the subarachnoid space
- To help detect arachnoiditis, spinal nerve root injury, or tumors in the posterior fossa of the skull

Description
Myelography uses fluoroscopy and radiography to evaluate the spinal subarachnoid space after contrast medium injection. Because the contrast medium is heavier than CSF, it flows through the subarachnoid space to the dependent area when the patient, lying prone on a fluoroscopic table, is tilted up or down. The fluoroscope allows the physician to see the contrast medium flow and the subarachnoid space outline. X-rays are taken to provide a permanent record.

Myelography can help locate a spinal lesion, a ruptured disk, spinal stenosis, or an abscess. Sometimes it's performed to confirm the need for surgery; in such cases, a neurosurgeon may stand by. If this test confirms a spinal tumor, the patient may be taken directly to the operating room. Immediate surgery also may be necessary when the contrast medium causes a total block of the subarachnoid space.

The procedure for myelography is as follows:

- The patient is positioned at the edge of the table on the side with the chin on the chest and the knees drawn up to the abdomen. (If the patient has a lumbar deformity or an infection at the puncture site, a cisternal puncture may be done.)
- After the lumbar puncture is performed, the fluoroscope is used to verify proper positioning of the needle in the subarachnoid space. Some CSF may be removed for routine laboratory analysis.
- The patient is turned to the prone position and secured with straps across the upper back, under the arms, and across the ankles. The chin is hyperextended to prevent the contrast medium from flowing into the cranium, and a towel is placed under the chin for comfort.
- If the patient complains of a headache or difficulty swallowing, or reports not breathing deeply enough,

the nurse will provide reassurance and explain that the patient can rest periodically during the procedure.

- Contrast medium is injected and the table tilted so that the dye flows through the subarachnoid space. (In rare circumstances, air is used as a negative contrast medium; however, this is typically reserved for a patient with suspected congenital abnormalities such as syringomyelia.)
- The contrast medium flow is observed by fluoroscope, and X-rays are taken. If an obstruction in the subarachnoid space blocks the upward flow of the contrast medium, a cisternal puncture may be performed.
- The contrast medium is withdrawn, if necessary, after satisfactory X-rays are obtained and the needle is removed.
- The puncture site is cleaned with povidone–iodine solution, and a small adhesive bandage is applied.

Interfering Factors

- Incorrect needle placement
- An uncooperative patient

▶ *Quality and Safety Nursing Alert*

Myelography is generally contraindicated in the patient with increased intracranial pressure, hypersensitivity to iodine or contrast media, or an infection at the puncture site.

Precautions

- Improper positioning after the test may affect recovery.

Nursing Considerations

Before the Test

- Confirm the patient's identity using two patient identifiers and confirmation of the patient's identification bracelet according to facility policy.
- Explain to the patient that myelography reveals obstructions in the spinal cord.
- Tell the patient that food and fluid intake will be restricted for 8 hours

before the test. If the test is scheduled for the afternoon and facility policy permits, the patient may have clear liquids before the test.

- Describe the test, including who will administer it and where it will take place.
- Explain that the patient may feel a transient burning sensation as the contrast medium is injected; a warm, flushed feeling; transient headache; a salty taste; or nausea and vomiting after the dye is injected. Explain that the patient may feel some pain caused by positioning, needle insertion, and, in some cases, removal of the contrast medium.
- Make sure that the patient or a responsible family member has signed an informed consent form.

▶ *Quality and Safety Nursing Alert*

Check the patient's history for hypersensitivity to iodine and iodine-containing substances (for example, shellfish), radiographic contrast media, and associated medications. Notify the radiologist if the patient has a history of epilepsy or phenothiazine use. If metrizamide is to be used as a contrast medium, discontinue phenothiazine 48 hours before the test.

- Instruct the patient to remove all jewelry and other metallic objects in the X-ray field.
- Advise the patient that the head of the bed must be elevated for 6 to 8 hours after the test and that the patient will remain on bed rest for an additional 6 to 8 hours. If an oil-based contrast agent is used, inform the patient that it will be manually removed after the test and that the patient will need to remain flat in bed for 6 to 24 hours.
- Perform pretest procedures and administer prescribed medications. If the puncture is to be performed in

the lumbar region, an enema may be prescribed. A sedative and anticholinergic (such as atropine sulfate) may be prescribed to reduce swallowing during the procedure. Make sure that pretest laboratory work (may include coagulation and kidney function studies) is present in the chart.

After the Test
- Based on the contrast medium used during the test, position the patient as follows: If metrizamide was used, tell the patient to stay in bed for the next 12 to 16 hours. Keep the head of the bed elevated for at least 8 hours. If an oil-based contrast medium was used, tell the patient to remain flat in bed for 24 hours.
- Monitor the patient's vital signs and neurologic status at least every 15 minutes for the first hour, every 30 minutes for the next 2 hours, and then every 4 hours for 24 hours, if not discharged. The patient may be discharged the same day.
- Encourage the patient to drink extra fluids to flush the contrast. The patient should void within 8 hours after returning to the room.
- If no complications or adverse reactions occur, tell the patient to resume a usual diet and activities the day after the test, as ordered.
- Monitor the patient for radicular pain, fever, back pain, or signs of meningeal irritation, such as headache, irritability, or stiff neck. If these signs or symptoms occur, keep the room quiet and dark, and administer an analgesic or antipyretic, as needed.

Myoglobin, Serum

Reference Values
5 to 70 ng/mL (SI, 5–70 mcg/L)

Abnormal Findings
Elevated Levels
- Myocardial infarction (MI)
- Acute alcohol intoxication
- Dermatomyositis
- Hypothermia (with prolonged shivering)
- Muscular dystrophy
- Polymyositis
- Rhabdomyolysis
- Severe burns
- Trauma
- Severe renal failure
- Systemic lupus erythematosus

Nursing Implications
- Report abnormal findings to the health care provider.
- Prepare to educate the patient about the diagnosis.
- Prepare the patient for further testing or surgery, as indicated.

Purpose
- As a nonspecific test, to estimate damage to skeletal or cardiac muscle tissue
- To predict flare-ups of polymyositis
- To determine if an MI has occurred

Description
Myoglobin, which is usually found in skeletal and cardiac muscle, functions as an oxygen-binding muscle protein. It's released into the bloodstream in ischemia, trauma, and muscle inflammation.

Myoglobin release into the bloodstream is especially important when trying to determine if cardiac muscle was damaged. Creatine kinase (CK) and its isoform CK-MB are released more slowly than myoglobin during an MI. Therefore, myoglobin, which can be detected as soon as 2 hours after the onset of chest pain and peaks in 4 hours, can be useful as an early indicator of an MI.

Interfering Factors
- Radioactive scans performed within 1 week of the test
- Recent angina, cardioversion, or improper timing of the test (possible increase)
- IM injection (possible false-positive result)

Precautions
- Handle the sample gently to prevent hemolysis.

Nursing Considerations

Before the Test

- Confirm the patient's identity using two patient identifiers and confirmation of the patient's identification bracelet according to facility policy.
- Explain the purpose of the test to the patient.
- Obtain a patient history, including disorders that may be associated with increased myoglobin levels.
- Advise the patient that the test requires a blood sample. Explain that slight discomfort from the tourniquet and needle puncture may be experienced.
- Inform the patient that the results need to be correlated with other tests for a definitive diagnosis.

During the Test

- Perform a venipuncture and collect the sample in a 4-mL tube with no additives.
- Apply direct pressure to the venipuncture site until bleeding stops.

After the Test

- If a hematoma develops at the venipuncture site, apply direct pressure.
- Expect to collect blood samples 4 to 8 hours after the onset of an acute MI.
- Send the sample to the laboratory immediately.

Myoglobin, Urine

Reference Values

No myoglobin

Abnormal Findings

Elevated Levels

- Acute or chronic muscular disease
- Alcoholic polymyopathy
- Familial myoglobinuria
- Extensive myocardial infarction (MI)
- Severe trauma to the skeletal muscles (crush injury, extreme hyperthermia, or severe burns)
- Strenuous or prolonged exercise (myoglobinuria disappears after rest)

Nursing Implications

- Report abnormal findings to the health care provider.
- Prepare to educate the patient about the diagnosis.
- Prepare the patient for further testing or surgery, as indicated.

Purpose

- To help diagnose rhabdomyolysis
- To detect extensive muscle tissue infarction
- To assess the extent of muscular damage from crushing trauma

Description

The myoglobin test detects the presence of myoglobin, a red pigment found in the cytoplasm of cardiac and skeletal muscle cells, in the urine. When muscle cells are extensively damaged by disease or severe crushing trauma, myoglobin is released into the blood, quickly cleared by renal glomerular filtration, and eliminated in the urine (myoglobinuria). For example, myoglobin appears in the urine within 24 hours after an MI.

Urine myoglobin and urine hemoglobin have marked structural similarities and must be differentiated, usually with the differential precipitation test. With the test, hemoglobin, bound to haptoglobin, precipitates when urine is mixed with ammonium sulfate, but myoglobin remains soluble and can be measured.

Interfering Factors

- Extremely dilute urine (reduces sensitivity)
- Contamination with iodine during surgery (positive results)
- Recent ingestion of large amounts of vitamin C (inhibits reaction if testing is performed with Chemstrip or other reagent strips)

Nursing Considerations

Before the Test

- Confirm the patient's identity using two patient identifiers and confirmation

of the patient's identification bracelet according to facility policy.

- Explain to the patient that the urine myoglobin test detects a red pigment found in muscle cells and helps evaluate muscle injury or disease.

- Inform the patient that there are no food or fluid restrictions for this test.

- Tell the patient that this test requires a random urine specimen and teach the proper collection technique.

During the Test

- Collect a random urine specimen.

After the Test

- Send the specimen to the laboratory immediately after collection.

Nasopharyngeal Culture

Normal Findings
- Nonhemolytic streptococci
- Alpha-hemolytic streptococci
- *Neisseria* species (except *N. meningitidis* and *N. gonorrhoeae*)
- Coagulase-negative staphylococci (such as *Staphylococcus epidermidis* and, occasionally, the coagulase-positive *S. aureus*)

Abnormal Findings
- Group A beta-hemolytic streptococci
- Groups B, C, and G beta-hemolytic streptococci
- *Bordetella pertussis*
- *Corynebacterium diphtheriae*
- *S. aureus*
- Pneumococci
- *Haemophilus influenzae*
- *Myxovirus influenzae*
- Paramyxoviruses
- *Candida albicans*
- *Mycoplasma* species
- *Mycobacterium tuberculosis*

Nursing Implications
- Report abnormal findings to the health care provider.
- Teach the patient about the diagnosis and treatment regimen.
- Prepare to administer antimicrobial therapy as indicated.
- Institute isolation precautions as applicable.

Purpose
- To identify pathogens causing upper respiratory tract symptoms
- To identify proliferation of normal nasopharyngeal flora, which may be pathogenic in debilitated and other immunocompromised patients
- To identify *B. pertussis* and *N. meningitidis*, especially in very young, elderly, or debilitated patients and asymptomatic carriers
- To isolate viruses (rarely), particularly to identify carriers of influenza virus A and B

Description
A nasopharyngeal culture is used to evaluate nasopharyngeal secretions for the presence of pathogenic organisms through direct microscopic examination of a Gram-stained specimen smear. Preliminary organism identification may be used to guide clinical management and determine additional testing needs. Cultured pathogens may then require susceptibility testing to determine appropriate antimicrobial therapy.

Nasopharyngeal cultures typically are useful for identifying *B. pertussis* and *N. meningitidis*, especially in very young, elderly, or debilitated patients. They also can be used to isolate viruses, especially carriers of influenza virus A and B, although the cost and complexity make this use infrequent.

Interfering Factors
- Recent antimicrobial therapy (decrease in bacterial growth)

Precautions
- Use standard precautions when performing the procedure and handling the specimen.
- To prevent specimen contamination, don't let the swab touch the sides of the patient's nostril or the patient's tongue.

Nursing Considerations

Before the Test

• Confirm the patient's identity using two patient identifiers and confirmation of the patient's identification bracelet according to facility policy.

• Ask patient about possible septal deviation.

• Explain to the patient that the nasopharyngeal culture is used to isolate the cause of nasopharyngeal infection.

• Tell the patient who will collect the specimen and that secretions will be obtained from the back of the nose and the throat using a flexible polyester swab.

• Warn the patient that slight discomfort and gagging may be experienced, but reassure that obtaining the specimen takes less than 15 seconds.

> ### Quality and Safety Nursing Alert
>
> **Make sure that resuscitation equipment is nearby. The patient with epiglottitis or diphtheria may experience laryngospasm after the culture is obtained.**

During the Test

• Use standard precautions, including mask, eye protection, and plastic gloves.

• Moisten the swab with sterile water or saline solution.

• Ask the patient to blow the nose before you begin collecting the specimen.

• Position the patient with the head tilted back.

• Using a penlight and a tongue blade, inspect the nasopharyngeal area.

• Gently pass the swab through the nostril and into the nasopharynx, keeping the swab near the septum and floor of the nose. Rotate the swab quickly and remove it.

• Alternatively, place a glass tube in the patient's nostril, and carefully pass the swab through the tube into the nasopharynx. Rotate the swab for 10 seconds and then place it in the culture tube with transport medium. Remove the glass tube.

• If B. pertussis is suspected, use Dacron or calcium alginate mini-tipped swabs for collection. Ideally, specimens for B. pertussis should be inoculated to a fresh culture medium at the patient's bedside because of the organism's susceptibility to environmental changes.

• If the specimen collection's purpose is to isolate a virus, follow the laboratory's recommended collection technique.

After the Test

• Label the specimen with the patient's name, health care provider's name, date and time of collection, origin of the material, and the suspected organism.

• Note if the patient is undergoing antimicrobial therapy or chemotherapy on the laboratory request.

• Keep the container upright.

• Inform the laboratory if the suspected organism is C. diphtheriae or B. pertussis because these need special growth media.

• Refrigerate viral specimens according to your laboratory's procedure.

• Specimens that can't be directly placed onto growth media should have media supplemented with antibiotics to reduce flora growth before transport.

Oral Glucose Tolerance Test

Reference Values

Fasting: 110 mg/dL (SI, 6.1 mmol/L)

30-minute: 110 to 170 mg/dL (SI, 26.1–9.4 mmol/L)

60-minute: less than 184 mg/dL (SI, less than 10.2 mmol/L)

120-minute: less than 138 mg/dL (SI, less than 7.7 mmol/L)

180-minute: 70 to 120 mg/dL (SI, 3.9–6.7 mmol/L)

Fasting levels or lower levels within 2 to 3 hours after OGTT; urine glucose remains negative throughout testing

Abnormal Findings

- Decreased glucose tolerance with levels peaking sharply before falling slowly to fasting levels (diabetes, Cushing disease, hemochromatosis, pheochromocytoma, or central nervous system lesions)
- Increased glucose tolerance with levels peaking at less than normal levels (insulinoma, malabsorption syndrome, adrenocortical insufficiency [Addison's disease], hypothyroidism, or hypopituitarism)

Nursing Implications

- Report abnormal findings to the health care provider.
- Educate the patient and family about the diagnosis.
- Prepare the patient for additional testing, as indicated.

Purpose

- To confirm diabetes in selected patients
- To help diagnose hypoglycemia and malabsorption syndrome

Description

The oral glucose tolerance test (OGTT) is the most sensitive method of evaluating borderline diabetes cases. Plasma and urine glucose levels are monitored for 3 hours after ingestion of a challenge dose of glucose to assess insulin secretion and the body's ability to metabolize glucose.

The OGTT isn't generally used in patients with fasting plasma glucose values greater than 140 mg/dL (SI, greater than 7.7 mmol/L) or postprandial plasma glucose values greater than 200 mg/dL (SI, greater than 11 mmol/L).

Interfering Factors

- Acute illness, such as myocardial infarction, fever, pregnancy, or recent infection (possible increase)
- Carbohydrate deprivation before the test (causing a diabetic response [abnormal increase with a delayed decrease] because the pancreas is unaccustomed to responding to high-carbohydrate load)
- Arginine, benzodiazepines, caffeine, epinephrine, chlorthalidone (Hygroton), corticosteroids, diazoxide (Hyperstat IV), furosemide (Lasix), hormonal contraceptives, recent IV glucose infusions, lithium, large doses of nicotinic acid, phenothiazines, large doses of salicylates, and estrogens
- Smoking

▶ *Quality and Safety Nursing Alert*

Patients age 50 and older experience decreasing carbohydrate tolerance, which causes increasing glucose tolerance to upper limits of about 1 mg/dL for every year after age 50.

Nursing Considerations

Before the Test

- Confirm the patient's identity using two patient identifiers and confirmation of the patient's identification bracelet according to facility policy.
- Explain to the patient that the OGTT is used to evaluate glucose metabolism.
- Instruct the patient to maintain a high-carbohydrate diet for 3 days and then to fast for 12 to 14 hours before the test, as instructed by the physician.
- Instruct the patient not to smoke, drink coffee or alcohol, or exercise strenuously for 8 hours before or during the test.
- Advise the patient that this test requires five blood samples and, usually, five urine specimens. Explain that slight discomfort from the needle punctures and the tourniquet may be experienced.
- Suggest that the patient bring a book or other quiet diversion to the test. The procedure usually takes 3 hours, but can last as long as 6 hours.
- Notify the laboratory and physician of medications the patient is taking that may affect test results; these may need to be restricted.
- Alert the patient to symptoms of hypoglycemia (weakness, restlessness, nervousness, hunger, and sweating), and tell the patient to report such symptoms immediately.

During the Test

- Between 7 AM and 9 AM, perform a venipuncture to obtain a fasting blood sample. Draw this sample into a 7-mL clot activator tube. A saline lock may be inserted and used to collect the multiple blood samples needed, as per facility protocol.
- Collect a urine specimen at the same time if your facility includes this as part of the test.
- After collecting these samples and specimens, administer the oral glucose test load and record the ingestion time. Encourage the patient to drink the entire glucose solution within 5 minutes.
- Draw blood samples 30 minutes, 1 hour, 2 hours, and 3 hours after giving the loading dose using 7-mL clot activator tubes. Collect urine specimens at the same intervals.
- Instruct the patient to lie down if feeling faint from the numerous venipunctures.
- Encourage the patient to drink water throughout the test to promote adequate urine excretion.

▶ **Quality and Safety Nursing Alert**

If the patient develops severe hypoglycemia during the test, notify the health care provider. Draw a blood sample, record the time on the laboratory request, and discontinue the test. Have the patient drink a glass of orange juice with sugar added or administer IV glucose to reverse the reaction.

After the Test

- Apply direct pressure to the venipuncture site until bleeding stops and to prevent hematoma formation.
- Specify on the laboratory slip when the patient last ate and the blood and urine collection times.
- As appropriate, record on the laboratory slip the time the patient received the last pretest dose of insulin or oral antidiabetic drug.
- Send blood samples and urine specimens to the laboratory immediately or refrigerate them.
- Provide a balanced meal or a snack, but observe for a hypoglycemic reaction.
- Instruct the patient to resume usual medications that were discontinued before the test, as ordered.

Oral Lactose Tolerance Test

Reference Values

20 mg/dL (SI, greater than 1.1 mmol/L) over fasting glucose levels within

15 to 60 minutes after ingesting the lactose loading dose is indicative of lactose tolerance.

Abnormal Findings

Elevated Levels

- Lactose tolerance (lactose intolerance is diagnosed when the serum glucose does not rise after ingesting 50–100 g of lactose)
- Crohn's disease

Nursing Implications

- Prepare the patient for a small-bowel biopsy with lactase assay to confirm the diagnosis.
- Report abnormal findings to the health care provider.
- Prepare to educate the patient about the diagnosis.
- Prepare the patient for further testing or surgery, as indicated.
- Provide emotional support to the patient and family.

Purpose

- To detect lactose intolerance

Description

The oral lactose tolerance test is used to measure plasma glucose levels after a challenge lactose dose is ingested. It's used to screen for lactose intolerance resulting from lactase deficiency.

Lactase absence or deficiency causes undigested lactose to remain in the intestinal lumen, producing such symptoms as abdominal cramps and watery diarrhea. True congenital lactase deficiency is rare. Usually, lactose intolerance is acquired because lactase levels generally decrease with age.

Interfering Factors

- Benzodiazepines, hormonal contraceptives, insulin, propranolol, and thiazide diuretics (possible false low)
- Delayed emptying of stomach contents (possible decrease)
- Glycolysis (possible false negative)

Precautions

- Send the blood sample and stool specimen to the laboratory immediately or refrigerate them if transport is delayed.
- Specify the collection time on the laboratory requests.

Nursing Considerations

Before the Test

- Confirm the patient's identity using two patient identifiers and confirmation of the patient's identification bracelet according to facility policy.
- Explain to the patient that the oral lactose tolerance test is used to determine if symptoms are due to an inability to digest lactose.
- Instruct the patient to fast and to avoid strenuous activity for 8 hours before the test.
- Advise the patient that this test requires four blood samples and that the test may take up to 2 hours. Explain that slight discomfort from the needle punctures and the tourniquet may be experienced.
- Notify the laboratory and health care provider of medications the patient is taking that may affect test results; these may need to be restricted.

During the Test

- After the patient has fasted for 8 hours, perform a venipuncture and collect a blood sample in a 4-mL tube with sodium fluoride and potassium oxalate added.
- Administer the lactose test load: for an adult, 50 g of lactose dissolved in 400 mL of water. Record the time of ingestion.

▶ *Quality and Safety Nursing Alert*

For a child, administer 50 g/m² of body surface area.

- Draw a blood sample 30, 60, and 120 minutes after giving the loading dose. Use a 4-mL tube with sodium fluoride and potassium oxalate added.

- If ordered, collect a stool specimen 5 hours after giving the loading dose.
- Watch for lactose intolerance symptoms, such as abdominal cramps, nausea, bloating, flatulence, and watery diarrhea, which may be caused by the loading dose.

After the Test

- Apply direct pressure to the venipuncture site until bleeding stops and to prevent hematoma formation.
- Instruct the patient to resume a usual diet, medications, and activities that were discontinued before the test, as ordered.

Orbital Radiography

Normal Findings

- Orbit composed of a roof, a floor, and medial and lateral walls
- Very thin roof and floor bones (floor may be less than 1 mm thick)
- Slightly thick medial walls (walls parallel to each other), except for ethmoid bone portion
- Thick lateral walls (thickest orbit part) that are strongest at the orbital rim
- Superior orbital fissure (gap at the back of orbit between the lateral wall and roof between the greater and lesser sphenoid bone wings)
- Optic canal (opening in the lesser wing of the sphenoid bone at the orbit apex containing the optic nerve and ophthalmic artery)

Abnormal Findings

- Abnormalities between affected side and the opposite side, indicating orbital fractures or lesions
- Orbital enlargement, suggesting pituitary tumors, benign tumor or cyst, malignant neoplasm, or vascular anomalies
- Optic canal enlargement, indicating retinoblastoma or optic nerve glioma in children
- Decreased orbital size, indicating congenital microphthalmia
- Orbital wall destruction, indicating infection
- Increased bone density, indicating possible osteoblastic metastasis, sphenoid ridge meningioma, or Paget's disease

Nursing Implications

- Report abnormal findings to the health care provider.
- Prepare to educate the patient about the diagnosis.
- Prepare the patient for further testing or surgery, as indicated.
- Provide emotional support to the patient and family.

Purpose

- To help diagnose orbital fractures and conditions
- To help locate intraorbital or intraocular foreign bodies

Description

Orbital radiography evaluates the orbit (the bony cavity that houses the eye and the lacrimal glands), as well as blood vessels, nerves, muscles, and fat. Special radiographic techniques can reveal foreign bodies in the orbit or eye that are invisible to an ophthalmoscope. In some cases, radiography is used in conjunction with computed tomographic scans and ultrasonography to better define an abnormality.

The procedure for orbital radiography is as follows:

- The patient is positioned reclining on the X-ray table or sitting in a chair and instructed to remain still while the X-rays are taken.
- A series of orbital X-rays are taken, including a lateral view, posteroanterior view, submentovertical (base) view, stereo Waters' views (views from both sides), Towne's (half-axial) projection, and optic canal projections. If enlargement of the superior orbital fissure is suspected, apical views are also obtained.
- The films are developed and inspected by the radiography department before the patient is released.

Nursing Considerations

Before the Test

- Confirm the patient's identity using two patient identifiers and confirmation of the patient's identification bracelet according to facility policy.
- Explain that orbital radiography involves taking several X-rays to assess the condition of the bones around the eye.
- Describe the test, including who will perform it, and when and where it will take place.
- Assure the patient that the procedure is usually painless unless the patient has suffered facial trauma, in which case positioning may cause some discomfort. Explain that the patient will be asked to turn the head from side to side and to flex or extend the neck, as instructed.
- Instruct the patient to remove all jewelry and other metallic objects from the X-ray field.

Osmolality, Urine

Reference Values

Random specimen: 50 to 1,400 mOsm/kg
24-hour urine specimen: 300 to 900 mOsm/kg

Abnormal Findings

Elevated Levels

- SIADH
- High-protein diet

Decreased Levels

- Tubular epithelial damage
- Decreased renal blood flow
- Functional nephrons loss
- Pituitary dysfunction
- Cardiac dysfunction
- Diabetes insipidus
- Glomerulonephritis

Nursing Implications

- Report abnormal findings to the health care provider.
- Prepare to educate the patient about the diagnosis.

- Prepare the patient for further testing or surgery, as indicated.
- Provide emotional support to the patient and family.

Purpose

- To evaluate renal tubular function
- To detect renal impairment

Description

The kidneys normally concentrate or dilute urine according to fluid intake. When intake is excessive, the kidneys excrete more water in the urine; when intake is limited, they excrete less. To make such variation possible, the distal segment of the tubule varies its permeability to water in response to antidiuretic hormone, which, with renal blood flow, determines urine concentration or dilution.

The urine osmolality test measures the concentrating ability of the kidneys in acute and chronic kidney disease. Osmolality is a more sensitive index of renal function than are dilution techniques that measure specific gravity. It measures the number of osmotically active ions or particles present per kilogram of water. Osmolality is high in concentrated urine and low in dilute urine. It's determined by the effect of solute particles on the freezing point of the fluid.

Interfering Factors

- Diabetes insipidus
- Diuretics (increase urine volume and dilution, thereby lowering specific gravity)
- Nephrotoxic drugs (cause tubular epithelial damage, thereby decreasing renal concentrating ability)
- Marked overhydration for several days before the test (may cause depressed concentration values)
- Dehydration or electrolyte imbalances (retention of fluids may cause inaccurate results)

Nursing Considerations

Before the Test

- Confirm the patient's identity using two patient identifiers and confirmation of the patient's identification bracelet according to facility policy.

- Explain to the patient that the urine osmolality test evaluates kidney function.
- Advise the patient that the test requires a urine specimen and collection of blood within 1 hour before or after the urine is collected. Withhold diuretics, as ordered.
- Emphasize to the patient that cooperation is necessary to obtain accurate results.
- If the patient can't urinate into the specimen containers, provide a clean bedpan, urinal, or toilet specimen pan. Rinse the collection device after each use.
- If the patient is catheterized, empty the drainage bag before the test. Obtain the specimen from the catheter.

During the Test

- Collect a random urine specimen and draw a blood sample within 1 hour of urine collection.
- If a 24-hour urine collection is ordered, record the total urine volume on the laboratory request. (Preservatives aren't required for a 24-hour container.)

After the Test

- Send each specimen or sample to the laboratory immediately after collection.
- After collecting the final specimen, provide the patient with a balanced meal or snack
- Make sure the patient voids within 8 to 10 hours after the catheter has been removed.

Otoacoustic Emissions Testing

Normal Findings

- 500- to 6,000-Hz otoacoustic emissions with at least 5-dB signal-to-noise ratio

- Emissions sufficiently above the background physiologic and ambient noise (provides evidence of functional outer hair cells in the cochlea, typically associated with normal or near-normal hearing)

Abnormal Findings

- Outer hair cell dysfunction and hearing loss of at least 25 dB hearing loss
- Significant conductive hearing loss

Nursing Implications

- Report abnormal findings to the health care provider.
- Prepare to educate the patient about the diagnosis.
- Prepare the patient for further testing or surgery, as indicated.
- Provide emotional support to the patient and family.

Purpose

- To screen and assess cochlea outer hair cell health
- To screen hearing of neonates

Description

Otoacoustic emissions testing is a rapid screening test that assesses the function of cochlea outer hair cells, which when damaged or lost can cause nonorganic hearing loss. Otoacoustic emissions (echoes normally produced by a healthy inner ear when an external sound is introduced) are absent when more than a slight to mild hearing loss is present. Subtle changes in otoacoustic emissions are sometimes present in normal-hearing carriers of recessive hearing loss genes; otoacoustic emission abnormalities may precede hearing loss.

This screening is commonly conducted on neonates and school-aged children and in certain occupational settings. However, hearing loss that develops after birth, such as from maternal cytomegalovirus infection, and some genetic hearing losses may not be identified with neonatal screening. Moreover, slight (minimal) hearing loss may go undetected.

The procedure for otoacoustic emissions testing is as follows:
- The probe is placed in the patient's ear after it's cleared of debris (vernix or cerumen).
- The audiologist adjusts signal levels and, in the case of distortion product otoacoustic emissions, the frequency characteristics.
- The emission level is monitored and compared with the background noise level.

Interfering Factors
- Screening by inexperienced technicians (possible high false-positive rates)
- Significant conductive hearing loss (possible failure during diagnostic testing)

- Cerumen obstruction
- Undetected auditory dyssynchrony (auditory neuropathy), such as from hyperbilirubinemia or kernicterus

Nursing Considerations

Before the Test
- Confirm the patient's identity using two patient identifiers and confirmation of the patient's identification bracelet according to facility policy.
- Inform the patient that the otoacoustic emissions test takes about 1 minute per ear (if the patient is quiet and has normal hearing) or slightly longer (if findings aren't immediately normal).
- Remove significant cerumen accumulation from the patient's ear canals.

O

Papanicolaou Test (Pap Smear)

Normal Findings
- No malignant cells or other abnormalities

Abnormal Findings
- Malignant cells
- Atypical squamous cells of undetermined significance (ASCUS)
- Low-grade squamous intraepithelial lesions (LSIL)
- High-grade squamous intraepithelial lesions (HSIL)
- Moderate, mild, or severe dysplasia
- Human papillomavirus (HPV)
- Carcinoma in situ (CIS)

Nursing Implications
- Report abnormal findings to the health care provider.
- Prepare to educate the patient about her diagnosis.
- Prepare the patient for further testing or surgery, as indicated.
- Provide emotional support to the patient and her family.

Purpose
- To detect malignant cells
- To detect inflammatory tissue changes
- To assess the patient's response to chemotherapy and radiation therapy
- To detect viral, fungal, and, occasionally, parasitic invasion

Description
The Papanicolaou test (Pap smear) is a widely known cytologic test for early detection of cervical cancer. The test can also be used to detect cancerous cells of the breast, lung, stomach, and renal system. A physician or specially trained nurse scrapes secretions from the patient's cervix and spreads them on a slide, which is sent to the laboratory for cytologic analysis. An alternative method is to use the ThinPrep preservative solution rather than a slide. The ThinPrep was introduced 1996 and allows testing for malignancy and HPV in one step. The test relies on the ready exfoliation of malignant cells from the cervix and shows cell maturity, metabolic activity, and morphology variations.

The American Cancer Society recommends a Pap test every 3 years for women between ages 20 and 40 who aren't in a high-risk category and who have had negative results from three previous Pap tests. Yearly tests (or tests at physician-recommended intervals) are advised for women older than age 40, for those in a high-risk category, and for those who have had a positive test previously. If a Pap test is positive or suggests malignancy, cervical biopsy can confirm the diagnosis. (See the *Testing for Cervical Cancer* box.)

The procedure for collecting a Pap smear is as follows:

- The health care provider puts on gloves and inserts an unlubricated speculum into the vagina. To make insertion easier, the speculum may be moistened with saline solution or warm water.
- After the health care provider locates the cervix, secretions are obtained from the cervix and material from the endocervical canal. The endocervical brush is placed inside the endocervix

Testing for Cervical Cancer

Tests used to detect cervical cancer include the ThinPrep test and the human papillomavirus (HPV) deoxyribonucleic acid (DNA) test.

ThinPrep Test

Cervical cells for ThinPrep test analysis may be collected in the same manner as those of a Papanicolaou (Pap) test, using a cytobrush and plastic spatula. The specimens are deposited in a bottle provided with a fixative and sent to the laboratory. A filter is then inserted into the bottle and excess mucus, blood, and inflammatory cells are filtered out by centrifuge. Remaining cells are then placed on a slide in a uniform, thin layer and read as a Pap test. This procedure causes fewer slides to be classified as unreadable, significantly reducing the incidence of false negatives and the need for repeat tests.

HPV DNA Test

When using the ThinPrep test, screening can also be easily done for HPV, of which certain strains have been identified as the primary cause of cervical cancer. The Digene hybrid capture 2 (hc2) HPV DNA test has been approved by the U.S. Food and Drug Administration to determine if those identified at high risk for developing cervical cancer have been exposed to HPV. The specimen is collected as a Pap smear but is dispersed with ThinPrep solution. Separate aliquots are used for each test, from brushings of the endocervix. The brush is then inserted into the specialized tube, snapped off at the shaft, and capped securely. The target solution in the tube disrupts the virus and releases target DNA, which combines with specific ribonucleic acid (RNA) probes, creating RNA:DNA hybrids. The hybrids are captured, bound, and magnified and measured using a luminometer.

If the patient is found to be positive for HPV, she has been infected with the virus. Depending on the type of HPV found through DNA testing, the patient harboring high-risk HPV strains has a higher risk of developing cervical cancer. It's recommended that the patient undergo colposcopy, in which the cervix is viewed under a microscope and a biopsy is taken from the tissue specimen.

and rolled firmly inside the canal. If using a Pap stick (wooden spatula), it's placed against the cervix with the longest protrusion in the cervical canal, then rotated clockwise 360 degrees while held firmly against the cervix.

- The specimen is then spread on the slide according to laboratory recommendations and the slide is immediately immersed in (or sprayed with) a fixative. If using the ThinPrep method, the brush and spatula are immediately immersed in the preservative solution with a swirling motion.
- Alternatively, posterior vaginal pool secretions and pancervical material may be collected and smeared on a single slide, which must be fixed immediately according to laboratory instructions.
- A bimanual examination may follow after the removal of the speculum.

During the procedure, the health care provider must consider these factors:

- The cervical specimen must be aspirated and scraped from the cervix. A vaginal pool specimen isn't recommended for cervical or endometrial cancer screening.
- The specimen should be thick enough that it isn't transparent.
- Scrapings taken directly from vaginal or vulval lesions are preferred.
- A small pipette may be used, if necessary, to aspirate cells from the squamocolumnar junction and the cervical canal in a patient whose uterus is involuting or atrophying from age.

Interfering Factors

- Douching within 48 hours or having intercourse within 24 hours before the test (can wash away cellular deposits)
- Excessive use of lubricating jelly on the speculum (false negative)
- Specimen collection during menstruation

• Exclusive use of a specimen collected from the vaginal fornix (possible false negative)
• Delay in fixing the specimen (difficult cytologic interpretation due to dehydration of cells)
• Too thin or thick a specimen

Precautions
• Preserve the slides immediately after the specimen is collected.
• Preserve the ThinPrep solution by immediately placing the lid back on the container because exposure to air or light can cause distortion of cells.

Nursing Considerations
Before the Test
• Confirm the patient's identity using two patient identifiers and confirmation of the patient's identification bracelet according to facility policy.
• Explain to the patient that the Pap test allows for the study of cervical cells.
• Stress its importance as an aid for cancer detection at a stage when the disease is commonly producing no symptoms and is still curable.
• Make sure the test isn't scheduled during the patient's menses; the best time is midcycle.
• Instruct the patient to avoid having intercourse for 24 hours, not to douche for 48 hours, and not to insert vaginal medications for 1 week before the test because doing so can wash away cellular deposits and change the vaginal pH.
• Tell the patient who will perform the procedure and where and when it will take place.
• Determine if the patient is on any medications, especially oral contraceptives, and record on the pathology sheet.
• Advise the patient that the test requires that the cervix be scraped and that she may experience slight discomfort but no pain from the speculum (but may feel some pain when the cervix is scraped). Inform her that the procedure takes 5 to 10 minutes or slightly longer if the vagina, pelvic cavity, and rectum are examined bimanually. Advise the patient that she may experience some slight spotting after the exam and that this is normal.
• Obtain an accurate patient history and ask these questions, noting pertinent data on the laboratory request:
  • When did you last have a Pap test?
  • Have you ever had an abnormal Pap test?
  • When was your last menses?
  • Are your menses regular? How many days do they last? Is bleeding heavy or light?
  • Have you taken or are you presently taking hormones or hormonal contraceptives?
  • Do you use an intrauterine device?
  • Do you have any vaginal discharge, pain, or itching?
  • Which, if any, gynecologic disorders have occurred in your family?
  • Have you ever had gynecologic surgery, chemotherapy, or radiation therapy? If so, describe it fully.
• Provide emotional support if the patient is anxious; tell her that test results should be available in a few weeks.
• Ask the patient to empty her bladder before the test is performed.

During the Test
• Instruct the patient to disrobe from the waist down and to drape herself.
• Ask the patient to lie on the examination table and to place her heels in the stirrups. (She may be more comfortable if she keeps her shoes or socks on.) Tell her to slide her buttocks to the edge of the table. Adjust the drape to minimize exposure.

P

- To avoid startling the patient, tell her when the examination will begin. Have her relax her legs and pelvic floor muscles.
- Immediately after the specimen is collected, label it appropriately, including the date, the patient's name, age, the date of her last menses, and the collection site and method.

After the Test

- Help the patient up and ask her to dress when the examination is completed.
- Supply the patient with a sanitary napkin if cervical bleeding occurs.
- Tell the patient when to return for her next Pap test.

Parathyroid Hormone

Reference Values

Parathyroid hormone (PTH): 10 to 50 pg/mL (SI, 1.1–5.3 pmol/L)
N-terminal fraction: 8 to 24 pg/mL (SI, 0.8–2.5 pmol/L)
C-terminal fraction: 0 to 340 pg/mL (SI, 0–35.8 pmol/L)

Abnormal Findings

Elevated Levels

- Primary, secondary, or tertiary hyperparathyroidism
- Calcium malabsorptions
- Chronic kidney disease
- Dietary vitamin D deficiency
- Osteomalacia
- Renal dialysis
- Parathyroid adenoma
- Parathyroid carcinoma
- Parathyroid hyperplasia
- Aging process
- Pregnancy
- Squamous cell carcinoma
- Hypocalcemia
- Malabsorption syndrome
- Rickettsia

Decreased Levels

- Hypoparathyroidism
- Malignant disease (See the *Clinical Implications of Abnormal Parathyroid Secretion* table.)
- Parathyroidectomy
- Vitamin A and D intoxication
- Hypomagnesemia
- Autoimmune disease or cancer
- Graves' disease
- Thiazide diuretics
- Hypercalcemia
- Sarcoidosis
- Milk–alkali syndrome
- DiGeorge's syndrome

Nursing Implications

- Report abnormal findings to the health care provider.
- Prepare to educate the patient about the diagnosis.
- Prepare the patient for further testing or surgery, as indicated.
- Provide emotional support to the patient and family.

Purpose

- To aid the differential diagnosis of parathyroid and hypothyroid disease or disorders
- To monitor patients with chronic kidney disease

Description

PTH, also known as *parathormone,* regulates calcium and phosphorus plasma concentration. Normally, PTH release is regulated by a negative feedback mechanism involving serum calcium. Normal or elevated circulating calcium levels (especially the ionized form) inhibit PTH release; decreased levels stimulate PTH release. The overall effect of PTH is to raise calcium plasma levels and lower phosphorus levels.

The clinical and diagnostic effects of PTH excess or deficiency are directly related to the effects of PTH on bone and the renal tubules and to its interaction with ionized calcium and biologically active vitamin D. Therefore, measuring serum calcium, phosphorus, and creatinine levels with serum PTH is helpful when

Clinical Implications of Abnormal Parathyroid Secretion

Conditions	Causes	Parathyroid Hormone Levels	Ionized Calcium Levels
Primary hyperparathyroidism	• Parathyroid adenoma or carcinoma	High	High to Normal
Secondary hyperparathyroidism	• Chronic kidney disease • Severe vitamin D deficiency • Calcium malabsorption • Pregnancy and lactation	High	Low
Tertiary hyperparathyroidism	• Progressive secondary hyperparathyroidism	High	High to Low
Hypoparathyroidism	• Accidental removal of the parathyroid glands • Autoimmune disease	Low	Low
Malignant tumors	• Squamous cell carcinoma of the lung • Renal, pancreatic, or ovarian carcinoma	High to Normal	High

trying to understand the causes and effects of pathologic parathyroid function. Suppression or stimulation tests may help confirm findings. N-terminal fragments are helpful in identifying acute conditions, whereas C-terminal fragments indicate chronic disturbances of the PTH metabolism.

Interfering Factors

• Failure to fast overnight before the test
• Radioisotope injection within 7 days prior to the test
• Medications that increase PTH: phosphates, anticonvulsants, steroids, isoniazid, lithium, and rifampin
• Medications that decrease PTH: cimetidine, pindolol, and propranolol

Precautions

• Handle the sample gently to prevent hemolysis.
• Send the sample to the laboratory immediately so the serum can be separated and frozen for assay.

Nursing Considerations

Before the Test

• Confirm the patient's identity using two patient identifiers and confirmation of the patient's identification bracelet according to facility policy.
• Explain to the patient that the PTH test helps evaluate parathyroid function.
• Instruct the patient to fast overnight because food may affect PTH levels and interfere with results.
• Advise the patient that the test requires a blood sample. Explain that slight discomfort from the needle puncture and the tourniquet may be experienced.

During the Test

• Sample should be collected at 8 AM because diurnal rhythm affects PTH levels. PTH levels are highest at 2 AM and lowest at 2 PM.
• Perform a venipuncture and collect 3 mL of blood into two separate 7-mL clot activator tubes.

P

- Apply direct pressure to the veni- puncture site until bleeding stops and to prevent hematoma formation.

After the Test
- Tell the patient to resume a usual diet.

Partial Thromboplastin Time (PTT)

Reference Values
21 to 35 seconds (SI, 21–35 seconds)
Therapeutic heparin therapy: 2 to 2.5 times normal limit

Abnormal Findings
Elevated Levels
- Certain plasma clotting factor deficiencies
- Presence of heparin
- Presence of fibrin split products, fibrinolysins, or circulating anticoagu- lants seen in liver cirrhosis, vitamin K deficiency, and disseminated intravas- cular coagulation (DIC)
- Genetic or acquired deficiency of clotting factors
- Hemophilia A

Decreased Levels
- Early stages of DIC
- Extensive cancer

Nursing Implications
- Report abnormal findings to the health care provider.
- Prepare to adjust the patient's antico- agulant therapy, as indicated.

Purpose
- To screen for clotting factor deficien- cies in the intrinsic pathways
- To monitor response to heparin therapy

Description
Also called the *activated partial thrombo- plastin test* (APTT), the partial thrombo- plastin time (PTT) test is used to evaluate all the clotting factors of the intrinsic pathway, except platelets, by measuring the time required for formation of a fibrin clot after calcium and phospholipid emul- sion is added to a plasma sample. An acti- vator, such as kaolin, is used to shorten clotting time.

Interfering Factors
- Anticoagulant therapy
- Antihistamines
- Ascorbic acid
- Chlorpromazine
- Salicylates

Precautions
- To prevent hemolysis, avoid excessive probing at the venipuncture site and handle the sample gently.

Nursing Considerations
Before the Test
- Confirm the patient's identity using two patient identifiers and confirma- tion of the patient's identification bracelet according to facility policy.
- Explain to the patient that the PTT test is used to determine if blood clots normally.
- Advise the patient that a blood sample will be taken. Explain that slight discomfort from the needle puncture and the tourniquet may be experienced.
- When appropriate, tell the patient receiving heparin therapy that this test may be repeated at regular inter- vals to assess the patient's response to treatment.
- Inform the patient that there are no food or fluid restrictions for this test.
- Do not draw from a closed-loop blood sampling system in an arterial line where heparin flush has been used. Do not draw from an arm into which heparin is infused.

During the Test
- Perform a venipuncture and collect the sample in a 7-mL tube with sodium citrate added. Sample must not be drawn from the arm with an IV infusion of heparin.

• Completely fill the collection tube, invert it gently several times, and send it on ice to the laboratory.

After the Test
• Ensure subdermal bleeding has stopped before removing pressure.
• For a patient on anticoagulant therapy, apply additional pressure at the venipuncture site to control bleeding and to prevent hematoma formation.
• If the hematoma is large, monitor pulses distal to the venipuncture site.

Percutaneous Liver Biopsy

Normal Findings
• Sheets of hepatocytes supported by a reticulin framework

Abnormal Findings
• Cirrhosis
• Hepatitis
• Granulomatous infections (such as tuberculosis)
• Hepatocellular carcinoma, cholangiocellular carcinoma, angiosarcoma
• Hepatic metastasis

Nursing Implications
• Report abnormal findings to the health care provider.
• Prepare to educate the patient about the diagnosis.
• Prepare the patient for further testing or surgery, as indicated.
• Provide emotional support to the patient and family.
• Inform the patient with a nonmalignant focal lesion that further studies (such as laparotomy or laparoscopy with biopsy) will be needed.

Purpose
• To diagnose hepatic parenchymal disease, malignant tumors, and granulomatous infections
• To determine prognosis for liver disease or to monitor response to treatment

Description
Percutaneous liver biopsy is the needle aspiration of a core of liver tissue for histologic analysis. This procedure is performed under local or general anesthesia using a special needle. Findings may help to identify hepatic disorders after ultrasonography, computed tomographic scan, and radionuclide studies have failed to detect them. Because many patients with hepatic disorders have clotting defects, testing for hemostasis should precede liver biopsy.

The procedure for percutaneous liver biopsy is as follows:

• For aspiration biopsy using the Menghini needle, the patient is positioned in a supine position with the right hand under the head. The patient is instructed to maintain this position and remain as still as possible during the procedure.
• The liver is palpated, the biopsy site is selected, marked, and prepped, and the local anesthetic is injected.
• The needle flange is set to control the penetration depth, and 2 mL of sterile normal saline solution is drawn into the syringe.
• The syringe is attached to the biopsy needle, and the needle is introduced into the subcutaneous tissue through the right eighth or ninth intercostal space at the midaxillary line and advanced up to the pleura.
• Next, 1 mL of normal saline solution is injected to clear the needle and the plunger, and then the plunger is drawn back to the 4-mL mark to create negative pressure.
• Then, the patient is asked to take a deep breath, exhale, and hold the breath at the end of expiration to prevent movement of the chest wall.
• As the patient holds the breath, the biopsy needle is quickly inserted into the liver and withdrawn in 1 second. For the patient who can't hold the breath, the biopsy needle is quickly inserted and withdrawn at the end of expiration.

P

- After the needle is withdrawn, the patient is told to resume normal respirations.
- The tissue specimen is then placed in a properly labeled specimen cup containing 10% formalin solution. This placement is done by releasing negative pressure while the point of the needle is in the formalin solution. The specimen is immediately sent to the laboratory.
- Then, 1 mL of normal saline solution is injected to clear the needle of the tissue specimen.
- Pressure is applied to the biopsy site to stop bleeding.
- The patient is positioned on the right side for 2 to 4 hours, with a small pillow or sandbag under the costal margin to provide extra pressure. Bed rest for at least 24 hours is advised.

Interfering Factors

- Inability to obtain a representative specimen
- Hemorrhage caused by inadvertent liver blood vessel puncture

Precautions

- Percutaneous liver biopsy is contraindicated in a patient with a platelet count below 100,000/μL; prothrombin (PT) time longer than 15 seconds; empyema of the lungs, pleurae, peritoneum, biliary tract, or liver; vascular tumor; hepatic angiomas; hydatid cyst; or tense ascites. If extrahepatic obstruction is suspected, ultrasonography or subcutaneous transhepatic cholangiography should rule out this condition before the biopsy is considered.
- Pain in the abdomen or dyspnea after the biopsy may indicate perforation of an abdominal organ or pneumothorax, respectively. In such cases, complete a thorough assessment and notify the health care provider immediately.

Nursing Considerations

Before the Test

- Confirm the patient's identity using two patient identifiers and confirmation of the patient's identification bracelet according to facility policy.
- Explain to the patient that this test is used to diagnose liver disorders. Describe the procedure and answer any questions.
- Instruct the patient to restrict food and fluids for 4 to 8 hours before the test.
- Inform the patient who will perform the biopsy and when and where it will be done.
- Make sure the patient or a responsible family member has signed an informed consent form.
- Check the patient's history for hypersensitivity to the local anesthetic.
- Make sure coagulation studies (PT time, partial thromboplastin time, INR, and platelet counts) have been performed and that the results are recorded on the patient's chart. A blood sample for baseline hematocrit assessment usually is obtained as well.
- Just before the biopsy, tell the patient to void, and then record the patient's vital signs.
- Inform the patient that a local anesthetic will be given, but that the patient may experience pain similar to that of a punch in the right shoulder as the biopsy needle passes the phrenic nerve.
- Instruct the patient to hold the breath when the needle is in place.

After the Test

- Check the patient's vital signs every 15 minutes for 1 hour, every 30 minutes for 4 hours, and every 4 hours thereafter for 24 hours. Observe carefully for signs of shock.
- If the patient is being discharged, instruct the patient to avoid coughing or straining. Bed rest with 24-hour observation is usually recommended. The patient should be advised not to do any heavy lifting. It is not advisable to operate machinery or drive for at least 24 hours. Instruct that it is not advised to take any aspirin, NSAIDs, or anticoagulants for approximately 1 week.

▶ Quality and Safety Nursing Alert

Immediately report bleeding or signs of bile peritonitis, such as tenderness and rigidity around the biopsy site. Watch for pneumothorax symptoms, such as rising respiratory rate, depressed breath sounds, dyspnea, persistent shoulder pain, and pleuritic chest pain. Report such complications promptly.

- If the patient experiences pain, which may persist for several hours after the test, administer an analgesic.
- Instruct the patient to resume a usual diet, as ordered.

Percutaneous Transhepatic Cholangiography

Normal Findings
- Biliary ducts of normal diameter that appear as regular channels homogeneously filled with contrast medium

Abnormal Findings
- Dilated biliary ducts, indicating obstructive jaundice, which may result from cholelithiasis, biliary tract carcinoma, or carcinoma of the pancreas or papilla of Vater

Nursing Implications
- Report abnormal findings to the health care provider.
- Prepare to educate the patient about the diagnosis.
- Prepare the patient for further testing or surgery, as indicated.
- Provide emotional support to the patient and family.

Purpose
- To determine the cause of upper abdominal pain following cholecystectomy
- To distinguish between obstructive and nonobstructive jaundice
- To determine the location, extent, and cause of mechanical obstruction

Description

Percutaneous transhepatic cholangiography is the fluoroscopic examination of the biliary ducts after injection of an iodinated contrast medium directly into a biliary radicle. This test is especially useful for evaluating patients with persistent upper abdominal pain after cholecystectomy or severe jaundice.

The procedure for percutaneous transhepatic cholangiography is as follows:

- After the patient is placed in a supine position on the X-ray table and adequately secured, the right upper quadrant of the abdomen is cleaned and draped; the skin, subcutaneous tissue, and liver capsule are infiltrated with a local anesthetic.
- With the patient holding the breath at the end of expiration, a flexible needle is inserted under fluoroscopic guidance through the tenth or eleventh intercostal space at the right midclavicular line.
- The needle is aimed toward the xiphoid process and advanced through the liver parenchyma. It's then slowly withdrawn, injecting the contrast medium to locate a biliary radicle. When fluoroscopy reveals placement in a radicle, the needle is held in position and the remaining contrast medium is injected.
- Using a fluoroscope and television monitor, biliary duct opacification is observed, and spot films of significant findings are taken with the patient in supine and lateral recumbent positions. When the required films have been taken, the needle is removed.
- A sterile dressing is applied to the puncture site.

Interfering Factors
- Marked obesity or gas overlying the biliary ducts (possible poor imaging)

Precautions
- Percutaneous transhepatic cholangiography is contraindicated in the

patient with cholangitis, massive ascites, uncorrectable coagulopathy, or hypersensitivity to iodine, as well as in the pregnant patient because of radiation's possible teratogenic effects.

Nursing Considerations

Before the Test

- Confirm the patient's identity using two patient identifiers and confirmation of the patient's identification bracelet according to facility policy.
- Explain to the patient that this test allows examination of the biliary ducts through X-ray films taken after a contrast medium is injected into the liver.
- Instruct the patient to fast for 8 hours before the test.
- Describe the test, including who will perform it and when and where it will take place.
- Explain that the patient may receive a laxative the night before and an enema on the morning of the test.
- Explain that the patient will be placed on a tilting X-ray table that rotates into vertical and horizontal positions during the procedure. Explain that the patient will be adequately secured to the table and assisted throughout the procedure.
- Warn the patient that the local anesthetic injection may sting the skin and produce transient pain when it punctures the liver capsule and that the contrast medium injection may produce a sensation of pressure and epigastric fullness and may cause transient upper back pain on the right side.
- Explain that the patient must rest for at least 6 hours after the procedure.
- Make sure that the patient or a responsible family member has signed an informed consent form.
- Check the patient's history for hypersensitivity to iodine, seafood, contrast media used in other diagnostic tests,

and the local anesthetic. Advise of possible adverse effects of contrast medium administration, such as nausea, vomiting, excessive salivation, flushing, urticaria, sweating, and, rarely, anaphylaxis; tachycardia and fever may accompany intraductal injection.
- Check the patient's history for normal bleeding, clotting, and prothrombin times, and a normal platelet count. If prescribed, administer 1 g of IV ampicillin every 4 to 6 hours for 24 hours before the procedure.
- Just before the procedure, administer a sedative, if prescribed.

After the Test

- Check the patient's vital signs until they're stable.
- Enforce bed rest for at least 6 hours after the test, preferably with the patient lying on the right side, to help prevent hemorrhage.
- Check the injection site for bleeding, swelling, and tenderness. Watch for signs of peritonitis, such as chills, temperature of 102° to 103°F (38.8°–39.4°C), and abdominal pain, tenderness, and distention. Notify the health care provider immediately if such complications develop.
- Tell the patient to resume a usual diet.

Pericardial Fluid Analysis

Normal Findings

- 10 to 50 mL of clear or straw-colored sterile fluid in the pericardium
- No evidence of pathogens, blood, or malignant cells
- Fewer than 1,000/μL (SI, less than 1×10^9/L) white blood cells (WBCs)
- Glucose concentration approximately equal to whole blood levels

Abnormal Findings

- Pericarditis
- Neoplasms
- Acute myocardial infarction
- Tuberculosis (TB)

- Rheumatoid disease
- Systemic lupus erythematosus

Elevated WBC Count or Neutrophil Fraction Levels
- Bacterial pericarditis

Elevated Lymphocyte Fraction Levels
- Fungal or tuberculous pericarditis

Bloody Pericardial Fluid
- Hemopericardium (myocardial rupture after infarction or aortic rupture secondary to a dissecting aortic aneurysm or thoracic trauma)
- Hemorrhagic pericarditis
- Traumatic paracentesis

Turbid or Milky Effusions
- Lymph or pus accumulation in the pericardial sac
- TB
- Rheumatoid disease

Hemorrhagic Effusions
- Malignant tumor
- Closed chest trauma (cardiac tamponade)
- Dressler's syndrome
- Postcardiotomy syndrome

Nursing Implications
- Report abnormal findings to the health care provider.
- Prepare to educate the patient about the diagnosis.
- Prepare the patient for further testing or surgery, as indicated.
- Provide emotional support to the patient and family.
- Prepare to administer antimicrobial therapy or other medications, as indicated.

Purpose
- To assist in identifying the cause of pericardial effusion and to help determine appropriate therapy and emergency therapy for pericardial tamponade

Description
Pericardial sac fluid analysis usually is done for the patient with pericardial effusion (an accumulation of excess pericardial fluid), which may result from inflammation (as in pericarditis), rupture, or penetrating trauma.

Obtaining a specimen requires pericardial fluid needle aspiration, a procedure called *pericardiocentesis*. This procedure must be performed cautiously because of potentially fatal complication risks, such as myocardial or coronary artery laceration, ventricular fibrillation or vasovagal arrest, pleural infection, or accidental puncture of the lung, liver, or stomach. If possible, echocardiography should be used before pericardiocentesis is performed to determine the effusion site and minimize complication risks. (See the *Aspirating Pericardial Fluid* box.)

The procedure for pericardial fluid analysis is as follows:

- The patient is placed in the supine position with the thorax elevated 60 degrees.
- A local anesthetic is administered at the insertion site after the skin is prepared with alcohol or povidone–iodine solution from the left costal margin to the xiphoid process.
- With the three-way stopcock open, a 50-mL syringe is aseptically attached to one end and the cardiac needle to the other end.
- The electrocardiogram (ECG) lead wire is attached to the needle hub with an alligator clip. The ECG is set to lead V and turned on (or the patient is connected to a bedside monitor).
- The needle is inserted through the chest wall into the pericardial sac, maintaining gentle aspiration until fluid appears in the syringe.
- The needle is angled 35 to 45 degrees toward the tip of the right scapula between the left costal margin and the xiphoid process. A Kelly clamp is attached at the skin surface after the needle is properly positioned so it won't advance further.
- While the fluid is being aspirated, the specimen tubes are labeled and numbered.

P

Aspirating Pericardial Fluid

In pericardiocentesis, a needle and syringe assembly is inserted through the chest wall into the pericardial sac, as illustrated here. Electrocardiographic (ECG) monitoring with a lead wire attached to the needle and electrodes placed on the limbs (right arm [RA], right leg [RL], left arm [LA], and left leg [LL]) helps to ensure proper needle placement and to avoid damage to the heart.

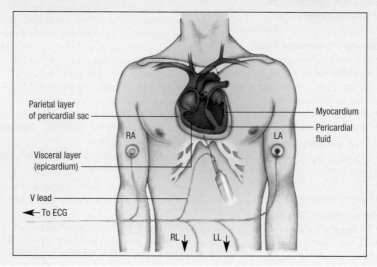

Parietal layer of pericardial sac

Visceral layer (epicardium)

V lead

To ECG

RA

RL

LL

LA

Myocardium

Pericardial fluid

- When the needle is withdrawn, pressure is applied immediately to the site with sterile gauze pads for 3 to 5 minutes. A bandage is then applied.

Interfering Factors
- Failure to use sterile collection technique, allowing skin contaminants to be mistaken for the causative organism
- Antimicrobial therapy (can prevent isolation of the causative organisms)

Precautions
- Use specimen tubes with the proper additives. Although fibrin isn't a normal component of pericardial fluid, it does appear in fluid in some pericardial diseases and in carcinoma, and clotting is possible.
- Before the specimen is obtained, clean the top of the culture and sensitivity tube with povidone–iodine solution or according to facility

policy to reduce the risk of extrinsic contamination.
- If anaerobic organisms are suspected, consult the laboratory concerning the proper collection technique to avoid exposing the aspirate to air. The aspirate may be placed in an anaerobic collection tube, or the syringe may be filled completely, displacing all air, and the collection tube capped tightly with a sterile rubber tip.
- Have resuscitation equipment on hand.

Nursing Considerations
Before the Test
- Confirm the patient's identity using two patient identifiers and confirmation of the patient's identification bracelet according to facility policy.
- Explain to the patient that pericardial fluid analysis detects excessive fluid around the heart, determines its

cause, and helps determine appropriate therapy.

- Inform the patient that there are no food or fluid restrictions for this test.
- Tell the patient who will perform the test and where and when it will take place.
- Advise the patient that a local anesthetic will be injected before the aspiration needle is inserted. Warn that although fluid aspiration isn't painful, the patient may experience pressure upon needle insertion into the pericardial sac and may be asked to briefly hold the breath to aid needle insertion and placement.
- Inform the patient that an IV line will be started at a slow rate in case medications need to be administered.
- Explain that someone will remain with the patient during the test and that the patient's pulse and blood pressure will be monitored after the procedure.
- Check the patient's history for current use of antimicrobial drugs and record such usage on the laboratory request form.
- Make sure that the patient or a responsible family member has signed an informed consent form.
- Explain the test to the family if pericardiocentesis is performed to relieve cardiac tamponade and the patient is in shock.

During the Test

- Watch for grossly bloody aspirate, a sign of inadvertent cardiac chamber puncture.
- Carefully observe the ECG tracing during cardiac needle insertion; an ST-segment elevation indicates that the needle has reached the epicardial surface and should be retracted slightly; an abnormally shaped QRS complex may indicate perforation of the myocardium. Also, premature ventricular contractions usually indicate that the needle has touched the ventricular wall.

After the Test

- Check blood pressure readings, pulse, respiration, and heart sounds every 15 minutes until stable, every 30 minutes for 2 hours, every hour for 4 hours, and then every 4 hours thereafter. Assure the patient that such monitoring is routine.
- Send all specimens to the laboratory immediately after collection.

> ▶ **Quality and Safety Nursing Alert**

Watch for respiratory or cardiac distress, especially signs of cardiac tamponade: muffled and distant heart sounds, distended neck veins, paradoxical pulse, and shock. Cardiac tamponade may result from rapid reaccumulation of pericardial fluid or puncture of a coronary vessel, causing bleeding into the pericardial sac.

Peritoneal Fluid Analysis

Normal Findings

- See the *Normal Findings in Peritoneal Fluid Analysis* table for specific information.

Abnormal Findings

- Milk-colored fluid, indicating malignant tumor, lymphoma, tuberculosis (TB), parasitic infestation, adhesion, or hepatic cirrhosis
- Cloudy or turbid fluid, indicating peritonitis, ruptured bowel (after trauma), pancreatitis, trauma, strangulated or infarcted intestine, or appendicitis
- Bloody fluid, indicating benign or malignant tumor, hemorrhagic pancreatitis, or a traumatic tap
- Bile-stained, green fluid, indicating a ruptured gallbladder, acute pancreatitis, a perforated intestine, or duodenal ulcer
- Red blood cell (RBC) count greater than 100/μL (SI, greater than 100/L), indicating a neoplasm or TB

Normal Findings in Peritoneal Fluid Analysis

This table outlines the normal findings in a specimen of peritoneal fluid.

Element	Normal Value or Finding
Gross appearance	Sterile, odorless, clear to pale yellow color; scant amount (<50 mL)
Red blood cells	None
White blood cells	<300/µL (SI, <300 × 10⁹/L)
Protein	0.3 to 4.1 g/dL (SI, 3–41 g/L)
Glucose	70 to 100 mg/dL (SI, 3.5–5 mmol/L)
Amylase	138 to 404 units/L (SI, 2.3–6.7 µkat/L)
Ammonia	<50 mcg/dL (SI, <29 µmol/L)
Alkaline phosphatase	Males > age 18: 90 to 239 units/L (SI, 1.5–3.9 µkat/L)
	Females < age 45: 76 to 196 units/L (SI, 1.2–3.2 µkat/L)
	Females > age 45: 87 to 250 units/L (SI, 1.4–4.1 µkat/L)
Cytology	No malignant cells present
Bacteria	None
Fungi	None

- RBC count greater than 100,000/µL (SI, greater than 100,000/L), indicating intra-abdominal trauma
- Elevated white blood cell count with more than 25% neutrophils, indicating spontaneous bacterial peritonitis (90% of cases) or cirrhosis (found in 50% of cases)
- Elevated granulocyte count greater than 250 cells/Ml is diagnostic for infection
- Elevated lymphocytes, indicating TB peritonitis or chylous ascites
- Protein levels greater than 3 g/dL (SI, greater than 3 g/L), indicating malignancy
- Protein levels greater than 4 g/dL (SI, greater than 4 g/L), indicating TB
- Decreased glucose levels, indicating TB peritonitis or peritoneal carcinomatosis
- Elevated amylase levels, indicating pancreatic trauma, pancreatic pseudocyst, acute pancreatitis, or intestinal necrosis or strangulation
- Alkaline phosphatase levels more than twice the normal serum level, indicating ruptured or strangulated small intestines
- Peritoneal ammonia levels more than twice the normal serum level, indicat-ing ruptured or strangulated large and small intestines, ruptured ulcer, or ruptured appendix
- Protein ascitic fluid-to-serum ratio of 0.5 or greater, indicating malignancy, TB, pancreatic ascites
- Albumin gradient between ascitic fluid and serum greater than 1 g/dL (SI, greater than 1 g/L), indicating chronic hepatic disease
- Albumin gradient between ascitic fluid and serum less than 1 g/dL (SI, less than 1 g/L), indicating malignancy
- Malignant cells upon cytologic examination
- Gram-positive cocci, indicating primary peritonitis
- Gram-negative organisms, indicating secondary peritonitis
- Fungi, indicating histoplasmosis, candidiasis, or coccidioidomycosis

Nursing Implications

- If a large amount of fluid was aspi-rated, watch the patient for signs of vascular collapse (color change, elevated pulse and respiratory rates, decreased blood pressure and central venous pressure, mental changes, and dizziness). Administer fluids orally if the patient is alert and can accept them.

- Observe the patient with severe hepatic disease for signs of hepatic coma, which may result from sodium and potassium loss accompanying hypovolemia. Watch the patient for mental changes, drowsiness, and stupor. Such a patient also is prone to uremia, infection, hemorrhage, and protein depletion.
- Administer IV infusions and albumin, as ordered. Check the laboratory report for electrolyte (especially sodium) and serum protein levels.

Purpose

- To determine the cause of ascites
- To detect abdominal trauma
- To relieve intra-abdominal pressure that accompanies ascites

Description

Peritoneal fluid analysis assesses a specimen of peritoneal fluid obtained by paracentesis. This procedure requires inserting a trocar and cannula through the abdominal wall as the patient receives a local anesthetic. If the fluid specimen is removed for therapeutic purposes, the trocar may be connected to a drainage system. However, if only a small amount of fluid is removed for diagnostic purposes, an 18G needle may be used in place of the trocar and cannula. In four-quadrant paracentesis, fluid is aspirated from each quadrant of the abdomen to verify abdominal trauma and confirm the need for surgery.

The procedure for peritoneal fluid analysis is as follows:

- The patient is seated on a bed or in a chair with the feet flat on the floor and the back well supported. If the patient can't tolerate being out of bed, he's placed in high Fowler's position and made as comfortable as possible.
- Except for the puncture site, the patient is kept covered to keep warm.

- A plastic sheet or absorbent pad is provided to collect spillage and to protect the patient and bed linens.
- Hair around the puncture site is clipped, the skin prepared, and the area draped.
- All medications, medication containers and syringes, and other solutions on and off the sterile field are labeled.
- The local anesthetic is injected.
- The health care provider inserts the needle or trocar and cannula 1 to 2 inches (2.5–5 cm) below the umbilicus. (However, it may also be inserted through the flank, the iliac fossa, the border of the rectus, or at each quadrant of the abdomen.)
- If a trocar and cannula are used, a small incision is made to facilitate insertion. When the needle pierces the peritoneum, it "gives" with an audible sound. The trocar is removed and a specimen of fluid is aspirated with a 50-mL Luer-lock syringe.
- If additional fluid is to be drained, one end of an IV tube is attached to the cannula and the other end to a collection bag. The fluid is then aspirated (no more than 1,500 mL). If aspiration is difficult, the patient is repositioned, as ordered.
- After aspiration, the trocar needle is removed and a pressure dressing is applied. Occasionally, the wound may be sutured first.
- The specimens are labeled in the order they were drawn. If the patient has received antibiotic therapy, it's noted on the laboratory request.

Interfering Factors

- Nonsterile collection technique or failure to send the specimen to the laboratory immediately after collection
- Contamination of the specimen with blood, bile, urine, or stools because of injury to underlying structures during paracentesis

P

Precautions

- Peritoneal fluid analysis should be performed cautiously in a pregnant patient and in the patient with bleeding tendencies or unstable vital signs.
- Avoid contamination of the specimens, which alters their bacterial content.

Nursing Considerations

Before the Test

- Confirm the patient's identity using two patient identifiers and confirmation of the patient's identification bracelet according to facility policy.
- Explain to the patient that peritoneal fluid analysis helps determine the cause of ascites or detects abdominal trauma.
- Inform the patient that there are no food or fluid restrictions for this test.
- Advise the patient that the test requires a peritoneal fluid specimen, that a local anesthetic will be administered to minimize discomfort, and that the procedure takes about 45 minutes to perform.
- Provide psychological support to decrease the patient's anxiety and assure that complications are rare.
- If the patient has severe ascites, explain that the procedure will relieve discomfort and allow for easier breathing.
- Make sure that the patient or a responsible family member has signed an informed consent form.
- Record the patient's baseline vital signs, weight, and abdominal girth.
- Inform the patient that a blood sample and X-rays may be taken as part of the procedure.
- Instruct the patient to void just before the test; voiding helps to prevent accidental bladder injury during needle insertion by decompressing the bladder.

During the Test

- Check the patient's vital signs every 15 minutes during the procedure. Watch for deviations from baseline findings. Observe for dizziness, pallor, perspiration, and increased anxiety.

> ◣ *Quality and Safety Nursing Alert*
>
> If rapid fluid aspiration induces hypovolemia and shock, reduce the vertical distance between the trocar and the collection bag to slow the drainage rate. If necessary, stop the drainage by turning off the stopcock or clamping the tubing.

After the Test

- Send the specimens to the laboratory immediately after collection.
- Carefully and properly dispose of needles and contaminated articles according to the Centers for Disease Control and Prevention guidelines; incinerate disposable items and return reusable ones to the central supply area.
- Apply a gauze dressing to the puncture site. Make sure it's thick enough to absorb all drainage. Check the dressing frequently (for example, whenever you check vital signs) and reinforce or apply a pressure dressing if needed.
- Weigh the patient.
- Monitor the patient's vital signs until they're stable. If the patient's recovery is poor, check vital signs every 15 minutes. Weigh and measure abdominal girth; compare these with baseline values.
- Allow the patient to rest and, if possible, withhold treatment or procedures that may cause undue stress, such as linen changes.
- Monitor the patient's urine output for at least 24 hours and watch for hematuria, which may indicate bladder trauma.

> ◣ *Quality and Safety Nursing Alert*
>
> Watch the patient for signs of hemorrhage or shock and for increasing pain or abdominal tenderness. These signs may indicate a perforated intestine or, depending on the site of the tap, puncture of the inferior epigastric artery, hematoma of the anterior cecal wall, or rupture of the iliac vein or bladder.

Persantine-Thallium Imaging

Normal Findings
- Characteristic isotope distribution throughout the left ventricle and no visible defects

Abnormal Findings
- ST-segment depression, indicating coronary artery disease (CAD) or myocardial infarction (if persistent)
- Cold spots, indicating sarcoidosis, myocardial fibrosis, or cardiac contusion

Nursing Implications
- Report abnormal findings to the health care provider.
- Prepare to educate the patient about the diagnosis.
- Prepare the patient for further testing or surgery, as indicated.
- Provide emotional support to the patient and family.
- Prepare to administer medication, as applicable.

Purpose
- To identify exercise- or stress-induced arrhythmias
- To assess the presence and degree of cardiac ischemia

Description
Persantine-thallium imaging is an alternative method of assessing coronary vessel function for the patient who can't tolerate exercise or stress electrocardiography (ECG). Dipyridamole (Persantine) infusion simulates the effects of exercise by increasing blood flow to the collateral circulation and away from the coronary arteries, thereby inducing ischemia. Thallium infusion allows the examiner to evaluate the cardiac vessels' response. The heart is scanned immediately after the thallium infusion and again 2 to 4 hours later. Diseased vessels can't deliver thallium to the heart, and thallium lingers in the myocardium's diseased areas.

The procedure for Persantine-thallium imaging is as follows:
- The patient reclines or sits while a resting ECG is performed. Persantine is given either orally or IV over 4 minutes. Blood pressure, pulse rate, and cardiac rhythm are monitored continuously.
- After Persantine administration, the patient is asked to get up and walk. After the Persantine takes effect, thallium is injected.
- The patient is placed in a supine position for about 40 minutes while the scan is performed. Then the scan is reviewed. If necessary, a second scan is performed.

Interfering Factors
- Artifacts, such as implants and electrodes (possible false positive)
- Absence of cold spots with CAD (possible delay in imaging)
- Recent nuclear scans
- Long-acting nitrates

Precautions
- The patient may experience arrhythmias, angina, ST-segment depression, or bronchospasm. Make sure resuscitation equipment is readily available.
- Common adverse reactions are nausea, headache, flushing, dizziness, and epigastric pain.

Nursing Considerations
Before the Test
- Confirm the patient's identity using two patient identifiers and confirmation of the patient's identification bracelet according to facility policy.
- Explain that the patient will need to restrict food and fluids before the test. Tell the patient to avoid caffeine and other stimulants (which may cause arrhythmias) for 24 hours.
- Instruct the patient to continue to take all regular medications, with the possible exception of beta-adrenergic blockers, as prescribed.
- Inform the patient that a painless, 5- to 10-minute baseline ECG will

P

precede Persantine-thallium imaging. Also explain that an IV line will infuse the medications for the study. Inform the patient who will start the IV, when and where the test will take place, and that slight discomfort from the needle insertion and the tourniquet may be experienced.

• Inform the patient that mild nausea, headache, dizziness, or flushing may be experienced after Persantine administration. Reassure the patient that these adverse reactions are usually temporary and rarely need treatment.

• Make sure that the patient or a responsible family member has signed an informed consent form.

After the Test
• If the patient must return for further scanning, have the patient rest and restrict food and fluids in the interim.

Phosphates, Serum

Reference Values
Adults: 2.7 to 4.5 mg/dL (SI, 0.87–1.45 mmol/L)
Children: 4.5 to 6.7 mg/dL (SI, 1.45–1.78 mmol/L)

Abnormal Findings

Elevated Levels
• Skeletal disease
• Healing fractures
• Hypoparathyroidism
• Acromegaly
• Diabetic ketoacidosis (DKA)
• High intestinal obstruction
• Lactic acidosis (due to hepatic impairment)
• Kidney failure
• Hypocalcemia

Decreased Levels
• Malnutrition
• Malabsorption syndromes
• Hyperparathyroidism
• Renal tubular acidosis
• Treatment of DKA

• Diuretics
• Chronic antacid ingestion
• Hypercalcemia
• Chronic alcoholism

Nursing Implications
• Report abnormal findings to the health care provider.
• Prepare to educate the patient about the diagnosis.
• Prepare the patient for further testing, as indicated.
• Prepare to administer insulin to the patient with DKA (elevated levels).
• Prepare to administer IV saline solution, as prescribed to patients with elevated levels.
• Instruct the patient with decreased levels to eat a high-phosphorous diet or to take phosphorous supplements. Provide written dietary instructions for the patient to follow.

Purpose
• To help diagnose renal disorders and acid–base imbalances
• To detect endocrine, skeletal, and calcium disorders

Description
The phosphate test is used to measure phosphate serum levels, the primary anion in intracellular fluid. Phosphates are essential in the storage and utilization of energy, calcium regulation, red blood cell function, acid–base balance, bone formation, and the metabolism of carbohydrates, protein, and fat. The intestines absorb most phosphates from dietary sources; the kidneys excrete phosphates and serve as a regulatory mechanism. Abnormal serum phosphate concentrations usually result from improper excretion rather than faulty ingestion or absorption from dietary sources.

Normally, calcium and phosphate have an inverse relationship; if one is increased, the other is decreased.

Interfering Factors
• Venous stasis caused by tourniquet use

- Sample obtained above an IV site that's receiving a solution containing phosphate
- Excessive vitamin D intake or therapy with anabolic steroids or androgens (possible increase)
- Use of acetazolamide, epinephrine, insulin, or phosphate-binding antacids; excessive excretion due to prolonged vomiting or diarrhea; vitamin D deficiency; and extended IV infusion of dextrose 5% in water (possible decrease)
- Oral contraceptives (possible decrease), injectable contraceptives (possible increase)
- Laxatives or enemas containing sodium phosphorus (possible increase)

Precautions
- Handle the sample gently to prevent hemolysis.

Nursing Considerations
Before the Test
- Confirm the patient's identity using two patient identifiers and confirmation of the patient's identification bracelet according to facility policy.
- Explain to the patient that the serum phosphate test is used to measure phosphate levels in the blood.
- Tell the patient that the test requires a blood sample. Explain that slight discomfort from the needle puncture and the tourniquet may be experienced.
- Patients should fast for 8 to 12 hours before the test; eating before the test may falsely lower the phosphate level.
- Notify the laboratory and health care provider of medications the patient is taking that may affect test results; these may need to be restricted.

During the Test
- Perform a venipuncture without using a tourniquet, if possible, and collect the sample in a 3- or 4-mL clot activator tube.

After the Test
- Apply pressure to the venipuncture site until bleeding stops and to prevent hematoma formation.
- Tell the patient to resume any medications that were discontinued before the test, as ordered.

Phospholipids
Reference Values
180 to 320 mg/dL (SI, 1.8–3.2 g/L)

Abnormal Findings
Elevated Levels
- Hypothyroidism
- Diabetes
- Nephrotic syndrome
- Chronic pancreatitis
- Obstructive jaundice

Decreased Levels
- Primary hypolipoproteinemia
- Dietary restriction of fat intake

Nursing Implications
- Report abnormal findings to the health care provider.
- Prepare to educate the patient about the diagnosis.
- Prepare the patient for further testing or surgery, as indicated.
- Provide emotional support to the patient and family.

Purpose
- To evaluate fat metabolism
- To help diagnose hypothyroidism, diabetes, nephrotic syndrome, chronic pancreatitis, obstructive jaundice, and hypolipoproteinemia

Description
The phospholipid test is a quantitative analysis of phospholipids, the major form of lipids in cell membranes. Phospholipids are involved in cellular membrane composition and permeability, and they help control enzyme activity within the membrane. They aid the transport of fatty acids and lipids across the intestinal barrier and from the liver

and other fat stores to other body tissues. Phospholipids are essential for pulmonary gas exchange.

Interfering Factors
- Antilipemics (possible decrease)
- Epinephrine, estrogens, and some phenothiazines (increase)

Precautions
- Send the sample to the laboratory immediately because spontaneous redistribution may occur among plasma lipids.

Nursing Considerations
Before the Test
- Confirm the patient's identity using two patient identifiers and confirmation of the patient's identification bracelet according to facility policy.
- Explain to the patient that the phospholipid test is used to determine how the body metabolizes fats.
- Advise the patient that the test requires a blood sample. Explain that slight discomfort from the needle puncture and the tourniquet may be experienced.
- Instruct the patient to abstain from drinking alcohol for 24 hours before the test and not to eat or drink anything after midnight before the test.
- Notify the laboratory and health care provider of medications the patient is taking that may affect test results; these may need to be restricted.

During the Test
- Perform a venipuncture and collect the sample in a 10- to 15-mL tube without additives.
- Apply direct pressure to the venipuncture site until bleeding stops and to prevent hematoma formation.

After the Test
- Tell the patient to resume a usual diet and medications that were discontinued before the test, as ordered.

Plasma Thrombin Time

Reference Values
10 to 15 seconds (SI, 10–15 seconds)
Less than 1.5 times the control value

Abnormal Findings
Prolonged Plasma Thrombin Time
- Heparin therapy
- Hepatic disease
- Disseminated intravascular coagulation (DIC)
- Hypofibrinogenemia
- Dysfibrinogenemia
- Acute leukemia
- Lymphoma
- Factor deficiency
- Shock

Nursing Implications
- Report abnormal findings to the health care provider.
- Prepare the patient for further testing, as indicated.
- The patient with a prolonged thrombin time may require fibrinogen levels measurement.
- If the patient is suspected of having DIC, the test for fibrin split products is also necessary.

Purpose
- To detect a fibrinogen deficiency or defect
- To help diagnose DIC and hepatic disease
- To monitor the effectiveness of heparin or thrombolytic agents

Description
Plasma thrombin time, or thrombin clotting time, measures how quickly a clot forms when a standard amount of bovine thrombin is added to a platelet-poor plasma sample from the patient and to a normal plasma control sample. After thrombin is added, the clotting time for each sample is compared and recorded. This test allows a quick but imprecise estimation of plasma fibrinogen levels, which are a function of clotting time. (See the *Understanding the*

Understanding the Antithrombin III Test

The antithrombin III test helps detect the cause of impaired coagulation, especially hypercoagulation, by measuring levels of antithrombin III (AT III), a protein that inactivates thrombin and inhibits coagulation. AT III may be evaluated by a functional clotting assay or synthetic substrates. Exogenous heparin is added to a fresh, citrated blood sample to accelerate activity, then excess thrombin (factor Xa) is added to the plasma. The amount of factor Xa not activated by AT III is quanti- tated and compared with a normal control sample. Reference values may vary for each laboratory, but should lie between 80% and 120% of normal.

Decreased AT III levels can indicate disseminated intravascular coagulation, fibrinolytic disorders, thrombophlebitis, or hepatic disorders. Slightly decreased levels can result from hormonal contraceptives. Elevated levels can result from kidney transplantation and the use of oral anticoagulants or anabolic steroids.

Antithrombin III Test box for information about another test that helps determine the cause of coagulation disorders.)

Interfering Factors
- Fibrin degradation products, fibrinogen, streptokinase, urokinase, tissue plasminogen activator (TPA), or heparin (possible increase)

Precautions
- To prevent hemolysis, avoid excessive probing during venipuncture and rough handling of the sample.

Nursing Considerations

Before the Test
- Confirm the patient's identity using two patient identifiers and confirmation of the patient's identification bracelet according to facility policy.
- Explain to the patient that the plasma thrombin time test is used to determine if blood clots normally.
- Notify the laboratory and physician of medications the patient is taking that may affect test results; these may need to be restricted.
- Advise the patient that a blood sample will be taken. Explain that slight discomfort from the needle puncture and the tourniquet may be experienced.
- Inform the patient that there are no food or fluid restrictions for this test.

During the Test
- Perform a venipuncture and collect the sample in a 3- to 4.5-mL siliconized tube.

- If the tube isn't filled to the correct volume, a citrate excess appears in the sample. Completely fill the collection tube and invert it gently several times to mix the sample and the anticoagulant thoroughly.
- Immediately put the sample on ice and send it to the laboratory.

After the Test
- Apply pressure to the venipuncture site until bleeding has stopped and to prevent hematoma formation.
- If a hematoma develops and is large, monitor pulses distal to the phlebotomy site.
- Tell the patient to resume any medications that were discontinued before the test, as ordered.

Plasminogen, Plasma

Reference Values
Males: 76% to 124% of normal
Females: 65% to 153% of normal
Infants: 27% to 59% of normal

Abnormal Findings

Elevated Levels
- Deep vein thrombosis
- Infection
- Malignancy
- Myocardial infarction
- Pregnancy
- Preeclampsia
- Eclampsia
- Stress
- Surgery

Decreased Levels
- Disseminated intravascular coagulation
- Tumors
- Cirrhosis

Nursing Implications
- Report abnormal findings to the health care provider.
- Prepare to educate the patient about the diagnosis.
- Prepare the patient for further testing or surgery, as indicated.
- Provide emotional support to the patient and family.
- Prepare to administer medication, as indicated.

Purpose
- To assess fibrinolysis
- To detect congenital and acquired fibrinolytic disorders

Description
Plasma plasminogen testing is used to assess plasminogen levels in a plasma sample. During fibrinolysis, plasmin dissolves fibrin clots to prevent excessive coagulation and impaired blood flow. Plasmin doesn't circulate in active form, however, so it can't be directly measured. Its circulating precursor, plasminogen, can be measured and used to evaluate the fibrinolytic system.

Interfering Factors
- Failure to use the proper collection tube, to adequately mix the sample and citrate, to send the sample to the laboratory immediately, or to have the sample separated and frozen
- Hemolysis resulting from excessive probing during venipuncture or too rough handling of the sample
- Hemoconcentration caused by prolonged tourniquet use before venipuncture (possible false decrease)
- Hormonal contraceptives (possible slight increase)
- Thrombolytic drugs, such as streptokinase and urokinase (possible decrease)

Precautions
- To prevent hemolysis, avoid excessive probing during venipuncture and rough handling of the sample.

Nursing Considerations
Before the Test
- Confirm the patient's identity using two patient identifiers and confirmation of the patient's identification bracelet according to facility policy.
- Explain to the patient that the plasma plasminogen test is used to evaluate blood clotting.
- Advise the patient that a blood sample will be taken. Explain that slight discomfort from the needle puncture and the tourniquet may be experienced.
- Notify the laboratory and physician of medications the patient is taking that may affect test results; these may need to be restricted.
- Inform the patient that there are no food or fluid restrictions for this test.

During the Test
- Perform a venipuncture and collect the sample in a 4.5-mL siliconized tube.
- Collect the sample as quickly as possible to prevent stasis, which can slow blood flow, causing coagulation and plasminogen activation.
- Invert the tube gently several times and immediately send the sample to the laboratory. If testing must be delayed, plasma must be separated and frozen at $-94°F$ ($-70°C$).

After the Test
- Apply pressure to the venipuncture site until bleeding has stopped and to prevent hematoma formation.
- If a hematoma develops and is large, monitor pulses distal to the venipuncture site.
- Tell the patient to resume medications that were discontinued before the test, as ordered.

Platelet Aggregation Test

Reference Values
60% to 100% in 3 to 5 minutes
(SI, 3–5 minutes)

Abnormal Findings
- Von Willebrand's disease
- Bernard-Soulier's syndrome
- Storage pool disease
- Glanzmann's thrombasthenia
- Polycythemia vera
- Severe liver disease
- Uremia
- Connective tissue disorders
- Recent cardiopulmonary or dialysis bypass

Nursing Implications
- Report abnormal findings to the health care provider.
- Prepare to educate the patient about the diagnosis.
- Prepare the patient for further testing, as indicated.

Purpose
- To assess platelet aggregation
- To detect congenital and acquired platelet bleeding disorders

Description
After vascular injury, platelets gather at the injury site and clump together to form an aggregate or plug that helps maintain hemostasis and promote healing. The platelet aggregation test is used to measure the rate at which the platelets in a plasma sample form a clump after the addition of an aggregating reagent.

Interfering Factors
- Antihistamines, anti-inflammatory drugs, aspirin and aspirin compounds, phenothiazines, phenylbutazone, tricyclic antidepressants, NSAIDs, Coumadin, and sulfinpyrazone (Anturane) (decrease)
- Ingestion of large amounts of garlic, blood storage temperature, hyperbilirubinemia, hemoglobinemia, hyperlipidemia, and platelet count (inhibits platelet aggregation)

Precautions
- Because the list of medications known to alter the results of this test is long and continually growing, the patient should be as drug free as possible before the test.
- Avoid excessive probing at the venipuncture site. Remove the tourniquet promptly to avoid bruising.
- Handle the sample gently to prevent hemolysis and keep it between 71.6°F and 98.6°F (22°C and 37°C) to prevent aggregation.

Nursing Considerations
Before the Test
- Confirm the patient's identity using two patient identifiers and confirmation of the patient's identification bracelet according to facility policy.
- Explain to the patient that the platelet aggregation test is used to determine if blood clots properly.
- Advise the patient that the test requires a blood sample. Explain that slight discomfort from the needle puncture and the tourniquet may be experienced.
- Instruct the patient to fast or to maintain a nonfat diet for 8 hours before the test because lipemia can affect the test results.
- Notify the laboratory and health care provider of medications the patient is taking that may affect test results; these may need to be restricted. Ask specifically about aspirin use within the past 14 days. Although the test can be postponed if the patient has used aspirin, ask the laboratory to verify aspirin presence in the plasma. If the sample's test results are abnormal, aspirin use must be discontinued and the test must be repeated in 2 weeks. (See the *Aspirin and Platelet Aggregation* box.)

P

Aspirin and Platelet Aggregation

Unlike other salicylates, aspirin inhibits platelet aggregation. This inhibition occurs in the second phase of platelet aggregation, when it prevents the release of adenosine diphosphate from platelets. Mean bleeding time may double in healthy individuals after ingestion of aspirin. In children or in patients with bleeding disorders, such as hemophilia, bleeding time may be even more prolonged.

Effect on Platelets

The effect of aspirin on platelets seems to result from the inhibition of prostaglandin synthesis. A single 325-mg oral dose of aspirin results in about 90% inhibition of the enzyme cyclooxygenase in circulating platelets, preventing the synthesis of compounds that induce platelet aggregation. The inhibition of cyclooxygenase is irreversible; thus, its effect lasts for 4 to 6 days—the life span of platelets. Bleeding time peaks within 12 hours.

Altered hemostasis persists about 36 hours after the last dose of aspirin, sometimes longer for the patient receiving long-term therapy.

Effect on Blood Vessels

Aspirin's action on blood vessels may oppose that seen in platelets because cyclooxygenase plays a different role in the vascular endothelium. Here, the enzyme produces prostacyclin, a compound that inhibits platelet aggregation and causes vasodilation. Inhibition of cyclooxygenase in the vascular endothelium, in effect, reverses aspirin's antithrombotic effect on platelets. However, studies suggest that cyclooxygenase in the platelets is more sensitive than that in the vascular endothelium; therefore, a low aspirin dosage (for example, 80 mg daily or 325 mg every other day) may prove more effective in preventing thrombosis than higher dosages.

During the Test

- Perform a venipuncture and collect the sample in a 4.5-mL siliconized tube.
- Completely fill the collection tube and invert it gently several times to mix the sample and the anticoagulant thoroughly.
- Apply the tourniquet only tightly enough to engorge the blood vessels in order to avoid bruising.

After the Test

- Apply pressure to the venipuncture site for 5 minutes or until bleeding stops and to prevent hematoma formation.
- Tell the patient to resume a usual diet and medications that were discontinued before the test, as ordered.

Platelet Count

Reference Values

Adults: 140,000 to 400,000/µL (SI, 140 to 400×10^9/L)

Children: 150,000 to 450,000/µL (SI, 150 to 450×10^9/L)

Critical Values

Less than 50,000/µL (can cause spontaneous bleeding)

Less than 5000/µL (possible fatal central nervous system bleeding or massive GI hemorrhage)

Abnormal Findings

Elevated Levels

- Hemorrhage
- Infectious or inflammatory disorders
- Iron deficiency anemia
- Splenectomy or other recent surgery
- Pregnancy
- Primary thrombocythemia
- Myelofibrosis with myeloid metaplasia
- Polycythemia vera
- Chronic myelogenous leukemia

Decreased Levels

- Aplastic or hypoplastic bone marrow
- Splenectomy
- Leukemia
- Disseminated infection
- Megakaryocytic hypoplasia
- Folic acid or vitamin B_{12}, deficiency
- Pooling of platelets in an enlarged spleen

- Increased platelet destruction caused by drugs or an immune disorder
- Disseminated intravascular coagulation
- Bernard-Soulier's syndrome
- Mechanical injury to platelets

Nursing Implications

- Prepare the patient for additional testing, including a complete blood count (CBC), bone marrow biopsy, direct antiglobulin test (direct Coombs' test), and serum protein electrophoresis.
- Report abnormal findings to the health care provider.
- Prepare to educate the patient about the diagnosis.

Purpose

- To evaluate platelet production
- To assess the effects of chemotherapy or radiation therapy on platelet production
- To diagnose and monitor severe thrombocytosis or thrombocytopenia
- To confirm a visual estimate of platelet number and morphology from a stained blood film

Description

Platelets, or thrombocytes, are the smallest formed elements in blood. They promote coagulation and the formation of a hemostatic plug in vascular injury. Platelet count is one of the most important screening tests of platelet function. Accurate counts are vital.

Interfering Factors

- Heparin (decrease)
- Acetazolamide (Dazamide), acetohexamide (Dymelor), antineoplastics, brompheniramine maleate, carbamazepine (Tegretol), chloramphenicol, ethacrynic acid (Edecrin), furosemide (Lasix), gold salts, hydroxychloroquine (Plaquenil), indomethacin (Indocin), isoniazid (INH), mefenamic acid, methazolamide (Glauc Tabs), methimazole (Tapazole), methyldopa (Aldomet), oral diazoxide (Proglycem), penicillamine (Cuprimine), penicillin, phenylbutazone, phenytoin (Dilantin), quinidine sulfate, quinine, salicylates, streptomycin, sulfonamides, thiazide and thiazidelike diuretics, and tricyclic antidepressants (possible decrease)
- Estrogens, oral contraceptives, excitement, high altitudes, persistent cold temperatures, or strenuous exercise (increase)

Precautions

- To prevent hemolysis, avoid excessive probing at the venipuncture site and handle the sample gently.

Nursing Considerations

Before the Test

- Confirm the patient's identity using two patient identifiers and confirmation of the patient's identification bracelet according to facility policy.
- Explain to the patient that the platelet count test is used to determine if the patient's blood clots normally.
- Advise the patient that a blood sample will be taken. Explain that slight discomfort from the needle puncture and the tourniquet may be experienced.
- Inform the patient that there are no food or fluid restrictions for this test.
- Notify the laboratory and health care provider of medications the patient is taking that may affect test results; these may need to be restricted.

During the Test

- Perform a venipuncture and collect the sample in a 3- or 4.5-mL EDTA tube.
- Completely fill the collection tube and invert it gently several times to mix the sample and the anticoagulant thoroughly.

After the Test

- Apply pressure to the venipuncture site until bleeding has stopped and to prevent hematoma formation.

P

- If a hematoma develops and is large, monitor pulses distal to the venipuncture site.
- Tell the patient to resume any medications that were discontinued before the test, as ordered.

Pleural Fluid Aspiration

Normal Findings
- Negative pressure
- Less than 20 mL of serous fluid

Abnormal Findings
- Transudative effusion, indicating ascites, systemic and pulmonary venous hypertension, heart failure, hepatic cirrhosis, or nephritis
- Exudative effusion, indicating lymphatic drainage interference, infection, pulmonary infarction, neoplasms, or pleurisy associated with rheumatoid arthritis
- Pathogens such as *Mycobacterium tuberculosis*, *Staphylococcus aureus*, *Streptococcus pneumoniae* and other streptococci, *Haemophilus influenzae*, and bacteroides (in ruptured pulmonary abscess)
- Serosanguineous fluid, indicating pleural extension of a malignant tumor
- Elevated lactate dehydrogenase level, indicating malignancy in nonpurulent, nonhemolyzed, nonbloody effusion
- Glucose level 30 to 40 mg/dL lower than blood glucose levels, indicating malignant tumor, bacterial infection, nonseptic inflammation, or metastasis
- Elevated amylase level, indicating pleural effusions associated with pancreatitis

Nursing Implications
- Report abnormal findings to the health care provider.
- Prepare to educate the patient about the diagnosis.
- Prepare the patient for further testing or surgery, as indicated.

- Provide emotional support to the patient and family.

Purpose
- To determine the cause and nature of pleural effusion
- To provide emergency relief of dyspnea related to pleural effusion
- To permit better radiographic visualization of a lung with large effusions
- To obtain specimens for cytologic, microbial, and pathologic examination

Description
The pleura, a two-layer membrane that covers the lungs and lines the thoracic cavity, maintains a small amount of lubricating fluid between its layers to minimize friction during respiration. Increased fluid in this space may result from such diseases as cancer or tuberculosis, or from blood or lymphatic disorders and can cause respiratory difficulty.

In pleural fluid aspiration (thoracentesis), the thoracic wall is punctured to obtain a specimen of pleural fluid for analysis or to relieve pulmonary (and possibly cardiac) compression and resultant respiratory distress.

The procedure for pleural fluid aspiration is as follows:

- The patient is positioned to widen the intercostal spaces and allow easier access to the pleural cavity. The patient must be well supported and comfortable, preferably seated at the edge of the bed with a chair or stool supporting the feet, and head and arms resting on a padded over-the-bed table. If the patient can't sit up, position on the unaffected side, with the arm on the affected side elevated above the head.
- After the patient is positioned, the health care provider disinfects the skin (when necessary, the needle insertion site is clipped), drapes the area, injects a local anesthetic into the subcutaneous tissue, and inserts the thoracentesis needle above the rib to avoid lacerating intercostal vessels. When

the needle reaches the pocket of fluid, the 50-mL syringe is attached and the stopcock and clamps are opened on the tubing to aspirate the fluid into the container.

- During aspiration, the patient is observed for signs of respiratory distress, such as weakness, dyspnea, pallor, cyanosis, changes in heart rate, tachypnea, diaphoresis, blood-tinged frothy mucus, and hypotension.
- After the needle is withdrawn, slight pressure and a small adhesive bandage is applied to the puncture site.

Interfering Factors

- Failure to use sterile technique
- Antimicrobial therapy before fluid aspiration for culture (possible decrease in numbers of bacteria, making it difficult to isolate the infecting organism)

Precautions

- Thoracentesis is contraindicated in the patient who has a history of bleeding disorders or anticoagulant therapy.
- Use strict sterile technique.

Nursing Considerations

Before the Test

- Confirm the patient's identity using two patient identifiers and confirmation of the patient's identification bracelet according to facility policy.
- Explain to the patient that pleural fluid analysis assesses the space around the lungs for fluid. Inform the patient who will perform the test and when and where it will be done.
- Inform the patient that there are no food or fluid restrictions for this test.
- Explain that chest X-rays or an ultrasound study may precede the test to help locate the fluid.
- Check the patient's history for hypersensitivity to local anesthetics.
- Warn the patient that a stinging sensation on injection of the anesthetic and some pressure during withdrawal

of the fluid may be experienced. Advise the patient not to cough, breathe deeply, or move during the test to minimize the risk of injury to the lung.

- Record the patient's baseline vital signs.
- Label all medications, medication containers, or other solutions on and off the sterile field.

After the Test

- Label the specimen container and record the date and time of the test and the amount, color, and character of the fluid (clear, frothy, purulent, bloody) on the laboratory request.
- Note on the laboratory request the patient's temperature and whether antimicrobial therapy is being administered.
- Send the specimen to the laboratory immediately after collection.
- Note any signs of distress exhibited during the procedure.
- Record the exact location from which the fluid was removed to aid diagnosis.
- Reposition the patient comfortably on the affected side. Tell the patient to remain on this side for at least 1 hour to seal the puncture site. Elevate the head of the bed to facilitate breathing.
- Monitor the patient's vital signs every 30 minutes for 2 hours and then every 4 hours until they're stable.
- Tell the patient to call a nurse immediately if experiencing difficulty breathing.

> ▶ *Quality and Safety Nursing Alert*

Watch the patient for signs of pneumothorax, tension pneumothorax, fluid reaccumulation, and, if a large amount of fluid was withdrawn, pulmonary edema or cardiac distress due to mediastinal shift. Usually, a posttest X-ray is ordered to detect these complications before clinical symptoms appear.

• Check the puncture site for fluid leakage. A large amount of leakage is abnormal. Also check the site and surrounding area for subcutaneous emphysema.

Pleural Tissue Biopsy

Normal Findings

• Mesothelial cells flattened in a uniform layer
• Areolar connective tissue layers containing blood vessels, nerves, and lymphatics below

Abnormal Findings

• Malignant disease
• Tuberculosis
• Viral, fungal, parasitic, or collagen vascular disease

Nursing Implications

• Report abnormal findings to the health care provider.
• Prepare to educate the patient about the diagnosis.
• Prepare the patient for further testing or surgery, as indicated.
• Provide emotional support to the patient and family.

Purpose

• To differentiate between nonmalignant and malignant disease
• To diagnose viral, fungal, or parasitic disease and collagen vascular disease of the pleura

Description

Pleural tissue biopsy is the removal of pleural tissue by needle biopsy or open biopsy for histologic examination. Needle pleural biopsy is performed under local anesthesia. It generally follows or is done in conjunction with thoracentesis (pleural fluid aspiration), which is performed when the effusion cause is unknown, but it can be performed separately.

Open pleural biopsy, performed in the absence of pleural effusion, permits direct visualization of the pleura and the underlying lung. It's performed in the operating room.

The procedure for pleural tissue biopsy is as follows:

• The patient is seated on the side of the bed, with the feet resting on a stool and the arms on the over-the-bed table or supported by the upper body. Inform the patient to hold this position and remain still during the procedure.
• The skin is prepped and draped.
• All medications, medication containers, or other solutions on and off the sterile field are labeled.
• The local anesthetic is administered.
• In a Vim-Silverman needle biopsy, a needle is inserted through the appropriate intercostal space into the biopsy site, with the outer tip distal to the pleura and the central portion pushed in deeper and held in place. The outer case is inserted about 3/8 inch (1 cm), the entire assembly is rotated 360 degrees, and the needle and tissue specimen are withdrawn. In Cope's needle biopsy, a trocar is introduced through the appropriate intercostal space into the biopsy site. To obtain the specimen, a hooked stylet is inserted through the trocar. As the outer tube is held stationary, the inner tube is twisted to cut off the tissue specimen, and the assembly is withdrawn.
• After the specimens are obtained, additional parietal fluid may be removed to treat the effusion.
• The specimen is immediately put into a 10% neutral buffered formalin solution in a labeled specimen bottle and sent to the laboratory.

Interfering Factors

• The patient's inability to remain still, keep from coughing, or follow instructions, such as "Hold your breath," during the procedure

Precautions

• Pleural biopsy is contraindicated in the patient with a severe bleeding disorder.

Nursing Considerations

Before the Test

- Confirm the patient's identity using two patient identifiers and confirmation of the patient's identification bracelet according to facility policy.
- Explain to the patient that the pleural tissue biopsy permits microscopic examination of pleural tissue.
- Describe the procedure to the patient and answer questions.
- Tell the patient who will perform the biopsy and when and where it will be done.
- Tell the patient that no fasting is required.
- Explain that blood studies will precede the biopsy, and chest X-rays will be taken before and after the biopsy.
- Make sure the patient or a responsible family member has signed an informed consent form.
- Advise the patient that a local anesthetic will be administered and that there should be minimal pain from the procedure. Check the patient's history for hypersensitivity to the anesthetic.
- Record the patient's vital signs just before the procedure.

After the Test

- Clean the skin around the biopsy site and apply an adhesive bandage.
- Make sure the chest X-ray is repeated immediately after the biopsy.
- Check the patient's vital signs every 15 minutes for 1 hour and then every hour for 4 hours or until stable.

▶ **Quality and Safety Nursing Alert**

Watch the patient for signs of respiratory distress (dyspnea), shoulder pain, and such complications as pneumothorax (immediate), pneumonia (delayed), and hemorrhage.

- Instruct the patient to lie on the unaffected side to promote healing of the biopsy site, as indicated.

Positron Emission Tomography (PET), Cardiac

Normal Findings

- No ischemic tissue areas
- Flow and distribution matching (if two tracers used)

Abnormal Findings

- Ischemia evidenced by reduced blood flow with increased glucose use
- Necrosis and scar tissue evidenced by reduced blood flow with decreased glucose use

Nursing Implications

- Anticipate the need for additional testing.
- Prepare the patient for follow-up and treatment.
- Provide emotional support to the patient and family.

Purpose

- To detect coronary artery disease
- To evaluate myocardial metabolism and contractility
- To distinguish viable from infarcted cardiac tissue, especially during the early stages of myocardial infarction

Description

Cardiac positron emission tomography (PET) scanning combines elements of computed tomographic scanning and conventional radionuclide imaging. Like radionuclide imaging, cardiac PET scans measure injected radioisotope emissions and convert these values to tomographic images. PET uses radioisotopes of biologically important elements—oxygen, nitrogen, carbon, and fluorine—which emit *positrons*. During positron emissions, gamma rays are detected by the PET scanner and reconstructed to form an image. One distinct advantage of PET scans is that positron emitters can be "tagged" chemically to biologically active molecules, such as carbon monoxide, neurotransmitters, hormones, and metabolites (particularly glucose), enabling study of their uptake and distribution in tissue.

P

The procedure for PET scans is as follows:

- The patient is placed in a supine position with the arms above the head.
- An attenuation scan, lasting about 30 minutes, is performed.
- The appropriate positron emitter is administered, and scanning is completed.
- An additional positron emitter may be given if comparative studies are needed.

Interfering Factors

- Patient's inability to maintain proper positioning

Nursing Considerations

Before the Test

- Confirm the patient's identity using two patient identifiers and confirmation of the patient's identification bracelet according to facility policy.
- Make certain that patient or a person responsible for the patient signs an informed consent form.
- Describe the procedure to the patient, including who will perform it, where it will take place, and the equipment to be used. Explain that the patient will undergo an attenuation scan for about 30 minutes, followed by the appropriate positron emitter and then the PET scan. The entire procedure may require from 1 to 3 hours or more.
- Tell the patient that the test is painless but slight discomfort from the tourniquet and the needle puncture may be experienced if an IV infusion is used.
- If fasting is ordered, describe food and fluid restrictions to the patient.
- Explain to the patient that a radioactive substance will be administered by injection or IV infusion and that a highly specialized camera will detect the radioactive decay of this substance and send data to a computer, which converts the data to an image.

▶ Quality and Safety Nursing Alert

Because the radioisotope may be harmful to a fetus, the female patient of childbearing age should be screened carefully before undergoing cardiac PET scanning.

- Stress to the patient the importance of remaining still during the study.

After the Test

- Instruct the patient to move slowly after the procedure to avoid postural hypotension.
- Encourage increased oral fluid intake to flush the radioisotope from the bladder.

Posturography

Normal Findings

- Normal vestibular, visual, and somatosensory balance (score of 100% indicates good stability; 0%, patient would have fallen without harness)
- Preference for visual, proprioceptive, or vestibular inputs
- Ankle or hip strategies (compensation for platform or visual surround motion)

Abnormal Findings

- Latency abnormalities, indicating extravestibular central nervous system lesions
- Strength differences between legs, indicating long-loop autonomic nervous system disorders and multiple sclerosis
- Spinocerebellar problems
- Range-of-motion limitations
- Ankle weakness
- Inability to suppress automatic reactions

Nursing Implications

- Report abnormal findings to the health care provider.
- Prepare to educate the patient about the diagnosis.

- Prepare the patient for further testing, as indicated.
- Provide emotional support to the patient and family.

Purpose

- To objectively determine the functional impairment associated with dizziness
- To determine the relative strengths and weaknesses of the vestibular system for establishing and monitoring the progress of a rehabilitation plan

Description

Balance involves the coordination of input from the vestibular system, from vision, and from proprioception. Posturography assesses the patient's ability to retain equilibrium when vision and proprioceptive input is removed.

A battery of tests is typically administered. Although the procedure for each test is somewhat specific to the equipment manufacturer, the general procedures are as follows:

Sensory Organization Test

- This test evaluates the person's ability to integrate information across the senses and to suppress information that results in sensory conflicts.
- The patient is placed in a harness, standing on a platform, while looking forward toward a screen that encompasses the entire visual field.
- The sensor on the platform measures the patient's sway and the strength and latency of leg movements that occur when the platform or visual field moves based on six test conditions:
    - The patient sees the screen in front, and the platform is fixed (eyes-open Romberg test).
    - The patient closes the eyes, and the platform remains fixed (eyes-closed Romberg test).
    - The visual field around the patient moves, and the platform remains fixed. The visual system information conflicts with the vestibular

and proprioceptive inputs. The patient with deficits in these areas experiences greater imbalance.
    - The platform moves, and the visual field remains fixed. The patient receives proprioceptive and vestibular input that differs from that of the visual system.
    - The patient's eyes are closed, and the platform moves. Proprioception and vestibular input are assessed.
    - The platform and screen in front move in concert. The three sensory systems work together to maintain balance.

Motor Control Test

- The platform makes a series of jerky motions, and the patient's responses are measured.

Adaptation Test

- The platform is tilted up or down, and the patient's ability to compensate for this movement during repetition of the platform tilt is analyzed.

Limit of Stability Test

- The patient leans as far as possible in different directions and responses are measured.

Interfering Factors

- Failure to consider orthopedic and musculoskeletal problems in interpreting the results and recommending a treatment plan
- Medications, such as vestibular suppressants or centrally acting medications

Nursing Considerations

Before the Test

- Confirm the patient's identity using two patient identifiers and confirmation of the patient's identification bracelet according to facility policy.
- Explain to the patient that posturography assesses how vision and motion affect the sense of balance. Advise of the need to stand on a platform during the test, that the platform can move, and that the

visual field in front will move. Assure that the patient won't fall during the test.

- Suggest that the patient wear comfortable, loose-fitting clothing; advise a woman to wear pants.
- Instruct the patient to refrain from taking nonessential medication for 48 hours before the test, as well as these agents, which can affect the results: alcoholic beverages, caffeine, tranquilizers, sleeping pills, antihistamines, antivertigo agents, opioids, and other medications that can create dizziness, including salicylates, antidepressants, diuretics, stimulants, and certain aminoglycoside antibiotics.
- Ask the patient to bring a list of medications to the evaluation.

After the Test
- Tell the patient to resume a usual diet and medications, as ordered.

Potassium, Serum
Reference Values
3.5 to 5 mEq/L (SI, 3.5–5 mmol/L)

Abnormal Findings
Elevated Levels
- Burn injuries
- Crush injuries
- Diabetic ketoacidosis
- Large blood transfusions
- Myocardial infarction
- Kidney failure
- Addison's disease (due to potassium buildup and sodium depletion)
- Anemia
- SIADH

Decreased Levels
- Aldosteronism
- Cushing syndrome
- Body fluids loss (such as long-term diuretic therapy, vomiting, or diarrhea)
- Excessive licorice ingestion
- Bartter's syndrome

- Draining wounds
- Cystic fibrosis
- Severe burns
- Alcoholism, chronic
- Osmotic hyperglycemia
- Respiratory alkalosis
- Diuretic, antibiotic, and mineralocorticoid administration
- Barium chloride poisoning
- Treatment of megaloblastic anemia with vitamin B_{12} or folic acid

Nursing Implications
- Report abnormal findings to the health care provider.
- Observe the patient with hyperkalemia (elevated levels) for weakness, malaise, nausea, diarrhea, colicky pain, muscle irritability progressing to flaccid paralysis, oliguria, and bradycardia.
- In patients with elevated levels, observe the electrocardiogram (ECG) for flattened P waves; a prolonged PR interval; a wide QRS complex; tall, tented T waves; and ST-segment depression.
- Observe the patient with hypokalemia (decreased levels) for decreased reflexes; a rapid, weak, irregular pulse; mental confusion; hypotension; anorexia; muscle weakness; and paresthesia.
- Monitor the ECG in a patient with decreased levels for a flattened T wave, ST-segment depression, and U-wave elevation.

Purpose
- To evaluate clinical signs of potassium excess (hyperkalemia) or potassium depletion (hypokalemia)
- To monitor renal function, acid–base balance, and glucose metabolism
- To evaluate neuromuscular and endocrine disorders
- To detect the origin of arrhythmias

Description
This test is used to measure serum levels of potassium, the major intracellular cation. Potassium helps to maintain

cellular osmotic equilibrium and regulate muscle activity, enzyme activity, and acid–base balance. It also influences renal function.

Potassium levels are affected by variations in the secretion of adrenal steroid hormones and by fluctuations in pH, serum glucose levels, and serum sodium levels. A reciprocal relationship appears to exist between potassium and sodium; a substantial intake of one element causes a corresponding decrease in the other. Although it readily conserves sodium, the body has no efficient method for conserving potassium. Even in potassium depletion, the kidneys continue to excrete potassium; therefore, potassium deficiency can develop rapidly and is quite common.

Because the kidneys excrete nearly all ingested potassium daily, a dietary intake of at least 40 mEq/day is essential. A normal diet usually includes 60 to 100 mEq of potassium. (See the *Treating Potassium Imbalance* box.)

Interfering Factors

• Repeated clenching of the fist before venipuncture (possible increase)
• Excessive or rapid potassium infusion, spironolactone or penicillin G potassium therapy, and renal toxicity from administration of amphotericin B or tetracycline (increase)
• Insulin and glucose administration; diuretic therapy (especially with thiazides but not with triamterene [Dyrenium], amiloride [Midamor], or spironolactone [Aldactone]); and IV infusions without potassium (decrease)

Precautions

• Draw the sample immediately after applying the tourniquet because a delay may increase the potassium level by allowing intracellular potassium to leak into the serum.
• Handle the sample gently to prevent hemolysis.
• In severe cases, ventricular fibrillation, respiratory paralysis, and cardiac

P

Treating Potassium Imbalance

Hypokalemia and hyperkalemia can cause serious problems if not treated promptly.

Hypokalemia

A patient with a potassium deficiency can be treated with oral potassium chloride replacement and increased dietary intake. In severe cases, potassium can cautiously be replaced by IV infusion at a rate not exceeding 20 mEq/hour and at a concentration of no more than 80 mEq/L of IV fluid. Mix the potassium well in the IV solution because it can settle near the neck of the bottle or plastic bag. Failure to mix the solution adequately or to infuse it properly can cause a burning sensation at the IV site and possibly even fatal hyperkalemia. If the patient complains of severe burning, slow the rate of the infusion.

Potassium is never administered by IV push or intramuscularly to avoid replacing potassium too quickly. IV potassium must be administered using an infusion pump. Monitor the electrocardiogram, urine output, and serum potassium levels frequently during the infusion. Never administer IV potassium replacement to a patient with inadequate urine flow because diminished excretion can rapidly lead to hyperkalemia.

Hyperkalemia

Dangerously high potassium levels may be reduced with sodium polystyrene sulfonate—a potassium-removing resin—administered orally, rectally, or through a nasogastric tube. Hyperkalemia may also be treated with an IV infusion of sodium bicarbonate or of glucose and insulin, which lowers blood potassium by causing it to move into cells.

A calcium IV infusion provides fast but transient relief from the cardiotoxic effects of hyperkalemia; however, it doesn't directly lower serum potassium levels. In kidney failure, dialysis may help remove excess potassium, but this procedure corrects the imbalance much more slowly.

arrest can develop. (Cardiac arrest may occur without warning.)

Nursing Considerations

Before the Test

- Confirm the patient's identity using two patient identifiers and confirmation of the patient's identification bracelet according to facility policy.
- Explain to the patient that the serum potassium test is used to determine the potassium content of blood.
- Advise the patient that the test requires a blood sample. Explain that slight discomfort from the needle puncture and the tourniquet may be experienced.
- Inform the patient that there are no food or fluid restrictions for this test.
- Notify the laboratory and physician of medications the patient is taking that may affect test results; these may need to be restricted.

During the Test

- Perform a venipuncture. Collect the sample in a 3- or 4-mL clot activator tube.

After the Test

- Apply direct pressure to the venipuncture site until bleeding stops and to prevent hematoma formation.
- Tell the patient to resume medications that were discontinued before the test, as ordered.

Potassium, Urine

Reference Values

Adults: 25 to 125 mmol/24 hours (SI, 25–125 mmol/day)

Children: 10 to 60 mmol/24 hours (SI, 10–60 mmol/day)

Abnormal Findings

Elevated Levels

- Dehydration
- Starvation
- Cushing disease
- Salicylate intoxication
- Renal loss of potassium (such as in aldosteronism), renal tubular acidosis, or chronic kidney disease (above 10 mmol/24 hours [SI, greater than 10 mmol/day] and lasting more than 3 days)

Decreased Levels

- Malabsorption syndrome
- Addison's disease
- Diarrhea
- Hyperkalemia
- Hypomagnesemia
- Nephrotic syndrome
- Kidney failure
- SIADH

Nursing Implications

- Report abnormal findings to the health care provider.
- Prepare to educate the patient about the diagnosis.
- Prepare the patient for further testing or surgery, as indicated.
- Prepare the patient with elevated levels for hemodialysis or charcoal administration to treat salicylate toxication, as indicated.

Purpose

- To determine whether hypokalemia is caused by renal or extrarenal disorders

Description

The urine potassium test quantitatively measures urine levels of potassium, a major intracellular cation that helps regulate acid–base balance and neuromuscular function. Potassium imbalance may cause such signs and symptoms as muscle weakness, nausea, diarrhea, confusion, hypotension, and electrocardiogram changes; severe imbalance may lead to cardiac arrest.

In most cases, a serum potassium test is performed to detect hyperkalemia (abnormally high levels) or hypokalemia (abnormally low levels). However, a urine potassium test may also be ordered to evaluate hypokalemia when a history and physical examination fail to uncover the cause. If results suggest a renal disorder, additional renal function tests may be ordered.

Interfering Factors

- Excess dietary potassium (increase)
- Contamination of the specimen with toilet tissue or stools
- Potassium-wasting medications, such as acetazolamide (Dazamide), ammonium chloride, and thiazide diuretics (increase)
- Excess vomiting or stomach suctioning

Precautions

- Warn the patient to avoid contaminating the specimen with toilet tissue or stools.
- Don't use a metallic bedpan for collection.
- Refrigerate the specimen or place it on ice during the collection period.

Nursing Considerations

Before the Test

- Confirm the patient's identity using two patient identifiers and confirmation of the patient's identification bracelet according to facility policy.
- Explain to the patient that the urine potassium test evaluates kidney function and that it requires collecting urine over a 24-hour period.
- If the specimen is to be collected at home, teach the patient the correct collection technique.
- Advise the patient that no special dietary restrictions are necessary.
- Notify the laboratory and health care provider of medications the patient is taking that may affect test results; these may need to be restricted.

During the Test

- Collect the patient's urine over a 24-hour period, discarding the first specimen and retaining the last.
- Send the specimen to the laboratory immediately after the collection is completed or refrigerate it.
- Administer potassium supplements and monitor serum levels, as appropriate.
- Provide dietary supplements and nutritional counseling, as necessary.
- Replace fluid volume loss with IV or oral fluids, as necessary.

After the Test

- Tell the patient to resume usual medications, as ordered.

Prostate-Specific Antigen

Reference Values

Ages 40 to 49: 0 to 2.5 ng/mL
   (SI, 0–2.5 mcg/L)
Ages 50 to 59: 0 to 3.5 ng/mL
   (SI, 0–3.5 mcg/L)
Ages 60 to 69: 0 to 4.5 ng/mL
   (SI, 0–4.5 mcg/L)
Ages 70 and older: 0 to 6.5 ng/mL
   (SI, 0–6.5 mcg/L)

Abnormal Findings

Elevated Levels (Greater Than 4 ng/mL)

- Prostate cancer (pretreatment level in 80% of patients)
- Benign prostatic hyperplasia (pretreatment level in 20% of patients)

Nursing Implications

- Report abnormal findings to the health care provider.
- Refer the patient for further assessment and testing, including tissue biopsy, to confirm prostate cancer because prostate-specific antigen (PSA) results alone don't confirm a diagnosis.

Purpose

- To screen for prostate cancer in men older than age 50
- To monitor prostate cancer's course and evaluate treatment

Description

Because PSA appears in normal, benign hyperplastic, and malignant prostatic tissue, as well as in metastatic prostatic carcinoma, serum PSA levels are used to monitor the presence, spread, or recurrence of prostate cancer and to evaluate the patient's response to treatment. Measurement of serum PSA levels, along with a digital rectal examination, is the recommended screening test for prostate cancer in men older than age 50, replacing the older prostatic acid phosphatase measurement. It's also useful in assessing response to treatment in a patient with stage B3 to D1 prostate cancer and in detecting the spread or recurrence of malignancy.

Interfering Factors
- Excessive doses of chemotherapeutic drugs, such as cyclophosphamide (Cytoxan), diethylstilbestrol, and methotrexate (MTX) (possible increase or decrease)
- Rectal or prostate exam within 24 hours prior to test

Precautions
- Collect the sample either before digital prostate examination or at least 48 hours after examination to avoid falsely elevated PSA levels.
- Handle the sample gently to prevent hemolysis.

Nursing Considerations
Before the Test
- Confirm the patient's identity using two patient identifiers and confirmation of the patient's identification bracelet according to facility policy.
- Explain to the patient that the PSA test is used to screen for prostate cancer or, if appropriate, to monitor the course of treatment.
- Advise the patient that the test requires a blood sample. Explain that he may experience slight discomfort from the needle puncture and the tourniquet.
- Inform the patient that he doesn't need to restrict food and fluids for the test.

During the Test
- Perform a venipuncture and collect the sample in a 7-mL clot activator tube.
- Immediately put the sample on ice and send it to the laboratory.

After the Test
- Apply direct pressure to the venipuncture site until bleeding stops and to prevent hematoma formation.

Protein Electrophoresis
Reference Values
Total serum protein levels: 6.4 to 8.3 g/dL (SI, 64–83 g/L)
Albumin fraction: 3.5 to 5 g/dL (SI, 35–50 g/L)
Alpha$_1$-globulin fraction: 0.1 to 0.3 g/dL (SI, 1–3 g/L)
Alpha$_2$-globulin: 0.6 to 1 g/dL (SI, 6–10 g/L)
Beta globulin: 0.7 to 1.1 g/dL (SI, 7–11 g/L)
Gamma globulin: 0.8 to 1.6 g/dL (SI, 8–16 g/L)

Abnormal Findings
- See the *Clinical Implications of Abnormal Protein Levels* box for specific information.

Nursing Implications
- Report abnormal results to the health care provider.
- Educate the patient and family about the diagnosis.
- Prepare the patient for additional testing, as necessary.
- Administer medications, as ordered.

Purpose
- To help diagnose hepatic disease, protein deficiency, renal disorders, and GI and neoplastic diseases

Description
Protein electrophoresis is used to measure serum albumin and globulin, the major blood proteins, by separating the proteins into five distinct fractions: albumin and alpha$_1$, alpha$_2$, beta, and gamma globulin proteins.

Interfering Factors
- Pretest administration of a contrast agent, such as sulfobromophthalein (false-high total protein)
- Cytotoxic drugs or pregnancy (possible decrease in serum albumin)
- Plasma use instead of serum

Clinical Implications of Abnormal Protein Levels

The clinical implications of abnormally increased and decreased protein levels are shown below.

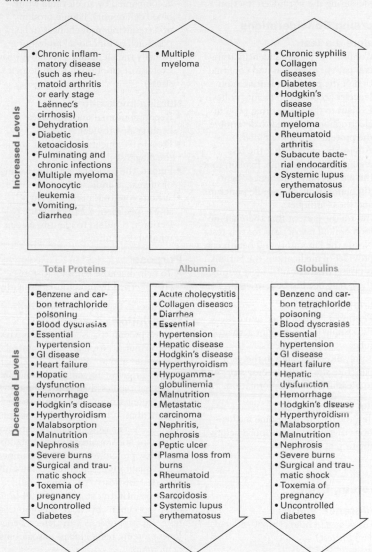

Increased Levels

Total Proteins
- Chronic inflammatory disease (such as rheumatoid arthritis or early stage Laënnec's cirrhosis)
- Dehydration
- Diabetic ketoacidosis
- Fulminating and chronic infections
- Multiple myeloma
- Monocytic leukemia
- Vomiting, diarrhea

Albumin
- Multiple myeloma

Globulins
- Chronic syphilis
- Collagen diseases
- Diabetes
- Hodgkin's disease
- Multiple myeloma
- Rheumatoid arthritis
- Subacute bacterial endocarditis
- Systemic lupus erythematosus
- Tuberculosis

Decreased Levels

Total Proteins
- Benzene and carbon tetrachloride poisoning
- Blood dyscrasias
- Essential hypertension
- GI disease
- Heart failure
- Hepatic dysfunction
- Hemorrhage
- Hodgkin's disease
- Hyperthyroidism
- Malabsorption
- Malnutrition
- Nephrosis
- Severe burns
- Surgical and traumatic shock
- Toxemia of pregnancy
- Uncontrolled diabetes

Albumin
- Acute cholecystitis
- Collagen diseases
- Diarrhea
- Essential hypertension
- Hepatic disease
- Hodgkin's disease
- Hyperthyroidism
- Hypogammaglobulinemia
- Malnutrition
- Metastatic carcinoma
- Nephritis, nephrosis
- Peptic ulcer
- Plasma loss from burns
- Rheumatoid arthritis
- Sarcoidosis
- Systemic lupus erythematosus

Globulins
- Benzene and carbon tetrachloride poisoning
- Blood dyscrasias
- Essential hypertension
- GI disease
- Heart failure
- Hepatic dysfunction
- Hemorrhage
- Hodgkin's disease
- Hyperthyroidism
- Malabsorption
- Malnutrition
- Nephrosis
- Severe burns
- Surgical and traumatic shock
- Toxemia of pregnancy
- Uncontrolled diabetes

P

Precautions
- Protein electrophoresis must be performed on a serum sample to avoid measuring the fibrinogen fraction.

Nursing Considerations
Before the Test
- Confirm the patient's identity using two patient identifiers and confirmation of the patient's identification bracelet according to facility policy.
- Explain to the patient that protein electrophoresis is used to determine the protein content of blood.
- Advise the patient that the test requires a blood sample. Explain that the patient may experience slight discomfort from the needle puncture and the tourniquet.
- Inform the patient that there are no food or fluid restrictions for this test.
- Notify the laboratory and health care provider of medications the patient is taking that may affect test results; these may need to be restricted.

During the Test
- Perform a venipuncture and collect the sample in a 7-mL clot activator tube.
- Apply direct pressure to the venipuncture site until bleeding stops and to prevent hematoma formation.

After the Test
- Tell the patient to resume medications that were discontinued before the test, as ordered.

Protein, Urine

Reference Values
50 to 80 mg/24 hours (SI, 50–80 mg/day) (at rest)

Abnormal Findings
- Presence of protein in urine, indicating chronic pyelonephritis, acute or chronic glomerulonephritis, amyloidosis, or toxic nephropathies in diseases where renal failure typically develops

as a late complication (such as diabetes or heart failure), nephrotic syndrome, urinary tract infection (when accompanied by an elevated white blood cell count), benign proteinuria (resulting from changes in body position), or functional proteinuria (usually transient and associated with exercise or emotional or physiologic stress)

Nursing Implications
- Report abnormal findings to the health care provider.
- Prepare to educate the patient about the diagnosis.
- Prepare the patient for further testing or surgery, as indicated.
- When proteinuria is present in a single specimen, a 24-hour urine collection is required to identify specific renal abnormalities.

Purpose
- To help diagnose pathologic states characterized by proteinuria, primarily renal disease

Description
A urine protein test is a quantitative test for proteinuria. Normally, the glomerular membrane allows only low-molecular-weight proteins to enter the filtrate. The renal tubules then reabsorb most of these proteins, normally excreting a small amount that's undetectable by a screening test. A damaged glomerular capillary membrane and impaired tubular reabsorption allow protein excretion in the urine.

A qualitative screening commonly precedes this test. A positive result requires quantitative analysis of a 24-hour urine specimen by acid precipitation tests. Electrophoresis can detect Bence Jones proteins, hemoglobins, myoglobins, or albumin.

Interfering Factors
- Contamination of the specimen with toilet tissue or stools
- Acetazolamide, cephalosporins, iodine-containing contrast media,

para-aminosalicylic acid, penicillin, sodium bicarbonate, sulfonamides, and tolbutamide (possible false positive or false negative)
• Very dilute urine, such as from forcing fluids, possibly depressing protein values and causing false-negative results

Precautions
• Warn the patient not to contaminate the urine with toilet tissue or stools.
• Refrigerate the specimen or place it on ice during the collection period.

Nursing Considerations
Before the Test
• Confirm the patient's identity using two patient identifiers and confirmation of the patient's identification bracelet according to facility policy.
• Explain to the patient that the urine protein test detects proteins in the urine.
• Inform the patient that there are no food or fluid restrictions for this test.
• Tell the patient that the test usually requires urine collection over a 24-hour period; random collection can be done.
• Notify the laboratory and health care provider of medications the patient is taking that may affect test results; these may need to be restricted.

During the Test
• Collect the patient's urine over a 24-hour period, discarding the first specimen and retaining the last. A special specimen container can be obtained from the laboratory.

After the Test
• Tell the patient to resume usual medications, as ordered.

Prothrombin Time

Reference Values
10 to 14 seconds (SI, 10–14 seconds)
For a patient receiving oral anticoagulants:
1 to 2½ times the normal control value

Abnormal Findings
• Prolonged prothrombin time (PT) (exceeding 2½ times the control value; may result from deficiencies in fibrinogen, prothrombin, vitamin K, or factor V, VII, or X)

Nursing Implications
• Report abnormal findings to the health care provider.
• Prepare to adjust the patient's anticoagulant dosage, as indicated.

Purpose
• To evaluate the extrinsic coagulation system (factors V, VII, and X, and prothrombin and fibrinogen)
• To monitor response to oral anticoagulant therapy

Description
PT measures the time required for a fibrin clot to form in a citrated plasma sample after the addition of calcium ions and tissue thromboplastin (factor III).

Interfering Factors
• Salicylates, more than 1 g/day (increase)
• Fibrin or fibrin split products in the sample or plasma fibrinogen levels greater than 100 mg/dL (possible prolonged PT)
• Antihistamines, chloral hydrate, corticosteroids, digoxin (Lanoxin), diuretics, glutethimide, griseofulvin, progestin–estrogen combinations, pyrazinamide, vitamin K, and xanthines, such as caffeine and theophylline (Theo-Dur) (possible decrease)
• Anabolic steroids, cholestyramine resin, corticotropin, heparin IV (within 5 hours of sample collection), indomethacin (Indocin), mefenamic acid (Ponstel), methimazole (Tapazole), phenylbutazone, phenytoin (Dilantin), propylthiouracil (PTU), quinidine, quinine, thyroid hormones, vitamin A, or alcohol in excess (prolonged PT)
• Antibiotics, barbiturates, hydroxyzine (Vistaril), mineral oil, or sulfonamides (possible increase or decrease)

Precautions

- To prevent hemolysis, avoid excessive probing during venipuncture and handle the sample gently.

Nursing Considerations

Before the Test

- Confirm the patient's identity using two patient identifiers and confirmation of the patient's identification bracelet according to facility policy.
- Explain to the patient that the PT test is used to determine if the blood clots normally. When appropriate, explain that this test is used to monitor the effects of oral anticoagulants; the test will be performed daily when therapy begins and will be repeated at longer intervals when medication levels stabilize.
- Advise the patient that a blood sample will be taken. Explain that the patient may feel slight discomfort from the needle puncture and the tourniquet.
- Inform the patient that there are no food or fluid restrictions for this test.
- Notify the laboratory and health care provider of medications the patient is taking that may affect test results; these may need to be restricted.

During the Test

- Perform a venipuncture and collect the sample in a 3- or 4.5-mL siliconized tube.
- Completely fill the collection tube and invert it gently several times to mix the sample and the anticoagulant thoroughly. If the tube isn't filled to the correct volume, an excess of citrate appears in the sample.

After the Test

- Apply direct pressure to the venipuncture site until bleeding stops and to prevent hematoma formation.
- If the hematoma is large, monitor pulses distal to the venipuncture site.
- Tell the patient to resume any usual medications discontinued before the test, as ordered.

Pulmonary Angiography

Normal Findings

- Symmetrical and uninterrupted contrast flow through the pulmonary circulatory system

Abnormal Findings

- Interruption of blood flow, indicating pulmonary emboli, vascular abnormalities, or tumors

Nursing Implications

- Report abnormal findings to the health care provider.
- Prepare to educate the patient about the diagnosis.
- Prepare the patient for further testing or surgery, as indicated.
- Provide emotional support to the patient and family.

Purpose

- To detect pulmonary embolism when less invasive studies are nondiagnostic
- To evaluate pulmonary circulation abnormalities
- To evaluate pulmonary circulation preoperatively in the patient with congenital heart disease
- To locate a large embolus before surgical removal

Description

Also called *pulmonary arteriography*, pulmonary angiography is the radiographic examination of the pulmonary circulation following injection of a radiopaque iodine contrast agent into the pulmonary artery or one of its branches.

The procedure for this test is as follows:

- After the patient is placed in a supine position, a local anesthetic is injected and the cardiac monitor is attached to the patient. Blood pressure and pulse oximeter are monitored, per facility protocol.
- A puncture is made at the procedure site, and a catheter is introduced into the antecubital or femoral vein. As the catheter passes through the right

atrium, the right ventricle, and the pulmonary artery, pressures are measured and blood samples are drawn from various regions of the pulmonary circulation.

- The contrast medium is injected and circulates through the pulmonary artery and lung capillaries while X-rays are taken.
- Pressure is applied over the catheter insertion site for 15 to 20 minutes or until bleeding stops.

This procedure carries certain risks and the patient should be monitored closely for possible complications, including arterial occlusion or rupture, myocardial perforation or rupture, ventricular arrhythmias from myocardial irritation, and acute kidney injury from hypersensitivity to the contrast agent.

Precautions

- Pulmonary angiography is contraindicated during pregnancy.
- Monitor the patient for ventricular arrhythmias caused by myocardial irritation from passage of the catheter through the heart chambers.

> ▶ *Quality and Safety Nursing Alert*
>
> Observe the patient for signs of hypersensitivity to the contrast agent, such as dyspnea, nausea, vomiting, sweating, increased heart rate, and numbness of extremities. Keep emergency equipment available in case of a hypersensitivity reaction to the contrast agent and procedural complications.

Nursing Considerations

Before the Test

- Confirm the patient's identity using two patient identifiers and confirmation of the patient's identification bracelet according to facility policy.
- Explain to the patient that this test permits evaluation of the blood vessels to help identify the cause of the patient's symptoms.

- Instruct the patient to fast for 8 hours before the test, or as prescribed. Tell the patient who will perform the test, where it will take place, and that laboratory work for kidney function and coagulation may precede the test.
- Advise the patient that a small puncture will be made in the blood vessel of the right arm where blood samples are usually drawn, or in the right groin at the femoral vein, and that a local anesthetic will be used to numb the area. Inform the patient that a small catheter will then be inserted into the blood vessel and passed into the right side of the heart to the pulmonary artery.
- Also advise the patient that contrast medium will then be injected into this artery. Explain that the patient may feel flushed, experience an urge to cough, or have a salty taste for approximately 3 to 5 minutes after the injection. Check the patient's history for hypersensitivity to anesthetics, iodine, seafood, or radiographic contrast agents.
- Explain that the patient's heart rate will be monitored continuously during the procedure and that the patient should tell the health care provider or nurse of any concerns.
- Make sure that the patient or a responsible family member has signed an informed consent form.
- Obtain or check laboratory tests (including prothrombin time, partial thromboplastin time, platelet count, INR, and blood urea nitrogen [BUN] and serum creatinine levels) and notify the radiologist of any abnormal results. IV hydration may need to be considered depending on the patient's renal and cardiac status. The radiologist may want to discontinue a heparin drip 3 to 4 hours before the test.

After the Test

- Maintain the patient on bed rest for about 6 hours.

- Observe the site for bleeding and swelling. If either occurs, maintain pressure at the insertion site for 10 minutes and notify the radiologist.
- Check the patient's blood pressure and pulse rate, distal pulses, and the catheter insertion site (arm or groin) every 15 minutes for 1 hour, every hour for 4 hours, and at regular intervals per facility policy.
- Observe the patient for signs of myocardial perforation or rupture by monitoring vital signs.
- Be alert for signs of acute kidney injury, such as sudden onset of oliguria, nausea, and vomiting. Check BUN and serum creatinine levels.
- Check the catheter insertion site for inflammation or hematoma formation, and report symptoms of a delayed hypersensitivity response to the contrast agent or local anesthetic (dyspnea, itching, tachycardia, palpitations, hypotension or hypertension, excitation, or euphoria).
- Advise the patient of any activity restrictions. Instruct the patient to resume a usual diet after the test (encourage drinking of fluids), or administer IV fluids (as ordered) to flush the contrast agent from the body, as ordered.
- Measure pulmonary artery pressures. Right ventricular end-diastolic pressure is usually less than or equal to 20 mm Hg, and pulmonary artery systolic pressure is usually less than or equal to 70 mm Hg. Pressures greater than this increase the risk of mortality associated with this procedure.

Pulmonary Function Tests

Reference Values
Values are based on age, height, weight, and sex (expressed as a percentage); values greater than 80% are considered normal.

Tidal volume (V_T): 5 to 7 mL/kg of body weight

Expiratory reserve volume (ERV): 25% of vital capacity (VC)

Inspiratory capacity (IC): 75% of VC

Forced expiratory volume (FEV_1): 83% of VC (after 1 second)

FEV_2: 94% of VC (after 2 seconds)

FEV_3: 97% of VC (after 3 seconds)

Abnormal Findings
- Values less than 80% (See the *Interpreting Pulmonary Function Tests* table for more information)

Nursing Implications
- Report abnormal findings to the health care provider.
- Prepare to educate the patient about the diagnosis.
- Prepare the patient for further testing, as indicated.
- Provide emotional support to the patient and family.
- Prepare to administer any medications or oxygen therapy, as indicated.

Purpose
- To determine the cause of dyspnea
- To assess the effectiveness of specific therapeutic regimens
- To determine whether a functional abnormality is obstructive or restrictive
- To measure pulmonary dysfunction
- To evaluate a patient before surgery
- To evaluate a person as part of a job screening (firefighting, for example)

Description
The pulmonary function tests series (volume, capacity, and flow rate) evaluates ventilatory function through spirometric measurements on patients with suspected pulmonary dysfunction.

Of the seven tests used to determine volume, V_T and ERV are direct spirographic measurements; minute volume, carbon dioxide response, inspiratory reserve volume, and residual volume are calculated from the results of other pulmonary function tests; and thoracic gas volume (TGV) is calculated from body plethysmography.

(text continues on page 440)

Interpreting Pulmonary Function Tests

This table includes the calculation method and implications of pulmonary function tests.

Pulmonary Function Test	Method of Calculation	Implications
Tidal Volume (V_T)		
Amount of air inhaled or exhaled during normal breathing	Determining the spirographic measurement for 10 breaths and then dividing by 10	Decreased V_T may indicate restrictive disease and requires further testing, such as full pulmonary function studies or chest X-rays.
Minute Volume (MV)		
Total amount of air expired per minute	Multiplying V_T by the respiratory rate	Normal MV can occur in emphysema; decreased MV may indicate other diseases, such as pulmonary edema. Increased MV can occur with acidosis, increased CO_2, decreased partial pressure of arterial oxygen, exercise, and low compliance states.
Carbon Dioxide (CO_2) Response		
Increase or decrease in MV after breathing various CO_2 concentrations	Plotting changes in MV against increasing inspired CO_2 concentrations	Reduced CO_2 response may occur in emphysema, myxedema, obesity, hypoventilation syndrome, and sleep apnea.
Inspiratory Reserve Volume (IRV)		
Amount of air inspired over above-normal inspiration	Subtracting V_T from inspiratory capacity (IC)	Abnormal IRV alone doesn't indicate respiratory dysfunction; IRV decreases during normal exercise.
Expiratory Reserve Volume (ERV)		
Amount of air exhaled after normal expiration	Direct spirographic measurement	ERV varies, even in healthy people, but usually decreases in obese people.
Residual Volume (RV)		
Amount of air remaining in the lungs after forced expiration	Subtracting ERV from functional residual capacity (FRC)	RV greater than 35% of total lung capacity (TLC) after maximal expiratory effort may indicate obstructive disease.

(continued on page 438)

Interpreting Pulmonary Function Tests (continued)

Pulmonary Function Test	Method of Calculation	Implications
Vital Capacity (VC)		
Total volume of air that can be exhaled after maximum inspiration	Direct spirographic measurement or adding V_T, IRV, and ERV	Normal or increased VC with decreased flow rates may indicate any condition that causes a reduction in functional pulmonary tissue, such as pulmonary edema. Decreased VC with normal or increased flow rates may indicate decreased respiratory effort resulting from neuromuscular disease, drug overdose, or head injury; decreased thoracic expansion; or limited diaphragm movement.
Inspiratory Capacity (IC)		
Amount of air that can be inhaled after normal expiration	Direct spirographic measurement or adding IRV and V_T	Decreased IC indicates restrictive disease.
Thoracic Gas Volume (TGV)		
Total volume of gas in the lungs from ventilated and nonventilated airways	Body plethysmography	Increased TGV indicates air trapping, which may result from obstructive disease.
Functional Residual Capacity (FRC)		
Amount of air remaining in the lungs after normal expiration	Nitrogen washout, helium dilution technique, or adding ERV and RV	Increased FRC indicates overdistention of the lungs, which may result from obstructive pulmonary disease.
Total Lung Capacity (TLC)		
Total volume of the lungs when maximally inflated	Adding V_T, IRV, ERV, and RV; FRC and IC; or VC and RV	Low TLC indicates restrictive disease; high TLC indicates overdistended lungs caused by obstructive disease.
Forced Vital Capacity (FVC)		
Amount of air exhaled forcefully and quickly after maximum inspiration	Direct spirographic measurement; expressed as a percentage of the total volume of gas exhaled	Decreased FVC indicates flow resistance in the respiratory system from obstructive disease, such as chronic bronchitis, or from restrictive disease, such as pulmonary fibrosis.

Pulmonary Function Test	Method of Calculation	Implications
Flow-Volume Curve (also called flow-volume loop)		
Greatest rate of flow (V_{max}) during FVC maneuvers versus lung volume change	Direct spirographic measurement at 1-second intervals; calculated from flow rates (expressed in L/second) and lung volume changes (expressed in liters) during maximal inspiratory and expiratory maneuvers	Decreased flow rates at all volumes during expiration indicate obstructive disease of the small airways, such as emphysema. A plateau of expiratory flow near TLC, a plateau of inspiratory flow at mid-VC, and a square wave pattern through most of VC indicate obstructive disease of large airways. Normal or increased PEFR, decreased flow with decreasing lung volumes, and markedly decreased VC indicate restrictive disease.
Forced Expiratory Volume (FEV)		
Volume of air expired in the first, second, or third second of an FVC maneuver	Direct spirographic measurement; expressed as a percentage of FVC	Decreased FEV_1 and increased FEV_2 and FEV_3 may indicate obstructive disease; decreased or normal FEV_1 may indicate restrictive disease.
Forced Expiratory Flow (FEF)		
Average rate of flow during the middle half of FVC	Calculated from the flow rate and the time needed for expiration of the middle 50% of FVC	Low FEF (25% to 75%) indicates obstructive disease of the small and medium-sized airways.
Peak Expiratory Flow Rate (PEFR)		
V_{max} during forced expiration	Calculated from the flow-volume curve or by direct spirographic measurement using a pneumotachometer or electronic tachometer with a transducer to convert flow to electrical output display	Decreased PEFR may indicate a mechanical problem, such as upper airway obstruction, or obstructive disease. PEFR is usually normal in restrictive disease but decreases in severe cases. Because PEFR is effort dependent, it's also low in a person who has poor expiratory effort or doesn't understand the procedure.

P

(continued on page 440)

Interpreting Pulmonary Function Tests (continued)

Pulmonary Function Test	Method of Calculation	Implications
Maximal Voluntary Ventilation (MVV) (also called maximum breathing capacity)		
Greatest volume of air breathed per unit of time	Direct spirographic measurement	Decreased MVV may indicate obstructive disease; normal or decreased MVV may indicate restrictive disease such as myasthenia gravis.
Peak Expiratory Flow Rate (PEFR)		
Milliliters of CO diffused per minute across the alveolocapillary membrane	Calculated from analysis of the amount of carbon monoxide exhaled compared with the amount inhaled	Decreased DLCO due to a thickened alveolocapillary membrane occurs in interstitial pulmonary diseases, such as pulmonary fibrosis, asbestosis, and sarcoidosis; DLCO is reduced in emphysema because of alveolocapillary membrane loss.

Of the pulmonary capacity tests, VC, IC, functional residual capacity (FRC), total lung capacity, and forced expiratory flow may be measured directly or calculated from the results of other tests. Forced vital capacity (FVC), flow–volume curve, FEV, peak expiratory flow rate, and maximal voluntary ventilation (MVV) are direct spirographic measurements. Diffusing capacity for carbon monoxide (DL_{CO}) is calculated from the amount of CO exhaled.

The procedures for pulmonary function tests are as follows:

V_T
- The patient is instructed to breathe normally into the mouthpiece 5 times.

ERV
- The patient is instructed to breathe normally for several breaths and then to exhale as completely as possible.

VC
- The patient is instructed to inhale as deeply as possible and to exhale into the mouthpiece as completely as possible.

- This procedure is repeated three times, and the test result showing the largest volume is used.

IC
- The patient is instructed to breathe normally for several breaths and then to inhale as deeply as possible.

FRC
- The patient is instructed to breathe normally into a spirometer that contains a known concentration of an insoluble gas (usually helium or nitrogen) in a known volume of air.
- After a few breaths, the gas concentrations in the spirometer and in the lungs reach equilibrium. Then the equilibrium point and the gas concentration in the spirometer are recorded.

TGV
- The patient is put in an airtight box (or body plethysmograph) and told to breathe through a tube connected to a transducer.

- At end expiration, the tube is occluded, the patient is told to pant, and changes in intrathoracic and plethysmographic pressures are measured. The results are used to calculate total TGV and FRC.

FVC and FEV

- The patient is instructed to inhale as slowly and deeply as possible, and then exhale into the mouthpiece as quickly and completely as possible.
- This procedure is repeated three times, and the largest volume is recorded. The volume of air expired at 1 second (FEV_1), at 2 seconds (FEV_2), and at 3 seconds (FEV_3) during all three repetitions also is recorded.

MVV

- The patient is instructed to breathe into the mouthpiece as quickly and deeply as possible for 15 seconds.

DL_{CO}

- The patient inhales a gas mixture with a low concentration of CO and then holds the breath for 10 seconds before exhaling.

Interfering Factors

- Hypoxia, metabolic disturbances, or lack of patient cooperation
- Gastric distention or pregnancy (possible lung volume displacement)
- Opioid analgesics or sedatives (possible decrease in inspiratory and expiratory forces)
- Bronchodilators (possible temporary improvement in pulmonary function)

Precautions

- Pulmonary function tests are contraindicated in the patient with acute

coronary insufficiency, angina, or recent myocardial infarction.
- Watch the patient for respiratory distress; changes in pulse rate, pulse oximetry, and blood pressure; and coughing or bronchospasm.

Nursing Considerations

Before the Test

- Confirm the patient's identity using two patient identifiers and confirmation of the patient's identification bracelet according to facility policy.
- Explain to the patient that these tests evaluate pulmonary function. Describe the testing procedure and equipment (such as a spirometer) used.
- Instruct the patient to eat only a light meal and not to smoke for 12 hours before the tests.
- Explain that the accuracy of the tests depends on the patient's cooperation. Assure the patient that the procedures are painless and that rest will be available between tests.
- Inform the laboratory if the patient is taking an analgesic that depresses respiration.
- Withhold bronchodilators for 4 to 8 hours, as ordered.
- Just before the test, tell the patient to void and to loosen tight clothing. Explain that if the patient wears dentures, they should be worn during the test to help form a seal around the mouthpiece. Advise the patient to put on the nose clip so that it can be adjusted before the test.

After the Test

- Instruct the patient to resume usual activities, diet, and medications, as ordered.

P

Q

Quantitative Immunoglobulins: IgA, IgG, and IgM

Reference Values

Adults
- IgA: 60 to 400 mg/dL (SI, 0.6–4 g/L)
- IgG: 700 to 1,500 mg/dL (SI, 7–15 g/L)
- IgM: 60 to 300 mg/dL (SI, 0.6–3 g/L)

Children (Varies According to Age)
- IgA: 6 to 377 mg/dL (SI, 0.06–3.77 g/L)
- IgG: 141 to 1,611 mg/dL (SI, 1.41–16.11 g/L)
- IgM: boys, 12 to 260 mg/dL (SI, 0.12–2.6 g/L); girls, 14 to 260 mg/dL (SI, 0.14–2.6 g/L)

Abnormal Findings
- Congenital and acquired hypogammaglobulinemias, myelomas, and macroglobulinemia (diagnosis confirmation)
- Hepatic and autoimmune diseases, leukemias, and lymphomas (diagnosis support with biopsies, white blood cell differential, and physical examination) (See the *Serum Immunoglobulin Levels in Various Disorders* table.)

Nursing Implications
- Report abnormal findings to the health care provider.
- Prepare to educate the patient about the diagnosis.
- Prepare the patient for further testing or surgery, as indicated.
- Provide emotional support to the patient and family.

- Be aware that alcohol or opioid abuse may affect results.

Purpose
- To document exposure to an infectious or foreign agent
- To evaluate immunity status
- To diagnose paraproteinemias, such as multiple myeloma and Waldenström's macroglobulinemia
- To detect hypogammaglobulinemia and hypergammaglobulinemia, as well as nonimmunologic diseases, such as cirrhosis and hepatitis, that are associated with abnormally high immunoglobulin levels
- To assess the effectiveness of chemotherapy and radiation therapy

Description

Immunoglobulin proteins can function as specific antibodies in response to antigen stimulation and are responsible for the humoral aspects of immunity. The most frequently measured immunoglobins—IgG, IgA, IgM, IgD, and IgE—are normally present in serum in predictable percentages. IgG and IgM are used primarily for diagnosing and monitoring infectious diseases. IgA is used in allergy testing.

IgG constitutes about 75% of total immunoglobulins and includes the warm-temperature type; IgA, about 15% of the total immunoglobins; and IgM, about 5% of total immunoglobins, including cold agglutinins, rheumatoid factor, and ABO blood group isoagglutinins. IgD and allergen-specific IgE are less than 2% of total immunoglobins.

Deviations from normal immunoglobulin percentages are characteristic in many immune disorders, including

Serum Immunoglobulin Levels in Various Disorders

Abnormal immunoglobulin levels are characteristic of many disorders, as shown below.

Disorder	IgG	IgA	IgM
Immunoglobulin Disorders			
Lymphoid aplasia	D	D	D
Agammaglobulinemia	D	D	D
Type I dysgammaglobulinemia (selective immunoglobulin [Ig] G and IgA deficiency)	D	D	N or I
Type II dysgammaglobulinemia (absent IgA and IgM)	N	D	D
IgA globulinemia	N	D	N
Ataxia-telangiectasia	N	D	N
Multiple Myeloma, Macroglobulinemia, Lymphomas			
Heavy chain disease (Franklin's disease)	D	D	D
IgG myeloma	I	D	D
IgA myeloma	D	I	D
Macroglobulinemia	D	D	I
Acute lymphocytic leukemia	N	D	N
Chronic lymphocytic leukemia	D	D	D
Acute myelocytic leukemia	N	N	N
Chronic myelocytic leukemia	N	D	N
Hodgkin's disease	N	N	N
Hepatic Disorders			
Hepatitis	I	I	I
Laënnec's cirrhosis	I	I	N
Biliary cirrhosis	N	N	I
Hepatoma	N	N	D
Other Disorders			
Rheumatoid arthritis	I	I	I
Systemic lupus erythematosus	I	I	I
Nephrotic syndrome	D	D	N
Trypanosomiasis	N	N	I
Pulmonary tuberculosis	I	N	N

Key: N = normal; I = increased; D = decreased.

cancer, hepatic disorders, rheumatoid arthritis, and systemic lupus erythematosus. Immunoelectrophoresis identifies IgG, IgA, and IgM in a serum sample; the level of each is measured by radial immunodiffusion or nephelometry. Some laboratories detect immunoglobulin by indirect immunofluorescence and radioimmunoassay.

Interfering Factors

- Chemotherapy or radiation therapy (possible decrease due to suppressive effects on bone marrow)
- Anticonvulsants, asparaginase, hormonal contraceptives, hydralazine, hydantoin derivatives, and phenylbutazone (possible increase)
- Methotrexate and severe hypersensitivity to bacille Calmette-Guérin vaccine (possible decrease)
- Dextran and methylprednisolone (decrease in IgM levels)
- Dextran and high doses of methylprednisolone and phenytoin (decrease in IgG and IgA levels)
- Methadone (increase in IgA levels)

Precautions

- Send the sample to the laboratory immediately to prevent immunoglobulin deterioration.

Nursing Considerations

Before the Test

- Confirm the patient's identity using two patient identifiers and confirmation of the patient's identification bracelet according to facility policy.
- Explain to the patient that the IgG, IgA, and IgM tests measure antibody levels and, if appropriate, evaluate treatment effectiveness.
- Instruct the patient to restrict food and fluids, except for water, for 12 to 14 hours before the test.
- Advise the patient that the test requires a blood sample. Explain that the patient may experience slight discomfort from the needle puncture and the tourniquet.
- Check the patient's history for drugs that may affect test results.

During the Test

- Perform a venipuncture and collect the sample in a 7-mL clot activator tube.

- Advise the patient with abnormally low immunoglobulin levels (especially IgG or IgM) to be careful to avoid bacterial infection. When caring for such a patient, watch for signs of infection, such as fever, chills, rash, and skin ulcers.
- Instruct the patient with abnormally high immunoglobulin levels and monoclonal gammopathy symptoms to report bone pain and tenderness. Such a patient has numerous antibody-producing malignant plasma cells in bone marrow, which hamper production of other blood components. Watch for signs of hypercalcemia, kidney failure, and spontaneous pathologic fractures.

After the Test

- Apply direct pressure to the venipuncture site until bleeding stops and to prevent hematoma formation.
- Tell the patient to resume a usual diet and medications that were discontinued before the test, as ordered.

Q

Radionuclide Renal Imaging

Normal Findings

- Renal perfusion (evident immediately after technetium 99m [^{99m}Tc] pertechnetate uptake in the abdominal aorta)
- Normal renal circulation pattern (evident within 1–2 minutes)
- Normal kidney delineation (simultaneous, symmetrical, equal intensity)
- Kidneys of normal size, shape, and position with defined collecting system and bladder
- Effective renal plasma flow (420 mL/ minute or greater, with greater than 66% of dose excreted in urine at 30 to 35 minutes)

Abnormal Findings

- Impeded renal circulation (caused by trauma and renal artery stenosis or renal infarction)
- Abnormal perfusion, indicating possible vascular graft obstruction in kidney transplant patients
- Abnormalities of the collecting system and urine extravasation
- Ureteral obstruction
- Tumors, infarctions, and inflammatory masses (abscesses, for example)
- Horseshoe kidney or polycystic kidney disease
- Lower than normal total concentration of the radionuclide, indicating acute tubular necrosis, severe infection, or ischemia
- Decreased radionuclide uptake in kidney transplant patients, indicating organ rejection
- Congenital ectopia or aplasia

Nursing Implications

- Report abnormal findings to the health care provider.
- Prepare to educate the patient about the diagnosis.
- Prepare the patient for further testing or surgery, as indicated.
- Provide emotional support to the patient and family.

Purpose

- To detect and assess functional and structural renal abnormalities (such as lesions and renovascular hypertension) and acute or chronic disease (such as pyelonephritis or glomerulonephritis)
- To assess renal transplantation or renal injury due to trauma to the urinary tract or obstruction

Description

Radionuclide renal imaging, which involves IV injection of a radionuclide followed by scintigraphy, provides a wealth of information for evaluating the kidneys. This test allows assessment of renal blood flow, renal structure, and nephron and collecting system function by observing the radionuclide uptake concentration and transit. Depending on the patient's clinical presentation, this procedure may include dynamic scans to assess renal perfusion and function or static scans to assess structure. This test also may be substituted for excretory urography in the patient with hypersensitivity to contrast agents.

The procedure for radionuclide renal imaging is as follows:

- The patient usually is placed in a prone position so that posterior views may be obtained. If the test is being performed to evaluate transplantation, the patient is placed in a supine position for anterior views.

- The patient is instructed not to change position.

- A perfusion study (radionuclide angiography) is performed first to evaluate renal blood flow. The ^{99m}Tc pertechnetate is administered IV, and rapid-sequence photographs (one per second) are taken for 1 minute.

- A function study is performed to measure the radionuclide transit time through the kidneys' functional units. After the iodine is administered IV, images are obtained at a rate of one per minute for 20 minutes. Alternatively, this entire procedure can be recorded on computer-compatible magnetic tape, and concurrent renogram curves can be plotted.

- Static images are obtained 4 or more hours later, after the radionuclide has drained through the pelvicaliceal system.

Interfering Factors

- Antihypertensives (possible masking of abnormality)
- Multiple organs imaged on the same day (possible poor imaging)

Precautions

- This test is contraindicated during pregnancy unless the benefits of the procedure outweigh the risk to the fetus.
- Lactating women may need to discard their breast milk for several days following the procedure, as directed by their pediatricians.

Nursing Considerations

Before the Test

- Confirm the patient's identity using two patient identifiers and confirmation of the patient's identification bracelet according to facility policy.

- Explain to the patient that radionuclide renal imaging permits the evaluation of the structure, blood flow, and function of the kidneys and that it involves taking several series of films of the bladder.

- Inform the patient who will perform the test and when and where it will be done. Make sure that the patient isn't scheduled for other radionuclide scans on the same day. (If static scans are ordered, there will be a delay of several hours before the images are taken.)

- Explain that the patient will receive an injection of a radionuclide and that transient flushing and nausea may be experienced. Emphasize that only a small amount of radionuclide is administered and that it's usually excreted within 24 hours. (If the patient is pregnant or a young child, a supersaturated solution of potassium iodide may be administered 1 to 3 hours before the test to block thyroid uptake of iodine.)

- If the patient receives antihypertensive medication, ask the health care provider if it should be withheld before the test.

- Make sure that the patient or a responsible family member has signed an informed consent form.

After the Test

- Instruct the patient to flush the toilet immediately after each voiding for 24 hours as a radiation precaution.

- If the patient is incontinent, change bed linens promptly and wear personal protective equipment to maintain standard precautions and prevent unnecessary skin contact.

- Monitor the injection site for signs of hematoma, infection, and discomfort. Apply warm compresses for comfort.

- Monitor the patient's intake and output and electrolyte, acid–base, blood urea nitrogen, and creatinine levels, as indicated.

- Resume usual medications.

Radionuclide Thyroid Imaging

Normal Findings

- Normal thyroid gland (butterfly-shaped with isthmus midline, measuring about 2 inches [5.1 cm] long and 1 inch [2.5 cm] wide, without nodules) showing a uniform uptake of the radioisotope
- Presence of third (pyramidal) lobe (normal variant)

Abnormal Findings

- See the *Results of Thyroid Imaging in Thyroid Disorders* table for more information.

Nursing Implications

- Report abnormal findings to the health care provider.
- Prepare to educate the patient about the diagnosis.
- Prepare the patient for further testing (thyroid ultrasonography to rule out cysts, fine-needle aspiration and

Results of Thyroid Imaging in Thyroid Disorders

This table shows the characteristic findings in radionuclide imaging tests that are associated with various thyroid disorders, as well as the possible causes of those disorders.

Condition	Findings	Causes
Hypothyroidism	• Glandular damage or absent gland	• Surgical removal of gland • Inflammation • Radiation • Neoplasm (rare)
Hypothyroid goiter	• Enlarged gland • Decreased uptake (of radioactive iodine) if glandular destruction is present • Increased uptake possible from congenital error in thyroxine synthesis	• Insufficient iodine intake • Hypersecretion of thyroid-stimulating hormone (TSH) caused by thyroid hormone deficiency
Myxedema	• Normal or slightly reduced gland size • Uniform pattern • Decreased uptake	• Defective embryonic development, resulting in congenital absence or underdevelopment of thyroid gland • Maternal iodine deficiency
Hyperthyroidism (Graves' disease)	• Enlarged gland • Uniform pattern • Increased uptake	• Unknown, but may be hereditary • Production of thyroid-stimulating immunoglobulins
Toxic nodular goiter	• Multiple hot spots	• Long-standing simple goiter
Hyperfunctioning adenomas	• Solitary hot spot	• Adenomatous production of triiodothyronine and thyroxine, suppressing TSH secretion and producing atrophy of other thyroid tissue
Hypofunctioning adenomas	• Solitary cold spot	• Cyst or nonfunctioning nodule
Benign multinodular goiter	• Multiple nodules with variable or no function	• Local inflammation • Degeneration
Thyroid carcinoma	• Usually a solitary cold spot with occasional or no function	• Neoplasm

R

biopsy, and triiodothyronine [T_3] thyroid suppression test) or surgery, as indicated.

- Provide emotional support to the patient and family.

Purpose

- To assess the size, structure, and position of the thyroid gland
- To evaluate thyroid function (in conjunction with other thyroid tests)

Description

In radionuclide thyroid imaging, the thyroid is studied by gamma camera after the patient receives a radioisotope (iodine-123 [^{123}I], technetium [^{99m}Tc] pertechnetate, or iodine-131 [^{131}I]). Thyroid imaging typically follows a palpable mass discovery, an enlarged gland, or an asymmetrical goiter and is performed concurrently with thyroid uptake tests and measurements of serum T_3 and serum thyroxine (T_4) levels. Later, thyroid ultrasonography may be performed.

The procedure for radionuclide thyroid imaging is as follows:

- The test is performed 24 hours after oral administration of ^{123}I or ^{131}I or 20 to 30 minutes after IV injection of ^{99m}Tc pertechnetate. Just before the test, the patient is asked to remove dentures and any jewelry that could interfere with thyroid visualization.
- The patient is placed in a supine position with the neck extended; the thyroid gland is palpated. The gamma camera is positioned above the anterior portion of the neck.
- Images of the patient's thyroid gland are projected on a monitor and are recorded on X-ray film. Three views of the thyroid are obtained: a straight-on anterior view and two bilateral oblique views.

Interfering Factors

- An iodine-deficient diet and phenothiazines (increased absorption of radioisotope, which affects imaging)
- Decreased uptake of radioactive iodine because of renal disease;

ingestion of iodized salt, iodine preparations, iodinated salt substitutes, or seafood; and use of aminosalicylic acid, corticosteroids, cough syrups containing inorganic iodine, multivitamins, thyroid hormones, or thyroid hormone antagonists (decreased absorption of radioisotope, which affects imaging)

- Severe diarrhea and vomiting, impairing GI absorption of radioiodine (decreased absorption of radioisotope, which affects imaging)

Precautions

- Radionuclide thyroid imaging is contraindicated during pregnancy and lactation and in the patient with a previous allergy to iodine, shellfish, or radioactive tracers.
- This study should be performed before radiographic contrast or iodine-containing thyroid drugs are administered.

Nursing Considerations

Before the Test

- Confirm the patient's identity using two patient identifiers and confirmation of the patient's identification bracelet according to facility policy.
- Inform the patient that radionuclide thyroid imaging helps determine the cause of thyroid dysfunction. Explain that after receiving the radiopharmaceutical, a gamma camera will be used to produce an image of the thyroid gland. Explain that the imaging procedure will take about 30 minutes and assure that exposure to radiation is minimal.
- Ask if the patient has undergone any tests that used radiographic contrast media within the past 60 days. Note previous radiographic contrast media exposure on the X-ray request.
- Check the patient's diet and medication history and instruct accordingly, as ordered. Medications such as thyroid hormones, thyroid hormone antagonists, and iodine preparations

(Lugol's solution, some multivitamins, and cough syrups) are typically discontinued 2 to 3 weeks before the test. Phenothiazines, corticosteroids, salicylates, anticoagulants, and antihistamines are discontinued 1 week before the test. Iodized salt, iodinated salt substitutes, and seafood are stopped 14 to 21 days before testing. Liothyronine (Cytomel), propylthiouracil (PTU), and methimazole (Tapazole) are discontinued 3 days before the test, and T_4 is stopped 10 days before.
- If ^{123}I or ^{131}I will be used, instruct the patient to fast after midnight the night before the test. (Fasting isn't required if an IV injection of ^{99m}Tc pertechnetate is used.) After receiving ^{123}I or ^{131}I orally or ^{99m}Tc pertechnetate IV, the patient should fast an additional 2 hours. Be sure to record the date and the time of administration.
- Just before the test, tell the patient to remove dentures, jewelry, and other materials that may interfere with the imaging process.
- Make sure the patient or a responsible family member has signed an informed consent form, if required.

After the Test
- Tell the patient to resume a usual diet and medications, as ordered.

Rapid Cytomegalovirus Antibody Test

Normal Findings
- No cytomegalovirus (CMV) in culture

Abnormal Findings
- Systemic CMV infection and disease

Nursing Implications
- Report abnormal findings to the health care provider.
- Prepare to educate the patient about the diagnosis.
- Provide emotional support to the patient and family.

Purpose
- To obtain rapid laboratory diagnosis of CMV infection, especially in the immunocompromised patient who has, or is at risk for developing, systemic infections caused by this virus

Description
CMV, a member of the herpes virus group, is usually asymptomatic and harmless; however, it can cause systemic infection in congenitally infected infants and in immunocompromised patients, such as transplant recipients, patients receiving chemotherapy for neoplastic disease, and those with acquired immune deficiency syndrome.

Interfering Factors
- Administration of antiviral drugs before collecting the specimen

Precautions
- Use gloves when obtaining and handling specimens.
- Women of childbearing age who previously have not been infected with CMV have the potential risk of passing CMV to their babies in utero.

Nursing Considerations

Before the Test
- Confirm the patient's identity using two patient identifiers and confirmation of the patient's identification bracelet according to facility policy.
- Explain the purpose of the test and describe the procedure for collecting the specimen, which will depend on the laboratory used.

During the Test
- Collect the specimens during the prodromal and acute stages of clinical infection to maximize the chances of detecting CMV.
- Use the proper specimen collection device:
  - For throat—microbiologic transport swab
  - For urine or cerebrospinal fluid—sterile screw-capped tube or vial

R

- For bronchoalveolar lavage tissue— sterile screw-capped jar
- For blood—sterile tube with an anticoagulant (heparin).

After the Test

- Transport the specimen to the laboratory as soon as possible after the collection. If the anticipated time between collection and inoculation into shell vial cell cultures is longer than 3 hours, store the specimen at 39.2°F (4°C). Don't freeze the specimen or allow it to become dry.

Red Blood Cell Count

Reference Values

Adult females: 4 to 5 million red blood cells (RBCs)/μL (SI, 4–5 × 10^{12}/L) of venous blood

Adult males: 4.5 to 5.5 million RBCs/μL (SI, 4.5–5.5 × 10^{12}/L) of venous blood

Children: 4.6 to 4.8 million RBCs/μL (SI, 4.6–4.8 × 10^{12}/L) of venous blood

Full-term neonates: 4.4 to 5.8 million RBCs/μL (SI, 4.4–5.8 × 10^{12}/L) of capillary blood at birth, decreasing to 3 to 3.8 million RBCs/μL (SI, 3–3.8 × 10^{12}/L) at age 2 months, and increasing slowly thereafter

Abnormal Findings

Elevated Levels

- Absolute or relative polycythemia

Decreased Levels

- Anemia
- Dilution caused by fluid overload
- Hemorrhage beyond 24 hours

Nursing Implications

- Report abnormal findings to the health care provider.
- Prepare to educate the patient about the diagnosis.
- Prepare the patient for further testing, as indicated.

Purpose

- To provide data for calculating mean corpuscular volume (MCV) and mean corpuscular hemoglobin (MCH), which reveal RBC size and hemoglobin (Hb) content
- To support other hematologic tests for diagnosing anemia or polycythemia

Description

The RBC count, also called an *erythrocyte count,* is part of a complete blood count. It's used to detect the number of RBCs in a microliter (μL) or cubic millimeter (mm^3) of whole blood. The RBC count itself provides no qualitative information regarding the size, shape, or concentration of Hb within the corpuscles, but it may be used to calculate two erythrocyte indices: MCV and MCH.

Interfering Factors

- Hemoconcentration caused by prolonged tourniquet constriction
- Hemodilution caused by drawing the sample from the same arm used for IV fluid infusion
- High white blood cell count (false-high test results in semiautomated and automated counters)
- Diseases that cause RBCs to agglutinate or form rouleaux (false decrease)
- Hemolysis resulting from rough handling of the sample or drawing the blood through a small-gauge needle for venipuncture

Precautions

- Handle the sample gently to prevent hemolysis.

Nursing Considerations

Before the Test

- Confirm the patient's identity using two patient identifiers and confirmation of the patient's identification bracelet according to facility policy.
- Explain to the patient that the RBC count is used to evaluate the number of RBCs and to detect possible blood disorders.
- Advise the patient that a blood sample will be taken. Explain that slight discomfort from the tourniquet and needle puncture may be experienced.

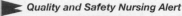

 Quality and Safety Nursing Alert

Explain to a pediatric patient (if old enough) and the parents that a small amount of blood will be taken from a finger or earlobe.

• Inform the patient that there are no food or fluid restrictions for this test.

During the Test
• For adults and older children, draw venous blood into a 3- or 4.5-mL EDTA–sodium metabisulfite solution tube.

 Quality and Safety Nursing Alert

For younger children, collect capillary blood in a microcollection device.

• Fill the collection tube completely.
• Invert the tube gently several times to mix the sample and the anticoagulant.

After the Test
• Apply pressure to the venipuncture site until bleeding stops and to prevent hematoma formation.

Red Cell Indices

Reference Values
Mean corpuscular volume (MCV): 84 to 99 μm^3
Mean corpuscular hemoglobin (MCH): 26 to 32 pg/cell
Mean corpuscular hemoglobin concentration (MCHC): 30 to 36 g/dL

Abnormal Findings

Elevated MCV
• Macrocytic anemias (megaloblastic anemias) (See the *Comparative Red Cell Indices in Anemias* table.)
• Folic acid or vitamin B$_{12}$ deficiency

Decreased MCV and MCH
• Microcytic, hypochromic anemias (iron deficiency anemia)
• Inadequate dietary intake or malabsorption of iron
• Increased iron loss
• Excessive blood loss
• Pyridoxine-responsive anemia, or thalassemia
• Inherited deoxyribonucleic acid synthesis, or reticulocytosis disorders

Nursing Implications
• Report abnormal findings to the health care provider.
• Prepare to educate the patient about the diagnosis.
• Prepare the patient for further testing, as indicated.

Purpose
• To help diagnose and classify anemias

Description
MCV, the ratio of hematocrit (HCT) (packed cell volume) to the red blood cell (RBC) count, expresses the average size of the erythrocytes and indicates whether they're undersized (microcytic), oversized (macrocytic), or normal (normocytic). MCH, the hemoglobin (Hb)-RBC ratio, gives the Hb weight in an average red cell. MCHC, the Hb ratio weight to HCT, defines the average

R

Comparative Red Cell Indices in Anemias

	Normal Values (Normocytic, Normochromic)	Iron Deficiency (Microcytic Hypochromic)	Pernicious Anemia (Macrocytic, Normochromic)
MCV	84 to 99 μm^3	60 to 80 μm^3	96 to 150 μm^3
MCH	26 to 32 pg/cell	5 to 25 pg/cell	33 to 53 pg/cell
MCHC	30 to 36 g/dL	20 to 30 g/dL	33 to 38 g/dL

Key: MCV = Mean corpuscular volume
MCH = Mean corpuscular hemoglobin
MCHC = Mean corpuscular hemoglobin concentration

Hb concentration in 100 mL of packed RBCs. It helps to distinguish normally colored (normochromic) RBCs from paler (hypochromic) RBCs.

Interfering Factors

- Hemoconcentration caused by prolonged tourniquet constriction
- High white blood cell count (false-high RBC count in semiautomated and automated counters, invalidating MCV and MCHC results)
- Falsely elevated Hb values, invalidating MCH and MCHC results
- Diseases that cause RBCs to agglutinate or form rouleaux (false-low RBC count)

Precautions

- Handle the sample gently to prevent hemolysis.

Nursing Considerations

Before the Test

- Confirm the patient's identity using two patient identifiers and confirmation of the patient's identification bracelet according to facility policy.
- Explain to the patient that red cell indices help determine if anemia is present.
- Tell the patient that a blood sample will be taken. Explain that slight discomfort from the tourniquet and needle puncture may be experienced.

During the Test

- Perform a venipuncture and collect the sample in a 3- or 5-mL EDTA tube.
- Completely fill the collection tube and invert it gently several times to adequately mix the sample and the anticoagulant.

After the Test

- Apply pressure to the venipuncture site until bleeding stops.
- If a hematoma develops at the venipuncture site, apply additional pressure. If the hematoma is large, monitor pulses distal to the phlebotomy site.

Renal Angiography

Normal Findings

- Normal vascular tree arborization and renal parenchyma architecture

Abnormal Findings

- Hypervascularity, indicating tumors
- Clearly delineated, radiolucent masses, indicating cysts
- Arteriosclerosis with noticeable blood vessel constriction, usually within the proximal portion of its length, indicating stenosis
- Arterial dysplasia (middle and distal portions of the vessel)
- Alternating aneurysms and stenotic regions (beads-on-a-string appearance)
- Absent or cutoff blood vessels with scar tissue and triangular areas near the periphery of the affected kidney, indicating infarction
- Aneurysms (saccular or fusiform) and renal arteriovenous fistula (abnormal widening and direct passage between the renal artery and renal vein)
- Renal tissue destruction, distortion, and fibrosis and tortuous vascularity, indicating severe or chronic pyelonephritis
- Increased capsular vessels with abnormal intrarenal circulation, indicating abscesses or inflammatory masses

Nursing Implications

- Report abnormal findings to the health care provider.
- Prepare to educate the patient about the diagnosis.
- Prepare the patient for further testing, as indicated.

Purpose

- To demonstrate total renal vasculature configuration before surgical procedures
- To determine the cause of renovascular hypertension, such as from stenosis, thrombotic occlusions, emboli, and aneurysms
- To evaluate chronic kidney disease or renal failure

- To investigate renal masses and renal trauma
- To detect complications following kidney transplantation, such as a nonfunctioning shunt or rejection of the donor organ
- To differentiate highly vascular tumors from avascular cysts

Description

Renal angiography is commonly used to evaluate renal trauma, intrarenal hematoma, parenchymal laceration, shattered kidneys, and areas of infarction. It may also be useful in distinguishing pseudotumors from tumors or cysts, evaluating the volume of residual functioning renal tissue in hydronephrosis, and evaluating donors and recipients before and after renal transplantation. It requires arterial injection of a contrast medium and permits renal vasculature and parenchyma radiographic examination.

The procedure for renal angiography is as follows:

- The patient is placed in a supine position and a peripheral IV infusion is started. The skin over the arterial puncture site is cleaned with antiseptic solution, and a local anesthetic is injected.
- The femoral artery is punctured and, under fluoroscopic visualization, cannulated. (If a femoral pulse is absent or the artery is convoluted or plaque-ridden, percutaneous transaxillary, transbrachial, or translumbar catheterization may be performed instead.)
- After passing the flexible guidewire through the artery, the cannula is withdrawn, leaving several inches of wire in the lumen.
- A polyethylene catheter is passed over the wire and advanced, under fluoroscopic guidance, up the femoroiliac vessels to the aorta. The guidewire is removed and the catheter is flushed with heparin solution.
- The contrast medium is injected, and screening aortograms are taken before

proceeding. When the aortographic study is completed, a renal catheter is exchanged for the vascular catheter.
- To determine the position of the renal arteries and to ensure that the tip of the catheter is in the lumen, a test bolus (3–5 mL) of contrast medium is injected immediately. If the patient has no adverse reaction to the contrast medium, 20 to 25 mL of the substance is injected just below the origin of the renal arteries.
- A series of rapid-sequence X-ray films of the filling of the renal vascular tree is exposed. If additional selective studies are required, the catheter remains in place while the films are examined. If the films are satisfactory, the catheter is removed.
- A sterile pad is applied firmly to the puncture site for 15 minutes.

Interfering Factors
- Patient movement
- Recent contrast studies, such as barium enema or an upper GI series (possible poor imaging)
- Presence of stools or gas in the GI tract (possible poor imaging)

Precautions
- Renal angiography is contraindicated during pregnancy and in the patient with bleeding tendencies, allergy to contrast media, or renal insufficiency caused by end-stage kidney disease.
- Consult with physician if diabetic patient is taking Glucophage (metformin). This drug must be held for several days, secondary to the risk of kidney failure and lactic acidosis.

Nursing Considerations
Before the Test
- Confirm the patient's identity using two patient identifiers and confirmation of the patient's identification bracelet according to facility policy.
- Explain to the patient that renal angiography permits visualization of the kidneys, blood vessels, and functional

R

units, and aids in diagnosing renal disease or masses. Explain the procedure, telling the patient when and where it will take place.

- Instruct the patient to fast for 8 hours before the test and to drink extra fluids the day before the test and the day after the test to maintain adequate hydration. (If necessary, an IV line may be started to maintain hydration.) Tell the patient that oral medication may be continued; a special order is needed if the patient is diabetic. Hold metformin for 24 hours before procedure and 48 hours after the procedure.
- Advise the patient that a laxative or an enema the evening before the test may be administered, and explain that transient discomfort (flushing, burning sensation, and nausea) during injection of the contrast medium may be experienced when testing begins.
- Make sure that the patient or a responsible family member has signed an informed consent form.

▶ *Quality and Safety Nursing Alert*

Check the patient's history for hypersensitivity to iodine, contrast media, or iodine-containing foods, such as shellfish. Mark sensitivities on the chart and inform the health care provider because the patient may require prophylactic antiallergenics (corticosteroids or diphenhydramine).

- Just before the test, administer prescribed medications (usually a sedative and an opioid analgesic). Take and record the patient's base line vital signs. Make sure that recent laboratory test results (blood urea nitrogen and serum creatinine levels and bleeding studies) are documented on the patient's chart. Verification of adequate renal function and adequate clotting ability is vital. Also evaluate peripheral pulse sites and mark them for easy access in postprocedure assessment.

- Instruct the patient to put on a gown, to remove all metallic objects that may interfere with test results, and to void before leaving the unit.

After the Test
- Before the patient is returned to the patient's room, observe the puncture site for a hematoma.
- Keep the patient flat in bed and instruct the patient to keep the punctured leg straight for at least 6 hours or as otherwise ordered.
- Check the patient's vital signs every 15 minutes for 1 hour, every 30 minutes for 2 hours, and then every hour until they stabilize.
- Monitor popliteal and dorsalis pedis pulses for adequate perfusion with vital signs and then at least every hour for 4 hours. Note the color and temperature of the involved extremity and compare with the uninvolved extremity. Watch for signs of pain or paresthesia in the involved limb.
- Watch for bleeding or hematomas at the injection site. Keep the pressure dressing in place and check for bleeding when you assess the patient's vital signs. If bleeding occurs, promptly notify the health care provider and apply direct pressure or a sandbag to the site.
- Apply cold compresses to the puncture site to reduce edema and lessen pain.

▶ *Quality and Safety Nursing Alert*

Provide the patient with extra fluids (2,000–3,000 mL) in the 24-hour period after the test to prevent nephrotoxicity from the contrast medium. Also monitor for anaphylaxis from the contrast medium. (Signs include cardiorespiratory distress, renal failure, and shock.)

- Monitor the patient for atrial arrhythmias and evaluate aspartate aminotransferase and lactate dehydrogenase activity if renal stenosis is observed.

Renal Venography

Normal Findings
- Immediate renal vein and tributaries opacification
- Venous blood content in a supine position of 1.5 to 1.6 ng/mL/hour

Abnormal Findings
- Occlusion near the inferior vena cava, indicating renal vein thrombosis
- Filling defect, indicating tumor, retroperitoneal fibrosis, obstruction, or compression
- Abnormally positioned or clustered vessel opacification
- Elevated renin content in both kidneys' renal venous blood, indicating essential renovascular hypertension
- Elevated renin levels in one kidney, indicating unilateral lesion

Nursing Implications
- Report abnormal findings to the health care provider.
- Prepare to educate the patient about the diagnosis.
- Prepare the patient for further testing, as indicated.

Purpose
- To detect renal vein thrombosis
- To evaluate renal vein compression due to extrinsic tumors or retroperitoneal fibrosis
- To assess renal tumors and detect invasion of the renal vein or inferior vena cava
- To detect venous anomalies and defects
- To differentiate renal agenesis from a small kidney
- To collect renal venous blood samples for evaluation of renovascular hypertension

Description
Renal venography permits radiographic examination of the main renal veins and their tributaries to evaluate renal vein thrombosis, tumors, and venous anomalies. In this test, contrast medium is injected by percutaneous catheter passed through the femoral vein and inferior vena cava into the renal vein.

The procedure for renal venography is as follows:

- The patient is placed in a supine position on the X-ray table with the abdomen centered over the film. The skin over the right femoral vein near the groin is cleaned with antiseptic solution and draped. (The left femoral vein or jugular veins may be used.)
- A local anesthetic is injected and the femoral vein is cannulated. Under fluoroscopic guidance, a guidewire is threaded a short distance through the cannula, which is then removed. A catheter is passed over the wire into the inferior vena cava. (When catheterization of the femoral vein is contraindicated, the right antecubital vein is punctured, and the catheter is inserted and advanced through the right atrium of the heart into the inferior vena cava.) A test bolus of contrast medium is injected to determine that the vena cava is patent. If it is, the catheter is advanced into the right renal vein and contrast medium (usually 20–40 mL) is injected.
- When studies of the right renal vasculature are completed, the catheter is withdrawn into the vena cava, rotated, and guided into the left renal vein.
- If visualization of the renal venous tributaries is indicated, epinephrine can be injected into the ipsilateral renal artery by catheter before contrast medium is injected into the renal vein. (Epinephrine temporarily blocks arterial flow and allows filling of distal intrarenal veins. Obstructing the artery briefly with a balloon catheter produces the same effect.)
- After anteroposterior films are made, the patient lies in a prone position for posteroanterior films.
- For renin assays, blood samples are drawn under fluoroscopy within 15 minutes after venography. After catheter removal, pressure is applied

R

to the site for 15 minutes and a dressing is placed.

Interfering Factors
- Recent contrast studies or stools or gas in the bowel
- Failure to restrict antihypertensive drugs, diuretics, estrogen, hormonal contraceptives, and salt

Precautions
- Renal venography is contraindicated in severe thrombosis of the inferior vena cava.
- The guidewire and catheter should be advanced carefully if severe renal vein thrombosis is suspected.
- Watch the patient for signs of hypersensitivity to the contrast medium.

Nursing Considerations

Before the Test
- Confirm the patient's identity using two patient identifiers and confirmation of the patient's identification bracelet according to facility policy.
- Explain to the patient that renal venography permits radiographic study of the renal veins. Describe the procedure and tell the patient when and where it will take place.
- Advise the patient that a catheter will be inserted into a vein in the groin area after the patient is given a sedative and a local anesthetic. Warn that mild discomfort during injection of the local anesthetic and contrast medium may be experienced and that transient burning and flushing from the contrast medium may be experienced. Warn that the X-ray equipment may make loud, clacking noises as the films are taken.

> **▶ Quality and Safety Nursing Alert**
>
> Check the patient's history for hypersensitivity to contrast media, iodine, or foods containing iodine, such as shellfish. Mark sensitivities on the chart and report them to the health care provider.

- Check the patient's history and coagulation studies for indications of bleeding disorders.
- If renin assays will be done, check the patient's diet and medications and consult with the health care team. As ordered, restrict the patient's sodium intake and discontinue antihypertensive drugs, diuretics, estrogen, and hormonal contraceptives.
- Instruct the patient to fast for 4 hours before the test, if ordered.
- Make sure that the patient or a responsible family member has signed an informed consent form.
- Administer a sedative, if necessary, just before the procedure.
- Record the patient's baseline vital signs. Make sure pretest blood urea nitrogen and urine creatinine levels are adequate because the kidneys clear contrast media.

After the Test
- Check the patient's vital signs and distal pulses every 15 minutes for the first hour, every 30 minutes for the second hour, and then every 2 hours for 24 hours. Keep the patient on bed rest for 2 hours.
- Observe the puncture site for bleeding or a hematoma when checking the patient's vital signs; if bleeding occurs, apply pressure. Report bleeding as soon as possible.

> **▶ Quality and Safety Nursing Alert**
>
> Report signs of vein perforation, embolism, and extravasation of contrast medium. These include chills, fever, rapid pulse and respiration, hypotension, dyspnea, and chest, abdominal, or flank pain. Also report complaints of paresthesia or pain in the catheterized limb— symptoms of nerve irritation or vascular compromise.

- Administer prescribed sedatives and antimicrobials.
- Prepare for further arteriography or surgery, as ordered.

- Instruct the patient to resume a usual diet and medications, as ordered. Advise the patient to increase fluid intake (unless contraindicated) to help clear contrast media.

Respiratory Syncytial Virus Antibodies

Normal Findings

- No detectable antibodies to the respiratory syncytial virus (RSV) (less than 1:5)

Abnormal Findings

- Active viral infection

Nursing Implications

- Report abnormal findings to the health care provider.
- Prepare to educate the patient about the diagnosis.
- Prepare the patient for further testing as indicated.
- Provide emotional support to the patient and family.
- Prepare to administer antimicrobial therapy as indicated.

Purpose

- To diagnose infections caused by RSV

Description

A member of the paramyxovirus group, RSV is the major viral cause of severe lower respiratory tract disease in infants (it's the most severe disease during the first 6 months of life), but may cause infections in people of any age. Infection involves viral replication in upper respiratory tract epithelial cells, but in younger children, especially, the infection spreads to the bronchi, the bronchioles, and even the parenchyma of the lungs.

In the RSV antibodies test, immunoglobulin (Ig) G and IgM class antibodies are quantified using indirect immunofluorescence.

Precautions

- Handle the sample gently to prevent hemolysis.

Nursing Considerations

Before the Test

- Confirm the patient's identity using two patient identifiers and confirmation of the patient's identification bracelet according to facility policy.
- Explain the purpose of the RSV antibodies test to the patient (or parents if the patient is a child).
- Advise the patient (or parents) that the test requires a blood sample. Explain that slight discomfort from the tourniquet and needle puncture may be experienced.

During the Test

- Perform a venipuncture and collect 5 mL of sterile blood in a clot activator tube.
- Transfer the serum to a sterile tube or vial and send it to the laboratory promptly.
- If transfer must be delayed, store the serum at 39.2°F (4°C) for 1 to 2 days or at −4°F (−20°C) for longer periods to avoid contamination.

After the Test

- Apply direct pressure to the venipuncture site until bleeding stops and to prevent formation of a hematoma.

R

Reticulocyte Count

Reference Values

Adults: 0.5% to 2.5% (SI, 0.005–0.025) of the total red blood cell (RBC) count

Infants: 2% to 6% (SI, 0.002–0.006) at birth, decreasing to adult levels in 1 to 2 weeks

Abnormal Findings

Elevated Levels

- Bone marrow response to anemia caused by hemolysis or blood loss
- After therapy for iron deficiency anemia or pernicious anemia

Decreased Levels

- Hypoplastic anemia
- Pernicious anemia

Nursing Implications

- Report abnormal findings to the health care provider.
- Prepare to educate the patient about the diagnosis.
- Prepare the patient for further testing as indicated.
- Prepare to administer parenteral vitamin B_{12}, as indicated in patients with decreased levels.

Purpose

- To help distinguish between hypoproliferative and hyperproliferative anemias
- To help assess blood loss, bone marrow response to anemia, and therapy for anemia

Description

Reticulocytes are nonnucleated, immature RBCs that remain in the peripheral blood for 24 to 48 hours as they mature. They're generally larger than mature RBCs. In the reticulocyte count test in a whole blood sample, they're counted and expressed as a percentage of the total RBC count. Because manual reticulocyte counting uses only a small sample, values may be imprecise and should be compared with the RBC count or hematocrit. The reticulocyte count is useful for evaluating anemia and is an index of effective erythropoiesis and bone marrow response to anemia.

Interfering Factors

- Prolonged tourniquet constriction
- Azathioprine (Imuran), chloramphenicol, dactinomycin (Cosmegen), and methotrexate (MTX) (possible false low)
- Antimalarials, antipyretics, corticotropin, furazolidone (Furoxone) (in infants), and levodopa (possible false high)
- Sulfonamides (possible false low or false high)
- Recent blood transfusion

Precautions

- Handle the sample gently to prevent hemolysis.

Nursing Considerations

Before the Test

- Confirm the patient's identity using two patient identifiers and confirmation of the patient's identification bracelet according to facility policy.
- Explain to the patient that the reticulocyte count is used to assist in the diagnosis of anemia or to monitor its treatment.
- Advise the patient that a blood sample will be taken. Explain that slight discomfort from the tourniquet and needle puncture may be experienced.

> ▶ **Quality and Safety Nursing Alert**
>
> If the patient is an infant or child, explain to the parents that a small amount of blood will be taken from the finger or earlobe.

- Notify the laboratory and health care provider of medications the patient is taking that may affect test results; these may need to be restricted.
- Inform the patient that there are no food or fluid restrictions for this test.

During the Test

- Perform a venipuncture and collect the sample in a 3- or 4.5-mL EDTA tube.
- Completely fill the collection tube and invert it gently several times to mix the sample and the anticoagulant.

After the Test

- Apply direct pressure to the venipuncture site until bleeding stops and to prevent hematoma formation.
- If a hematoma develops and is large, monitor pulses distal to the phlebotomy site.
- Instruct the patient to resume medications discontinued before the test, as ordered.
- Monitor the patient with an abnormal reticulocyte count for trends or significant changes in repeated tests.

Rh Typing

Reference Values
Classified as Rhesus (Rh)-positive or Rh-negative

Abnormal Findings
• None

Nursing Implications
• If an Rh-negative woman delivers an Rh-positive neonate or aborts a fetus whose Rh type is unknown, she should receive an $Rh_o(D)$ immune globulin injection within 72 hours to prevent hemolytic disease of the neonate in future births.
• Donor blood may be transfused only if it's compatible with the recipient's blood.

Purpose
• To establish blood type according to the Rh system
• To help determine the donor's compatibility before transfusion
• To determine if the patient will require an $Rh_o(D)$ immune globulin injection

Description
The Rh system classifies blood by the presence or absence of Rh antigen, called Rh_o (D) factor, on the surface of red blood cells (RBCs). In Rh typing, a patient's RBCs are mixed with serum containing anti-$Rh_o(D)$ antibodies and are observed for agglutination. If agglutination occurs, the $Rh_o(D)$ antigen is present and the patient's blood is typed Rh positive; if agglutination doesn't occur, the antigen is absent and the patient's blood is typed Rh negative.

Prospective blood donors are tested fully to exclude the D^u variant, a weak variant of the D antigen, before being classified as having Rh-negative blood. People who have this antigen are considered Rh-positive donors, but are generally transfused as Rh-negative recipients.

Interfering Factors
• Recent administration of dextran or IV contrast media (cellular aggregation resembling antibody-mediated agglutination)
• Cephalosporins, levodopa (Dopar), and methyldopa (Aldomet) (possible false positive for the D^u antigen due to positive direct antiglobulin [Coombs'] test)

Precautions
• Handle the sample gently and send it to the laboratory immediately.

Nursing Considerations
Before the Test
• Confirm the patient's identity using two patient identifiers and confirmation of the patient's identification bracelet according to facility policy.
• Explain to the patient that Rh typing determines or verifies blood group to ensure safe blood transfusion.
• Inform the patient that there are no food or fluid restrictions for this test.
• Tell the patient that the test requires a blood sample. Explain that slight discomfort from the tourniquet and needle puncture may be experienced.
• Check the patient's history for recent administration of dextran, IV contrast media, or drugs that may alter test results.

During the Test
• Perform a venipuncture and collect the sample in a 7-mL EDTA tube.
• Label the sample with the patient's name, the hospital or blood bank number, the date, and your initials.
• If a transfusion is ordered, make sure a transfusion request form accompanies the sample to the laboratory.

After the Test
• Apply direct pressure to the venipuncture site until bleeding stops and to prevent hematoma formation.
• If necessary, give the pregnant patient a card identifying that she may need to receive an $Rh_o(D)$ injection.

R

Rheumatoid Factor

Reference Values
Less than 1:20 (nonreactive)

Abnormal Findings
- Nonreactive titer (25% of rheumatoid arthritis [RA] patients)
- Reactive at greater than 39 international units/mL (8% of non-RA patients)
- Reactive at greater than 80 international units/mL (3% of non-RA patients)

Nursing Implications
- Report abnormal findings to the health care provider.
- Prepare to educate the patient about the diagnosis.
- Prepare the patient for further testing, as indicated.
- Provide emotional support to the patient and family.

Purpose
- To diagnose rheumatoid arthritis (RA) and Sjögren's syndrome

Description
The rheumatoid factor (RF) test is the most useful immunologic test for supporting the diagnosis of RA in conjunction with clinical symptoms and history. In this disease, autoantibodies of immunoglobulin (Ig) G and IgA antibodies are produced by lymphocytes in the synovial joints and react with IgM antibody to produce immune complexes, complement activation, and tissue destruction. How IgG molecules become antigenic is still unknown, but they may be altered by aggregating with viruses or other antigens. Techniques for detecting RF include the sheep cell agglutination test and the latex fixation test. Although the presence of this autoantibody is diagnostically useful, it is nonspecific and can be found in some bacterial and viral infections, as well as in a small percentage of healthy people. Increased RF occurs with other diseases such as systemic lupus erythematosus, tuberculosis, syphilis, sarcoidosis, cancer, and some viral infections.

Interfering Factors
- Inadequately activated complement (possible false positive)
- Serum with high lipid or cryoglobulin levels (possible false positive, requiring a repeat test after restricting fat intake)
- Serum with high IgG levels (possible false negative due to competition with IgG on the surface of latex particles or sheep red blood cells used as substrate)

Nursing Considerations

Before the Test
- Confirm the patient's identity using two patient identifiers and confirmation of the patient's identification bracelet according to facility policy.
- Explain to the patient that the test helps confirm RA.
- Inform the patient that there are no food or fluid restrictions for this test.
- Advise the patient that the test requires a blood sample. Explain that slight discomfort from the tourniquet and needle puncture may be experienced.

During the Test
- Perform a venipuncture and collect the sample in a 7-mL clot activator tube.

After the Test
- Apply direct pressure to the venipuncture site until bleeding stops and to prevent hematoma formation.
- Because a patient with RA may be immunologically compromised, keep the venipuncture site clean and dry for 24 hours.
- Check regularly for signs of infection.

Rubella Antibodies

Reference Values
Immunity: Titer more than 1:10 (positive)
No immunity: Titer 1:8 or less (negative)

Abnormal Findings
- Recent infection in an adult
- Congenital rubella in an infant

Nursing Implications
- Instruct the patient to return for an additional blood test when appropriate.
- If a woman of childbearing age is found to be susceptible to rubella, explain that vaccination can prevent rubella and that she must wait at least 3 months after the vaccination to become pregnant or risk permanent damage or death to the fetus.
- If the pregnant patient is found to be susceptible to rubella, instruct her to return for follow-up rubella antibody tests to detect possible subsequent infection. Immunization is contraindicated in pregnancy because of the risk of permanent damage or death to the fetus.
- If the test confirms rubella in a pregnant patient, provide emotional support. Refer her for appropriate counseling as needed.

Purpose
- To confirm the presence of immunity against rubella virus; may be ordered on newborn infants who may have been affected during pregnancy
- To detect a past rubella infection, especially congenital infection
- To identify those who have never been exposed to or vaccinated against rubella
- To verify that pregnant women and those planning to become pregnant have sufficient immunity to rubella to protect them and their unborn children from rubella infection

Description
Although rubella (German measles) is generally a mild viral infection in children and young adults, it can produce severe infection in the fetus, resulting in spontaneous abortion, stillbirth, or congenital rubella syndrome. Because rubella infection normally induces immunoglobulin (Ig) G and IgM antibody production, measuring rubella antibodies can determine present infection as well as immunity resulting from past infection. The hemagglutination inhibition test is the most commonly used serologic test for rubella antibodies.

Suspected cases of congenital rubella may be confirmed if rubella-specific IgM antibodies are present in the infant's serum. Immune status in adults can be confirmed by an existing IgG-specific titer.

Exposure risk (when the immunity status is unknown) may be evaluated using two serum samples. The first sample should be drawn in the acute phase of clinical symptoms. If clinical symptoms aren't apparent, the sample should be drawn as soon as possible after the suspected exposure. The second sample should be drawn 3 to 4 weeks later, during the convalescent phase.

Precautions
- Handle the sample gently to prevent hemolysis.

Nursing Considerations
Before the Test
- Confirm the patient's identity using two patient identifiers and confirmation of the patient's identification bracelet according to facility policy.
- Explain to the patient that the rubella antibodies test diagnoses or evaluates susceptibility to rubella.
- Inform the patient that there are no food or fluid restrictions for the test.
- Advise the patient that this test requires a blood sample and that if a current infection is suspected, a second blood sample will be needed in 2 to 3 weeks to identify a rise in the titer. Explain that the patient may experience slight discomfort from the tourniquet and needle puncture.

During the Test
- Perform a venipuncture and collect the sample in a 7-mL clot activator tube.

After the Test
- Apply direct pressure to the venipuncture site until bleeding stops and to prevent hematoma formation.

Severe Acute Respiratory Syndrome Viral Testing

Normal Findings
- Negative for severe acute respiratory syndrome (SARS) virus antibodies

Abnormal Findings
- SARS infection

Nursing Implications
- Report abnormal findings to the health care provider.
- Prepare to educate the patient about the diagnosis.
- Prepare the patient for further testing, as indicated.
- Provide emotional support to the patient and family.

Purpose
- To identify the SARS coronavirus (CoV) as the cause of the infection

Description
The SARS-CoV causes a pneumonia-like infection. The incubation period is approximately 8 to 10 days. Typically, a patient being tested has traveled to or lives in an area where the infection has been identified. Usually, SARS testing isn't performed unless there's a high index of suspicion, such as when groups of infections have developed and other causes have been ruled out.

Three different tests are available for SARS viral testing:

- enzyme-linked immunosorbent assay (ELISA), which identifies SARS virus antibodies, usually about 20 days after the onset of symptoms

- immunofluorescence assay, which identifies SARS virus antibodies as early as 10 days after infection (a time-consuming test because the virus is grown in the laboratory)
- reverse transcriptase–polymerase chain reaction (RT-PCR), which identifies the genetic information of ribonucleic acid in the virus as early as within 2 days.

Specimens for SARS testing may be obtained from the nasopharyngeal, oropharyngeal, or bronchoalveolar area; trachea; pleural fluid; sputum; or postmortem tissue. Testing with RT-PCR usually involves serum and blood samples.

Precautions
- Use standard precautions when performing the procedure and handling specimens; adhere to your facility's infection control policies at all times.
- Because the patient may cough violently during suctioning, wear gloves, a mask, and, if necessary, a gown to avoid exposure to pathogens.

Nursing Considerations

Before the Test
- Confirm the patient's identity using two patient identifiers and confirmation of the patient's identification bracelet according to facility policy.
- Explain to the patient that the SARS viral test is used to identify the organism causing respiratory tract infection and describe the types of specimens that will be collected and how the collections will be done.
- If the specimen will be collected by expectoration, encourage fluid intake

the night before collection to help sputum production, unless contraindicated by a fluid restriction. Teach the patient how to expectorate by taking three deep breaths and forcing a deep cough; emphasize that sputum isn't the same as saliva, which is unacceptable for culturing. Tell the patient to brush the teeth and gargle with water before the specimen collection to reduce contaminating oropharyngeal bacteria.

- If the specimen will be collected by swabbing the area, warn the patient that a slight itching sensation may be felt.
- If the specimen will be collected by tracheal suctioning, tell the patient that some discomfort may be experienced as the catheter passes into the trachea.
- If the specimen will be collected by bronchoscopy, instruct the patient to fast for 6 hours before the procedure.
- Make sure the patient or a responsible family member has signed an informed consent form.

During the Test
- Put on gloves.
- Proceed with the specimen collection as outlined here. Make sure that all specimens are placed in the appropriate sterile container for transport.

Washing or Aspirating the Nasopharyngeal Area
- Have the patient sit with the head tilted slightly back.
- Insert a syringe filled with 1 to 1.5 mL of nonbacteriostatic saline solution into one nostril and instill the saline.
- Attach a small plastic catheter or tubing to the syringe and flush it with 2 to 3 mL of saline.
- Insert the tubing into the nostril and aspirate the secretions; then repeat in the other nostril.

Swabbing the Nasopharyngeal or Oropharyngeal Area
- Obtain sterile swabs that have plastic sticks and Dacron or rayon tips.

▶ **Quality and Safety Nursing Alert**

Never use cotton-tipped applicators or swabs with wooden sticks. Some viruses can become inactivated by the substances contained in these swabs, thereby interfering with RT-PCR testing.

- Insert the swab into the nostril and let it remain there for several seconds to absorb the secretions; if swabbing the oropharyngeal area, run the swab along the posterior pharynx and tonsils. Avoid touching the tongue.

Expectorating Sputum
- Have the patient rinse the mouth with water.
- Instruct the patient to cough deeply and expectorate into the sterile dry container.

Collecting Blood and Plasma Samples
- Perform a venipuncture and collect 5 to 10 mL of whole blood in a serum separator tube (for serum RT-PCR or ELISA antibody testing) or an EDTA tube (for plasma testing).

Collecting Other Specimens
- Assist with tracheal suctioning, bronchoscopy, or thoracentesis, as appropriate.

After the Test
- Label the container with the patient's name. Include on the test request form the nature and origin of the specimen, the date and time of collection, the initial diagnosis, and any current antimicrobial therapy.
- Seal the container in a biohazard bag and send it to the laboratory immediately.
- Dispose of equipment properly.
- Provide mouth care as indicated.
- Report evidence of positive SARS tests to local, state, and federal health departments.

S

Sickle Cell Test

Normal Findings
- Absence of hemoglobin (Hb) S (negative result)
- Presence of Hb S (positive result)

Abnormal Findings
- Presence of sickle cells or elevated Hb S levels

Nursing Implications
- Report abnormal findings to the health care provider.
- Prepare to educate the patient about the diagnosis.
- Prepare the patient for further testing, such as Hb electrophoresis, to further diagnose the sickling tendency of cells.
- Provide emotional support to the patient and family.

Purpose
- To identify sickle cell disease and sickle cell trait (See the *Identifying Sickle Cell Trait* box.)

Description
The sickle cell test, also known as the *Hb S test*, is used to detect sickle cells, which are severely deformed, rigid erythrocytes that may slow blood flow. Sickle cell trait (characterized by heterozygous

---

Identifying Sickle Cell Trait

Sickle cell trait is a relatively benign condition that results from heterozygous inheritance of the abnormal hemoglobin (Hb) S producing gene. Like sickle cell anemia, it's most common in blacks.

In persons with sickle cell trait, 20% to 40% of their total Hb is Hb S; the rest is normal. Such persons, called carriers, usually have no symptoms. They have normal Hb and hematocrit values and can expect a normal lifespan. Nevertheless, they must avoid situations that provoke hypoxia, which occasionally causes a sickling crisis similar to that in sickle cell anemia.

Genetic counseling is essential for sickle cell carriers. Every child of two sickle cell carriers has a 25% chance of inheriting sickle cell anemia and a 50% chance of being a carrier.

Hb S) is found almost exclusively in African Americans; 0.2% of African Americans born in the United States have sickle cell disease.

Although the sickle cell test is useful as a rapid screening procedure, it may produce erroneous results. Hb electrophoresis should be performed to confirm the diagnosis if sickle cell disease is strongly suspected.

Interfering Factors
- Hb concentration less than 10%, elevated Hb S levels in infants younger than age 6 months, or transfusion within 3 months of the test (possible false negative)
- Transfusion within 3 months with RBCs having the sickle cell trait (possible false positive)

Precautions
- Handle the sample gently to prevent hemolysis.

Nursing Considerations

Before the Test
- Confirm the patient's identity using two patient identifiers and confirmation of the patient's identification bracelet according to facility policy.
- Explain to the patient that the Hb S test is used to detect sickle cell disease.
- Advise the patient that a blood sample will be taken. Explain that slight discomfort from the tourniquet and the needle puncture may be experienced.

> ▶ *Quality and Safety Nursing Alert*
>
> **If the patient is an infant or child, explain to the parents that a small amount of blood will be taken from the finger or earlobe.**

- Check the patient's history for a blood transfusion within the past 3 months.
- Inform the patient that there are no food or fluid restrictions.

During the Test

- Perform a venipuncture and collect the sample in a 3- or 4.5-mL EDTA tube.

 Quality and Safety Nursing Alert

For young children, collect capillary blood in a microcollection device.

- Completely fill the collection tube and invert it gently several times to thoroughly mix the sample and the anticoagulant.

After the Test

- If a hematoma develops at the venipuncture site, apply direct pressure. If the hematoma is large, monitor pulses distal to the phlebotomy site. Make sure subdermal bleeding has stopped before removing pressure.
- Patients with a positive sickle cell diagnosis may need genetic counseling and patient education to avoid acute exacerbations.

Skin Biopsy
Normal Findings

- Normal skin consisting of squamous epithelium (epidermis) and fibrous connective tissue (dermis)

Abnormal Findings

- Benign tumors or growths, such as cysts, seborrheic keratoses, warts, pigmented nevi (moles), keloids, dermatofibromas, multiple neurofibromas
- Malignant tumors, such as basal cell carcinoma, squamous cell carcinoma, malignant melanoma

Nursing Implications

- Report abnormal findings to the health care provider.
- Prepare to educate the patient about the diagnosis.
- Prepare the patient for further testing or surgery as indicated.
- Provide emotional support to the patient and family.

Purpose

- To provide differential diagnosis among basal cell carcinoma, squamous cell carcinoma, malignant melanoma, and benign growths
- To diagnose chronic bacterial or fungal skin infections

Description

Skin biopsy involves the removal of a small piece of tissue, under local anesthesia, from a lesion suspected of being malignant or from other dermatoses. One of three techniques may be used: shave biopsy, punch biopsy, or excisional biopsy. Shave biopsy uses a scalpel to slice a superficial specimen from the site. Punch biopsy removes an oval core from the center of a lesion down to the dermis or subcutaneous tissue. Excisional biopsy removes the entire lesion with a small border of normal skin.

Lesions suspected of being malignant usually have changed color, size, or appearance or have failed to heal properly after injury. Fully developed lesions should be selected for biopsy whenever possible because they provide more diagnostic information than lesions that are resolving or in early developing stages.

The procedure for skin biopsy starts with cleaning the biopsy site and administering a local anesthetic. The biopsy then proceeds as follows, depending on the method used:

Shave Biopsy

- The protruding growth is cut off at the skin line with a #15 scalpel, and the tissue is placed immediately in a properly labeled specimen bottle containing 10% formalin solution.
- Pressure is applied to the area to stop the bleeding.

Punch Biopsy

- The skin surrounding the lesion is pulled taut, and the punch is firmly introduced into the lesion and rotated to obtain a tissue specimen. The plug is lifted with forceps or a needle and

S

severed as deeply into the fat layer as possible.

• The specimen is placed in a properly labeled specimen bottle containing 10% formalin solution or in a sterile container, if indicated.

• Closing the wound depends on the size of the punch: A 3-mm punch requires only an adhesive bandage, a 4-mm punch requires one suture, and a 6-mm punch requires two sutures.

Excisional Biopsy

• A #15 scalpel is used to excise the entire lesion; an elliptical incision is made as wide and as deep as necessary.

• The tissue specimen is removed and placed immediately in a properly labeled specimen bottle containing 10% formalin solution.

• Pressure is applied to the site to stop bleeding.

• The wound is closed using 4-0 suture. If the incision is large, skin grafting may be required.

Interfering Factors

• Improper biopsy site selection
• Inability to obtain an appropriate specimen

Precautions

• Send the specimen to the laboratory immediately.

Nursing Considerations

Before the Test

• Confirm the patient's identity using two patient identifiers and confirmation of the patient's identification bracelet according to facility policy.

• Explain to the patient that the biopsy provides a specimen for microscopic study. Describe the procedure to the patient and answer questions. Tell the patient who will perform the procedure and where and when it will be done.

• Inform the patient that there are no food or fluid restrictions for this test.

• Advise the patient that a local anesthetic will be administered to minimize pain during the procedure. Check the patient's history for hypersensitivity to the anesthetic.

• Make sure the patient or a responsible family member has signed an informed consent form.

After the Test

• Check the biopsy site for bleeding.

• If the patient experiences pain, administer an analgesic as ordered.

• Advise the patient with sutures to keep the area as clean and dry as possible. Facial sutures are removed in 3 to 5 days; trunk sutures in 7 to 14 days. Tell the patient with adhesive strips to leave them in place for 14 to 21 days or until they fall off.

Skull Radiography

Normal Findings

• Age-appropriate size, shape, thickness, and position of the cranial bones, as well as vascular markings, sinuses, and sutures

Abnormal Findings

• Fractures of the vault or base
• Congenital anomalies
• Erosion, enlargement, or decalcification of the sella turcica resulting from increased intracranial pressure
• Osteomyelitis
• Chronic subdural hematomas
• Oligodendrogliomas
• Meningiomas
• Space-occupying lesions
• Acromegaly
• Paget's disease

Nursing Implications

• Report abnormal findings to the health care provider.

• Prepare to educate the patient about the diagnosis.

• Prepare the patient for further testing or surgery, as indicated.

• Provide emotional support to the patient and family.

Purpose

- To detect fractures in the patient with head trauma
- To help diagnose pituitary tumors
- To detect congenital anomalies
- To detect metabolic and endocrinologic disorders

Description

Although skull radiography is of limited value in assessing patients with head injuries, skull X-rays are extremely valuable for studying abnormalities of the skull base and cranial vault, congenital and perinatal anomalies, and systemic diseases that produce bone defects of the skull. For more accurate head injury, as well as skull and head abnormality assessments, nonenhanced computed tomographic studies of the head are done.

Skull radiography evaluates the three groups of bones that comprise the skull: the calvaria (vault), the mandible (jaw bone), and the facial bones. The calvaria and the facial bones are closely connected by immovable joints with irregular serrated edges called *sutures*. The skull bones form an anatomic structure so complex that a complete skull examination requires several radiologic views of each area.

The procedure for skull radiography is as follows:

- The patient is asked to recline on the X-ray table or sit in a chair and is instructed to remain still during the procedure.
- Foam pads, sandbags, or a headband are used to immobilize the patient's head and increase comfort.
- Five views of the skull are routinely taken: left and right lateral, anteroposterior Towne's, posteroanterior Caldwell, and axial (or base).
- Films are developed and checked for quality before the patient leaves the area.

Interfering Factors

- Improper patient positioning or excessive head movement (possible poor imaging)

- Failure to remove radiopaque objects from the X-ray field (possible poor imaging)

Nursing Considerations

Before the Test

- Confirm the patient's identity using two patient identifiers and confirmation of the patient's identification bracelet according to facility policy.
- Inform the patient that skull radiography helps to determine the presence of anomalies and helps establish a diagnosis. Explain that the head will be immobilized and that several X-rays of the skull will be taken from various angles. Tell the patient who will perform the test and when and where it will take place.
- Tell the patient that there are no food or fluid restrictions and that the test will cause no discomfort.
- Instruct the patient to remove glasses, dentures, jewelry, or any metallic objects that would be in the X-ray field.

Sodium, Serum

Reference Values

Adults and children: 135 to 145 mEq/L (SI, 135–145 mmol/L)
Infants: 132 to 142 mEq/L (SI, 132–142 mmol/L)

Critical Values

- Less than 120 mEq/L (SI, 120 mmol/L) or greater than 160 mEq/L (SI, greater than 160 mmol/L)

Abnormal Findings

Elevated Levels

- Diabetes insipidus
- Impaired renal function
- Prolonged hyperventilation
- Aldosteronism
- Excessive sodium intake

Decreased Levels

- Sweating
- GI suctioning
- Diuretic therapy
- Diarrhea

S

- Vomiting
- Adrenal insufficiency
- Burns
- Chronic renal insufficiency with acidosis

Nursing Implications

- Report abnormal findings to the health care provider.
- Observe the patient with elevated levels for hypernatremia (Na^+ greater than 135) and associated water loss, signs of thirst, restlessness, dry and sticky mucous membranes, flushed skin, oliguria, and diminished reflexes.
- If increased total body sodium causes water retention, observe patients with elevated levels for hypertension, dyspnea, edema, and heart failure.
- In the patient with decreased levels and hyponatremia, watch for apprehension, lassitude, headache, decreased skin turgor, abdominal cramps, and tremors that may progress to seizures.
- Prepare the patient for further testing as indicated.

Purpose

- To evaluate fluid, electrolyte, and acid–base balance and related neuromuscular, renal, and adrenal functions

Description

The sodium test is used to measure serum sodium levels in relation to the amount of water in the body. Sodium, the major extracellular cation, affects body water distribution, maintains extracellular fluid osmotic pressure, and helps promote neuromuscular function. It also helps maintain acid–base balance and influences chloride and potassium levels.

Because extracellular sodium concentration helps the kidneys to regulate body water (decreased sodium levels promote water excretion and increased levels promote retention), serum sodium levels are evaluated in relation to the amount of water in the body. For example, a sodium deficit (hyponatremia) refers to a decreased level of sodium in relation to the body's water level. (See the *Fluid Imbalances* table.)

The body normally regulates this sodium–water balance through aldosterone, which inhibits sodium excretion and promotes its reabsorption (with water) by the renal tubules to maintain balance. Low sodium levels stimulate aldosterone secretion; elevated sodium levels depress it.

Interfering Factors

- Most diuretics (decrease by promoting sodium excretion)
- Chlorpropamide, lithium, and vasopressin (decrease by inhibiting water excretion)
- Corticosteroids (increase by promoting sodium retention)
- Antihypertensives, such as hydralazine, methyldopa, and reserpine (possible increase due to sodium and water retention)

Precautions

- Handle the sample gently to prevent hemolysis.

Nursing Considerations

Before the Test

- Confirm the patient's identity using two patient identifiers and confirmation of the patient's identification bracelet according to facility policy.
- Explain to the patient that the serum sodium test is used to determine the sodium content of the blood.
- Advise the patient that the test requires a blood sample. Explain that slight discomfort from the tourniquet and the needle puncture may be experienced.
- Inform the patient that there are no food or fluid restrictions.
- Notify the laboratory and health care provider of medications the patient is taking that may affect test results; these may need to be restricted.

During the Test

- Perform a venipuncture and collect the sample in a 3- or 4-mL clot activator tube.

Fluid Imbalances

This table lists the causes, signs and symptoms, and diagnostic test findings associated with hypervolemia (increased fluid volume) and hypovolemia (decreased fluid volume).

Causes	Signs and Symptoms	Laboratory Findings
Hypervolemia		
• Increased water intake • Decreased water output due to renal disease • Heart failure • Excessive ingestion or infusion of sodium chloride • Long-term administration of adrenocortical hormones • Excessive infusion of isotonic solutions	• Increased blood pressure, pulse rate, body weight, and respiratory rate • Bounding peripheral pulses • Moist pulmonary crackles • Moist mucous membranes • Moist respiratory secretions • Edema • Weakness • Seizures and coma due to swelling of brain cells	• Decreased red blood cell (RBC) count, hemoglobin (Hb) concentration, packed cell volume, serum sodium concentration (dilutional decrease), and urine specific gravity
Hypovolemia		
• Decreased water intake • Fluid loss due to fever, diarrhea, or vomiting • Systemic infection • Impaired renal concentrating ability • Fistulous drainage • Severe burns • Hidden fluid in body cavities	• Increased pulse and respiratory rates • Decreased blood pressure and body weight • Weak and thready peripheral pulses • Thick, slurred speech • Thirst • Oliguria • Anuria • Dry skin	• Increased RBC count, Hb concentration, packed cell volume, serum sodium concentration, and urine specific gravity

After the Test
• Apply direct pressure to the venipuncture site until bleeding stops and to prevent hematoma formation.
• Instruct the patient to resume any medications that were discontinued before the test, as ordered.

Stool Culture
Normal Findings
• Bacteria not associated with enteric disease, non–spore-forming bacilli, clostridia, anaerobic streptococci
• Gram-negative bacilli (predominantly *Escherichia coli* and other Enterobacteriaceae, plus small amounts of *Pseudomonas* gram-positive cocci (mostly enterococci)
• Yeasts

Abnormal Findings
• Bacteria associated with enteric disease
• *Shigella*
• *Salmonella*
• *Bacillus cereus*
• *Campylobacter jejuni*
• *Vibrio cholerae*
• *V. parahaemolyticus*
• *Clostridium botulinum* (food poisoning)
• *Clostridium difficile*
• *Campylobacter perfringens*
• *Staphylococcus aureus* (possible infection)
• Enterotoxigenic *E. coli*
• *Yersinia enterocolitica*

Nursing Implications
• Report abnormal findings to the health care provider.

S

- Prepare to educate the patient about the diagnosis.
- Prepare the patient for further testing as indicated.
- Prepare to administer antimicrobial therapy, as indicated.

Purpose

- To identify pathogenic organisms caused by GI disease
- To identify healthy persons infected with pathogenic bacteria in a carrier state

Description

Normal bacterial flora in stools include several potentially pathogenic organisms. Bacteriologic examination is valuable for identifying pathogens that cause overt GI disease, such as typhoid and dysentery, and carrier states. A sensitivity test may follow isolation of the pathogen. The most common pathogenic organisms of the GI tract are *Shigella*, *Salmonella*, and *Campylobacter jejuni*. Less common pathogenic organisms include *V. cholerae*, *Clostridium botulinum*, *C. difficile*, *C. perfringens*, *S. aureus*, enterotoxigenic *E. coli*, *B. cereus*, *Y. enterocolitica*, and *V. parahaemolyticus*. (See the *Pathogens of the GI Tract* box.) Identifying these organisms is vital to treating the patient, to prevent possibly fatal complications (especially in a debilitated patient), and

to confine these severe infectious diseases. A sensitivity test may follow isolation of the pathogen.

Some viruses, such as rotavirus and parvovirus, may also cause GI symptoms. However, these viruses can be detected only by immunoassay or electron microscopy. Stool culture may detect other viruses, such as enterovirus, which can cause aseptic meningitis.

Interfering Factors

- Contamination of the specimen by urine (possible injury to or destruction of enteric pathogens)
- Antimicrobial therapy (possible decrease in bacterial growth)
- Recent barium studies (possible interference in detecting parasites)

Precautions

- Use standard precautions when performing the procedure and handling the specimen.
- If the patient uses a bedpan or a diaper, avoid contaminating the stool specimen with urine or toilet paper.
- Do not collect stool if the patient has defecated into the toilet.
- The specimen must represent the first, middle, and last portion of the stools passed. Be sure to include mucoid and bloody portions.
- Specimens should be collected before antimicrobial therapy is started.

Pathogens of the GI Tract

The presence of the following pathogens in a stool culture may indicate certain disorders.

Aeromonas hydrophila: gastroenteritis, which causes diarrhea, especially in children
Bacillus cereus: food poisoning, acute gastroenteritis (rare)
Campylobacter jejuni: gastroenteritis
Clostridium botulinum: food poisoning and infant botulism (a possible cause of sudden infant death syndrome)
Toxin-producing Clostridium difficile: pseudomembranous enterocolitis
Clostridium perfringens: food poisoning
Enterotoxigenic Escherichia coli: gastroenteritis (resembles cholera or shigellosis)

Salmonella: gastroenteritis, typhoid fever, nontyphoidal salmonellosis, paratyphoid fever
Shigella: shigellosis, bacillary dysentery
Staphylococcus aureus: food poisoning, suppression of normal bowel flora from antimicrobial therapy
Vibrio cholerae: cholera
Vibrio parahaemolyticus: food poisoning, especially seafood
Yersinia enterocolitica: gastroenteritis, enterocolitis (resembles appendicitis), mesenteric lymphadenitis, ileitis

Nursing Considerations

Before the Test

- Confirm the patient's identity using two patient identifiers and confirmation of the patient's identification bracelet according to facility policy.
- Explain to the patient that the stool culture is used to determine the cause of GI distress or to determine if the patient is a carrier of infectious organisms and that it requires collecting a stool specimen on 3 consecutive days.
- Advise the patient that there are no food or fluid restrictions for this test.
- Special measures must be undertaken with infants who wear diapers to prevent the contamination of the stool specimen with urine and to keep stool from touching the inside of disposable diapers that may have a bacteriostatic agent.
- Check the patient's history for dietary patterns, recent antimicrobial therapy, and recent travel that might suggest endemic infections or infestations.

During the Test

- Collect a stool specimen directly into the container. If the patient isn't ambulatory, collect the specimen in a clean, dry bedpan and, using a tongue blade, transfer the specimen to the container.
- If you must collect the specimen by rectal swab, insert the swab past the anal sphincter, rotate it gently, and withdraw it. Then place the swab in the appropriate container.
- Check with the laboratory for the proper collection procedure before obtaining a specimen for a virus test.
- Label the specimen with the patient's name, health care provider's name, facility number, and date and time of collection.
- Put the specimen container in a leak-proof bag.
- Send the specimen to the laboratory immediately. Trophozoites and cysts may be destroyed if exposed to heat, cold, or a delay in delivery to the laboratory.
- Indicate the suspected enteritis cause and current antimicrobial therapy on the laboratory request.

Stool Examination

Normal Findings

- No parasites or ova in stools

Abnormal Findings

- *Entamoeba histolytica* (confirms amebiasis)
- *Giardia lamblia* (confirms giardiasis)
- Helminth ova or larvae
- Hookworms
- *Diphyllobothrium latum*

Nursing Implications

- Report abnormal findings to the health care provider.
- Prepare to educate the patient about the diagnosis.
- Prepare the patient for further testing as indicated.

Purpose

- To confirm or rule out intestinal parasitic infection and disease

Description

Stool specimen examination is frequently used to diagnose the cause of prolonged diarrhea and to detect several types of intestinal parasites. Some of these parasites live in nonpathogenic symbiosis; others cause intestinal disease. In the United States, the most common parasites include the roundworms *Ascaris lumbricoides* and *Necator americanus* (commonly called *hookworm*); the tapeworms *D. latum*, *Taenia saginata*, and, rarely, *T. solium*; the amoeba *E. histolytica*; and the flagellate *G. lamblia*. Cyclospora can also be detected in stool examination for ova and parasites.

Detection of pinworm requires a different collection method. (See the *Collection Procedure for Pinworm* box.)

S

Collection Procedure for Pinworm

The ova of the pinworm *Enterobius vermicularis* seldom appear in stools because the female migrates to the anus and deposits her ova there. To collect them, place a piece of cellophane tape, sticky side out, on the end of a tongue blade, and press it firmly on the anal area. Then transfer the tape, sticky side down, to a slide. (Kits with tape and a slide or a sticky paddle are available.) Because the female usually deposits her ova at night, collect the specimen early in the morning, before the patient bathes or defecates.

Interfering Factors
- Presence of urine (false-negative results)
- Excessive heat or cold
- Recent barium studies (possible interference with detection of organism)

Precautions
- Don't contaminate the stool specimen with urine, which can destroy trophozoites.
- Don't collect stools from a toilet bowl because water is toxic to trophozoites and may contain organisms that interfere with test results.
- If the entire stool can't be sent to the laboratory, include macroscopic worms or worm segments, as well as bloody and mucoid portions of the specimen.
- Use gloves when performing the procedure and handling the specimen, disposing of equipment, sealing the container, and transporting the specimen. Dispose of gloves after specimen collection and transport.

Nursing Considerations
Before the Test
- Confirm the patient's identity using two patient identifiers and confirmation of the patient's identification bracelet according to facility policy.
- Explain to the patient that the stool examination detects intestinal parasitic infection and that it requires three separate stool specimens—one every other day or every third day. Up to six specimens may be required to confirm the presence of *E. histolytica*.
- Instruct the patient to avoid treatments with castor or mineral oil, bismuth, magnesium or antidiarrheal compounds, barium enemas, and antibiotics for 7 to 10 days before the test.
- If the patient has diarrhea, assess recent dietary and travel history.
- Check the patient's history for use of antiparasitic drugs, such as tetracycline, paromomycin (Humatin), metronidazole (Flagyl), and iodoquinol (Yodoxin), within 2 weeks of the test.

During the Test
- Put on gloves and collect a stool specimen directly in the container. If the patient is bedridden, collect the specimen in a clean, dry bedpan, and then, using a tongue blade, transfer it into a properly labeled container.
- Note on the laboratory request the date and time of collection and the specimen consistency. Also record recent or current antimicrobial therapy and any pertinent history.
- Send the specimen to the laboratory immediately. If a liquid or soft stool specimen can't be examined within 30 minutes of passage, place it in a preservative; if a formed stool specimen can't be examined immediately, refrigerate it or place it in preservative.

After the Test
- Instruct the patient to resume usual medications, as ordered.

Stool Examination for Rotavirus Antigen
Normal Findings
- Absence of rotavirus

Abnormal Findings
- Rotavirus infection

Nursing Implications

- Report abnormal findings to the health care provider.
- Prepare to educate the patient about the diagnosis.
- Prepare the patient for further testing or surgery, as indicated.
- Provide emotional support to the patient and family.

Purpose

- To obtain a laboratory diagnosis of rotavirus gastroenteritis

Description

Rotaviruses are the most common cause of infectious diarrhea in infants and young children. They're most prevalent in children ages 3 months to 2 years during the winter months and in adults with HIV infection. Clinical features include diarrhea, vomiting, fever, and abdominal pain. Infection symptoms may range from mild in adults to severe in young children, especially hospitalized infants.

Human rotavirus detection typically requires sensitive, specific enzyme immunoassays that provide results within minutes or hours (depending on the assay) because human rotaviruses don't replicate efficiently in laboratory cell cultures. Specimens are collected during the prodromal and acute stages of clinical infection to ensure detection of the viral antigens by enzyme immunoassay.

Interfering Factors

- Collection of a specimen in containers with preservatives, such as detergents, metal ions, or serum (decreased number of pathogens)

Precautions

- Avoid using collection containers with preservatives, metal ions, detergents, and serum, which may interfere with the assay.
- Store stool specimens for up to 24 hours at 35° to 46°F (1.6° to 7.7°C). If a longer storage period or shipment is necessary, freeze specimens at –4°F (–20°C) or colder. Repeated freezing and thawing will cause the specimen to deteriorate and yield misleading results.
- Don't store the specimen in a self-defrosting freezer.
- Use gloves when obtaining or handling all specimens.

Nursing Considerations

Before the Test

- Confirm the patient's identity using two patient identifiers and confirmation of the patient's identification bracelet according to facility policy.
- Explain the purpose of stool examination to the patient or parents (if the patient is a child) and inform them that the test requires a stool specimen.

During the Test

- Collect the specimens by placing 1 g of stools in a screw-capped tube or vial (usual collection method). If a microbiological transport swab is used, it must be heavily stained with stools to be diagnostically productive for rotavirus.

After the Test

- Monitor the patient's intake and output, and provide the patient with fluids to avoid dehydration caused by vomiting and diarrhea. Severe dehydration will require parenteral fluid therapy.

Sweat Test

Reference Values

Sodium: 10 to 30 mEq/L (SI, 10–30 mmol/L)
Chloride: 10 to 35 mEq/L (SI, 10–35 mmol/L)

Abnormal Findings

Elevated Levels

- Cystic fibrosis (sodium concentrations 50–60 mEq/L [SI, 50–60 mmol/L] strongly suggests disease; concentrations above 60 mEq/L [SI, greater than

60 mmol/L] along with typical clinical features confirms diagnosis)
- Untreated adrenal insufficiency (Addison's disease)
- Type I glycogen storage disease
- Vasopressin-resistant diabetes insipidus, meconium ileus, renal failure, and alcoholic pancreatitis

Nursing Implications
- Report abnormal findings to the health care provider.
- Prepare to educate the patient about the diagnosis.
- Prepare the patient for further testing or surgery as indicated.
- Provide emotional support to the patient and family.

Purpose
- To confirm or exclude the cystic fibrosis (CF) diagnosis in persons suspicious of having CF and in siblings of CF patients

Description
The sweat test is a quantitative measurement of electrolyte concentrations (primarily sodium and chloride) in sweat, usually performed using pilocarpine iontophoresis (pilocarpine is a sweat inducer). Although this test is used primarily to confirm CF in children, it's also performed on adults to determine if they're homozygous or heterozygous for the disorder. Genetic testing for CF also has become available. (See the *Tag-It Cystic Fibrosis Kit* box.)

Interfering Factors
- Dehydration or edema, especially in the collection area
- Failure to obtain an adequate amount of sweat, a common problem in neonates
- Presence of pure salt depletion, common during hot weather (possible false normal)
- Failure to clean the skin thoroughly or to use sterile gauze pads (possible false high)
- Failure to seal the gauze pad or filter paper carefully (possible false high electrolyte levels due to evaporation)

Precautions
- Always perform iontophoresis on the right arm (or right thigh). Never perform iontophoresis on the chest, especially in a child, because the current can induce cardiac arrest.
- Use battery-powered equipment, if possible, to prevent electric shock.
- Stop the test immediately if the patient complains of a burning sensation, which usually indicates that the positive electrode is exposed or positioned improperly. Adjust the electrode and continue the test.

Nursing Considerations
Before the Test
- Confirm the patient's identity using two patient identifiers and confirmation of the patient's identification bracelet according to facility policy.

Tag-It Cystic Fibrosis Kit

The U.S. Food and Drug Administration approved the use of a DNA test for diagnosing cystic fibrosis (CF). The test, called the *Tag-It Cystic Fibrosis Kit,* is a blood test that screens for genetic mutations and variations in the CF transmembrane conductance regulator (CFTR) gene. This test identifies 23 genetic mutations and four variations in the CFTR gene. It also screens for 16 additional mutations in the gene that are involved in many cases of CF.

The test is recommended for use in detecting and identifying these mutations and variations in the gene as a means for determining carrier status in adults, screening neonates, and confirming diagnostic testing in neonates and children. There are more than 1,300 genetic variations in the CFTR gene responsible for causing CF. Therefore, the test isn't recommended as the only means for diagnosing CF. Test results need to be viewed along with the patient's condition, ethnic background, and family history. Additionally, genetic counseling is suggested to help patients understand the results and their implications.

- Explain the sweat test to the child (if old enough to understand), using clear, simple terms. Explain that the patient may feel a slight tickling sensation during the procedure, but won't feel any pain.
- Inform the child and parents that there are no restrictions on diet, medication, or activity before the test.
- Encourage the parents to assist with preparations and to stay with their child during the test. Their presence will minimize the child's anxiety.

During the Test

- Wash the area that will undergo iontophoresis with distilled water and dry it. (The flexor surface of the right forearm is commonly used or, when the patient's arm is too small to secure electrodes [as with an infant], the right thigh.)
- Place a gauze pad saturated with premeasured pilocarpine solution on the positive electrode; place the pad saturated with normal saline solution on the negative electrode.
- Apply both electrodes to the area to undergo iontophoresis and secure them with straps. Lead wires to the analyzer are given a current of 4 mA in 15 to 20 seconds. Iontophoresis will continue at 15- to 20-second intervals for 5 minutes.
- Try to distract the child with a book, television, toy, or another diversion if nervous or frightened during the test.

- Remove both electrodes after iontophoresis.
- Discard the pads, clean the skin with distilled water, and then dry it.
- Using forceps, place a dry gauze pad or filter paper (previously weighed on a gram scale) on the area that underwent iontophoresis. Cover the pad or filter paper with a slightly larger piece of plastic, and seal the edges of the plastic with waterproof adhesive tape.
- Leave the gauze pad or filter paper in place for about 30 to 40 minutes. (The appearance of droplets on the plastic usually indicates induction of an adequate amount of sweat.)
- Remove the pad or filter paper with the forceps, place it immediately in the weighing bottle, and insert the stopper in the bottle. (The difference between the first and second weights indicates the weight of the sweat specimen collected.)
- Be sure to collect at least 100 mg of sweat for analysis.
- Carefully seal the gauze pad or filter paper in the weighing bottle and immediately send the bottle to the laboratory.

After the Test

- Wash the area that underwent iontophoresis with soap and water, and dry it thoroughly. If the area looks red, assure the patient that this reaction is normal and will disappear within a few hours.
- Tell the patient or parents that usual activities may be resumed.

S

T- and B-Lymphocyte Assays

Reference Values
T cells: 68% to 75% of total lymphocytes (1,400–2,700/mcL)
B cells: 10% to 20% of total
lymphocytes (270–640/mcL)
Null cells: 5% to 20% of total
lymphocytes
Total lymphocyte count: 1,500 to
3,000/mcL

Abnormal Findings

Elevated T-Cell Count
- Multiple myeloma
- Acute lymphocytic leukemia
- Graves' disease

Elevated B-Cell Count
- Chronic lymphocytic leukemia
- Multiple myeloma
- Waldenström's macroglobulinemia
- DiGeorge's syndrome

Decreased T-Cell Count
- DiGeorge's, Nezelof's, and Wiskott-
  Aldrich's syndromes
- Chronic lymphocytic leukemia
- Waldenström's macroglobulinemia
- Acquired immune deficiency syndrome
- Systemic lupus erythematosus

Decreased B-Cell Count
- Acute lymphocytic leukemia
- Congenital or acquired immunoglob-
  ulin deficiency diseases

Nursing Implications
- Report abnormal findings to the
  health care provider.
- Prepare to educate the patient about
  the diagnosis.
- Prepare the patient for further testing,
  as indicated.

Purpose
- To help diagnose primary and secondary immunodeficiency diseases
- To distinguish between benign and
  malignant lymphocytic proliferative
  diseases
- To monitor the patient's response to
  therapy

Description
Lymphocytes, key cells in the immune
system, have the capacity to recognize
antigens through special receptors
on their surfaces. The two primary
kinds of lymphocytes, T and B cells,
originate in the bone marrow. T cells
mature under the influence of the thy-
mus gland; B cells evolve without thymic influence.

The procedure for T- and B-lymphocyte
assays recovers approximately 80% of
the lymphocytes, but doesn't differentiate between T and B cells. The percentage of T and B cells is determined by
attaching a label or marker and by using
different identification techniques. The
rosette assay identifies T cells, which
tend to form unstable clusterlike shapes
(or rosettes) after exposure to sheep red
blood cells at 39.2°F (4°C). Direct immunofluorescence detects B cells, which
have monoclonal immunoglobulin on
their surfaces; unlike T cells, B cells present receptors for complement, as well as
for Fc portions of immunoglobulin.

Interfering Factors
- Exposing the sample to temperature
  extremes
- Changes in health status from the
  effects of chemotherapy, radiography,
  steroid or immunosuppressive therapy,

stress, or surgery (possible rapid change in T- and B-cell counts)

• Immunoglobulins, such as autologous antilymphocyte antibodies, that sometimes occur in autoimmune disease (possible change in results)

Precautions

• If antilymphocyte antibodies are suspected, as in autoimmune disease, notify the laboratory.

Nursing Considerations

Before the Test

• Confirm the patient's identity using two patient identifiers and confirmation of the patient's identification bracelet according to facility policy.

• Explain to the patient that the T- and B-lymphocyte assays measure certain white blood cells.

• Advise the patient that this test requires a blood sample. Explain that slight discomfort from the tourniquet and the needle puncture may be experienced.

During the Test

• Perform a venipuncture and collect the sample in a 7-mL green-topped tube.

• Fill the collection tube completely and invert it gently several times to mix the sample and the anticoagulant adequately.

• Send the sample to the laboratory immediately to ensure viable lymphocytes.

After the Test

• Apply direct pressure to the venipuncture site until bleeding stops and to prevent hematoma formation.

• Because the patient with T- and B-cell changes may have a compromised immune system, keep the venipuncture site clean and dry.

Thallium Imaging

Normal Findings

• Normal distribution of the isotope throughout the left ventricle

• No defects (cold spots)

• Improved regional perfusion after coronary artery bypass surgery, indicating graft patency

• Increased perfusion after taking antianginal drugs, indicating ischemia relief

• Improved perfusion after balloon angioplasty

Abnormal Findings

• Persistent defects, indicating myocardial infarction (MI)

• Transient defects that disappear after 3 to 6 hours, indicating ischemia from coronary artery disease (CAD)

Nursing Implications

• Report abnormal findings to the health care provider.

• Prepare to educate the patient about the diagnosis.

• Prepare the patient for further testing or surgery, as indicated.

Purpose

• To assess myocardial scarring and perfusion

• To demonstrate the location and extent of acute or chronic MI, including transmural and postoperative infarction (resting imaging)

• To diagnose CAD (stress imaging)

• To evaluate the patency of grafts after coronary artery bypass grafting (CABG)

• To evaluate the effectiveness of antianginal therapy or balloon angioplasty (stress imaging)

• To measure efficacy of certain pharmacotherapeutic agents.

Description

Also called *cold spot myocardial imaging* or *thallium scintigraphy*, thallium imaging evaluates myocardial blood flow after radioisotope thallium-201 or Cardiolite IV injection. The main difference between these tracers is that Cardiolite has a better energy spectrum for imaging. Cardiolite requires living myocardial cells for uptake and allows for imaging the myocardial

T

blood flow before and after reperfusion. This sequence allows for better myocardial salvage estimation. Because thallium, the physiologic potassium analogue, concentrates in healthy myocardial tissue but not in necrotic or ischemic tissue, areas of the heart with a normal blood supply and intact cells rapidly take it up. Areas with poor blood flow and ischemic cells fail to take up the isotope and appear as "cold spots" on a scan.

This test is performed in a resting state or after stress. Resting imaging can detect acute MI within the first few hours of symptoms, but doesn't distinguish an old from a new infarction. Stress imaging, performed after the patient exercises on a treadmill until experiencing angina or rate-limiting fatigue, can assess known or suspected CAD and can evaluate the effectiveness of antianginal therapy or balloon angioplasty and the patency of grafts after CABG. Possible complications of stress testing include arrhythmias, angina pectoris, and MI.

The procedure for thallium imaging is as follows:

Resting Imaging
- Optimally, the patient receives an injection of IV thallium or Cardiolite within the first few hours of MI symptoms and scanning begins after 10 minutes.
- If further scanning is required, the patient is told to rest and restrict food and beverages other than water.

Stress Imaging
- The patient, wired with electrodes, walks on a treadmill at a regulated pace that's gradually increased while the electrocardiogram (ECG), blood pressure, and heart rate are monitored.
- When the patient reaches peak stress, the examiner injects 1.5 to 3 millicuries of thallium into the antecubital vein and then flushes it with 10 to 15 mL of normal saline solution or an infusion of Cardiolite.
- The patient exercises an additional 45 to 60 seconds to permit circulation

and uptake of the isotope and then lies on the back under the scintillation camera.
- If the patient is asymptomatic, the precordial leads are removed. Scanning begins after 10 minutes with the patient in the anterior, left anterior oblique, and left lateral positions.
- Additional scans may be taken after the patient rests and, rarely, after 24 hours. Taking a scan after the patient rests is helpful in differentiating between an ischemic area and an infarcted or scarred area of the myocardium.

Interfering Factors
- Cold spots (possible result of sarcoidosis, myocardial fibrosis, cardiac contusion, attenuation due to soft tissue, apical cleft, coronary spasm, and artifacts, such as implants and electrodes)
- The absence of a cold spot in the presence of CAD (possibly because of insignificant obstruction, inadequate stress, delayed imaging, collateral circulation, or single-vessel disease, particularly of the right or left circumflex coronary arteries)

Precautions
- Contraindications to testing include impaired neuromuscular function, pregnancy, locomotor disturbances, acute MI or myocarditis, aortic stenosis, acute infection, unstable metabolic conditions (such as diabetes), digoxin toxicity, and recent pulmonary infarction.
- Have emergency medical equipment readily available if needed.

> ### ▶ Quality and Safety Nursing Alert
>
> Stop stress imaging at once if the patient develops chest pain, dyspnea, fatigue, syncope, hypotension, ischemic ECG changes, significant arrhythmias, or critical signs and symptoms (pale, clammy skin, confusion, or staggering) or significant hypertension.

Nursing Considerations

Before the Test

- Confirm the patient's identity using two patient identifiers and confirmation of the patient's identification bracelet according to facility policy.
- Explain to the patient that thallium imaging helps determine if any areas of the heart muscle aren't receiving an adequate blood supply. Describe the test, including who will perform it and when and where it will take place. Explain that the patient will receive an IV radioactive tracer, that multiple images of the heart will be scanned, and that it's important to lie still while the images are taken. Advise that additional scans may be required.
- Remove any topical vasodilators, as ordered by the patient's primary health care provider.
- Warn the patient that discomfort from skin abrasion during preparation for electrode placement may be experienced. Assure the patient that the test involves minimal radiation exposure.
- Instruct the patient undergoing stress imaging to restrict alcohol, tobacco, and nonprescribed medications for 24 hours before the test, as ordered, and to have nothing by mouth for 3 hours before the test. Also instruct the patient to wear walking shoes during the test and to report any fatigue, pain, or shortness of breath immediately.
- Make sure that the patient or a responsible family member has signed an informed consent form.

Thoracoscopy

Normal Findings

- Small amount of lubricating fluid (facilitates movement of the lung and chest wall)
- Lesion-free parietal and visceral layers that can separate from each other

Abnormal Findings

- Lesions, such as tumors, ulcers, and bleeding sites
- Carcinoma
- Empyema
- Pleural effusion
- Tuberculosis

Nursing Implications

- Report abnormal findings to the health care provider.
- Prepare to educate the patient about the diagnosis.
- Prepare the patient for further testing or surgery, as indicated.

Purpose

- To diagnose pleural disease
- To obtain biopsy specimens
- To treat pleural conditions, such as cysts, blebs, and effusions
- To perform wedge resections (e.g., to remove diseased lung tissue)

Description

In thoracoscopy, an endoscope is inserted directly into the chest wall to view the pleural space, thoracic walls, mediastinum, and pericardium. It's used for diagnostic and therapeutic purposes and can sometimes replace traditional thoracotomy. Thoracoscopy reduces morbidity (by reducing the use of open chest surgery) and postoperative pain, decreases surgical and anesthesia time, and allows faster recovery.

The procedure for thoracoscopy is as follows:

- The patient is anesthetized and a double-lumen endobronchial tube is inserted.
- The operative side lung is collapsed, and a small intercostal incision (approximately 1 inch [2.5 cm] long) is made through which a trocar is inserted.
- A lens is then inserted to view the area and assess thoracoscopy access.
- Two or three more small incisions (approximately 1 inch long) are made, and trocars are placed to insert suction and dissection instruments.

T

- The camera lens and instruments are moved from site to site as needed.
- After thoracoscopy, the lung is reexpanded, a chest tube is placed through one incision site, and a water-sealed drainage system is attached. The other incisions are closed with adhesive strips and dressed.

Interfering Factors
- Extensive disease or inaccessibility (may prevent thoracoscopy)
- Excessive bleeding during the procedure (may require open thoracotomy)
- Use of antiseptic mouthwash

Precautions
- If specimens are obtained, send them to the laboratory immediately.
- Thoracoscopy is contraindicated in the patient who has coagulopathies or lesions near major blood vessels, has extensive pleural disease or pleural adhesions, or can't be adequately oxygenated with one lung.

> **Quality and Safety Nursing Alert**
>
> Be alert for complications, although rare, including hemorrhage, nerve injury, perforation of the diaphragm, air emboli, and tension pneumothorax.

Nursing Considerations
Before the Test
- Confirm the patient's identity using two patient identifiers and confirmation of the patient's identification bracelet according to facility policy.
- Describe the procedure and explain to the patient that thoracoscopy permits visual examination of the chest wall to view the pleural space, thoracic wall, mediastinum, and pericardium.
- Explain that the patient will have a chest tube and drainage system in place after surgery and that analgesics will be available for control of pain.
- Instruct the patient not to eat or drink for 10 to 12 hours before the procedure.

- Make sure that the appropriate preoperative tests (such as pulmonary function and coagulation tests, electrocardiography, and chest X-ray) have been performed and that an informed consent form has been signed.

After the Test
- Monitor the patient's postoperative vital signs as per facility policy or every 15 minutes for 1 hour, every 30 minutes for 2 hours, every hour for 2 hours, and then every 4 hours.
- Assess the patient's respiratory status, the chest drainage system patency, and the drainage amount in the drainage chamber of the chest drainage system.
- Patient must remain NPO until gag reflex returns.
- Give analgesics, as needed, for pain, and monitor the patient for adverse effects.

Throat Culture
Normal Findings
- Nonhemolytic and alpha-hemolytic streptococci
- *Neisseria* species
- Staphylococci
- Diphtheroids
- Some *Haemophilus* species
- Pneumococci
- Yeasts
- Enteric gram-negative rods
- Spirochetes
- *Veillonella* species
- *Micrococcus* species

Abnormal Findings
- Group A beta-hemolytic streptococci (*Streptococcus pyogenes*) (scarlet fever and pharyngitis)
- *Candida albicans* (thrush)
- *Corynebacterium diphtheriae* (diphtheria)
- *Bordetella pertussis* (whooping cough)
- *N. gonorrhoeae*
- *Neisseria meningitidis*
- *Mycoplasma* and *Chlamydia*

Nursing Implications
- Report abnormal findings to the health care provider.
- Prepare to educate the patient about the diagnosis.
- Prepare the patient for further testing, as indicated.
- Provide emotional support to the patient and family.
- Prepare to institute isolation precautions, as indicated.
- Prepare to administer antimicrobial therapy, as indicated.

Purpose
- To isolate and identify group A beta-hemolytic streptococci
- To screen asymptomatic carriers of pathogens, especially *N. meningitidis*

Description
A throat culture is used primarily to isolate and identify pathogens, thus allowing early treatment of pharyngitis and prevention of sequelae, such as rheumatic heart disease and glomerulonephritis. It's also used to screen for carriers of *N. meningitidis*. In rare instances, a throat culture may be used to identify *C. diphtheriae* or *B. pertussis*. Although a throat culture may also be used to identify *C. albicans*, direct potassium hydroxide preparation usually provides the same information more quickly.

A throat culture requires swabbing the back of the throat, streaking a culture plate, and allowing the organisms to grow for pathogen isolation and identification. A Gram-stained smear may provide preliminary identification, which may guide clinical management and determine the need for further tests. Culture results are considered in relation to the patient's clinical status, recent antimicrobial therapy, and normal flora amount.

Interfering Factors
- Failure to report recent or current antimicrobial therapy on the laboratory request (possible false negative)
- More than a 15-minute delay in sending the specimen to the laboratory

Precautions
- Obtain the throat specimen before beginning antimicrobial therapy.
- Wear personal protective equipment when performing the procedure and handling specimens.

> **Quality and Safety Nursing Alert**
>
> Laryngospasm may occur after the throat culture is obtained if the patient has epiglottitis or diphtheria. Keep resuscitation equipment nearby.

Nursing Considerations

Before the Test
- Confirm the patient's identity using two patient identifiers and confirmation of the patient's identification bracelet according to facility policy.
- Explain to the patient that the throat culture is used to identify microorganisms that may be causing symptoms or to screen for asymptomatic carriers.
- Inform the patient that there are no food or fluid restrictions for this test.
- Advise the patient that a specimen will be collected from the throat. Describe the procedure and warn that gagging during the swabbing may occur.
- Check the patient's history for recent antimicrobial therapy. Determine immunization history if it's pertinent to the preliminary diagnosis.

During the Test
- Tell the patient to tilt the head back and close the eyes.
- With the throat well illuminated, check for inflamed areas using a tongue blade.
- Swab the tonsillar areas from side to side; include inflamed or purulent sites.
- Don't touch the tongue, cheeks, or teeth with the swab.
- Immediately place the swab in the culture tube.
- If a commercial sterile collection and transport system is used, crush the

ampule and force the swab into the medium to keep the swab moist.

- Note recent antimicrobial therapy on the laboratory request; label the specimen with the patient's name, physician's name, date, and time of collection, and origin of the specimen; indicate the suspected organism, especially *C. diphtheriae* (requires two swabs and a special growth medium), *B. pertussis* (requires a nasopharyngeal culture and a special growth medium), and *N. meningitidis* (requires enriched selective media).
- Follow procedures for nonculture antigen testing, if used. This method can be used to detect group A streptococcal antigen in as few as 5 minutes. Cultures then are performed on negative specimens.

After the Test
- Send the specimen to the laboratory immediately. Unless a commercial sterile collection and transport system is used, keep the container upright during transport.

Thyroid Biopsy
Normal Findings
- Gland divided into pseudolobules made up of fibrous networks of follicles and capillaries
- Follicle walls lined with cuboidal epithelium containing protein thyroglobulin, which stores triiodothyronine (T_3) and thyroxine (T_4)

Abnormal Findings
- Well-encapsulated, solitary nodules of uniform but abnormal structure, indicating papillary carcinoma
- Follicular carcinoma (which may resemble normal thyroid cells)
- Hypertrophic, hypervascular, hyperplastic cells, indicating nontoxic nodular goiter
- Specific histologic patterns characteristic of subacute granulomatous thyroiditis or lymphocytic thyroiditis,

Hashimoto's thyroiditis (chronic thyroiditis), or hyperthyroidism

Nursing Implications
- Report abnormal findings to the health care provider.
- Prepare to educate the patient about the diagnosis.
- Prepare the patient for further testing or surgery, as indicated.

Purpose
- To differentiate between benign and malignant thyroid disease
- To help diagnose Hashimoto's disease, hyperthyroidism, and nontoxic nodular goiter

Description
Thyroid biopsy is the excision of a thyroid tissue specimen for histologic examination. This procedure is indicated in patients with thyroid enlargement or nodules (even if serum T_3 and T_4 levels are normal), breathing and swallowing difficulties, vocal cord paralysis, weight loss, hemoptysis, and a sensation of fullness in the neck. It's commonly performed when noninvasive tests, such as thyroid ultrasonography and scans, are abnormal or inconclusive. Coagulation studies should always precede thyroid biopsy.

Thyroid tissue may be obtained with a hollow needle under local anesthesia or during open (surgical) biopsy under general anesthesia. Fine-needle or coreneedle aspiration with a cytologic smear examination can aid in diagnosis and replace an open biopsy. Open biopsy, performed in the operating room, provides more information than needle biopsy; it also permits direct examination and immediate excision of suspicious tissue.

Interfering Factors
- Inability to obtain a representative tissue specimen

Precautions
- Proceed cautiously in the patient with coagulation defects, as indicated by a prolonged prothrombin time (PT),

partial thromboplastin time (PTT), or international normalized ratio (INR).

- Patient should be in euthyroid state prior to any type of thyroid surgery to prevent thyroid storm.
- Immediately place the specimen in formalin solution because cell breakdown in the tissue specimen begins immediately after excision.

Nursing Considerations
Before the Test
- Confirm the patient's identity using two patient identifiers and confirmation of the patient's identification bracelet according to facility policy.
- Explain to the patient that thyroid biopsy permits microscopic thyroid tissue specimen examination. Describe the procedure to the patient and answer any questions. Inform the patient who will perform the procedure and when and where it will take place.
- Inform the patient that foods containing iodine, such as seafood, should be avoided, but that there are no food or fluid restrictions unless the patient is receiving a general anesthetic.
- Make sure the patient or a responsible family member has signed an informed consent form.
- Explain that the patient will receive a local anesthetic to minimize pain during the procedure but may experience some pressure when the tissue specimen is procured. Check the patient's history for hypersensitivity to anesthetics or analgesics.
- Check the results of the patient's coagulation studies and make sure they're in the chart.
- Advise the patient that a sore throat the day after the test may be experienced.
- Administer a sedative to the patient 15 minutes before the biopsy.

During the Test
- For needle biopsy, place the patient in the supine position with a pillow under the shoulder blades. (This position pushes the trachea and thyroid forward and allows the neck veins to fall backward.)
- Prepare the skin over the biopsy site.
- Label all medications, medication containers, or other solutions on and off the sterile field.
- As the health care provider prepares to inject the local anesthetic, warn the patient not to swallow. After the anesthetic is injected, the carotid artery is palpated and the biopsy needle is inserted parallel to the thyroid cartilage to prevent damage to the deep structures and the larynx. When the specimen is obtained, the needle is removed and the specimen is placed in formalin immediately.
- Apply pressure to the biopsy site to stop bleeding. If bleeding continues for more than 5 minutes, press on the site for up to an additional 15 minutes. Apply an adhesive bandage. (Bleeding may persist in a patient with a prolonged PT or PTT or in a patient with a large, vascular thyroid with distended veins.)

After the Test
- Place the patient in semi-Fowler's position for comfort; tell the patient to avoid straining the biopsy site by putting both hands behind the neck when sitting up.

> **Quality and Safety Nursing Alert**
> Watch for tenderness, swelling, or redness, and report signs of bleeding at the biopsy site immediately. Check the back of the patient's neck and the pillow for bleeding every hour for 8 hours. Observe for difficult breathing caused by edema or hematoma, with resultant tracheal collapse.

- Keep the biopsy site clean and dry.

Thyroid-Stimulating Hormone, Serum

Reference Values

0 to 15 microinternational units/mL (SI, 0–15 microinternational units/L)

Abnormal Findings

Elevated Levels

- Euthyroid status with thyroid cancer
- Primary hypothyroidism or endemic goiter (levels greater than 20 microinternational units/mL [SI, greater than 20 microinternational units/L])

Decreased Levels

- Secondary hypothyroidism
- Hyperthyroidism (Graves' disease)
- Thyroiditis (See the *TRH Challenge Test* box.)

Nursing Implications

- Report abnormal findings to the health care provider; be aware that decreased levels may be normal for some patients.
- Prepare to educate the patient about the diagnosis.
- Prepare the patient for further testing or surgery, as indicated.

Purpose

- To confirm or rule out primary hypothyroidism and distinguish it from secondary hypothyroidism
- To monitor drug therapy in the patient with primary hypothyroidism

Description

Thyroid-stimulating hormone (TSH), or *thyrotropin,* promotes increases in the size, number, and activity of thyroid cells and stimulates the release of triiodothyronine and thyroxine. These hormones affect total body metabolism and are essential for normal growth and development.

This test measures serum TSH levels by radioimmunoassay. It can detect primary hypothyroidism and determine whether the hypothyroidism results from thyroid gland failure or from pituitary or hypothalamic dysfunction. Normal serum TSH levels rule out primary hypothyroidism. This test may not distinguish between low-normal and subnormal levels, especially in secondary hypothyroidism.

Interfering Factors

- Aspirin, steroids, or thyroid hormone use (possible alteration in test results)
- Diseases of the esophagus

Precautions

- Handle the sample gently to prevent hemolysis.

Nursing Considerations

Before the Test

- Confirm the patient's identity using two patient identifiers and confirmation of the patient's identification bracelet according to facility policy.

TRH Challenge Test

The thyrotropin-releasing hormone (TRH) challenge test, which evaluates thyroid function and is the first direct test of pituitary reserve, is a reliable diagnostic tool in thyrotoxicosis (Graves' disease). The challenge test requires an injection of TRH.

Procedure

After a venipuncture is performed to obtain a baseline thyroid-stimulating hormone (TSH) reading, synthetic TRH (protirelin) is administered by IV bolus in a dose of 200 to 500 mcg. As many as five samples (5 mL each) are then drawn at 5, 10, 15,

20, and 60 minutes after the TRH injection to assess thyroid response. To facilitate blood collection, an indwelling catheter can be used to obtain the required samples.

Test Results

A sudden spike above the baseline TSH reading indicates a normally functioning pituitary, but suggests hypothalamic dysfunction. If the TSH level fails to rise or remains undetectable, pituitary failure is likely. In thyrotoxicosis and thyroiditis, TSH levels fail to rise when challenged by TRH.

- Explain to the patient that the serum thyroid-stimulating hormone test helps assess thyroid gland function.
- Advise the patient that the test requires a blood sample. Explain that slight discomfort from the tourniquet and the needle puncture may be experienced.
- Withhold steroids, thyroid hormones, aspirin, and other medications that may influence test results, as ordered. If they must be continued, note this on the laboratory request.
- Keep the patient relaxed and recumbent for 30 minutes before the test.

During the Test
- Perform a venipuncture and collect the sample in a 5-mL clot activator tube in the morning, preferably between 6 AM and 8 AM.
- Apply direct pressure to the venipuncture site until bleeding stops and to prevent hematoma formation.

After the Test
- Tell the patient to resume medications that were discontinued before the test, as ordered.

Thyroxine, Serum
Reference Values
5 to 13.5 mcg/dL (SI, 60–165 mmol/L)

Abnormal Findings
Elevated Levels
- Primary and secondary hyperthyroidism

Decreased Levels
- Primary or secondary hypothyroidism

Nursing Implications
- Report abnormal findings to the health care provider.
- Prepare to educate the patient about the diagnosis.
- Prepare the patient for further testing or surgery, as indicated.

Purpose
- To evaluate thyroid function
- To help diagnose hyperthyroidism and hypothyroidism

- To monitor the patient's response to antithyroid medication in hyperthyroidism or to thyroid replacement therapy in hypothyroidism (Thyroid-stimulating hormone [TSH] estimates are needed to confirm hypothyroidism.)
- To assess nutritional efficacy

Description
Thyroxine (T_4) is an amine secreted by the thyroid gland in response to TSH and, indirectly, thyrotropin-releasing hormone. The secretion rate normally is regulated by a complex system of negative and positive feedback involving the thyroid, anterior pituitary, and hypothalamus. The suspected precursor, or prohormone, of tri-iodothyronine (T_3), T_4 is believed to convert to T_3 by monodeiodination, which occurs mainly in the liver and kidneys.

Only a fraction of T_4 (about 0.05%) circulates freely in the blood; the rest binds strongly to plasma proteins, primarily thyroxine-binding globulin (TBG). This minute fraction is responsible for the clinical effects of thyroid hormone. TBG binds so tenaciously that T_4 survives in the plasma for a relatively long time, with a half-life of about 6 days. This immunoassay, one of the most common thyroid diagnostic tools, measures the total circulating T_4 level when TBG is normal. An alternative test is the Murphy-Pattee or T_4 (D), based on competitive protein binding.

Interfering Factors
- Hereditary factors and hepatic disease (possible increase or decrease in TBG)
- Protein-wasting disease (such as nephrotic syndrome) and androgens (possible decrease in TBG)
- Estrogens, levothyroxine, methadone, and progestins (increase)
- Free fatty acids, heparin, iodides, liothyronine sodium, lithium, phenytoin, propylthiouracil, nonsteroidal anti-inflammatory drugs (high doses), steroids, sulfonamides, and sulfonylureas (decrease)

Precautions
• Handle the sample gently to prevent hemolysis.

Nursing Considerations
Before the Test
• Confirm the patient's identity using two patient identifiers and confirmation of the patient's identification bracelet according to facility policy.
• Inform the patient that the serum T_4 test helps evaluate thyroid gland function. Explain that the test requires a blood sample and that the patient may experience slight discomfort from the tourniquet and needle puncture.
• Inform the patient that there are no food or fluid restrictions for this test.
• Withhold medications that may interfere with test results, as ordered. If they must be continued, note this on the laboratory request. If this test is being performed to monitor thyroid therapy, the patient should continue to receive daily thyroid supplements.

During the Test
• Perform a venipuncture and collect the sample in a 7-mL clot activator tube.
• Send the sample to the laboratory immediately so that the serum can be separated.
• Apply direct pressure to the venipuncture site until bleeding stops.
• If a hematoma develops at the venipuncture site, continue direct pressure.

After the Test
• Tell the patient to resume medications that were discontinued before the test, as ordered.

Thyroxine-Binding Globulin, Serum

Reference Values
16 to 32 mcg/dL (SI, 120–180 mg/mL)

Abnormal Findings
Elevated Levels
• Hypothyroidism or congenital (genetic) excess
• Some forms of hepatic disease
• Acute intermittent porphyria

Decreased Levels
• Hyperthyroidism
• Congenital deficiency
• Active acromegaly
• Nephrotic syndrome
• Malnutrition associated with hypoproteinemia, acute illness, or surgical stress

Nursing Implications
• Report abnormal findings to the health care provider.
• Prepare to educate the patient about the diagnosis.
• Prepare the patient for additional testing, such as the serum free triiodothyronine (FT_3) and free thyroxine (FT_4) tests, to evaluate thyroid function more precisely.

Purpose
• To evaluate abnormal thyrometabolic states that don't correlate with thyroid hormone (T_3 or T_4) values (for example, a patient with overt signs of hypothyroidism and a low FT_4 level with a high total T_4 level due to a marked increase of thyroxine-binding globulin [TBG] secondary to hormonal contraceptives)
• To identify TBG abnormalities

Description
The TBG test measures the serum TBG level, the predominant protein carrier for circulating T_4 and T_3. TBG values may be identified by saturating the sample for TBG determination with radioactive T_4, then subjecting this to electrophoresis and measuring the amount of TBG by the amount of radioactive T_4 by radioimmunoassay.

Any condition that affects TBG levels and subsequent binding capacity also affects the amount of FT_4 in circulation.

An underlying TBG abnormality renders tests for total T_3 and T_4 inaccurate, but doesn't affect the accuracy of tests for FT_3 and FT_4.

Interfering Factors

- Estrogens, including hormonal contraceptives, and phenothiazines such as perphenazine (increase)
- Androgens, prednisone, phenytoin, and high doses of salicylates (decrease)

Precautions

- Handle the sample gently to prevent hemolysis.

Nursing Considerations

Before the Test

- Confirm the patient's identity using two patient identifiers and confirmation of the patient's identification bracelet according to facility policy.
- Explain to the patient that the serum TBG test helps evaluate thyroid function.
- Tell the patient that the test requires a blood sample. Explain that slight discomfort from the tourniquet and the needle puncture may be experienced.
- Withhold medications that may affect the accuracy of test results, such as estrogens, anabolic steroids, phenytoin, salicylates, or thyroid preparations, as ordered. If they must be continued, note this on the laboratory request. (They may be continued to determine if prescribed drugs are affecting TBG levels.)

During the Test

- Perform a venipuncture and collect the sample in a 7-mL clot activator tube.
- Apply direct pressure to the venipuncture site until bleeding stops and to prevent hematoma formation.

After the Test

- Tell the patient to resume medications that were discontinued before the test, as ordered.

Total Carbon Dioxide Content

Reference Values

22 to 26 mEq/L (SI, 22–26 mmol/L)

Abnormal Findings

Elevated Levels

- Metabolic alkalosis
- Respiratory acidosis
- Primary aldosteronism
- Cushing syndrome
- Severe vomiting and continuous gastric drainage

Decreased Levels

- Metabolic acidosis
- Respiratory alkalosis

Nursing Implications

- Report abnormal findings to the health care provider.
- Prepare to educate the patient about the diagnosis.
- Prepare the patient for further testing as indicated.
- With elevated levels, monitor the patient's intake and output and prepare to administer IV replacement fluids, as indicated.

Purpose

- To help evaluate acid–base balance

Description

When carbon dioxide (CO_2) pressure in red blood cells exceeds 40 mm Hg, CO_2 spills out of the cells and dissolve in plasma. There, it may combine with water to form carbonic acid, which in turn may dissociate into hydrogen and bicarbonate ions.

The total CO_2 content test is used to measure the total concentration of all CO_2 forms in serum, plasma, or whole blood samples. It's commonly ordered for patients with respiratory insufficiency and is usually included in an arterial blood gas and/or electrolyte balance assessment. Test results are most significant when considered with pH and arterial blood gas values.

Because about 90% of CO_2 in serum is in bicarbonate form, this test closely

T

assesses bicarbonate levels. Total CO_2 content reflects adequacy of gas exchange in the lungs and efficiency of the carbonic acid–bicarbonate buffer system, which maintains acid–base balance and normal pH.

Interfering Factors

- Excessive corticotropin, cortisone, or thiazide diuretics use; excessive alkali or licorice ingestion (increase)
- Acetazolamide, ammonium chloride, dimercaprol, paraldehyde, and salicylates; ethylene glycol or methyl alcohol ingestion (decrease)

Precautions

- Fill the tube completely to prevent diffusion of CO_2 into the vacuum.

Nursing Considerations

Before the Test

- Confirm the patient's identity using two patient identifiers and confirmation of the patient's identification bracelet according to facility policy.
- Explain to the patient that the total CO_2 content test is performed to measure the amount of CO_2 in the blood.
- Advise the patient that the test requires a blood sample. Explain that discomfort from the tourniquet and the needle puncture may be experienced.
- Inform the patient that there are no food or fluid restrictions for this test.
- Notify the laboratory and health care provider of medications the patient is taking that may affect test results; these may need to be restricted.

During the Test

- Perform a venipuncture and collect the sample in the proper tube. When CO_2 content is measured along with electrolytes, a 3- or 4-mL clot activator tube may be used. When this test is performed as an arterial blood gas, a heparinized tube is appropriate.
- Apply direct pressure to the venipuncture site until the bleeding has stopped and to prevent hematoma formation.

After the Test

- Tell the patient to resume any medications that were discontinued before the test, as ordered.

Total Cholesterol

Reference Values

Females: Less than 190 mg/dL (SI, less than 4.9 mmol/L)
Males: Less than 205 mg/dL (SI, less than 5.3 mmol/L)
Children ages 12 to 18: Less than 170 mg/dL (SI, less than 4.4 mmol/L)

Abnormal Findings

Elevated Levels

- Coronary artery disease (CAD) risk
- Incipient hepatitis
- Lipid disorders
- Bile duct blockage
- Nephrotic syndrome
- Obstructive jaundice
- Pancreatitis
- Hypothyroidism

Decreased Levels

- Malnutrition
- Cellular necrosis of the liver
- Hyperthyroidism

Nursing Implications

- Report abnormal findings to the health care provider.
- Prepare to educate the patient about the diagnosis.
- Prepare the patient for further testing or surgery, as indicated.

Purpose

- To assess CAD risk
- To evaluate fat metabolism
- To help diagnose nephrotic syndrome, pancreatitis, hepatic disease, hypothyroidism, and hyperthyroidism
- To assess lipid-lowering drug therapy efficacy

Description

The total cholesterol test, the quantitative analysis of serum cholesterol, is used to measure circulating levels of free cholesterol and cholesterol esters; it reflects

Skin Test for Cholesterol

A new 3-minute test that measures the amount of cholesterol in the skin rather than in the blood is the first noninvasive test of its kind. It measures how much cholesterol is present in other tissues in the body and provides additional data about a person's risk of heart disease.

The skin test, which doesn't require patients to fast, involves placing a bandagelike applicator pad on the palm of the hand. Drops of a special solution that reacts to skin cholesterol are then added to the pad; 3 minutes later, a handheld computer interprets the information into a skin cholesterol reading.

Because the test measures the amount of cholesterol that has accumulated in the tissues over time, results don't correlate with blood cholesterol levels; therefore, the test isn't meant to be a substitute or surrogate for a cholesterol test that measures the amount of cholesterol in the blood. In addition, the Food and Drug Administration cautions that the test isn't intended for use as a screening tool for heart disease in the general population. Instead, it has been approved for use among adults with severe heart disease—those with at least a 50% blockage of two or more heart arteries.

the level of the two forms in which this biochemical compound appears in the body. High serum cholesterol levels may be associated with an increased CAD risk.

A 3-minute skin test for cholesterol is now available. (See the *Skin Test for Cholesterol* box.)

Interfering Factors
• Cholestyramine, colestipol, dextrothyroxine, haloperidol, neomycin, and niacin (decrease)
• Chlorpromazine, epinephrine, hormonal contraceptives, and trifluoperazine (increase)
• Androgens (possible variable effect)

Precautions
• Send the sample to the laboratory immediately.

Nursing Considerations
Before the Test
• Confirm the patient's identity using two patient identifiers and confirmation of the patient's identification bracelet according to facility policy.
• Explain to the patient that the total cholesterol test is used to assess the body's fat metabolism.
• Tell the patient that the test requires a blood sample. Explain that slight discomfort from the tourniquet and the needle puncture may be experienced.

• Instruct the patient not to eat or drink for 12 hours before the test. Water is permitted.
• Notify the laboratory and health care provider of medications the patient is taking that may affect test results; these may need to be restricted.

During the Test
• After the patient has been seated for 5 minutes, perform a venipuncture and collect the sample in a 4-mL EDTA tube. (Finger sticks can also be used for initial screening when using an automated analyzer.)

After the Test
• Apply direct pressure to the venipuncture site until bleeding stops and to prevent hematoma formation.
• Tell the patient to resume a usual diet and medications that were discontinued before the test as ordered.

Transesophageal Echocardiography

Normal Findings
• No cardiac abnormalities

Abnormal Findings
• Endocarditis
• Congenital heart disease
• Intracardiac thrombi

T

- Tumors
- Aortic dissection or aneurysm
- Valvular disease (e.g., mitral valve disease)
- Congenital defects such as patent ductus arteriosus

Nursing Implications
- Report abnormal findings to the referring health care provider.
- Prepare to educate the patient about the diagnosis.
- Prepare the patient for further testing or surgery, as indicated.
- Provide emotional support to the patient and family.

Purpose
- To visualize and evaluate thoracic and aortic disorders (such as dissection and aneurysm), valvular disease (especially in the mitral valve and in prosthetic devices), endocarditis, congenital heart disease, intracardiac thrombi, cardiac tumors, and valvular repairs

Description
Transesophageal echocardiography combines ultrasound with endoscopy to give a better view of the heart's structures. In this procedure, a small transducer is attached to the end of a gastroscope and inserted into the esophagus, allowing images to be taken from the posterior aspect of the heart. This method causes less tissue penetration and interference from chest wall structures and produces high-quality thoracic aorta images, except of the superior ascending aorta, which is shadowed by the trachea.

Transesophageal echocardiography is appropriate for inpatients and outpatients, for patients under general anesthesia, and for critically ill, intubated patients. The usual procedure is as follows:

- The patient is connected to a cardiac monitor, automated blood pressure cuff, and pulse oximetry probe so that all parameters can be assessed during the procedure.

- The patient is helped to lie down on the left side and administered the prescribed sedative.
- The back of the patient's throat is sprayed with a topical anesthetic.
- A bite block is placed in the mouth and the patient is instructed to close the lips around it.
- A gastroscope is introduced and advanced 12 to 14 inches (30–35 cm) to the level of the right atrium. To visualize the left ventricle, the scope is advanced 16 to 18 inches (40–45 cm).
- Ultrasound images are recorded and then reviewed after the procedure.

Interfering Factors
- Patient's inability to cooperate
- Use of a transesophageal approach (restricts visualization of the left atrial appendage and ascending or descending aorta)
- Hyperinflation of lungs caused by conditions such as chronic obstructive pulmonary disease or mechanical ventilation (possible poor imaging)

Precautions
- Keep resuscitation equipment readily available.
- Have suction equipment nearby to avoid aspiration if vomiting occurs.
- Watch the cardiac monitor closely for evidence of vasovagal responses, which may occur with coughing and gagging.
- Use pulse oximetry to monitor for hypoxia.
- If bleeding occurs, stop the procedure immediately.
- Laryngospasm, arrhythmias, or bleeding increase the risk of complications. If any of these occurs, postpone the test.

Nursing Considerations
Before the Test
- Confirm the patient's identity using two patient identifiers and confirmation

of the patient's identification bracelet according to facility policy.

- Explain to the patient that transesophageal echocardiography allows visual examination of heart structures and their function. Describe the procedure and tell the patient who will perform the test, where and when it's scheduled, and the need to fast for 6 hours before the test.
- The patient should avoid alcohol for a day or two prior to the test because of potential interaction with the sedation for the test.
- Review the patient's medical history for possible contraindications to the test, such as esophageal obstruction or varices, GI bleeding, previous mediastinal radiation therapy, or severe cervical arthritis.
- Ask the patient about allergies and note them on the chart.
- Before the test, instruct the patient to remove dentures or oral prostheses and note any loose teeth.
- Explain to the patient that the throat will be sprayed with a topical anesthetic and that it may cause coughing or gagging when the tube is inserted. Inform the patient that an IV line will be inserted to administer sedation before the procedure and that slight discomfort from the tourniquet and the needle puncture may be experienced. Explain that the patient will be made as comfortable as possible and that blood pressure, heart rate, and pulse oximetry readings will be monitored continuously.
- Make sure that the patient or a responsible family member has signed an informed consent form.

After the Test

- Monitor the patient's vital signs and oxygen levels for any changes.
- Keep the patient in a supine position until the sedative wears off.
- Encourage the patient to cough after the procedure while lying on the side or sitting upright.

> ⚑ **Quality and Safety Nursing Alert**
>
> **Don't give the patient food or water until the gag reflex returns.**

- If the procedure is done on an outpatient basis, make sure someone is available to drive the patient home.
- Treat sore throat symptomatically with warm saline gargles or throat lozenges.
- Advise the patient to avoid alcohol for a day or two following the test because of potential interaction with the sedation used for the test.

Triglycerides

Reference Values

Females: 10 to 190 mg/dL (SI, 0.11–2.21 mmol/L)
Males: 44 to 180 mg/dL (SI, 0.44–2.01 mmol/L)

Abnormal Findings

Elevated Levels

- Biliary obstruction
- Diabetes
- Nephrotic syndrome
- Endocrinopathies
- Alcohol overconsumption
- Congenital hyperlipoproteinemia

Decreased Levels

- Malnutrition
- Abetalipoproteinemia

Nursing Implications

- Report abnormal findings to the health care provider.
- Prepare to educate the patient about the diagnosis.
- Be aware that decreased serum triglyceride levels suggest a clinical abnormality; prepare the patient for additional tests for a definitive diagnosis.
- Be aware that increased serum triglyceride levels suggest a clinical abnormality. Prepare the patient for additional tests, such as lipoprotein phenotyping, for a definitive diagnosis.

Purpose
- To screen for hyperlipidemia or pancreatitis
- To help identify nephrotic syndrome and poorly controlled diabetes
- To assess coronary artery disease (CAD) risk
- To calculate the low-density lipoprotein cholesterol level using the Friedewald equation

Description
Serum triglyceride analysis provides quantitative analysis of triglycerides, the main storage form of lipids, which constitute about 95% of fatty tissue. Although not in itself diagnostic, the triglyceride test permits early identification of hyperlipidemia and the risk of CAD.

Interfering Factors
- Use of a glycol-lubricated collection tube
- Antilipemics (decreased serum lipid levels)
- Cholestyramine and colestipol (decreased cholesterol levels; possible increased triglyceride levels)
- Alcohol, corticosteroids (long-term use), estrogen, ethyl furosemide, hormonal contraceptives, and miconazole (increase)
- Dextrothyroxine, gemfibrozil, and niacin (decreased cholesterol and triglyceride levels)

Precautions
- Avoid prolonged venous occlusion; remove the tourniquet within 1 minute of application.

Nursing Considerations
Before the Test
- Confirm the patient's identity using two patient identifiers and confirmation of the patient's identification bracelet according to facility policy.
- Explain to the patient that the triglyceride test is used to detect fat metabolism disorders.

- Advise the patient that the test requires a blood sample. Explain that slight discomfort from the tourniquet and the needle puncture may be experienced.
- Instruct the patient to fast for at least 12 hours before the test and to abstain from alcohol for 24 hours. Water is permitted.
- Notify the laboratory and health care provider of medications the patient is taking that may affect test results; these may need to be restricted.

During the Test
- Perform a venipuncture and collect a sample in a 4-mL EDTA tube.
- Send the sample to the laboratory immediately.

After the Test
- Apply direct pressure to the venipuncture site until bleeding stops and to prevent hematoma formation.
- Tell the patient to resume a usual diet and medications that were discontinued before the test, as ordered.

Troponin

Reference Values
Cardiac troponin I (cTnI) levels:
Less than 0.35 mcg/L (SI, less than 0.35 mcg/L)
Cardiac troponin T (cTnT) levels: Less than 0.1 mcg/L (SI, less than 0.1 mcg/L)

Abnormal Findings
Elevated Levels
- Possible cardiac injury (cTnI levels greater than 2.0 mcg/L [SI, greater than 2.0 mcg/L])
- Cardiac injury (qualitative cTnT rapid immunoassay greater than 0.1 mcg/L [SI, greater than 0.1 mcg/L])

Nursing Implications
- Report abnormal findings to the health care provider.
- Prepare to educate the patient about the diagnosis.

- Prepare the patient for further testing or surgery, as indicated.
- Provide emotional support to the patient and family.

Purpose

- To detect and diagnose acute myocardial infarction (MI) and reinfarction
- To evaluate possible causes of chest pain

Description

- The cTnI and cTnT proteins in striated cells are extremely specific cardiac damage markers that are released into the bloodstream after an injury. Elevations in troponin levels can be seen within 1 hour of MI and will persist for a week or longer.

Interfering Factors

- Sustained vigorous exercise (increase in absence of significant cardiac damage)
- Cardiotoxic drugs, such as doxorubicin (increase)
- Renal disease and certain surgical procedures (possible increase)

Precautions

- Obtain each sample on schedule.

Nursing Considerations

Before the Test

- Confirm the patient's identity using two patient identifiers and confirmation of the patient's identification bracelet according to facility policy.
- Explain to the patient that the troponin test helps assess myocardial injury and that multiple samples may be drawn to detect fluctuations in serum levels.
- Inform the patient that there are no food or fluid restrictions for this test.
- Advise the patient that the test requires multiple blood samples. Explain that slight discomfort from the tourniquet and the needle puncture may be experienced.

During the Test

- Perform a venipuncture and collect the sample in a 7-mL clot activator tube.
- Note the date and collection time on each sample.

After the Test

- Apply direct pressure to the venipuncture site until bleeding stops and to prevent hematoma formation.

T

U

Ultrasonography

Normal Findings
- See the *Ultrasonography Findings* table.

Abnormal Findings
- See the *Ultrasonography Findings* table.

Nursing Implications
- Report abnormal findings to the health care provider.
- Prepare to educate the patient about the diagnosis.
- Prepare the patient for further testing or surgery, as indicated.
- Provide emotional support to the patient and family.

Purpose
- See the *Ultrasonography Findings* table.

Description
In ultrasonography, a transducer directs high-frequency sound waves into the area being tested. The echoing sound waves are converted to images on a screen, indicating the size, shape, and position of various structures. Appropriate views are photographed or videotaped. The procedure for ultrasonography varies depending on the area being tested.

Abdominal Aorta
- The patient is placed in a supine position, and conductive gel or mineral oil is applied to the abdomen.
- Longitudinal scans are made at ¼- to ¾-inch (0.5–2-cm) intervals left and right of the midline until the entire abdominal aorta is outlined; trans-

verse scans are made at ⅜- to ¾-inch (1–2-cm) intervals from the xiphoid process to the bifurcation at the common iliac arteries.
- The patient may be placed in the right and left lateral positions.
- Appropriate views are photographed or videotaped.

Eye
- The patient is placed in a supine position on an X-ray table.
- For the B-scan, the patient is asked to close the eyes, and a water-soluble gel (such as Goniosol) is applied to the eyelid. The transducer is placed on the eyelid. (See the *Eye Scans* box, p. 499.)
- For the A-scan, the patient's eye is numbed with anesthetizing drops and a clear plastic eyecup is placed directly on the eyeball. A water-soluble gel is applied to the eyecup, and the transducer is positioned on the medium.

Gallbladder and Biliary System
- The patient is placed in a supine position.
- Water-soluble conductive gel is applied to the face of the transducer.
- Transverse and longitudinal oblique scans of the gallbladder are taken at ⅜-inch (1-cm) intervals, starting at the xiphoid process level and moving laterally to the right subcostal area. Longitudinal oblique scans are taken at 5-mm intervals parallel to the long axis of the gallbladder marked on the patient's skin, beginning medial to the gallbladder and continuing through to its lateral border.

(*text continues on page 498*)

Ultrasonography Findings

This table identifies normal and abnormal findings for various types of ultrasonography.

Area	Test Purpose	Normal Findings	Abnormal Findings
Abdominal aorta	• Detect and measure a suspected or known abdominal aortic aneurysm	• Abdominal aorta that's about ⅜- to 1-inch to (1.5–2.5 cm) in diameter and tapered along its length from the diaphragm to the bifurcation	• Aneurysm (luminal diameter greater than 1½ inches [4 cm]; high risk of rupture if greater than 2½ inches [7 cm])
Eye	• Evaluate the eye's fundus • Help diagnose vitreous disorders and retinal detachment • Diagnose and differentiate between intraocular and orbital lesions and follow their progression • Locate intraocular foreign bodies	• Characteristic forms on A- and B-scan images (optic nerve, posterior lens capsule) • Smooth, concave curve on posterior wall with identifiable retrobulbar fat, lens, and vitreous humor • Normal orbital echo patterns (depending on transducer position, patient's gaze position)	• Vitreous hemorrhage (variations in density) • Massive vitreous organization and vitreous bands • Retinal or choroidal detachment (sheetlike echo on B-scan) • Metastatic tumors, melanomas, hemangiomas, retinoblastomas, meningiomas, neurofibromas, gliomas, or neurilemomas
Gallbladder and biliary system	• Confirm cholelithiasis • Diagnose acute cholecystitis • Distinguish between obstructive and nonobstructive jaundice	• Sonolucent gallbladder that's circular on transverse scans and pear-shaped on longitudinal scans, with sharp, smooth outer gallbladder walls • Indistinct intrahepatic radicles and cystic duct • Common bile duct with a linear appearance (may be obscured by overlying bowel gas)	• Cholelithiasis (acoustic shadow in the gallbladder fossa) • Polyps (sharply defined echogenic areas) • Carcinoma (poorly defined mass commonly appearing with a thickened gallbladder wall) • Acute cholecystitis (enlarged gallbladder with thickened, double-rimmed walls) • Chronic cholecystitis (thickened gallbladder walls and contracted gallbladder) • Obstructive jaundice (dilated biliary system and gallbladder) • Biliary obstruction, carcinoma, or pancreatitis

U

(continues on page 496)

Ultrasonography Findings (continued)

This table identifies normal and abnormal findings for various types of ultrasonography.

Area	Test Purpose	Normal Findings	Abnormal Findings
Liver	• Distinguish between obstructive and nonobstructive jaundice • Screen for hepatocellular disease • Detect hepatic metastases and hematomas • Define cold spots as tumors, abscesses, or cysts	• Homogeneous, low-level echo pattern, interrupted only by echo patterns of portal and hepatic veins, the aorta, and the inferior vena cava • Completely sonolucent hepatic veins • Highly echogenic portal vein margins	• Obstructive jaundice (dilated intrahepatic biliary radicles and extrahepatic ducts) • Nonobstructive jaundice • Cirrhosis (variable liver size, dilated portal branches, irregular echo pattern with increased amplitude) • Fatty infiltration of the liver (hepatomegaly, regular echo pattern that doesn't alter attenuation) • Metastatic lymphomas or sarcomas (hypoechoic areas) • Mucin-secreting adenocarcinoma of the colon (highly echogenic) • Abscesses (sonolucent masses with ill-defined, slightly thickened borders) or ascitic fluid • Hepatic cysts (spherical, sonolucent areas with well-defined borders) • Intrahepatic hematoma (poorly defined, sonolucent mass) or subcapsular hematoma (focal, sonolucent mass on liver's periphery) • Hepatoblastomas (most common in children)
Pancreas	• Help diagnose pancreatitis, pseudocysts, and pancreatic carcinoma	• Coarse, uniform echo pattern, usually more echogenic than the adjacent liver	• Pancreatitis (enlarged pancreas with decreased echogenicity and distinct borders) • Pseudocyst (defined mass with echo-free interior) • Pancreatic carcinoma (ill-defined mass with scattered internal echoes or a mass in the pancreas head)

U

| Renal structures | • Determine size, shape, and position of the kidneys, their internal structures, and perirenal tissues
• Evaluate urinary obstruction and abnormal fluid accumulation
• Assess and diagnose complications after kidney transplantation
• Detect renal or perirenal masses
• Differentiate between renal cysts and solid masses
• Verify placement of a nephrostomy tube | • Sharply outlined renal capsule
• More cortex echoes than medulla echoes
• Irregular renal collecting system with a higher density than surrounding tissue
• Visualization of renal veins and some internal structures | • Cysts (fluid-filled structures that don't reflect sound waves)
• Tumors (irregularly shaped masses that produce multiple echoes)
• Abscesses (masses with irregular boundaries that echo sound waves poorly)
• Acute pyelonephritis and glomerulonephritis (scarred and atrophied renal parenchyma with increased echoes)
• Hydronephrosis (large, echo-free mass that compresses the renal cortex)
• Congenital anomalies (horseshoe, ectopic, or duplicated kidneys)
• Transplant rejection (kidney hypertrophy)
• Bladder outlet obstruction (increased urine volume or residual urine after voiding) |
| Spleen | • Demonstrate splenomegaly
• Monitor primary and secondary splenic disease
• Evaluate the effectiveness of therapy
• Evaluate the spleen after abdominal trauma
• Help detect splenic cysts and subphrenic abscesses | • Homogeneous, low-level echo pattern of splenic parenchyma
• Clearly defined superior and lateral splenic borders (each having a convex margin)
• Indentations on the undersurface and medial borders from surrounding organs
• Highly reflective echoes in the hilar region
• Concave medial surface (differentiates left upper-quadrant masses and an enlarged spleen)
• Medially concave spleen (even with splenomegaly, unless distorted by a space-occupying lesion) | • Splenomegaly (increased echogenicity)
• Splenic rupture (irregular, sonolucent area accompanied by splenomegaly, indicating splenic rupture)
• Subcapsular hematoma (splenomegaly with altered splenic position and a sonolucent area on the spleen's periphery)
• Subphrenic abscess (sonolucent area beneath the diaphragm) |

U

(continues on page 498)

Ultrasonography Findings (continued)

This table identifies normal and abnormal findings for various types of ultrasonography.

Area	Test Purpose	Normal Findings	Abnormal Findings
Thyroid	• Evaluate thyroid structure • Differentiate between a cyst and a solid tumor • Monitor thyroid gland size during suppressive therapy	• Uniform echo pattern throughout the gland	• Cysts (smooth-bordered, echo-free areas) • Adenomas and carcinomas (solid and well-demarcated areas)
Vagina	• Establish early pregnancy (fifth to sixth week of gestation) with fetal heart motion • Identify ectopic pregnancy • Monitor follicular growth during infertility treatment • Evaluate abnormal pregnancy • Visualize retained products of conception • Diagnose fetal abnormalities, placental location, and cervical length • Evaluate adnexal pathology • Evaluate the uterine lining (in dysfunctional uterine bleeding and postmenopausal bleeding)	***Nonpregnant patient*** • Uterus and ovaries of normal size and shape • Body of uterus lying on the superior surface of the bladder; uterine tubes attached laterally • Ovaries located on lateral pelvic walls; external iliac vessels above the ureter posteroinferiorly, covered by fimbria of the uterine tubes medially ***Pregnant patient*** • Gestational sac and fetus of normal size for gestational date	• Empty uterus (if patient was pregnant) • Peritonitis • Ectopic pregnancy

• During each scan, the patient is asked to inhale deeply and hold the breath. (If the gallbladder is positioned deeply under the right costal margin, a scan may be taken through the intercostal spaces while the patient holds the breath.)

• The patient is placed in a left lateral decubitus position and is scanned beneath the right costal margin. (This position and scanning angle may displace and allow the detection of stones lodged in the gallbladder neck and cystic duct region.)

• Scanning with the patient erect helps demonstrate mobility or fixity of suspicious echogenic areas.

• Views may be photographed for later study.

Liver

• The patient is placed in a supine position.

Eye Scans

Ultrasonography of the eye involves two types of scans: A and B. An A-scan converts the resulting echoes into waveforms whose crests represent the positions of different structures, providing a linear dimensional picture. The B-scan converts the echoes into dot patterns that form a two-dimensional, cross-sectional image of the ocular structure.

Because the B-scan is easier to interpret than the A-scan, it's used more commonly to evaluate eye structures and to diagnose abnormalities. However, the A-scan is more valuable in measuring the eye's axial length and characterizing the tissue texture of abnormal lesions. Thus, a combination of A- and B-scans produces the most useful test results.

The image below is a normal B-scan using the lid contact method. The posterior lens capsule is visible, but the cornea and iris aren't because of obscuring echoes from the eyelid.

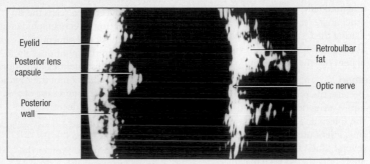

Eyelid

Posterior lens capsule

Posterior wall

Retrobulbar fat

Optic nerve

- Water-soluble conductive gel is applied to the face of the transducer.
- Transverse scans are taken at ⅜-inch (1-cm) intervals, using a single-sweep technique between the costal margins, to visualize the liver's left lobe and part of the right lobe. Sector scans through the intercostal spaces are used to view the remainder of the right lobe.
- Scans are taken longitudinally from the right border of the liver to the left.
- For better demonstration of the right lateral dome, oblique cephalad-angled scans may be taken beneath the right costal margin.
- Scans are then taken parallel to the hepatic portal, at a 45-degree angle toward the superior right lateral dome, to examine the peripheral anatomy, portal venous system, common bile duct, and biliary tree. Clear images are photographed for later study.
- During each scan, the patient is asked to hold the breath briefly in deep inspi-

ration to displace the liver caudally from the costal margin and the ribs.

Pancreas
- The patient is placed in a supine position.
- A water-soluble conductive gel or mineral oil is applied to the abdomen and, with the patient at full inspiration, transverse scans are taken at ⅜-inch (1-cm) intervals, starting from the xiphoid and moving caudally; longitudinal scans are taken to view the head, body, and tail of the pancreas in sequence; scanning the right anterior oblique view allows imaging of the head and body of the pancreas; oblique sagittal scans are used to view the portal vein; and scanning from the sagittal view images the vena cava.
- Good ultrasonography views are photographed for later study.

Renal Structures
- The patient is placed in a prone position, the area to be scanned is exposed,

and conductive gel is applied to the transducer.

- The longitudinal axis of the kidneys is located by using measurements from excretory urography or by performing transverse scans through the upper and lower renal poles. These points are marked on the skin and connected with straight lines. Sectional images ⅜- to ¾-inch (1–2 cm) apart can then be obtained by moving the transducer longitudinally, transversely, or at any other angle required.
- During the test, the patient may be asked to breathe deeply to visualize upper portions of the kidney.

Spleen

- Because the procedure for ultrasonography varies depending on the size of the spleen and the patient's physique, the patient usually is repositioned several times; the transducer scanning angle or path also is changed.
- Generally, the patient is placed first in a supine position, with the chest uncovered.
- A water-soluble conductive gel is applied to the face of the transducer, and transverse scans of the spleen are taken at ⅜- to ¾-inch (1–2-cm) intervals, beginning at the level of the diaphragm and moving posteriorly while the transducer is angled anteromedially.
- The patient is then placed in a right lateral decubitus position, and transverse scans are taken through the intercostal spaces using a sectoring motion.
- A pillow may be placed under the patient's right side to help separate the intercostal spaces, making it easier to position the transducer face between them.
- Longitudinal scans are taken from the axilla toward the iliac crest.
- To prevent rib artifacts and to obtain the best view of the splenic parenchyma, oblique scans are taken by passing the transducer face along the intercostal spaces.

- During each scan, the patient may be asked to hold the breath briefly at various stages of inspiration.
- Good views are photographed for later study.

Thyroid

- The patient is placed in a supine position with a pillow under the shoulder blades to hyperextend the neck.
- The neck is coated with water-soluble conductive gel.
- The transducer then scans the thyroid, projecting its echographic image on the oscilloscope screen.
- The image on the monitor is photographed for subsequent examination.
- Accurate visualization of the thyroid's anterior portion requires use of a short-focused transducer.

Vaginal Structures

- The patient is placed in the lithotomy position. Protect the patient's privacy with a sheet or blanket to decrease exposure. If the sonographer is a male, a female assistant should be present during the examination.
- Water-soluble conductive gel is placed on the transducer tip to allow better sound transmission, and a protective sheath is placed over the transducer.
- More lubricant may need to be placed on the sheathed transducer tip to allow for its gentle insertion into the vagina by the patient or the sonographer. Allowing the patient to introduce the probe may decrease her anxiety.
- To observe the pelvic structures, the probe is rotated 90 degrees to one side and then the other.

Interfering Factors

Abdominal Aorta

- Bowel gas and motility, excessive body movement, severe dyspnea, and surgical wounds
- Residual barium from GI contrast studies within the past 24 hours

- Air introduced during endoscopy within the past 12 to 24 hours
- Mesenteric fat in the obese patient

Gallbladder and Biliary System
- Failure to observe pretest dietary restrictions
- Overlying bowel gas or retained barium from a previous test (possible poor imaging)
- Deficiency of body fluids in a dehydrated patient, obscuring boundaries between organs and tissue structures (possible poor imaging)

Liver
- Overlying ribs and gas or residual barium in the stomach or colon (possible misleading results)
- Body fluid deficiency in a dehydrated patient, obscuring boundaries between organs and tissue structures (possible misleading results)

Pancreas
- Gas or residual barium in the stomach and intestine (possible poor imaging)
- Body fluid deficiency in a dehydrated patient, obscuring boundaries between organs and tissue structures (possible poor imaging)
- Obesity (possible poor imaging)
- Fatty infiltration of the pancreas (possible poor imaging)

Renal Structures
- Retained barium from a previous test (possible poor imaging)
- Obesity (possible poor imaging)

Spleen
- Overlying ribs, an aerated left lung, or gas or residual barium in the colon or stomach (possible poor imaging)
- Body fluid deficiency in a dehydrated patient, obscuring boundaries between organs and tissue structures (possible poor imaging)
- Body physique affecting the spleen's shape or adjacent masses, displacing the spleen (possible poor imaging; may be mistaken for splenomegaly)
- Splenic trauma (possible difficulty in tolerating the procedure)

Vagina
- Mistaking the bowel for the ovaries
- Small tubal mass (possible difficulty in detecting ectopic pregnancy)

Precautions
- Keep the patient undergoing ultrasonography of the gallbladder and biliary system in a fasting state to prevent bile excretion in the gallbladder. Even smelling greasy foods, such as popcorn, can cause the gallbladder to empty.

Nursing Considerations

Before the Test
- Confirm the patient's identity using two patient identifiers and confirmation of the patient's identification bracelet according to facility policy.
- Explain the purpose of ultrasonography to the patient.
- Tell the patient who will perform the test, when and where it will be done, and that the lights may be lowered to help visualize the monitor.
- Inform the patient that mineral oil or a gel, which may feel cool, will be applied to the area being tested and that a transducer will pass over the skin, directing safe, painless, and inaudible sound waves into the area.
- Instruct the patient to remain still during scanning and to hold the breath when requested.

Abdominal Aorta
- Tell the patient to fast for 12 hours before the test to minimize bowel gas and motility. If ordered, administer simethicone to reduce bowel gas.

Eye
- Inform the patient that there are no food or fluid restrictions for this test.
- Explain that the patient may be asked to move the eyes or change the gaze during the procedure.

Gallbladder and Biliary System
- Instruct the patient to eat a fat-free meal in the evening and then to fast for 8 to 12 hours before the procedure

to promote bile accumulation in the gallbladder and enhance ultrasonic visualization.

- Instruct the patient to remain as still as possible during the procedure and to hold the breath when requested. This will ensure that the gallbladder is in the same position for each scan.

Liver

- Instruct the patient to fast for 8 to 12 hours before the test to reduce bowel gas, which hinders ultrasound transmission.

Pancreas

- Instruct the patient to fast for 8 to 12 hours before the test to reduce bowel gas, which hinders ultrasound transmission.
- Ask the patient who is a smoker to abstain before the test to eliminate the risk of swallowing air while inhaling, which interferes with test results.

Renal Structures

- Inform the patient that there are no food or fluid restrictions for this test.

Spleen

- Instruct the patient to fast for 8 to 12 hours before the procedure, if possible, to reduce the amount of gas in the bowel, thus improving sound wave transmission.

After the Test

- Remove the conductive gel from the patient's skin.
- Instruct the patient to resume a usual diet and medications, as ordered.

▶ Quality and Safety Nursing Alert

Aneurysms requiring ultrasonography of the aorta may expand and dissect rapidly. Check the patient's vital signs frequently. Sudden onset of constant abdominal or back pain accompanies rapid expansion of the aneurysm; sudden, excruciating pain with weakness, sweating, tachycardia, and hypotension signals rupture.

- If rejection of a transplanted kidney is suspected or diagnosed by renal ultrasonography, monitor the patient's intake and output, blood pressure, blood urea nitrogen and creatinine levels, and vital signs. In addition, monitor for adrenal dysfunction (hypotension, decreased urine output, and electrolyte imbalances) if a tumor is detected on the gland.
- If ultrasonography is used as a guide for nephrostomy tube placement or abscess drainage, monitor the amount and characteristics of drainage and tube patency.
- After vaginal ultrasonography, provide the patient with a paper towel to remove the lubricant and offer a sanitary pad.

Upper GI and Small-Bowel Series

Normal Findings

- Barium suspension propelled by a peristaltic wave through the entire esophagus in about 2 seconds
- Even filling and distention of pharynx and esophagus lumen by bolus, revealing smooth, regular mucosa
- Opening and closing of cardiac sphincter as bolus enters stomach
- Normal-appearing stomach, with longitudinal folds (rugae), smooth, regular contour, and no evidence of flattened, rigid areas suggestive of intrinsic or extrinsic lesions
- Relatively smooth duodenal bulb mucosa and appearance of circular folds in the duodenal loop; folds deepen and become more numerous in the jejunum; folds become less prominent in ileum, resembling those in duodenum except for their broadness (Temporary lodging of barium between folds reveals a speckled pattern on X-ray.)
- Gradual tapering of the small intestine's diameter from the duodenum to ileum

Abnormal Findings

Esophagus
- Strictures, tumors, diverticula, varices, and ulcers
- Hiatal hernia (particularly in the distal esophagus)
- Achalasia (cardiospasm)
- Gastric reflux

Stomach
- Adenocarcinoma
- Adenomatous polyps and leiomyomas
- Stomach and duodenal ulcers

Pancreas
- Inflammation, indicating pancreatitis
- Pancreatic carcinoma

Small Intestine
- Inflammation and ulceration, possibly indicating regional enteritis
- Tumors
- Lymphosarcoma

Nursing Implications
- Report abnormal findings to the health care provider.
- Prepare to educate the patient about the diagnosis.
- Prepare the patient for further testing, biopsy, or surgery as indicated.

Purpose
- To detect hiatal hernia, diverticula, and varices
- To help diagnose strictures, blockages, ulcers, tumors, regional enteritis, and malabsorption syndrome
- To help detect motility disorders

Description
The upper GI and small-bowel series is the fluoroscopic examination of the esophagus, stomach, and small intestine after ingestion of barium sulfate, a contrast agent. As the barium passes through the digestive tract, fluoroscopy outlines peristalsis and the mucosal contours of the respective organs, and spot films record significant findings. This test is indicated for patients who have upper GI symptoms (difficulty swallowing, regurgitation, burning or gnawing epigastric pain), signs of small-bowel disease (diarrhea, weight loss), and signs of GI bleeding (hematemesis, melena—bright-red to black, tarry stools).

Although this test can detect various mucosal abnormalities, subsequent biopsy is typically necessary to rule out malignancy or distinguish specific inflammatory diseases. Oral cholecystography, barium enema, and routine X-rays should always precede this test because retained barium clouds anatomic detail on X-ray films.

The procedure for the upper GI and small-bowel series is as follows:

- After the patient is secured in a supine position on the X-ray table, the table is tilted until the patient is erect, and the heart, lungs, and abdomen are examined fluoroscopically.
- The patient is instructed to take several swallows of the barium suspension, and its passage through the esophagus is observed. (Occasionally, the patient is given a thick barium suspension, especially when esophageal disease is strongly suspected.)
- During fluoroscopic examination, spot films of the esophagus are taken from lateral angles and from right and left posteroanterior angles.
- When barium enters the stomach, the patient's abdomen is palpated or compressed to ensure adequate coating of the gastric mucosa.
- To perform a double-contrast examination, the patient is instructed to sip the barium through a perforated straw. As the patient does so, a small amount of air also is introduced into the stomach, permitting detailed examination of the gastric rugae, and spot films of significant findings are taken. The patient is then instructed to ingest the remaining barium suspension and the filling of the stomach and emptying into the duodenum are observed fluoroscopically.
- Two series of spot films of the stomach and duodenum are taken

U

from posteroanterior, anteroposterior, lateral, and oblique angles, with the patient erect and then in a supine position.

- The passage of barium into the remainder of the small intestine is then observed fluoroscopically, and spot films are taken at 30- to 60-minute intervals until the barium reaches the ileocecal valve region. If abnormalities in the small intestine are detected, the area is palpated and compressed to help clarify the defect, and a spot film is taken. The examination ends when the barium enters the cecum.

Interfering Factors

- Excess air in the small bowel (possible poor imaging)
- Failure to remove metallic objects in the X-ray field (possible poor imaging)

Precautions

- The upper GI and small-bowel series may be contraindicated in the patient with digestive tract obstruction or perforation. Barium may intensify the obstruction or seep into the abdominal cavity. Sometimes a small-bowel series is performed to find a "transition zone." If a perforation is suspected, Gastrografin (a water-soluble contrast medium) rather than barium may be used.
- The test is contraindicated during pregnancy because of radiation's possible teratogenic effects.

Nursing Considerations

Before the Test

- Confirm the patient's identity using two patient identifiers and confirmation of the patient's identification bracelet according to facility policy.
- Explain to the patient that the upper GI and small-bowel series uses ingested barium and X-ray films to examine the esophagus, stomach, and small intestine. Describe the test, including who will perform it and

when and where it will take place. Encourage the patient to bring reading material.

- Explain that the patient will be placed on an X-ray table that rotates into various positions but that the patient will be adequately secured and assisted throughout. Warn the patient that the abdomen may be compressed to ensure proper coating of the stomach or intestinal walls with barium or to separate overlapping bowel loops.
- Describe the milkshake consistency and chalky taste of the barium mixture. Explain that the patient must drink 16 to 20 oz (473–591 mL) for a complete examination.
- Instruct the patient to consume a low-residue diet (no seeds, juices with pulp, raw vegetables, or whole grain products) for 2 to 3 days before the test and then to fast and avoid smoking after midnight the night before the test.
- As ordered, withhold most oral medications after midnight and anticholinergics and opioids for 24 hours; these drugs affect small intestinal motility. Antacids, histamine-2 receptor antagonists, and proton pump inhibitors also are sometimes withheld for several hours if gastric reflux is suspected.
- Just before the procedure, instruct the patient to put on a gown without snap closures and to remove jewelry, dentures, hair clips, or other objects that might obscure anatomic detail on the X-ray films.

After the Test

- Make sure additional X-rays haven't been ordered before allowing the patient food, fluids, and oral medications (if applicable).
- Instruct the patient to drink plenty of fluid (unless contraindicated) to help eliminate the barium.
- Administer a cathartic or enema. Explain that the patient's stools will be light colored for 24 to 72 hours.

Record and describe any stools passed by the patient in the health care facility. Barium retention in the intestine may cause obstruction or fecal impaction, so notify the physician if the patient doesn't pass the barium within 2 to 3 days. Also, barium retention may affect scheduling of other GI tests.

- Instruct the patient to tell the physician of abdominal fullness or pain or a delay in return to brown stools.

Urea Clearance

Reference Values

With maximal clearance: 64 to 99 mL/minute

Flow rate less than 2 mL/minute: 41 to 68 mL/minute

Abnormal Findings

Decreased Levels

- Decreased renal blood flow (caused by shock or renal artery obstruction)
- Acute or chronic glomerulonephritis
- Advanced bilateral chronic pyelonephritis
- Acute tubular necrosis
- Nephrosclerosis
- Polycystic kidney disease
- Renal tuberculosis
- Cancer
- Bilateral ureteral obstruction
- Heart failure
- Dehydration

Nursing Implications

- Report abnormal findings to the health care provider.
- Prepare to educate the patient about the diagnosis.
- Prepare the patient for further testing or surgery, as indicated.

Purpose

- To assess overall renal function

Description

The urea clearance test is a quantitative analysis of urine levels of urea, the main nitrogenous component in urine and the end product of protein metabolism. (See the *How Urea Is Formed* box.)

After filtration by the glomeruli, roughly 40% of the urea is reabsorbed by the renal tubules. Because of this reabsorption, urea clearance was once considered a precise fraction (60%) of the glomerular filtration rate (GFR). However, because the reabsorption rate of urea varies with the amount of water reabsorbed, this test actually assesses overall renal function; the creatinine clearance test provides a more accurate evaluation of the GFR.

In urea clearance, blood urea content and the total amount of urea excreted in the urine are proportional only when the rate of urine flow is 2 mL/minute or higher (maximal clearance). At lower flow rates, the test's accuracy decreases. The equation for determining urea clearance is $C = (U \times V) \div P$; it's similar to the equation used for creatinine clearance.

How Urea Is Formed

Urea, the main nitrogenous component in urine, is the final product of protein metabolism. Amino acids absorbed by the intestinal villi pass from the portal vein into the liver. Because the liver stores only small amounts of amino acids—which are later returned to the blood for use in the synthesis of enzymes, hormones, or new protoplasm—the excess is converted into other substances, such as glucose, glycogen, and fat.

Before this conversion, the amino acids are deaminated—they lose their nitrogenous amino groups. These amino groups are then converted to ammonia. Because ammonia is extremely toxic, especially to the brain, it must be removed as quickly as it's formed. (Serious liver disease causes elevated blood ammonia levels and eventually leads to hepatic coma.)

In the liver, ammonia combines with carbon dioxide to form urea, which is released into the blood and ultimately secreted in urine.

Interfering Factors

- Failure of patient to empty the bladder completely (the most common error in this test)
- Caffeine, milk, or small doses of epinephrine (increase)
- Antidiuretic hormone or large doses of epinephrine (decrease)
- Amphotericin B, corticosteroids, streptomycin, and thiazide diuretics

Precautions

- Because this is a clearance test, make sure the patient empties the bladder completely and that the total amount of urine is collected from each hour's specimen.
- Send each specimen to the laboratory as soon as it's collected.
- If the patient is catheterized, empty the drainage bag before beginning the specimen collection.
- Handle the blood sample gently to prevent hemolysis and send it to the laboratory immediately.

Nursing Considerations

Before the Test

- Confirm the patient's identity using two patient identifiers and confirmation of the patient's identification bracelet according to facility policy.
- Explain to the patient that the urea clearance test evaluates kidney function.
- Advise the patient that the test requires two timed urine specimens and one blood sample. Explain how the urine specimens will be collected, who will perform the venipuncture and when, and that slight discomfort from the tourniquet and the needle puncture may be experienced.
- Instruct the patient to fast from midnight before the test and to abstain from exercise before and during the test.
- Check the patient's medication history for drugs that may affect urea clearance. Review your findings with the laboratory and then notify the health care provider; these medications may need to be restricted.

During the Test

- Instruct the patient to empty the bladder and discard the urine. Then give the patient water to drink to ensure adequate urine output.
- Collect two specimens 1 hour apart, and mark the collection time on the laboratory request.
- Perform a venipuncture anytime during the collection period and collect the sample in a 7-mL red-topped tube.

After the Test

- If a hematoma develops at the venipuncture site, apply direct pressure.
- Tell the patient to resume usual diet, activities, and medications, as ordered.

Uric Acid, Serum and Urine

Reference Values

Serum Uric Acid

Females: 2.3 to 6 mg/dL (SI, 143–357 mcmol/L)
Males: 3.4 to 7 mg/dL (SI, 202–416 mcmol/L)

Urine Uric Acid

250 to 750 mg/24 hours (SI, 1.48–4.43 mmol/day)

Abnormal Findings

Elevated Levels

Serum Uric Acid

- Gout
- Impaired kidney function
- Heart failure
- Glycogen storage disease (type I, von Gierke's disease)
- Infections
- Hemolytic and sickle cell anemia
- Polycythemia
- Neoplasms
- Psoriasis

Urine Uric Acid

- Chronic myeloid leukemia
- Polycythemia vera
- Multiple myeloma

- Early remission in pernicious anemia
- Lymphosarcoma
- Lymphatic leukemia during radiotherapy
- Fanconi's syndrome
- Wilson's disease

Decreased Levels
Serum Uric Acid
- Defective tubular absorption (such as Fanconi's syndrome)
- Acute hepatic atrophy

Urine Uric Acid
- Gout
- Chronic glomerulonephritis
- Diabetic glomerulosclerosis
- Collagen disorders

Nursing Implications
- Report abnormal findings to the health care provider.
- Prepare to educate the patient about the diagnosis.
- Prepare the patient for further testing or surgery, as indicated.

Purpose
- To confirm gout diagnosis
- To help detect renal dysfunction
- To detect enzyme deficiencies and metabolic disturbances that affect uric acid production, such as gout (urine uric acid)

Description
The uric acid test is used to measure serum uric acid levels, the major end metabolite of purine. Disorders of purine metabolism, rapid destruction of nucleic acids, and conditions marked by impaired renal excretion characteristically raise serum uric acid levels.

A quantitative analysis of urine uric acid levels may supplement serum uric acid testing when seeking to identify disorders that alter production or excretion of uric acid (such as gout, leukemia, and renal dysfunction).

The most specific laboratory method for detecting uric acid is spectrophotometric absorption after treatment of the specimen with the enzyme uricase.

Interfering Factors
Serum Uric Acid
- Low doses of aspirin, ethambutol, loop diuretics, pyrazinamide, thiazides, and vincristine (possible increase)
- Acetaminophen, ascorbic acid, and levodopa (possible false high if using colorimetric method)
- Aspirin in high doses (possible decrease)
- Alcohol abuse, high-purine diet, starvation, and stress (possible increase)

Urine Uric Acid
- Diuretics, such as benzthiazide, ethacrynic acid, and furosemide (decrease); alcohol, allopurinol, phenylbutazone, probenecid, pyrazinamide, salicylates, vitamin C, and warfarin (Coumadin) (increase)
- High-purine diet (increase)
- Low-purine diet (decrease)

Precautions
- Handle the blood sample gently to prevent hemolysis.
- Send the urine specimen to the laboratory immediately after collection is completed.

Nursing Considerations
Before the Test
- Confirm the patient's identity using two patient identifiers and confirmation of the patient's identification bracelet according to facility policy.
- Explain to the patient that the uric acid test is used to detect gout and kidney dysfunction. Advise the patient that the test requires a blood sample or urine specimen. Explain who will perform the test, and how and when the serum or urine will be collected.
- Notify the laboratory and health care provider of medications the patient is taking that may affect test results; these may need to be restricted.

U

Serum Uric Acid

- Explain to the patient that slight discomfort from the tourniquet and the needle puncture may be experienced.
- Instruct the patient to fast for 8 hours before the test.

Urine Uric Acid

- Anticipate the need for a diet low or high in purine before or during urine collection, as appropriate.
- Tell the patient that the test requires urine collection over a 24-hour period and instruct on proper collection technique.

During the Test
Serum Uric Acid

- Perform a venipuncture. Collect the sample in a 3- or 4-mL clot activator tube.

Urine Uric Acid

- Collect the patient's urine over a 24-hour period, discarding the first specimen and retaining the last.

After the Test

- Instruct the patient to resume a usual diet or dietary restrictions ordered by the health care provider and to resume medications that were discontinued before the test, as ordered.
- For the serum uric acid test, apply direct pressure to the venipuncture site until bleeding stops. If a hematoma develops at the venipuncture site, continue direct pressure.

Urinalysis

Reference Values

Color: Clear, straw-colored to dark yellow urine
Odor: Slightly aromatic
Specific gravity: 1.005 to 1.035
pH: 4.5 to 8.0
Red blood cells (RBCs): 0 to 2 per high-power field

White blood cells (WBCs) or epithelial cells: 0 to 5 per high-power field
Casts: None except one to two hyaline casts per low-power field
Crystals: Present

Abnormal Findings
Color

- Orange (concentrated urine, bilirubin, phenazopyridine [Pyridium], carrots, rifampicin [Rifampin] may cause an orange-red color)
- Green (*Pseudomonas*, indican, chlorophyll)

Odor

- Fruity (diabetes, starvation, dehydration, fetid urine, urinary tract infections [*Escherichia coli*])
- Musty (phenylketonuria)
- Fishy or cabbagelike (tyrosinemia)

Appearance

- Turbid (renal infection)

Specific Gravity

- Low specific gravity (characteristic of diabetes insipidus, acute tubular necrosis, and pyelonephritis)
- Fixed specific gravity (doesn't changes despite fluid intake), indicating chronic glomerulonephritis and severe renal damage
- High specific gravity, indicating nephrotic syndrome, dehydration, acute glomerulonephritis, heart failure, liver failure, and shock

pH

- Alkaline, possibly resulting from Fanconi's syndrome, upper urinary tract infection caused by urea-splitting bacteria (*Proteus* and *Pseudomonas*), and metabolic or respiratory acidosis
- Acidic, suggesting renal tuberculosis, pyrexia, phenylketonuria, alkaptonuria, or acidosis

Casts

- Hyaline: renal parenchymal disease, inflammation, or trauma to the glomerular capillary membrane

U

- Epithelial: renal tubular damage, nephrosis, eclampsia, amyloidosis, or heavy metal poisoning
- Coarse and fine: acute or chronic renal failure, pyelonephritis, or chronic lead intoxication
- Fatty and waxy: chronic renal failure, nephrotic syndrome, or diabetes

RBCs and Casts
- Glomerulonephritis
- Lupus nephritis
- Pyelonephritis
- Subacute bacterial endocarditis
- Malignant hypertension
- Periarteritis nodosum
- Goodpasture's syndrome
- Renal calculi
- Cystitis
- Prostatitis

WBCs and Casts
- Acute pyelonephritis
- Nephrotic syndrome
- Pyogenic infection
- Lupus nephritis

Crystals
- Calcium oxalate (hypercalcemia, ethylene glycol ingestion)
- Cystine crystals (inborn error of metabolism)

Nursing Implications
- Report abnormal findings to the health care provider.
- Prepare to educate the patient about the diagnosis.
- Prepare the patient for further testing or surgery, as indicated.
- Provide emotional support to the patient and family.
- Anticipate the need for antibiotic therapy, as indicated.

Purpose
- To screen the patient's urine for kidney or urinary tract disease
- To help detect metabolic or systemic disease unrelated to renal disorders
- To detect the presence of drugs

Description
Urinalysis evaluates the physical characteristics of urine; determines specific gravity and pH; detects and measures protein, glucose, and ketone bodies; and examines sediment for blood cells, casts, and crystals. It includes visual examination, reagent strip screening, refractometry for specific gravity, and microscopic inspection of centrifuged sediment.

Nursing Considerations
Before the Test
- Confirm the patient's identity using two patient identifiers and confirmation of the patient's identification bracelet according to facility policy.
- Explain that this analysis helps to diagnose kidney or urinary tract disease and to evaluate overall body function.
- Inform the patient that there are no food or fluid restrictions for this test.
- Notify the laboratory and health care provider of drugs the patient is taking that may affect laboratory results.

During the Test
- Collect a random urine specimen of at least 15 mL. Obtain a first-voided morning specimen if possible.
- Strain the specimen to catch calculi or calculus fragments if the patient is being evaluated for renal colic. Carefully pour the urine through an unfolded 4 × 4-inch gauze pad or a fine-mesh sieve placed over the specimen container.

After the Test
- Instruct the patient to resume a usual diet and medications.

Urine Culture
Normal Findings
- Sterile urine with no bacterial growth

Abnormal Findings
- Bacterial count of 100,000 mL or more, indicating urinary tract infection (UTI)

- Presence of *Mycobacterium tuberculosis*, indicating tuberculosis of the urinary tract

Nursing Implications
- Report abnormal findings to the health care provider.
- Prepare to educate the patient about the diagnosis.
- Prepare the patient for further testing or surgery, as indicated.
- Provide emotional support to the patient and family.
- Anticipate administration of antibiotics, as applicable.

Purpose
- To diagnose UTI
- To monitor microorganism colonization after urinary catheter insertion

Description
A urine culture is used to evaluate UTIs, most commonly bladder infections, and to identify pathogenic fungi such as *Coccidioides immitis*. Testing may involve a quick urine screen to determine if urine contains high bacteria or white blood cell (WBC) counts; only urine with bacteria or WBCs is processed for culture. A clean-voided midstream collection, rather than suprapubic aspiration or catheterization, is the method of choice for obtaining a urine specimen.

To distinguish between true bacteriuria and contamination, it's necessary to know the number of organisms in a milliliter of urine, estimated by a culture technique known as a *colony count;* an additional quick centrifugation test determines where a UTI originates. Specimen collection may be required on three consecutive mornings for a patient with suspected urogenital tuberculosis.

 Quality and Safety Nursing Alert

Isolation of more than two species of organisms or of vaginal or skin organisms usually suggests contamination and requires a repeat culture.

Interfering Factors
- Antibiotics and diuretics

Precautions
- Possible infection when specimens are obtained by catheterization.

Nursing Considerations
Before the Test
- Confirm the patient's identity using two patient identifiers and confirmation of the patient's identification bracelet according to facility policy.
- Explain to the patient that the test requires a urine specimen. Instruct the patient to collect a clean-voided midstream specimen, stressing the importance of cleaning the external genitalia thoroughly with the cleansing cloth provided and maintaining asepsis throughout the procedure.
- Note and report all allergies, and check the patient's history for current use of antimicrobial drugs.
- Make sure the specimen is collected before beginning antibiotic therapy.

During the Test
- Record the suspected diagnosis, the collection time and method, current antimicrobial therapy, and fluid- or drug-induced diuresis on the laboratory request.
- Collect the first-voided urine specimen. Be sure to collect at least 3 mL of urine, but don't fill the specimen cup more than halfway.
- Seal the cup with a sterile lid and send it to the laboratory at once.

After the Test
- If transport is delayed for more than 30 minutes, store the specimen at 39.7°F (4.3°C) or place it on ice unless the urine transport tube contains a preservative.

Urine Hydroxyproline

Reference Values
1 to 9 mg/24 hours (SI, 1–3.4 international units/day)

Abnormal Findings

Elevated Levels
- Bone disease
- Metastatic bone tumors
- Endocrine disorders that stimulate hormonal secretion
- Growth hormone use
- Parathyroid hormone use
- Phenobarbital use
- Sulfonylurea use

Decreased Levels
- Therapy for bone resorption disorders
- Ascorbic acid, vitamin D, aspirin, glucocorticoids, antineoplastic agents, calcium gluconate, corticosteroids, estradiol, propranolol, calcitonin, and mithramycin use
- Psoriasis and burns (possible increase caused by collagen turnover)

Nursing Implications
- Report abnormal findings to the health care provider.
- Prepare to educate the patient about the diagnosis.
- Prepare the patient for further testing or surgery, as indicated.
- Provide emotional support to the patient and family.

Purpose
- To monitor treatment for disorders characterized by bone resorption, including Paget's disease, metastatic bone tumors, certain endocrine disorders (hyperthyroidism), rheumatoid arthritis, and osteoporosis
- To help diagnose disorders characterized by bone resorption

Description
This test determines hydroxyproline levels colorimetrically on a timed urine specimen or by ion exchange or gas–liquid chromatography. Total urine levels of hydroxyproline, an amino acid found mainly in collagen (a component of skin and bone), are a good index of bone matrix turnover because levels increase when collagen breaks down during bone resorption. Bone matrix turnover and hydroxyproline levels normally rise in children during periods of rapid skeletal growth. However, they also rise in disorders that increase bone resorption, such as Paget's disease, metastatic bone tumors, and certain endocrine disorders.

A collagen-restricted diet is essential for this test because hydroxyproline levels reflect collagen intake. Free hydroxyproline, a small component of total hydroxyproline and a sensitive indicator of dietary collagen intake, may be measured to validate results.

Interfering Factors
- Failure to observe restrictions
- Failure to collect all urine during the collection period, to store the specimen properly, or to send the specimen to the laboratory immediately after the collection is complete

Nursing Considerations

Before the Test
- Confirm the patient's identity using two patient identifiers and confirmation of the patient's identification bracelet according to facility policy.
- Explain to the patient that the urine hydroxyproline test helps to monitor treatment or to detect an amino acid disorder related to bone formation. Tell the patient that the test requires urine collection over a 2- or 24-hour period and teach the correct collection technique.
- Inform the patient of the need to follow a collagen-free diet and to avoid eating ice cream, candy, meat, fish, poultry, jelly, and any foods containing gelatin for 24 hours before the test and during the test period itself.
- Notify the laboratory and health care provider of drugs the patient is taking that may affect test results; it may be necessary to restrict these.

U

During the Test

- Collect the patient's urine over a 2- or 24-hour period. In a 24-hour collection, discard the first specimen and retain the last.
- Use a container that has a preservative to prevent hydroxyproline degradation.
- Refrigerate the specimen or keep it on ice during the collection period.

- Note the patient's age and sex on the laboratory request.
- Send the specimen to the laboratory immediately after the collection is complete.

After the Test

- Instruct the patient to resume a usual diet and medications, as ordered.

V

Vanillylmandelic Acid, Urine

Reference Values
2 to 7 mg/24 hours (SI, 1–35 mcmol/day)

Abnormal Findings
Elevated Levels
- Catecholamine-secreting tumor

Nursing Implications
- Report abnormal findings to the health care provider.
- Prepare to educate the patient about the diagnosis.
- Prepare the patient for further testing or surgery, as indicated.
- Provide emotional support to the patient and family.

Purpose
- To help detect pheochromocytoma, neuroblastoma, and ganglioneuroma
- To evaluate the function of the adrenal medulla

Description
Using spectrophotofluorimetry, the vanillylmandelic acid (VMA) test determines urine levels of VMA, a phenolic acid. VMA, normally the most prevalent catecholamine metabolite in urine, is the product of epinephrine and norepinephrine hepatic conversion; urine VMA levels reflect these major catecholamines' endogenous production. Like the urine total catecholamines test, this test helps detect catecholamine-secreting tumors—especially pheochromocytoma—and helps evaluate adrenal medulla function, the primary catecholamine production site.

Ideally, the VMA test should be performed on a 24-hour urine specimen (not a random specimen) to overcome the effects of diurnal variation in catecholamine secretion. Other catecholamine metabolites—metanephrine, normetanephrine, and homovanillic acid—may be measured at the same time. If evaluating hypertension, specimen collection may be of greatest value during the hypertensive episode.

Interfering Factors
- Excessive exercise or emotional stress (increase), pain
- Epinephrine, lithium carbonate, methocarbamol, and norepinephrine (increase); chlorpromazine, clonidine, guanethidine, monoamine oxidase inhibitors, and reserpine (decrease); levodopa and salicylates (increase or decrease)
- Hypoglycemia
- Many types of foods, such as caffeine products, vanilla, fruit, licorice

Precautions
- Refrigerate the specimen or keep it on ice during the collection period.

Nursing Considerations
Before the Test
- Confirm the patient's identity using two patient identifiers and confirmation of the patient's identification bracelet according to facility policy.
- Explain to the patient that the urine VMA test evaluates hormonal secretion. Advise that it requires collection of urine over a 24-hour period and teach the proper collection technique.

- Instruct the patient to restrict foods and beverages containing phenolic acid, such as coffee, tea, bananas, citrus fruits, chocolate, vanilla, and carbonated beverages, for 3 days before the test.
- Advise the patient to avoid stressful situations and excessive physical activity during the urine collection period.
- Notify the laboratory and health care provider of medications the patient is taking that may affect test results; these may need to be restricted.

During the Test
- Collect the patient's urine over a 24-hour period, discarding the first specimen and retaining the last. Use a bottle containing a preservative to keep the specimen at a pH of 3.0.
- Send the specimen to the laboratory immediately after the collection is completed.

After the Test
- Tell the patient to resume all usual activities, diet, and medications, as ordered.

Venereal Disease Research Laboratory Test

Reference Values
No flocculation in serum (reported as nonreactive test, although syphilis is undetectable for 14 to 21 days after infection)

Abnormal Findings

Reactive Test
- Primary syphilis (50% of patients)
- Secondary syphilis (nearly all patients)
- Neurosyphilis (in test using a cerebrospinal fluid [CSF] specimen)

Biologic False-Positive Reactions
- Infectious mononucleosis
- Malaria
- Leprosy

- Hepatitis
- Systemic lupus erythematosus
- Rheumatoid arthritis
- Nonsyphilitic treponemal diseases (pinta and yaws)

Nursing Implications
- If the test is nonreactive or borderline, but syphilis hasn't been ruled out, instruct the patient to return for follow-up testing. Explain that borderline test results don't necessarily mean that the patient is free from the disease.
- If the test is reactive, explain the importance of proper treatment. Provide the patient with further information about sexually transmitted diseases and how they're spread, and stress the need for antibiotic therapy. Report the results to state public health authorities and prepare the patient for mandatory inquiries.
- If the test is reactive but the patient shows no clinical signs of syphilis, explain that many uninfected people show false-positive reactions. Stress the need for further specific tests to rule out syphilis.

Purpose
- To screen for primary and secondary syphilis
- To confirm primary or secondary syphilis in the presence of syphilitic lesions
- To monitor the patient's response to treatment

Description
The Venereal Disease Research Laboratory (VDRL) test, a flocculation test, is used widely to screen for primary and secondary syphilis. Although the test has diagnostic significance during the first two stages of syphilis, transient or permanent biologic false-positive reactions can make accurate interpretation difficult. A biologic false-positive reaction can result from viral or bacterial infection, chronic systemic illness, or nonsyphilitic treponemal disease.

Rapid Plasma Reagin Test

The rapid plasma reagin (RPR) test is quick, macroscopic serologic test that's an acceptable substitute for the Venereal Disease Research Laboratory (VDRL) test in diagnosing syphilis. The RPR test, available as a kit, uses a cardiolipin antigen to detect reagin, the antibody relatively specific for *Treponema pallidum,* the causative agent of syphilis.

In the RPR test, the patient's serum is mixed with cardiolipin on a plastic-coated card, rotated mechanically, and then examined with the unaided eye. If flocculation occurs, the test sample is diluted until no visible reaction occurs. The last dilution to show visible floccula-tion is the titer of the reagin antibody.

In the RPR test, as in the VDRL test, normal serum shows no flocculation.

Usually, a serum sample is used in the VDRL test, but this test may also be performed on a CSF specimen obtained by lumbar puncture to test for tertiary syphilis. The VDRL test of CSF is less sensitive than the fluorescent trepone-mal antibody absorption test. The rapid plasma reagin test can also be used to diagnose syphilis. (See the *Rapid Plasma Reagin Test* box.)

Interfering Factors
* Alcohol ingestion within 24 hours of the test (possible transient nonreactive results)
* Immunosuppression (possible nonre-active results)

Precautions
* Handle the specimen carefully to prevent hemolysis.

Nursing Considerations
Before the Test
* Confirm the patient's identity using two patient identifiers and confirma-tion of the patient's identification bracelet according to facility policy.
* Explain to the patient that the VDRL test detects syphilis, a disease that usually goes undetected and untreated in the general population because

the majority of infected people don't know they're infected.
* Advise the patient that the test requires a blood sample. Explain that the patient may experience slight discomfort from the tourniquet and the needle puncture.
* Inform the patient that there are no food, fluid, or medication restrictions, but the patient should abstain from alcohol for 24 hours before the test.

During the Test
* Perform a venipuncture and collect the sample in a 7-mL clot activator tube.

After the Test
* Apply direct pressure to the veni-puncture site until bleeding stops and to prevent hematoma formation.

Vertebral Radiography

Normal Findings
* No vertebral fractures, subluxations, dislocations, curvatures, or other abnormalities
* Alignment of vertebrae forming four alternately concave and convex curves (lateral view in adults); cervi-cal and lumbar curves are convex anteriorly, and thoracic and sacral curves are convex anteriorly
* Coccyx pointing forward and downward
* Only one vertebral curve (concave anteriorly) in neonates

Abnormal Findings
* Spondylolisthesis
* Fractures, dislocations
* Subluxations
* Wedging
* Kyphosis, scoliosis, or lordosis

Nursing Implications
* Depending on X-ray results, definitive diagnosis may also require additional tests, such as myelography, magnetic resonance imaging, or computed tomographic scanning.

- Report abnormal findings to the health care provider.
- Prepare to educate the patient about the diagnosis.
- Prepare the patient for further testing or surgery, as indicated.

Purpose

- To detect vertebral fractures, dislocations, subluxations, and deformities
- To detect vertebral degeneration, infection, and congenital disorders
- To detect disorders of the intervertebral disks
- To determine the vertebral effects of arthritic and metabolic disorders

Description

Vertebral radiography visualizes all or part of the vertebral column. A commonly performed test, it's used to evaluate the vertebrae for deformities, fractures, dislocations, tumors, and other abnormalities. Bone films determine bone density, texture, erosion, and changes in bone relationships. Bone cortex X-rays reveal the presence of any widening or narrowing and signs of irregularity. Joint X-rays can reveal the presence of fluid, spur formation, narrowing, and changes in the joint structure.

The type and extent of vertebral radiography depend on the patient's clinical condition. For example, a patient with lower back pain requires only lumbar and sacral segment studies. The exact procedure varies considerably, depending on the vertebral segment being examined, but usually includes these steps:

- Initially, the patient is placed in a supine position on the X-ray table for an anteroposterior view.
- The patient may be repositioned for lateral or right and left oblique views; specific positioning depends on the vertebral segment or adjacent structure of interest.

Interfering Factors

- Improper positioning of the patient or patient movement (possible poor imaging)

Precautions

- Vertebral radiography is contraindicated during the first trimester of pregnancy, unless the benefits outweigh the risk of fetal radiation exposure.

> ▶ *Quality and Safety Nursing Alert*
>
> **Exercise extreme caution when handling a trauma patient with suspected spinal injuries, particularly of the cervical area. The patient should be filmed while on the stretcher to avoid further injury during transfer to the radiographic table.**

Nursing Considerations

Before the Test

- Confirm the patient's identity using two patient identifiers and confirmation of the patient's identification bracelet according to facility policy.
- Explain to the patient that vertebral radiography involves taking X-rays to examine the spine. Tell the patient who will perform the test, and when and where it will take place.
- Explain that the patient will be placed in various positions for the X-rays. Tell the patient that although some positions may cause slight discomfort, cooperation is needed to ensure accurate results. Stress that the patient must keep still and hold the breath as instructed during the procedure.
- Inform the patient that there are no food or fluid restrictions for this test.

After the Test

- Provide analgesics or local heat applications, as ordered, to relieve pain.

Voiding Cystourethrography

Normal Findings

- Normal structure and function of the bladder and urethra

- No regurgitation of contrast medium into the ureters

Abnormal Findings

- Urethral stricture
- Vesical or urethral diverticula
- Ureterocele
- Cystocele
- Prostate enlargement
- Vesicoureteral reflux
- Neurogenic bladder

Nursing Implications

- Report abnormal findings to the health care provider.
- Prepare to educate the patient about the diagnosis.
- Prepare the patient for further testing or surgery, as indicated.
- Provide emotional support to the patient and family.
- If stricture is present, prepare for surgery, as indicated.

Purpose

- To detect abnormalities of the bladder and urethra, such as vesicoureteral reflux, neurogenic bladder, prostatic hyperplasia, urethral strictures, or diverticula

Description

In voiding cystourethrography, a contrast medium is instilled by gentle syringe pressure or gravity into the bladder through a urethral catheter. Fluoroscopic films or overhead radiographs demonstrate bladder filling and then show contrast medium excretion as the patient voids.

The procedure for voiding cystourethrography is as follows:

- The patient is placed in a supine position, and an indwelling urinary catheter is inserted into the bladder.
- The contrast medium is instilled through the catheter until the bladder is full.
- The catheter is clamped, and X-rays are exposed with the patient in supine, oblique, and lateral positions.
- The catheter is removed, and the patient assumes the right oblique

position (right leg flexed to 90 degrees, left leg extended, penis parallel to right leg) and begins to void.

- Four high-speed exposures of the bladder and urethra, coned down to reduce radiation exposure, are usually made on one film during voiding.
- If the right oblique view doesn't delineate both ureters, the patient is asked to stop urinating and to begin again in the left oblique position.
- The most reliable voiding cysto-urethrograms are obtained with the patient recumbent. The patient who can't void recumbent may do so standing (not sitting).

 Quality and Safety Nursing Alert

Expression cystourethrography may have to be performed, under a general anesthetic, for a young child who can't void on command.

 Quality and Safety Nursing Alert

Observe and record the time, color, and volume of the patient's voidings. Report hematuria, if present, after the third voiding.

Interfering Factors

- Embarrassment (inhibits the patient from voiding on command)
- Interrupted or less vigorous voiding, muscle spasm, or incomplete sphincter relaxation (due to urethral trauma during catheterization)
- Contrast media presence from recent tests, stools, or gas in the bowel (possible poor imaging)

Precautions

- Voiding cystourethrography is contraindicated in the patient with an acute or exacerbated urethral or bladder infection or an acute urethral injury.
- Hypersensitivity to the contrast medium also may be a contraindication for testing.

V

Nursing Considerations

Before the Test

- Confirm the patient's identity using two patient identifiers and confirmation of the patient's identification bracelet according to facility policy.
- Explain to the patient that voiding cystourethrography permits assessment of the bladder and urethra. Explain who will perform the test and when and where it will be done.
- Inform the patient that a catheter will be inserted into the bladder and that a contrast medium will be instilled through the catheter. Advise that a feeling of fullness and an urge to void may be experienced when the contrast medium is instilled. Explain that X-rays will be taken of the bladder and urethra and that the patient will be asked to assume various positions.
- Inform the patient that there are no food or fluid restrictions for this test.

- Make sure that the patient or a responsible family member has signed an informed consent form.

 Quality and Safety Nursing Alert

Check the patient's history for hypersensitivity to contrast media/dye or iodine-containing foods such as shellfish; note sensitivities on the chart and notify the health care provider.

- Administer a sedative, if prescribed, just before the procedure.

After the Test

- Encourage the patient to drink large quantities of fluids to reduce burning on urination and to flush out residual contrast medium.

 Quality and Safety Nursing Alert

Monitor the patient for chills and fever related to contrast material extravasation or urinary sepsis. Also monitor for symptoms of urinary tract infection.

V

White Blood Cell Count and Differential

Reference Values

4,000 to 10,000/mcL (SI, 4 to 10 × 10⁹/L)

For an accurate diagnosis, differential test results always must be interpreted in relation to the total white blood cell (WBC) count. (See the *Interpreting WBC Differential Values* box for normal WBC differential values for adults and children.)

Abnormal Findings

Elevated Levels

- Infection
- Abscess
- Meningitis
- Appendicitis
- Tonsillitis
- Leukemia
- Tissue necrosis due to burns, myocardial infarction, or gangrene

Decreased Levels

- Bone marrow depression
- Viral infections
- Following treatment with antineoplastics
- Ingestion of mercury or other heavy metals
- Exposure to benzene or arsenicals
- Influenza
- Typhoid fever
- Measles
- Infectious hepatitis
- Mononucleosis
- Rubella
- Abnormal differential patterns indicative of other diseases or conditions (See the *Influence of Disease on Blood Cell Count* table.)

Nursing Implications

- Report any abnormal findings to the health care provider.
- Prepare to educate the patient about the diagnosis.
- Prepare the patient for further testing or surgery, as indicated.
- Provide emotional support to the patient and family.
- Prepare to administer antimicrobial therapy, as indicated.
- Institute isolation precautions, as applicable.

Purpose

WBC Count

- To determine infection or inflammation
- To determine the need for further tests, such as bone marrow biopsy
- To monitor response to chemotherapy or radiation therapy

WBC Differential

- To evaluate the body's capacity to resist and overcome infection
- To detect and identify various types of leukemia (See the *Performing a LAP Stain* box, p. 522.)
- To determine the stage and severity of an infection
- To detect allergic reactions and parasitic infections and assess their severity (eosinophil count)
- To distinguish viral from bacterial infections

Description

A WBC count, also called a *leukocyte count*, is part of a complete blood count. It indicates the number of white cells in a microliter (mcL, or cubic millimeter) of

(text continues on page 522)

Interpreting WBC Differential Values

The differential count measures the types of white blood cells (WBCs) as a percentage of the total WBC count (the relative value). The absolute value is obtained by multiplying the relative value of each cell type by the total WBC count. The relative and absolute values must be considered to obtain an accurate diagnosis.

For example, consider a patient whose WBC count is 6,000/mcL (SI, 6 × 10^9/L) and whose differential shows 30% (SI, 0.3) neutrophils and 70% (SI, 0.7) lymphocytes. His relative lymphocyte count seems to be quite high (lymphocytosis), but when this figure is multiplied by his WBC count (6,000 × 70% = 4,200 lymphocytes/mcL) (SI, [6 × 10^9/L] × 0.7 = 4.2 × 10^9/L lymphocytes), it's well within the normal range.

However, this patient's neutrophil count (30%; SI, 0.3) is low; when this figure is multiplied by the WBC count (6,000 × 30% = 1,800 neutrophils/mL) (SI, [6 × 10^9/L] 0.30 = 1.8 × 10^9/L neutrophils), the result is a low absolute number, which may mean depressed bone marrow.

The normal percentages of WBC type in adults are:
- Neutrophils: 54% to 75% (SI, 0.54–0.75)
- Eosinophils: 1% to 4% (SI, 0.01–0.04)
- Basophils: 0% to 1% (SI, 0–0.01)
- Monocytes: 2% to 8% (SI, 0.02–0.08)
- Lymphocytes: 25% to 40% (SI, 0.25–0.4)

Influence of Disease on Blood Cell Count

This table shows how abnormal blood cell counts can affect various diseases or conditions.

Cell Type	How Affected
	Neutrophils
	Increased by: • Infections: osteomyelitis, otitis media, salpingitis, septicemia, gonorrhea, endocarditis, smallpox, chickenpox, herpes, Rocky Mountain spotted fever • Ischemic necrosis resulting from myocardial infarction, burns, carcinoma • Metabolic disorders: diabetic acidosis, eclampsia, uremia, thyrotoxicosis • Stress response caused by acute hemorrhage, surgery, excessive exercise, emotional distress, third trimester of pregnancy, childbirth • Inflammatory diseases: rheumatic fever, rheumatoid arthritis, acute gout, vasculitis, myositis **Decreased by:** • Bone marrow depression resulting from radiation or cytotoxic drugs • Infections: typhoid, tularemia, brucellosis, hepatitis, influenza, measles, mumps, rubella, infectious mononucleosis • Hypersplenism: hepatic disease and storage diseases • Collagen vascular disease such as systemic lupus erythematosus (SLE) • Folic acid or vitamin B$_{12}$ deficiency

W
X
Y

Cell Type	How Affected
	Eosinophils

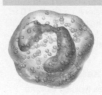

Increased by:
• Allergic disorders: asthma, hay fever, food or drug sensitivity, serum sickness, angioneurotic edema
• Parasitic infections: trichinosis, hookworm, roundworm, amebiasis
• Skin diseases: eczema, pemphigus, psoriasis, dermatitis, herpes
• Neoplastic diseases: chronic myelocytic leukemia (CML), Hodgkin's disease, metastasis, and necrosis of solid tumors

Decreased by:
• Stress response
• Cushing syndrome

Basophils

Increased by:
• CML, Hodgkin's disease, ulcerative colitis, chronic hypersensitivity states

Decreased by:
• Hyperthyroidism
• Ovulation, pregnancy
• Stress

Lymphocytes

Increased by:
• Infections: tuberculosis (TB), hepatitis, infectious mononucleosis, mumps, rubella, cytomegalovirus
• Thyrotoxicosis, hypoadrenalism, ulcerative colitis, immune diseases, lymphocytic leukemia

Decreased by:
• Severe debilitating illnesses: heart failure, kidney failure, advanced TB
• Defective lymphatic circulation, high levels of adrenal corticosteroids, immunodeficiency due to immunosuppressives

Monocytes

Increased by:
• Infections: subacute bacterial endocarditis, TB, hepatitis, malaria
• Collagen vascular disease: SLE, rheumatoid arthritis
• Carcinomas
• Monocytic leukemia
• Lymphomas

Performing a LAP Stain

Levels of leukocyte alkaline phosphatase (LAP), an enzyme found in neutrophils, may be altered by infection, stress, chronic inflammatory diseases, Hodgkin's disease, and hematologic disorders. Most of these conditions elevate LAP levels; only a few—notably chronic myelogenous leukemia (CML)—depress them. Thus, this test is usually used to differentiate CML from other disorders that produce an elevated white blood cell count.

Procedure

To perform the LAP stain, a blood sample is obtained by venipuncture or fingerstick. The venous blood sample is collected in a 7-mL green-top tube and transported immediately to the laboratory, where a blood smear is prepared; the peripheral blood sample is smeared on a 3-inch glass slide and fixed in cold formalin-methanol. The blood smear is then stained to show the amount of LAP present in the cytoplasm of the neutrophils. One

hundred neutrophils are counted and assessed; each is assigned a score of 0 to 4, according to the degree of LAP staining. Normally, values for LAP range from 40 to 100, depending on the laboratory's standards.

Implications of Results

Depressed LAP values typically indicate CML; however, values may also be low in paroxysmal nocturnal hemoglobinuria, aplastic anemia, and infectious mononucleosis. Elevated levels may indicate Hodgkin's disease, polycythemia vera, or a neutrophilic leukemoid reaction—a response to such conditions as infection, chronic inflammation, or pregnancy.

After a diagnosis of CML, the LAP stain may also be used to help detect onset of the blastic phase of the disease, when LAP levels typically rise. However, LAP levels also increase toward normal in response to therapy; because of this, test results must be correlated with the patient's condition.

whole blood. WBC counts may vary by as much as 2000 cells/mcL (SI, 2×10^9/L) on any given day due to strenuous exercise, stress, or digestion. The WBC count may increase or decrease significantly in certain diseases, but it's diagnostically useful only when the patient's white cell differential and clinical status are considered.

The WBC differential is used to evaluate the distribution and morphology of WBCs, providing more specific information about a patient's immune system than a WBC count alone.

WBCs are classified as one of five major types of leukocytes—neutrophils, eosinophils, basophils, lymphocytes, and monocytes—and the percentage of each type is determined. The differential count is the percentage of each type of WBC in the blood. The total number of each WBC type is obtained by multiplying its percentage by the total WBC count.

High levels of these leukocytes are associated with various allergic diseases and reactions to parasites. An eosinophil count is sometimes ordered as a follow-up

test when an elevated or depressed eosinophil level is reported.

Interfering Factors

WBC Count

- Digestion, exercise, or stress
- Anticonvulsants, such as phenytoin derivatives; anti-infectives, such as flucytosine (Ancobon) and metronidazole (Flagyl); most antineoplastics; nonsteroidal anti-inflammatory drugs such as indomethacin (Indocin); and thyroid hormone antagonists (decrease)
- Elderly patients with overwhelming sepsis (decrease)

WBC Differential

- Anticonvulsants, capreomycin (Capastat sulfate), cephalosporins, D-penicillamine, desipramine (Norpramin), gold compounds, indomethacin, isoniazid, methysergide (increase or decrease eosinophil count), nalidixic acid (NegGram), novobiocin, paraaminosalicylic acid, paromomycin (Humatin), penicillins, phenothiazines, procainamide

W
X
Y

(Procanbid) (decrease eosinophil count), rifampin, streptomycin, sulfonamides, and tetracyclines (increase count by provoking an allergic reaction)

Precautions
- Completely fill the sample collection tube.
- Invert the sample gently several times to mix the sample and the anticoagulant.

Nursing Considerations

Before the Test
- Confirm the patient's identity using two patient identifiers and confirmation of the patient's identification bracelet according to facility policy.
- Explain to the patient that the WBC count and differential test is used to detect an infection or inflammation (WBC count) or evaluate the immune system (WBC differential).
- Advise the patient that a blood sample will be taken. Explain that slight discomfort from the tourniquet and needle puncture may be experienced.
- Explain that there are no food or fluid restrictions but that the patient should avoid strenuous exercise for 24 hours before the test and eating a heavy meal before the test.
- Advise the patient being treated for an infection that this test will be repeated to monitor progress.
- Notify the laboratory and physician of medications the patient is taking that may affect test results; these may need to be restricted.

During the Test
- Perform a venipuncture and collect the sample in a 3- or 4.5-mL EDTA tube.

After the Test
- If a hematoma develops at the venipuncture site, apply pressure. If the hematoma is large, monitor pulses distal to the venipuncture site.
- Make sure subdermal bleeding has stopped before removing pressure.
- Instruct the patient to resume usual diet, activity, and medications

discontinued before the test, as ordered.
- Be aware that a patient with severe leukopenia may have little or no resistance to infection and requires infection control precautions.

Wound Culture

Normal Findings
- No pathogenic organisms

Abnormal Findings
- *Staphylococcus aureus*
- Group A beta-hemolytic streptococci
- *Proteus*
- *Escherichia coli* and other Enterobacteriaceae
- Some *Pseudomonas* species
- *Clostridium*
- *Peptococcus*
- *Bacteroides*
- *Streptococcus*

Nursing Implications
- Report any abnormal findings to the health care provider.
- Prepare to educate the patient about the diagnosis.
- Prepare the patient for further testing or surgery, as indicated.
- Provide emotional support to the patient and family.
- Prepare to administer antimicrobial therapy, as indicated.
- Institute isolation precautions, as applicable.

Purpose
- To identify an infectious microbe in a wound

Description
Performed to confirm infection, a wound culture is a microscopic analysis of a specimen from a lesion. Wound cultures may be aerobic, for detection of organisms that usually appear in a superficial wound, or anaerobic, for organisms that need little or no oxygen and appear in areas of poor tissue perfusion, such as postoperative

wounds, ulcers, and compound fractures. Indications for wound culture include fever, as well as inflammation and drainage in damaged tissue.

Interfering Factors

- Failure to report recent or current antimicrobial therapy (possible false negative)
- Use of inappropriate transport medium, allowing the specimen to dry and the bacteria to deteriorate.
- Improper culture technique.

Precautions

- Clean the area around the wound thoroughly to limit contamination of the culture by normal skin flora, such as diphtheroids, *Staphylococcus epidermidis*, and alpha-hemolytic streptococci. Don't clean the area around a perineal wound.
- Make sure no antiseptic enters the wound.
- Obtain exudate from the entire wound, using more than one swab if necessary.
- Because some anaerobes die in the presence of even a small amount of oxygen, place the specimen in the culture tube quickly; take care that no air enters the tube and check that double stoppers are secure.
- Keep the specimen container upright and send it to the laboratory within 15 minutes to prevent growth or deterioration of microbes.
- Wear gloves during the procedure and when handling the specimen; take necessary isolation precautions when sending the specimen to the laboratory.

Nursing Considerations

Before the Test

- Confirm the patient's identity using two patient identifiers and confirmation of the patient's identification bracelet according to facility policy.
- Explain to the patient that the wound culture is used to identify infectious microbes.
- Describe the procedure, informing the patient that a drainage specimen from the wound is withdrawn by a syringe or removed on sterile cotton swabs.
- Be sure that the specimen has been collected before starting antibiotic therapy.

During the Test

- Put on gloves, prepare a sterile field, and clean the area around the wound with antiseptic solution.
- For an aerobic culture, express the wound and swab as much exudate as possible or insert the swab deeply into the wound and gently rotate. Immediately place the swab in the aerobic culture tube.
- For an anaerobic culture, insert the swab deeply into the wound, gently rotate, and immediately place the swab in the anaerobic culture tube. (See the box describing anaerobic specimen collection, page 16).
- Alternatively, insert the needle into the wound, aspirate 1 to 5 mL of exudate into the syringe, and immediately inject the exudate into the anaerobic culture tube. If the needle is covered with a rubber stopper, the aspirate may be sent to the laboratory in the syringe.

After the Test

- Record on the laboratory request recent antimicrobial therapy, the source of the specimen, and the suspected organism. Label the specimen container with the patient's name, the physician's name, the facility number, the wound site, and the time of collection.
- Dress the wound.

Zinc, Serum

Reference Values
70 to 120 mcg/dL (SI,
  10.7–18.4 mcmol/L)

Abnormal Findings

Elevated Levels
- Accidental ingestion or industrial exposure to zinc

Decreased Levels
- Insufficient dietary intake
- Hereditary deficiency
- Alcoholic cirrhosis of the liver
- Myocardial infarction
- Ileitis
- Chronic kidney disease
- Rheumatoid arthritis
- Hemolytic or sickle cell anemia
- Leukemia

Nursing Implications
- Report abnormal findings to the health care provider.
- Prepare to educate the patient about the diagnosis.
- Prepare the patient for further testing or surgery, as indicated.
- Provide emotional support to the patient and family.

Purpose
- To detect zinc deficiency or toxicity

Description
This test measures serum zinc levels through atomic absorption spectroscopy analysis. Zinc is an integral component of more than 80 enzymes and proteins and plays a critical role in enzyme catalytic reactions. An important trace element, zinc occurs naturally in water and in most foods; high levels are found in meat, seafood, dairy products, whole grains, nuts, and legumes. Zinc deficiency can seriously impair body metabolism, growth, and development.

Interfering Factors
- Failure to use a metal-free collection tube
- Time of day and time of last meal (possible increase or decrease)
- Zinc-chelating agents, such as penicillinase, and corticosteroids (decrease)
- Estrogens; penicillamine; antineoplastics, such as cisplatin; antimetabolites; and diuretics (possible decrease)

Precautions
- Handle the sample gently to prevent hemolysis.

Nursing Considerations

Before the Test
- Confirm the patient's identity using two patient identifiers and confirmation of the patient's identification bracelet according to facility policy.
- Explain to the patient that this test determines the level of zinc in blood.
- Advise the patient that the test requires a blood sample. Explain that slight discomfort from the tourniquet and the needle puncture may be experienced.
- Inform the patient that there are no food or fluid restrictions for this test.

During the Test
- Perform a venipuncture and collect a 7- to 10-mL sample in a zinc-free collection tube.
- Send the sample to the laboratory immediately. Reliable analysis must begin before platelet disintegration can alter test results.

After the Test
- Apply direct pressure to the venipuncture site until bleeding stops.

Selected References

American Association of Clinical Chemistry. (n.d.). Lab tests online. Available at: www.labtestsonline.org

American Chemical Society. Available at: www.acs.org

American Society of Clinical Neurophysiology. (2006). Guideline 9A: Guidelines on evoked potentials. Available at: http://www.acns.org/pdf/guidelines/Guideline-9A.pdf

American Society of Gastrointestinal Endoscopy. Available at: www.asge.org

American Society of Neurophysiological Monitoring. Intraoperative monitoring using somatosensory evoked potentials: A position statement by the American Society of Neurophysiological Monitoring. Available at: http://www.asnm.org/resource/resmgr/position_statements/sep.pdf

Bard, Inc. (2007). The power PICC: Nursing—instructions for use. Pamphlet. Bard Access Systems. Available at: http://www.bardaccess.com/powerpicc/assets/pdfs/BAW0715354_PowerPICC_Nursing_IFU_web.pdf

Beers, M.H., et al., eds (2011). The Merck manual of diagnosis and therapy. Whitehouse Station, NJ: Merck Research Laboratories.

Black, J.M., and Hawks, J.H. (2008). Medical–surgical nursing: Clinical management for positive outcomes (8th ed.) St. Louis: Elsevier Saunders.

Bridgen, M.L. (1999). Clinical utility of erythrocyte sedimentation rate. American Family Physician. Available at: www.aafp.org/afp/991001ap/1443.html

Centers for Disease Control and Prevention. About CMV. Available at: http://www.cdc.gov/cmv/overview.html

Chernecky, C., & Berger, B. (2012). Laboratory tests and diagnostic procedures (6th ed.). St. Louis: Saunders.

Corbett, J. (2012). Laboratory tests and diagnostic procedures with nursing diagnoses (8th ed.). Upper Saddle River, NJ: Prentice Hall.

Cooper, N. (2002). Evidence-based lumbar puncture: Best practice to prevent headache. Hospital Medicine, 63(10), 598–599.

Dunning, M.B., & Fischbach, F. (2011). Nurses' quick reference to common laboratory & diagnostic tests (5th ed.). Philadelphia: Wolters Kluwer | Lippincott Williams & Wilkins.

Ferri, F.F. (2010). Ferri's best test: A practical guide to clinical laboratory medicine and diagnostic imaging (2nd ed.). Philadelphia: Elsevier Mosby.

Fischbach, F., & Dunning, M.B. (2015). A manual of laboratory and diagnostic tests (9th ed.). Philadelphia: Wolters Kluwer | Lippincott Williams & Wilkins.

French, M.A., Lewin, S.R., Dykstra, C., et al. (2004). Graves' disease during immune reconstitution after highly active antiretroviral therapy for HIV infection: Evidence of thymic dysfunction. AIDS Research and Human Retroviruses, 20(2),157–162.

Ginsburg, B.H. (2009). Factors affecting blood glucose monitoring: Sources of errors in measurement. Journal of Diabetes Science and Technology, 3(4),903–913.

Health A to Z. Available at: www.healthatoz.com

Hinkle, J.L., & Cheever, K.H. (2014). Brunner and Suddarth's textbook of medical-surgical nursing (13th ed.). Philadelphia: Lippincott Williams & Wilkins.

Hudson, T.L., Dukes, S.F., Reilly, K. (2006). Use of local anesthesia for arterial punctures. *American Journal of Critical Care*, 15(6),595–599.

Kee, J.L. (2013). *Laboratory and diagnostic tests with nursing implications* (9th ed.). Upper Saddle River, NJ: Pearson Prentice Hall.

Kee, J.L. (2012). *Pearson handbook of laboratory & diagnostic tests: With nursing implications* (7th ed.). Upper Saddle River, NJ: Pearson.

King, C., et al. (2007). *Textbook of pediatric emergency procedures*. Philadelphia: Lippincott Williams & Wilkins.

Kress, T., Krueger, D., & Ziccardi, S. (2008). Creatine kinases: An assay with muscle. *Nursing*, 38(10), 62.

Maradit-Kremers, H., Nicola, P.J., Crowson, C.S., et al. (2007). Raised erythrocyte sedimentation rate signals heart failure in patients with rheumatoid arthritis. *Annals of the Rheumatic Diseases*, 66(1), 76–80.

Mason, R.J., Broaddus, V.C., Martin, T.R., et al. (2010). *Murray and Nadel's textbook of respiratory medicine* (5th ed.). Philadelphia: Saunders.

Mayo Clinic Mayo Medical Laboratories. Unit Code 88886: Porphyrins evaluation, erythrocytes. Available at: www.mayomedicallaboratories.com/test-catalog/Overview/88886

McPherson, R.A., & Pincus, M.R. (2011). *Henry's clinical diagnosis and management by laboratory methods* (22nd ed.). Philadelphia: Elsevier Saunders.

MDAdvice.com. Available at: www.mdadvice.com

Medline Industries, Inc. Medline. Available at: www.medline.com

National Institutes of Health Office of Dietary Supplements. Dietary supplement fact sheet: Calcium. Available at: http://Dietary-supplements.info.nih.gov/factsheets/calcium.asp

National Kidney Foundation. Clinical practice guidelines for chronic kidney disease: Evaluation, classification, and stratification. Available at: http://www.kidney.org/professionals/kdoqi/pdf/ckd_evaluation_classification_stratification.pdf

Pagana, K.D., & Pagana, T.J. (2009). *Mosby's manual of diagnostic and laboratory tests* (4th ed.). Baltimore: Elsevier/Mosby.

PathologyOutlines.com. Available at: www.pathologyoutlines.com

Shellock, F.G. Pregnant patients and MR procedures. Available at: www.mrisafety.com/safety_article.asp?subject=50

Society of Gastroenterology Nurses and Associates. Available at: www.sgna.org

Springhouse, ed. (2008). *Diagnostic test facts made incredibly quick!*. Philadelphia: Lippincott, Williams & Wilkins.

Tarzi, M., et al. (2007). An evaluation of tests used for the diagnosis monitoring of C1 inhibitor deficiency: Normal serum C4 does not exclude hereditary angio-edema. *Clinical and Experimental Immunology*, 149, 513–516.

Trauma.Org (2000). Neurotrauma radiology for traumatic brain injury. Available at: www.trauma.org/archive/neuro/neuroradiology.html

U.S. National Library of Medicine and National Institutes of Health. Erythropoietin test. Available at: www.nlm.nih.gov/medlineplus/ency/article/003683.htm

U.S. National Library of Medicine and National Institutes of Health. ESR. Available at: www.nlm.nih.gov/medlineplus/ency/article/003638.htm

U.S. National Library of Medicine and National Institutes of Health. Euglobulin lysis time. Available at: www.nlm.nih.gov/medlineplus/ency/article/003654.htm

U.S. National Library of Medicine and National Institutes of Health. Fetal–maternal erythrocyte distribution. Available at: www.nlm.nih.gov/medlineplus/ency/article/003407.htm

Venes, D. (2013). *Taber's cyclopedic medical dictionary* (22nd ed.). Philadelphia: F.A. Davis.

WebMD. Available at: www.webmd.com

Whiteman, K. (2006). ACTH stimulation: Testing the adrenals. *Nursing*, 37(7), 24–25.

Index